RC681.A2 I488 1982   MAIN
Myocardial injury /

3 3073 00263757 5

MYOCARDIAL INJURY

ADVANCES IN EXPERIMENTAL MEDICINE AND BIOLOGY

Editorial Board:

NATHAN BACK, *State University of New York at Buffalo*

NICHOLAS R. DI LUZIO, *Tulane University School of Medicine*

EPHRAIM KATCHALSKI-KATZIR, *The Weizmann Institute of Science*

DAVID KRITCHEVSKY, *Wistar Institute*

ABEL LAJTHA, *Rockland Research Institute*

RODOLFO PAOLETTI, *University of Milan*

Recent Volumes in this Series

Volume 155
MACROPHAGES AND NATURAL KILLER CELLS: Regulation and Function
Edited by Sigurd J. Normann and Ernst Sorkin

Volume 156
KININS – III
Edited by Hans Fritz, Nathan Back, Günther Dietze,
and Gert L. Haberland

Volume 157
HYPERTHERMIA
Edited by Haim I. Bicher and Duane F. Bruley

Volume 158
STABILITY AND SWITCHING IN CELLULAR DIFFERENTIATION
Edited by R. M. Clayton and D. E. S. Truman

Volume 159
OXYGEN TRANSPORT TO TISSUE – IV
Edited by Haim I. Bicher and Duane F. Bruley

Volume 160
PORPHYRIN PHOTOSENSITIZATION
Edited by David Kessel and Thomas J. Dougherty

Volume 161
MYOCARDIAL INJURY
Edited by John J. Spitzer

Volume 162
HOST DEFENSES TO INTRACELLULAR PATHOGENS
Edited by Toby K. Eisenstein, Paul Actor, and Herman Friedman

Volume 163
FOLYL AND ANTIFOLYL POLYGLUTAMATES
Edited by I. David Goldman, Joseph R. Bertino, and Bruce A. Chabner

MYOCARDIAL INJURY

Edited by

John J. Spitzer

Louisiana State University Medical Center
New Orleans, Louisiana

PLENUM PRESS • NEW YORK AND LONDON

SETON HALL UNIVERSITY
McLAUGHLIN LIBRARY
SO. ORANGE. N. J.

Library of Congress Cataloging in Publication Data

International Society for Heart Research. American Section. Meeting (4th: 1982: New
    Orleans, La.)
    Myocardial injury.

    (Advances in experimental medicine and biology; v. 161)
    Bibliography: p.
    Includes index.
    1. Heart — Muscle — Diseases — Congresses. I. Spitzer, John J. II. Title. III. Series.
RC681.I488 1982   616.1'2   82-24624
ISBN 0-306-41253-5

RC
681
A2
I488
1982

Proceedings of the Fourth Annual Meeting of the American Section of the International
Society for Heart Research, held May 26–29, 1982, in New Orleans, Louisiana

© 1983 Plenum Press, New York
A Division of Plenum Publishing Corporation
233 Spring Street, New York, N.Y. 10013

All rights reserved

No part of this book may be reproduced, stored in a retrieval system, or transmitted
in any form or by any means, electronic, mechanical, photocopying, microfilming,
recording, or otherwise, without written permission from the Publisher

Printed in the United States of America

PREFACE

The chapters of this book represent contributions by plenary lecturers and invited symposium speakers of the Fourth Annual Meeting of the American Section of the International Society for Heart Research, held on May 26-29, 1982 in New Orleans, Louisiana. The aim of the Organizing Committee was to present an up-to-date picture of our knowledge of myocardial injury which would be equally useful to basic scientists and clinicians.

The papers of this volume are divided into two groups: a) those dealing primarily with techniques to study myocardial injury, and b) those that discuss the different types of myocardial injury. The grouping of the papers within each of these headings roughly corresponds to the symposia presented at the meeting.

I wish to acknowledge the financial support of the National Institutes of Health. Without grant HL 29149, the program could not have been financed. Contributions from the following companies were also gratefully received: Ayerst Laboratories, Ciba-Geigy, Merck Sharp and Dome, Pfizer Laboratories Division, A.H. Robbin Co., Smith-Kline Corporation, U.S.V. Pharmaceutical Co., and The Upjohn Co. My thanks are due to the members of The Organizing Committee (Drs. Gregory J. Bagby, Gerald S. Berenson, Alastair H. Burns, Harvey I. Miller, Robert Roskoski, Jr., and Judy A. Spitzer) for their help and support, and to the Secretary of the Meeting, Ms. L. Beatrice Abene for her excellent assistance.

John J. Spitzer, M.D.

CONTENTS

PART I: TECHNIQUES TO STUDY MYOCARDIAL INJURY

Propagation Mechanisms in Normal and Injured Myocardium

The Possibility of Propagation Between Myocardial
    Cells not Connected by Low-resistance Pathways   1
  N. Sperelakis

Effects of Injury on the Structure of Intercellular
    Junctions in Cardiac Muscle   25
  K.M. Baldwin

Modulation of Junctional Permeability in Cardiac Fibers . . .   37
  W.C. De Mello

The Role of Cell-to-Cell Coupling in Cardiac
    Conduction Disturbances   61
  M.S. Spach

A Model Study of the Effect of the Intercalated
    Discs on Discontinuous Propagation
    in Cardiac Muscle   79
  P.J. Diaz, Y. Rudy, and R. Plonsey

                Adrenergic and Cholinergic Receptors

Beta-adrenergic Stimulation of Adenylate Cyclase
    and Alpha-adrenergic Inhibition of Adenylate
    Cyclase: GTP-binding Proteins as Macromolecular
    Messengers   91
  L.E. Limbird

Agonist Regulation of the Muscarinic Cholinergic
    Receptor in Embryonic Chick Heart   113
  J.B. Galper, L.C. Dziekan, and T.W. Smith

Development and Regulation of Cardiac Muscarinic
    Acetylcholine Receptor Number, Function
    and Guanyl Nucleotide Sensitivity   143
    S.W. Halvorsen, B. Engel, D.D. Hunter,
    and N.M. Nathanson

Regional Distribution of Choline Acetyltransferase
    Activity and Multiple Affinity Forms of
    the Muscarinic Receptor in Heart   159
    R. Roskoski, Jr.

Neurochemical Indices of Autonomic Innervation of
    Heart in Different Experimental Models of
    Heart Failure   179
    D.D. Lund, P.G. Schmid, and R. Roskoski, Jr.

            Isolated Myocardial Cells and Cell Cultures

Mechanical and Contractile Properties of
    Isolated Single Intact Cardiac Cells   199
    M. Tarr

Studies of Substrate Metabolism in Isolated Myocytes   217
    J.J. Spitzer

Ion Movements in Adult Rat Heart Myocytes   231
    G.P. Brierley, C. Hohl, and R.A. Altschuld

Cardiac Muscle Cell Proliferation and Cell
    Differentiation In Vivo and In Vitro   249
    W.C. Claycomb

                    Miscellaneous Methods

Radionuclide Ventriculography to Evaluate
    Myocardial Function   267
    R.L. Huxley, J.R. Corbett, S.E. Lewis,
    and J.T. Willerson

Energy Production and Utilization in Contractile
    Failure Due to Intracellular
    Calcium Overload   305
    N.S. Dhalla, J.N. Singh, D.B. McNamara,
    A. Bernatsky, A. Singh, and J.A.C. Harrow

Aortic Perfusion Pressure and Protein Synthesis   317
    Y. Kira, P. Kochel, and H.E. Morgan

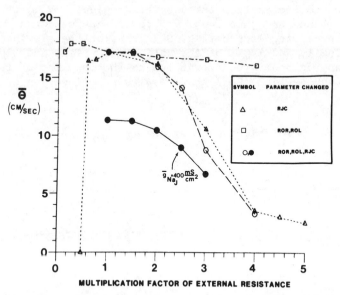

Propagation Velocity as a Function of External Resistance

Fig. 8. Graphic summary of data for average propagation velo-
         city ($\bar{\theta}$) as a function of the external resistances
         along the entire chain of 6 cells. The value of 1.0
         on the abscissa represents the standard resistance
         parameters used in the model. When ROL, ROR, and RJC
         were increased simultaneously to 1.5x, 2.0x, 2.5x,
         3.0x, and 4.0x times the standard values, $\bar{\theta}$ was
         greatly decreased (circle symbols in figure). When
         only ROL and ROR were increased, there was only a
         slight decrease in $\bar{\theta}$ (square symbols). Decrease in
         ROL and ROR to 1/2x, 1/4x, and 1/8x times also had
         little effect on $\bar{\theta}$. When RJC alone was increased
         (triangle symbols), the decrease in $\bar{\theta}$ was about as
         great as when all three external resistances were
         varied. Lowering RJC to 0.7x and 0.6x had little
         effect, but lowering to 0.5x produced an abrupt
         failure of propagation. Thus, there was only a
         relatively small effect of RJC between 6 MΩ (0.6x)
         and 20 MΩ (2x). When $\bar{g}_{Na}$ of the junctional membranes
         ($\bar{g}_{Na_J}$) was set equal to that for the surface membranes
         (400 mS/cm^2), $\bar{\theta}$ was slowed (filled circles). Figure
         modified from Sperelakis, Marschall and Mann, unpub-
         lished observations.

In a sucrose-gap type of simulation, raising the resistance of the extracellular fluid bathing the middle two cells, up to 3 times the normal value, slowed down propagation velocity in the sucrose-gap region (Fig. 9). Raising the resistance to 4 times the higher blocked propagation through this region. $+\dot{V}_{max}$ of both the surface membrane and junctional membrane decreases as a function of the external resistance (Fig. 9). Part of the slowing of propagation velocity and $+\dot{V}_{max}$ of the action potentials and block in the sucrose gap region may be attributed to the lowering of the Na$^+$ equilibrium potential (E_{Na}) that results from lowering of [Na]$_o$ (in

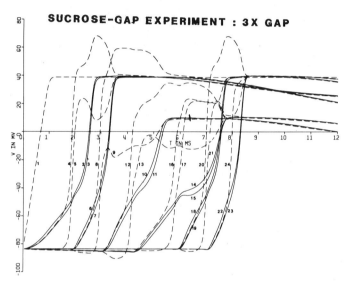

Fig. 9.   Sucrose-gap-type of experiment in which the external resistances (ROL, ROR, RJC) were increased by 3-fold along only the middle two cells (Cells 3 and 4) of the 6-cell chain. The external resistances were raised by the equivalent of replacing half of the NaCl in the solution bathing the sucrose-gap region with an equi-osmolar amount of sucrose. Since the Na$^+$ equilibrium potential (E_{Na}) was decreased in the sucrose-gap region (assumes that [Na]$_i$ remained constant), this accounts for the smaller overshoot of the action potentials in Cells 3 and 4. Note that propagation velocity ($\bar{\theta}$) and $+\dot{V}_{max}$ were decreased in the two cells in the sucrose gap. $\bar{\theta}$ in the sucrose gap was 6.7 cm/sec, compared to 19.8 cm/sec for the cells outside of the sucrose gap. Increasing the gap resistances to 4x caused failure of propagation in the sucrose gap region (not depicted). Figure modified from Sperelakis, Marschall and Mann, unpublished observations.

order to raise r_o). This lowers the electrochemical driving force
($E_m - E_{Na}$) for inward fast Na^+ current during the rising phase of
the action potential, and hence lowers $+\dot{V}_{max}$ and peak "overshoot"
potential of the action potentials (APs). (For simplicity, r_o was
increased by lowering $[Na]_o$ and $[Cl]_o$ only; $[K]_o$, and hence E_K, was
not changed.) The other reason for the lowering of propagation
velocity in the sucrose-gap region is the fact that RJC of the
junction in the center of the gap (between cells 3 and 4) was increased proportionally to ROL and ROR, and hence this acts to slow
propagation, as described above for the experiment in which the
external resistances were varied uniformly along the entire chain
of 6 cells.

Thus, the electric field model allows propagation of excitation at constant velocity down a chain of cells not connected by
low-resistance tunnels, and propagation velocity is dependent on
the extracellular resistance, and particularly on RJC. Hence, this
model can account for many of the biologically-observed facts.

Combined K^+ Accumulation and Electric Field Models

We are currently in the process of attempting to combine the
K^1 accumulation model with the electric field model. By incorporating the likely possibility of rapid K^+ accumulation in the junctional cleft into the electric field model, we expect that this
will facilitate the transmission process. In turn, this should
allow all electrical properties of the junctional membranes to be
identical to those of the surface membrane and yet achieve successful transmission. The safety factor for transmission should also
be enhanced.

SUMMARY AND DISCUSSION

The results with our electric field model demonstrate that
propagation of action potentials can occur at a constant velocity
of about 17.1 cm/sec down a chain of excitable cells that are not
interconnected by low-resistance tunnels. Transmission of excitation across the cell junctions occurs by an electrical mechanism,
namely when the pre-junctional membrane fires an action potential,
the electric field that develops in the narrow junctional cleft
depolarizes the post-junctional membrane to threshold. The key
assumption in the model is that the junctional membranes are
ordinary excitable membranes.

Raising the extracellular resistances, ROL and ROR, along the
entire chain of 6 cells by up to 4-fold slowed propagation velocity
slightly. However, when the radial cleft resistance, RJC, was
increased either alone, or concomitantly with ROL and ROR, then

there was a marked slowing of propagation velocity. In a real
biological experiment, raising the ROL and ROR (e.g., by partial
replacement of NaCl in the bathing solution by isosmotic sucrose)
should also cause a proportional increase in RJC. These results
indicate that RJC is the most important parameter of the external
resistances in determining velocity of propagation. In addition,
it is clear that the model is relatively insensitive to the actual
values of ROL and ROR selected, since lowering of ROL and ROR by
up to 8-fold also had relatively little effect.

Although we don't know whether the electric field model applies
to actual biological cells, it does provide a possible alternative
mechanism for electrical interactions among excitable cells; this
mechanism does not require low-resistance connections between the
cells.

The other possible mechanism, namely the local-circuit current
hypothesis, requires that there by low-resistance tunnels between
the cells. A theoretical analysis of the potential in the junctional
cleft between myocardial cells, assuming that the junctional membranes were non-excitable and low in resistance, was done by Heppner
and Plonsey (1970) and by Woodbury and Crill (1970). For such a
modified cable situation, they found that the maximum resistivity
of the junctional membranes that would allow successful transmission
(for a cleft thickness of 80 $\overset{o}{A}$) was about 3 Ω-cm^2, i.e., about
1/100 - 1/1000 times that of the surface membrane. The value of
3 Ω-cm^2 is in good agreement with values calculated for a similar
arrangement by Weidmann (1966), Sperelakis (1969), and Sperelakis
and Mann (1977); for other references, see the review by Sperelakis
(1979).

The electric field hypothesis can account for a number of
experimental facts concerning propagation in cardiac muscle, namely
that (a) propagation velocity is about 0.3 m/sec; (b) propagation
is bi-directional; (c) the transmission process is labile and often
can exhibit partial or complete block; (d) increasing the separation
of the junctional membranes under pathological or experimental
conditions, thus decreasing RJC, impedes and blocks transmission;
(e) there is a prepotential step on the rising phase of the action
potential; (f) synaptic-like vesicles are not observed at the
intercalated disks. In addition, and more importantly, the electric
field hypothesis is consistent with the lack of measurement of low
resistance between myocardial cells in adult heart tissue by a
number of different approaches (for a summary of these, see
Sperelakis (1969) and Sperelakis (1979), as well as the Background
section above.)

The electric field model is also consistent with recent observations of Spach et al. (1981) who found that the rate of rise of
the cardiac action potential was greater with transverse propagation,

although propagation in the transverse direction was much slower
than in the longitudinal direction, i.e., propagation velocity
could be separated from rate of rise. They also reported that
propagation in cardiac muscle is saltatory or discontinuous in
nature. These findings are consistent with the predictions given
by Sperelakis and colleagues (e.g., see Sperelakis, 1969), namely
that myocardial cells behave as truncated cables with little or
no low-resistance coupling between the cells.

Diaz, Rudy and Plonsey (1981) also concluded, from a theoretical analysis of a model based on resistive couplings between cells,
that "continuous cable theory does not adequately describe propagation in cardiac muscle" and that excitation jumps from intercalated
disk to intercalated disk, i.e., saltatory propagation occurs.
They found that propagation inside a single cell was ten times
faster than the average velocity over many cells, i.e., most propagation time is consumed at the cell junctions. This is also consistent with the predictions given by Sperelakis and colleagues for
truncated cables (see Sperelakis, 1969). In the model of Diaz et
al., propagation velocity was greatly slowed at r_{jc} values below
170 MΩ, and failed at r_{jc} values below 17 MΩ. These r_{jc} values
are considerably higher than those required in our electric field
model (>5 MΩ).

A study highly quoted in support of low-resistance coupling
in cardiac muscle is that of Barr et al. (1965) showing that a
sucrose gap of about 100-200 μm blocked propagation in frog atrial
strands unless a low shunt resistance was placed across the sucrose
gap region. However, it seems this experiment shows only that in
a biological system, current must flow in order to produce a potential change. Regardless of interpretation, the fact that the sucrose
gap region had to be short in order for the experiment to work, indicates that the length constant (λ) cannot be long, as claimed by
some investigators. Another study highly quoted in support of low-
resistance coupling is that of Weidmann (1966), who showed that
the steady-state distribution of ^{42}K along ventricular muscle
bundles (across a membrane separating a loading compartment) was
exponential with a length constant of about 1.55 mm whereas that
for ^{82}Br was only 0.55 mm. However, it seems difficult to conclude
what the resistivity of the intercalated disk is from this experiment
because of the anistropic muscle bundle acting as a cable (problem
discussed above) and because longitudinal diffusion can occur through
capillaries, etc. A number of other studies have been done using
dye diffusion as a presumed indicator of low-resistance coupling
(for references, see the 1979 review by Sperelakis). However, it
is interesting that no evidence of electrotonic coupling was found
among pyramidal cells of the guinea pig hippocampus, although the
fluorescent dye Lucifer Yellow injected into one soma spread to
neighboring cells (dye coupling) (Knowles et al., 1982). Therefore,
dye studies must be interpreted with caution.

Although the parameters of the electric field model were selected specifically for cardiac muscle, the principles of this model have general applicability to interactions between other types of closely-apposed excitable cells. The only requirements are that their cell membranes be in close apposition over a small fraction of the total surface area, and that the junctional membranes be ordinary excitable membranes. The model might also apply to intracellular interactions between the cell membrane and SR membrane. Electrical field interactions between neurons in vertebrate brain, both excitatory and inhibitory, have been described by Korn and Faber (1980), but these are ephaptic in nature, depending on current flow through the second neuron and on the resistance of the extracellular space.

ACKNOWLEDGMENTS

The work of the author reviewed in this article was supported in part by research grant HL-18711 from the National Institutes of Health and by grant support from the Academic Computing Center of the University of Virginia. I also wish to acknowledge the collaboration with recent colleagues, namely Dr. James E. Mann, Jr., Mr. James A. Ruffner, and Mr. Richard A. Marschall.

REFERENCES

Baldwin, K.M. Cell-to-cell tracer movement in cardiac muscle: Ruthenium red vs lanthanum. Cell Tiss. Res. 221, 279-294 (1981).

Barr, L., Dewey, M.M., and W. Berger. Propagation of action potentials and the structure of the nexus in cardiac muscle. J. Gen. Physiol. 48, 797-823 (1965).

Beder, S.D. and Skinner, J.E. Cardiac cellular electrophysiology in awake conscious pigs: membrane cable properties. Circulation 64, IV-116, Abstr. #428 (1981).

Beeler, G.W. and Reuter, H. Reconstruction of the action potential of ventricular myocardial fibers. J. Physiol. 268, 177-210 (1977).

De Mello, W.C. The healing-over process in cardiac and other muscle fibers. In: Electrical Phenomena in Heart (W.C. De Mello, ed.), Academic Press, New York, pp. 323-351 (1972).

De Mello, W.C. Effect of intracellular injection of calcium and strontium on cell communication in heart. J. Physiol. 250, 231-245 (1975).

Diaz, P.J., Rudy, Y., and Plonsey, R. A cardiac propagation model with intercalated discs. (Abstr.) 34th ACEMB meeting, Houston, Sept. 21-23, p. 217 (1981).

Forbes, M.S. and Sperelakis, N. Ultrastructure of lizard ventricular muscle. J. Ultrastruct. Res. 34, 439-451 (1971).

Heppner, D.B. and Plonsey, R. Simulation of electrical interaction of cardiac cells. Biophys. J. 10, 1057-1075 (1970).

Hoshiko, T. and Sperelakis, N. Prepotentials and unidirectional propagation in myocardium. Am. J. Physiol. 201, 873-880 (1961).

Hoshiko, T. and Sperelakis, N. Components of the cardiac action potential. Am. J. Physiol. 203, 258-260 (1962).

Kline, R. and Morad, M. Potassium efflux and accumulation in heart muscle. Biophys. J. 16, 367-372 (1976).

Knowles, W.D., Funch, P.G., and Schwartzkroin, P.A. Electrotonic and dye coupling in hippocampal CAI pyramidal cells in vitro. (in press).

Korn, H. and Faber, D.S. Electrical field effect interactions in the vertebrate brain. Trends in Neuroscience 3(1), 6-9 (1980).

Macdonald, R.L., Hsu, D., Mann, J.E., and Sperelakis, N. An analysis of the problem of K^+ accumulation in the intercalated disk clefts of cardiac muscle. J. Theor. Biol. 51, 455-473 (1975).

Mann, J.E., Jr., Foley, E., and Sperelakis, N. Resistance and potential profiles in the cleft between two myocardial cells: electrical analog and computer simulations. J. Theor. Biol. 68, 1-15 (1977).

Mann, J.E. and Sperelakis, N. Further development of a model for electrical transmission between myocardial cells not connected by low-resistance pathways. J. Electrocardiol. 12, 23-33 (1979).

Mann, J.E., Sperelakis, N., and Ruffner, J.A. Alteration in sodium channel gate kinetics of the Hodgkin-Huxley equations applied to an electric field model for interaction between excitable cells. IEEE Trans. Biomed. Eng. 28, 655-661 (1981).

McLean, M.J. and Sperelakis, N. Difference in degree of electrotonic interactions between highly differentiated and reverted cultured heart cell reaggregates. J. Memb. Biol. 57, 37-50 (1980).

Noble, D. A modification of the Hodgkin-Huxley equations applicable to Purkinje fiber action and pacemaker potentials. J. Physiol. 160, 317-352 (1962).

Page, E., McCallister, L.P. Studies on the intercalated disk of rat left ventricular myocardial cells. J. Ultastruct. Res. 43, 388-411 (1973).

Plonsey, R. and Rudy, Y. Electrocardiogram sources in a 2-dimensional anisotropic activation model. Med. Biol. Eng. Comput. 18, 87-94 (1980).

Ruffner, J., Sperelakis, N., and Mann, J.E., Jr. Application of the Hodgkin-Huxley equations to an electric field model for interactions between excitable cells. J. Theor. Biol. 87, 129-152 (1980).

Spach, M.S., Miller, W.T., III, Geselowitz, D.B., Barr, R.C., Kootsey, J.M., and Johnson, E.A. The discontinuous nature of propagation in normal canine cardiac muscle. Evidence for recurrent discontinuity of intracellular resistance that affects the membrane currents. Circ. Res. 48, 39-54 (1981).

Sperelakis, N. Additional evidence for high-resistance intercalated
    discs in the myocardium. Circulation Res. 12, 676-683 (1963).
Sperelakis, N. Lack of electrical coupling between contiguous
    myocardial cells in vertebrate hearts. In: Comparative Phys-
    iology of the Heart: Current Trends, (F.V. McCann, ed.),
    Birkhauser-Verlag, Basel, Switzerland, pp. 135-165 (1969).
Sperelakis, N. Propagation mechanisms in heart. Ann. Rev. Physiol.
    41, 441-457 (1979).
Sperelakis, N. and Macdonald, R.L. Ratio of transverse to longi-
    tudinal resistivities of isolated cardiac muscle fiber bundles.
    J. Electrocardiol. 7, 301-314 (1974).
Sperelakis, N. and Hoshiko, T. Electrical impedance of cardiac
    muscle. Circ. Res. 9, 1280-1283 (1961).
Sperelakis, N. and Lehmkuhl, D. Effect of current on transmembrane
    potentials in cultured chick heart cells. J. Gen. Physiol.
    47, 895-927 (1964).
Sperelakis, N. and Mann, J.E., Jr. Evaluation of electric field
    changes in the cleft between excitable cells. J. Theor. Biol.
    64, 71-96 (1977).
Sperelakis, N. and Rubio, R. Ultrastructural changes produced by
    hypertonicity in cat cardiac muscle. J. Mol. Cell. Cardiol.
    3, 139-156 (1971).
Sperelakis, N. and Shumaker, K. Phase-plane analysis of cardiac
    action potentials. J. Electrocardiology 1, 31-42 (1968).
Sperelakis, N., Hoshiko, T., and Berne, R.M. Non-syncytial nature
    of cardiac muscle: membrane resistance of single cells. Am.
    J. Physiol. 198, 531-536 (1960).
Sperelakis, N., Marschall, R.A., and Mann, J.E. Propagation down
    a chain of excitable cells by electric field interactions in
    the junctional clefts: Effect of variation in extracellular
    resistances, including a "sucrose gap" simulation. (submitted
    for publication).
Sperelakis, N., Mayer, G., and MacDonald, R. Velocity of propaga-
    tion in vertebrate cardiac muscles as functions of tonicity
    and $[K^+]_o$. Amer. J. Physiol. 219, 952-963 (1970).
Sperelakis, N., Rubio, R., and Redick, J. Sharp discontinuity in
    sarcomere lengths across intercalated disks of fibrillating
    cat hearts. J. Ultrastruct. Res. 30, 503-532 (1970).
Sperelakis, N., Hoshiko, T., Keller, R.F., Jr. and Berne, R.M.
    Intracellular and external recordings from frog ventricular
    fibers during hypertonic perfusion. Am. J. Physiol. 198,
    135-140 (1960).
Tarr, M. and Sperelakis, N. Weak electrotonic interaction between
    contiguous cardiac cells. Am. J. Physiol. 207, 691-700 (1964).
Tarr, M. and Sperelakis, N. Decreased intercellular resistance
    during spontaneous depolarization in myocardium. Am. J.
    Physiol. 212, 1503-1511 (1967).
Weidmann, S. The diffusion of radiopotassium across intercalated
    disks of mammalian cardiac muscle. J. Physiol. 187, 323-342
    (1966).

Weidmann, S.   Electrical coupling between myocardial cells.   Prog. Brain Res. 31, 275-281 (1969).

Woodbury, J.W. and Crill, W.E.   The potential in the gap between two abutting cardiac muscle cells.   Biophys. J. 10, 1076-1083 (1970).

Yarom, Y. and Spira, M.E.   Extracellular potassium ions mediate specific neuronal interaction.   Science 216, 80-82 (1982).

EFFECTS OF INJURY ON THE STRUCTURE OF

INTERCELLULAR JUNCTIONS IN CARDIAC MUSCLE

Kate M. Baldwin

Department of Anatomy
Howard University
Washington, D.C.

INTRODUCTION

Since the discovery that cardiac muscle was composed of discrete cellular units (Sjostrand and Anderson, 1954) and was not a structural syncytium, much has been published about cardiac intercellular junctions (see Sommer and Johnson, 1979 for a review). Therefore, the structure of normal cardiac intercellular junctions will be described briefly and then the effects of injury upon them will be discussed.

NORMAL INTERCELLULAR JUNCTIONS

Three different intercellular junctions can be distinguished in mammalian ventricular muscle: fasciae adherentes, desmosomes (maculae adherentes), and gap junctions (nexuses) (Fig. 1).

Fasciae adherentes are the sites where the 5 - 7 nm thick actin myofilaments insert into the cell membrane. In addition to the actin filaments, there is a diffuse density of unknown composition associated with both the cytoplasm and the intercellular cleft at the junction (Fig. 1). Fasciae adherentes are generally oriented perpendicular to the long axis of themyofibrils, but the cell membrane is curved elaborately within the junction so that the forces on the cell membrane are tangential, rather than perpendicular to it.

Desmosomes (maculae adherentes) differ from the fasciae adherentes in several ways. They are smaller in area (maculae instead of fasciae). In addition to the diffuse density associated with

25

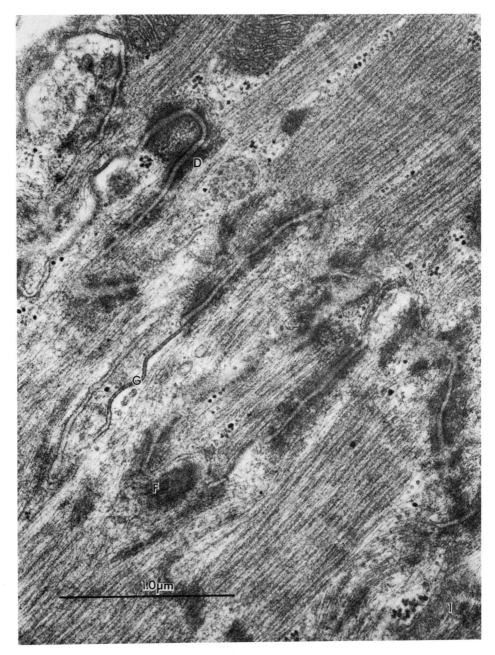

Fig. 1.   Intercellular junctions in rabbit ventricle. Fasciae adher-
          entes (F), desmosomes (D), and gap junctions (G) are asso-
          ciated with the highly tortuous membranes of the interca-
          lated disc.

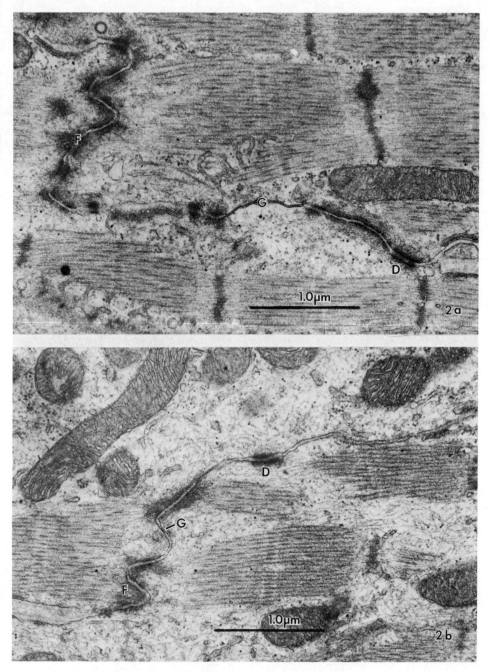

Fig. 2.   Intercellular junctions in rabbit atrium (a) and sinoatrial
          node (b). Fasciae adherentes (F), desmosomes (D) and gap
          junctions (G) join these cells, but the intercellular
          boundaries are less complex than in the ventricles.

both the cytoplasm and the intercellular cleft, there are distinct intracellular plaques associated with the junctional membranes; this makes desmosones appear darker then fasciae adherentes in micrographs (Fig. 1). The filaments which insert into the membrane at this junction are of the intermediate (10 nm) type.

It is the fasciae adherentes and the desmosomes which together form the intercalated discs seen by light microscopy.

Gap junctions (nexuses) are sites where the membranes of two adjacent cells are closely opposed, leaving only a 1.5 nm "gap" between them (Fig. 1). The junctional membrane of each cell contains a cluster of connexon units. It has been proposed that each connexon contains a central, permeable pore and that the central pores of the connexons of one cell line up with those in the adjacent cell. Thus there is one continuous permeable channel between the two cells (see Sommer and Johnson, 1979; Page and Shibata, 1981; Peracchia, 1980 for reviews). Evidence from several studies suggests that ions and molecules up to about 1000 daltons can pass from cell to cell through the connexon pores (Sheridan, 1974; Simpson et al., 1977; Brink and Dewey, 1978) and thus the gap junctions are the presumed sites of low resistence between cardiac and other cells. Gap junctions usually are found where the cell membranes run parallel to the long axis of the cell (on the "risers" of the intercalated disc "staircase", Fig. 1).

The same three junctions are found in mammalian atrial cells (Fig. 2a) or cells of the conducting system (Fig. 2b), but often along the lateral surfaces of the cells; the elaborate intercalated discs typical of ventricular cells are uncommon.

EFFECTS OF INJURY

Bullfrog Atrium

I first studied the effects of injury on cardiac intercellular junctions while trying to discover the cause of the relatively rapid decline of cardiac injury potentials. It was known that if a strip of frog cardiac muscle was crushed at one end, the injury potential decreased to near zero within 20 minutes. It was also known that during this 20 minutes the injured cells did not recover and the uninjured cells did not depolarize (Baldwin, 1970), so the injury potential decrease must have been due to an increase in resistance between the injured and uninjured cells. This seemed a good system in which to study structural correlates of electrical coupling and uncoupling in cardiac cells.

There are only two types of junctions between normal frog atrial cells: fasciae adherentes (although they are really too small to be

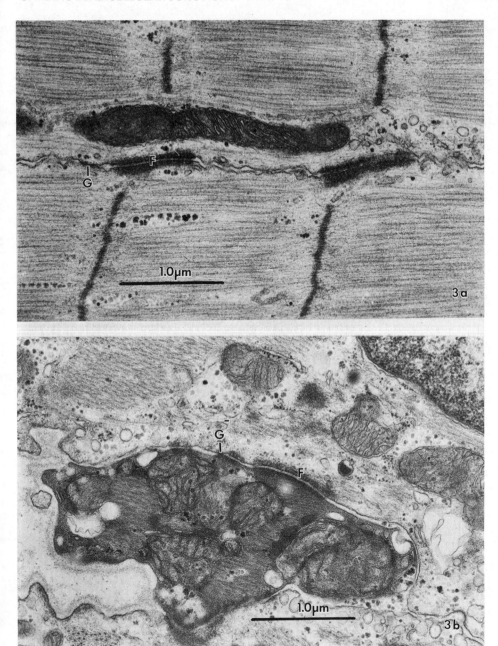

Fig. 3. Bullfrog atrium. In control samples (a) fasciae adherentes
        (F) and small gap junctions (G) are present along the lateral
        surfaces of the cells. Injured cell (b) is very dense, but
        its junctions with adjacent uninjured cells remain intact.

true fasciae) and very infrequent gap junctions (Fig. 3a). Surprisingly, cells injured by crushing and allowed time to uncouple exhibit no detectable changes in their intercellular junctions (Fig. 3b). Fasciae adherentes are intact and gap junctions are found at least as frequently as in control preparations.

Sheep Purkinje Fibers

Since frog heart has few and small gap junctions, and gap junctions are the proposed sites of electrical coupling between cells, it seemed appropriate to study the effects of injury on the large gap junctions in mammalian cardiac cells. Hence, another series of experiments were performed, this time using Purkinje fibers in sheep heart false tendons. Injury was produced by cutting the false tendons and the injured cells were allowed time to uncouple from the uninjured cells prior to fixation.

Control cells have the same three types of junctions as other mammalian cardiac cells (Fig. 4a) and in particular have large and frequent gap junctions. But here again, we can detect no changes in the intercellular junctions after injury (Fig. 4b). Even at very high magnification, the width of the gap of the gap junctions shows no detectable change (Baldwin, 1977) and the packing of connexon units in lanthanum impregnated specimens is similar in control (Fig. 4c) and injured (Fig. 4d) cells (Baldwin, 1981).

Freeze Fracture of Rabbit Ventricle

The next approach tried was to compare injured and control gap junctions using freeze fracture electron microscopy. The particular advantage of this technique is that frozen cell membranes fracture preferentially along an internal plane so that they split into two parts: one which lies adjacent to the cytoplasm (P face) and one which lies adjacent to the extracellular fluid (E face) (Fig. 5). These exposed membrane faces allow examination of structures normally embedded within the membrane. Connexon particles of gap junctions remain attached to the P membrane face and gap junctions are thus readily identifiable as a cluster of particles on the P membrane face. The E face at gap junctions has pits into which, presumably, the connexon particles fit. Very briefly, the freeze fracture technique involves: aldehyde fixation of the tissue, cryoprotection by soaking it in glycerol solutions, rapid freezing of it in liquid nitrogen-cooled Freon 22, and maintenance of the tissue at -100° C. or less. The frozen tissue is placed in a vacuum, fractured, and a thin metal replica of the fractured surface is made. The tissue is then digested away and the replica is examined in the electron microscope.

In the experiments described here, blocks were cut from rabbit ventricle and the cut surfaces were allowed to heal over prior to fixation. Control samples taken from the interior of the blocks

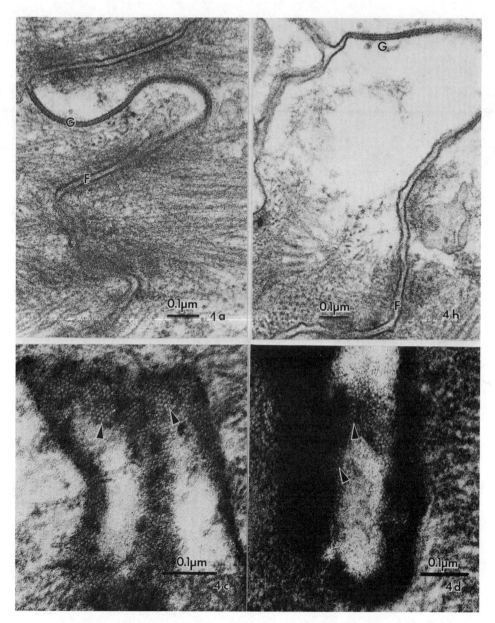

Fig. 4. Control sheep Purkinje fibers (a) with fasciae adherentes
(F) and a gap junction (G). After uncoupling injuries (b),
there are no detectable changes in the junctions. After
lanthanum impregnation, connexon units of tangentially
cut gap junctions (arrows) form similar hexagonal arrays
in control (c) and injured (d) tissues.

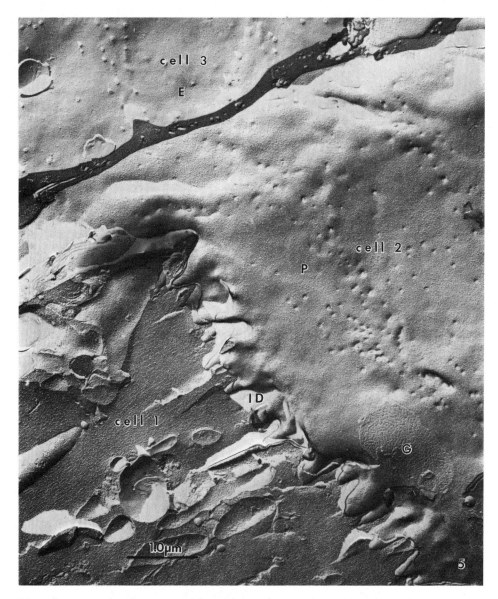

Fig. 5.   Freeze fracture of rabbit ventricle. The fracture plane
          has passed through the cytoplasm of cell 1; over cell 2,
          exposing the P-face (P) of its cell membrane; and under
          cell 3, leaving only the E-face (E) of its cell membrane
          behind. An intercalated disc (ID) with an associated gap
          junction (G) is present between cells 1 and 2. Note that
          the fascia adherens of the intercalated disc is not demon-
          strated by this technique.

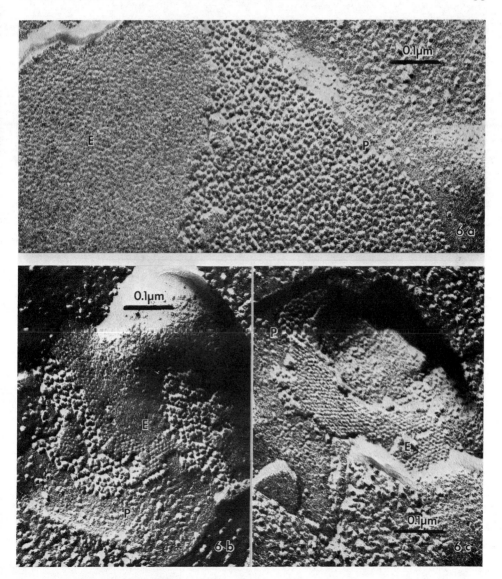

Fig. 6.   Freeze fracture of rabbit ventricle gap junctions. In con-
          trol samples (a) the P-face (P) particles and the E-face
          (E) pits have an irregular packing pattern. The average
          center-to-center spacing of the particles is 10.5 nm. In
          samples fixed one to five minutes after injury (b), the par-
          ticles and pits tend to be in clumps, and the packing within
          the clumps is hexagonal. The average interparticle spacing
          is 9.5 nm. In samples fixed 15 - 30 minutes after injury
          (c) particles and pits form a homogeneous unit with hexa-
          gonal packing and an average interparticle spacing of
          9.5 nm.

(away from the cut edges) were compared to injured tissue near the
cut edges.

In control gap junctions (Fig. 6a) the P-face connexon particles and the E-face pits are clustered together into a compact structure with an average center-to-center spacing of the particles of
10.5 nm. The packing of the particles and pits seems to be irregular. Injured cell gap junctions from tissue fixed one to five minutes after injury show a clumping of P-face particles and E-face
pits and within the clumps the packing shows considerable geometric
regularity (Fig. 6b). Furthermore, the average center-to-center
spacing of the particles is decreased to 9.5 nm. Gap junctions in
tissue fixed 15 - 30 minutes after injury no longer show particle
clumping, but consist of homogeneous units with hexagonally packed
particles and pits. The average center-to-center spacing of particles in these junctions is also 9.5 nm (Baldwin, 1979).

Uncoupling treatments (usually metabolic poisoning) have led
to a decrease in particle spacing and an increase in regularity of
particle packing in gap junctions of a number of non-cardiac tissues
(Peracchia, 1977) and other cardiac tissue as well (Dahl and Isenberg,
1980). Some reports have described a decrease in particle spacing
without the increase in regularity of particle packing (Page and
Shibata, 1981; Ashraf and Halverson, 1978).

CONCLUSIONS

In summary, the effects of injury on the structure of cardiac
intercellular junctions are surprisingly slight. In sectioned material, no detectable changes in junction ultrastructure were found.
In freeze fracture replicas of gap junctions, a decrease in P-face
particle spacing and an increase in regularity of particle and pit
packing were observed. These changes in junction structure, particularly those related to the packing pattern of the junctional particles and pits, appear to be convenient markers for gap junctions
which have been uncoupled by injury.

There is no evidence that the changes in gap junction structure
are related in any causal way to the uncoupling process. In fact,
some recent reports have indicated that uncoupling precedes any
changes in junction ultrastructure (Anderson et al., 1981; Hanna
et al., 1981). Attempts to discover changes in the structure of the
connexon particles themselves after uncoupling treatments have led
to somewhat conflicting results (Dahl and Isenberg, 1980; Peracchia,
1980; Hanna et al., 1981). Thus we shall have to await further developments before discovering the structural changes which are directly responsible for functional uncoupling of cell junctions.

REFERENCES

Anderson, S. K., Atkinson, M. M., Sheridan, J. D., and Johnson,
    R. G., 1981, Freeze fracture studies of gap junctions in cells
    infected with a temperature-sensitive mutant of avian sarcoma
    virus, J. Cell Biol., 91:121a.
Baldwin, K. M., 1970, the fine structure and electrophysiology of
    heart muscle cell injury, J. Cell Biol., 46:455-476.
Baldwin, K. M., 1977, The fine structure of healing over in mammalian
    cardiac muscle, J. Mol. Cell. Cardiol., 9:959-966.
Baldwin, K. M., 1979, Cardiac gap junction configuration after an
    uncoupling treatment as a function of time, J. Cell Biol.,
    82:66-75.
Baldwin, K. M., 1981, Cell-to-cell tracer movement in cardiac muscle,
    Cell Tissue Res., 221:279-294.
Brink, P. R., and Dewey, M. M., 1978, Nexal membrane permeability to
    anions, J. Gen. Physiol., 72:67-86.
Dahl, G., and Isenberg, G., 1980, Decoupling of heart muscle cells:
    correlation with increased cytoplasmic calcium activity and
    with changes of nexus ultrastructure, J. Membr. Biol., 53:
    63-75.
Hanna, R. B., Reese, T. S., Ornberg, R. L., Spray, D. C. and
    Bennett, M. V. L., 1981, Fresh frozen gap junctions: resolu-
    tion of structural detail in the coupled and uncoupled states,
    J. Cell Biol., 91:125a.
Page, E. and Shibata, Y., 1981, Permeable junctions between cardiac
    cells, Ann. Rev. Physiol., 43:431-441.
Peracchia, C., 1977, Gap junctions. Structural changes after uncoup-
    ling procedures, J. Cell Biol., 72:628-641.
Peracchia, C., 1980, Structural correlates of gap junction permeation,
    Int. Rev. Cytol., 66:81-146.
Sheridan, J., 1974, Electrical coupling of cells and cell communica-
    tion, in "Cell Communication", R. P. Cox ed., John Wiley and
    Sons, New York.
Simpson, I., Rose, B., and Lowenstein, W. R., 1977, Size limit of
    molecules permeating the junctional membrane channels, Science,
    195:294-296.
Sjostrand, F. S., and Anderson, E., 1954, Electron microscopy of the
    intercalated discs of cardiac muscle tissue, Experientia, 10:
    369-371.
Sommer, J. R., and Johnson, E. A., 1979, Ultrastructure of cardiac
    muscle, in "Handbook of Physiology - The Cardiovascular System
    1," R. M. Berne ed., Williams and Wilkins, Baltimore.

MODULATION OF JUNCTIONAL PERMEABILITY IN CARDIAC FIBERS

Walmor C. De Mello

Department of Pharmacology, Medical Sciences Campus
G.P.O. Box 5067
San Juan, Puerto Rico 00936

The concept of cardiac muscle as an anatomical syncytium prevailed for years. In a detailed analysis of heart structure made at the beginning of the century, Heidenheim (1901) referring to Godlewsky's (1901) observations emphasized the finding that no cell boundary was found in sections of embryonic heart muscle (..."dass sich damals trotz genauer Untersuchungen Keine Zellengrenzen fanden"). At that time intercalated discs were usually considered contraction artifacts or even sites of sarcomere differentiation (see Godlewsky, 1901, 1902).

The development of electron microscopy enabled Sjöstrand and Andersson (1954) to demonstrate that cardiac muscle fibers consist of single cells which are surrounded by a cell membrane and isolated from each other by clefts which have been considered as a part of the extracellular space (Sjöstrand and Andersson, 1954; Pöche and Lindner, 1955).

The plasma cell membrane is, however, modified at the intercellular region and shows not only desmosomes but areas in which the two apposing cell membranes are in intimate contact -the nexus or gap junction (Dewey and Barr, 1964).

Freeze-cleave preparations of liver and other cells (see McNutt and Weinstein, 1970; Gilula and Satir, 1971) show particles distributed extensively throughout the non-junctional membrane. The intramembranous particles in the area of cell contact are distributed in a hexagonal array and closely packed (McNutt and Weinstein, 1973), establishing patches which, in the heart, are small in diameter (see Peracchia, 1980). The particles (70-80 A in diameter) have dots in its center. Electron-dense channels have been identified in negative stains of gap junctions (Gilula, 1978).

37

The formation of intercytoplasmic channels involves the contact of particles or hemichannels with similar structures located in the plasma membrane of the apposing cell (see Fig. 1). This process is achieved in a relatively short time since the time required for the synchronization of the beat in cultured heart cells varies from a few minutes to 1 h (Mark and Strasser, 1966; De Haan and Hirakow, 1972; Sperelakis, 1972). In cultured heart cells the coupling resistance is quite high (>100 MΩ) at the moment of cell contact but begins to fall immediately after reaching values of about 20 MΩ at the moment of synchronization (Clapham et al.,1980). Assuming a resistance of 1 x 10^{10} Ω for a single hydrophilic channel the rate of channel synthesis was found to be one channel per cell per minute (Clapham et al., 1980).

SPREAD OF ELECTRICAL ACTIVITY IN HEART MUSCLE

As cardiac fibers consist of separated cells surrounded by a membrane with a high electrical resistance it became difficult to understand how the activation of a cell initiates activity in its neighbors. We know today that hydrophilic channels connect the cytosol of cardiac cells providing the conditions for a morphological "continuum". This means that although cardiac fibers are composed of separated units the classification of the heart as a functional syncytium is valid.

In syncytial tissues the most probable mechanism of impulse propagation is local circuit current flow. During the passage of an electrical impulse action current flows in local circuit from the active areas along the myoplasm and gap junctions, outward through the resting adjacent cell membrane, back along the extra-cellular fluid and inward through the active region so completing the local circuit (see Fig. 2).

The potential change across the non-junctional cell membrane (V_m) is given by the difference between the potential on the inside (V_1) and the potential on the outside of the cell (V_o).

$V_m = (V_1 - V_o)$. The current flowing along the outside of the cell membrane is $i_o = \dfrac{-1}{r_o} \dfrac{dV_o}{dx}$, where $\dfrac{dV_o}{dx}$ is the extra-cellular potential gradient and r_o the resistance per unit length of the extracellular fluid.

The current flowing along the core of the cardiac fiber is given by

$i_i = \dfrac{-1}{r_i} \dfrac{dV_i}{dx}$, where $\dfrac{dV_i}{dx}$ is the intracellular

potential gradient and r_i the intracellular resistance per unit length, which represents the myoplasmic and junctional resistances.

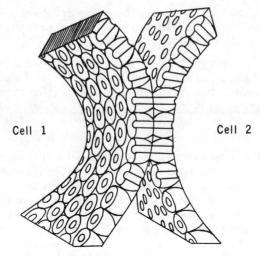

Figure 1. Diagrammatic visualization of the gap junction. Hemichannels from apposing plasma membranes are fused together at the central part of the Figure establishing
intercellular channels.

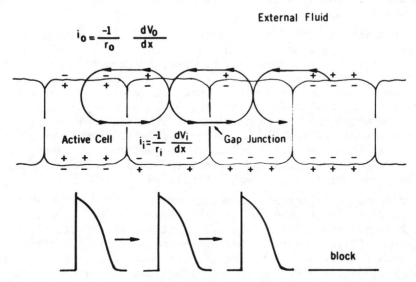

Figure 2. Diagram illustrating the flow of local circuit current
in a cardiac fiber and emphasizing the role of juntional
conductance in the spread of propagated activity. At
right - block of impulse conduction due to a marked
increase in junctional resistance.

Contrary to nerve cells, cardiac myocytes have a highly structured intracellular medium in which the sarcoplasmic reticulum is probably the most refinely organized system.

Although it is reasonable to think that these structures may enhance the myoplasmic resistance (Kushmerick and Podolsky, 1969) experimental evidence has been provided that the cytoplasm of muscle fibers has a specific resistance of the same order of magnitude of the resistance of the extracellular fluid (Fatt and Katz, 1951; Falk and Fatt, 1964).

The hypothesis that activity spreads in cardiac muscle by local circuit flow has been intensively investigated (see Weidmann, 1970). A conclusive test of the hypothesis is the injection of a current pulse into the cell and the study of its effect on the membrane potential of neighboring cells. When subthreshold current pulses are used electrotonic potentials can be recorded from cells located nearby. In cardiac Purkinje fibers evidence has been provided that electric current flows freely between the cells (Weidmann, 1952). The electrotonus in these fibers can be precisely described by the cable equations and the steady-state distribution of the electrotonic potentials closely follows the predict results for a uniform cable. The core resistivity in Purkinje fibers is quite low (105 Ωcm; Weidmann, 1952) and the space constant is large (1.9 mm - Weidmann, 1952) in comparison with the length of a single cell (125 μm) which means that the electrical resistance of the inter-cellular junctions is very low (Kamiyama and Matsuda, 1966; Weidmann, 1970; see Fig. 3).

In rat atrium, the depolarization of one cell causes appreciable changes in the membrane potential of adjacent cells (Woodbury and Crill, 1961). In these studies, however, a steep decrement of the electrotonic potentials is found (λ = 130 μm) when the cell is polarized through an intracellular microelectrode. A high intra-cellular or extracellular resistance, or a low non-junctional resistance might explain these results. The enormous decrement of the electrotonic potential, however, is related to the three-dimensional characteristics of the rat trabecula. The decay is abrupter than exponential and is better fitted by a Bessel function (Woodbury and Crill, 1961; Noble, 1962).

Widespread of electrotonic potential, however, can be observed in myocardial fibers when the current is applied to the tissue through large extracellular electrodes (Trautwein et al., 1956; Sakamoto, 1969; Weidmann, 1970). When the polarizing current influences many cells synchronously, the space constant ranges from 880 μm (Weidmann, 1970) to 1.300 μm (Kamiyama and Matsuda, 1966 and Sakamoto, 1969).

Barr et al. (1965) demonstrated that impulse conduction along a thin bundle of atrial muscle is blocked by immersing its

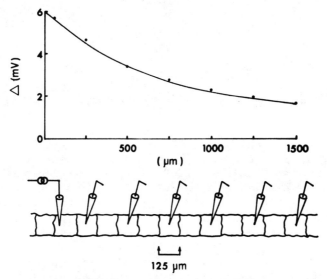

Fig. 3.   Spread of voltage along a cardiac Purkinje fiber
showing a space constant much larger than the length
of a single cell.

central portion in isotonic sucrose solution while keeping the two
ends of the muscle strip in Ringer's solution. The suppression of
impulse conduction is due to the increase of the extracellular
resistance produced by the sucrose solution. Consequently the
longitudinal flow of current through the myoplasm and extracellular
fluid is abolished. The conduction is re-established, however, if
an electrical shunt is produced between the two pools of Ringer's
solution. These findings indicate that a low internal and external
resistance are necessary are necessary for the propagation of the
action potential.

The velocity of impulse conduction (θ) depends on the intracellular longitudinal resistance (r_i) and is closely related to
fiber diameter (a)

$$\theta \quad \alpha \quad \frac{1}{\sqrt{r_i a}}$$

Therefore, one way of achieving a higher speed of impulse conduction
is reducing r_i. This can be obtained by increasing the diameter of
the fiber or the number or conductance of the intercellular channels.
The role of r_i in the control of conduction velocity in heart has
been neglected in the past because it was assumed that the intracellular resistance was low and fixed. We know today that the
junctional resistance can be modulated by variation of free $\{Ca^{++}\}_i$
or by pH_i (De Mello, 1975, 1980a, 1982; Rose and Loewenstein, 1975b).

Evidence has been provided, for instance, that ouabain decreases
the junctional conductance in Purkinje fibers (De Mello, 1976) or
myocardial fibers (Weingart, 1977) and concurrently reduces the
conduction velocity. Complete suppression of impulse conduction
can be accomplished by markedly enhancing the junctional resistance
(De Mello, 1975; see Fig. 2).

The slow conduction in the atrioventricular node has been associated with a high intracellular resistance (De Mello, 1977a; Ikeda
et al., 1980). In this tissue, the cells are electrically coupled
but the space constant measured using a suction electrode to
polarize the cells is quite small (430 μm - De Mello, 1977a). The
high value of r_i is probably related to the small diameter of the
node cells and also to the small number of gap junctions (Maekawa
et al., 1967; James and Sherf, 1968; De Felice and Challice, 1969).

Recently, an increase in conduction velocity has been found in
rat trabeculae simultaneously with a decline in r_i (Estapé and
De Mello, 1982). In these experiments in which the fibers are
exposed to theophylline (0.4 mM), no change in resting potential
or membrane resistance are found supporting the view that
variations in junctional resistance, per se, can indeed, control
the conduction velocity in cardiac fibers.

Interestingly, in Purkinje fibers showing spontaneous rhythmicity the space constant is greatly increased during the pacemaker potential. This means that the electrical coupling of the pacemaker cells is gradually increased in diastole, a factor certainly important in the synchronization of these cells. The increase in the space constant is not only due to a rise membrane resistance, but also to a fall in r_i during diastolic depolarization (De Mello, 1981).

JUNCTIONAL PERMEABILITY

The intercellular channels in several tissues are permeable to Na^+, Cl^-, SO_4^- and I^- (see Bennett, 1977).

In heart evidence has been provided that K ions move freely from cell-to-cell through the gap junctions. When one half of a bundle of ventricular fibers is exposed to radioactive K and the other half is continously washed with radioinactive Tyrode, a steady-state with respect to tissue ^{42}K is reached in about 6 hours (Weidmann, 1966). At the end of this time an appreciable amount of ^{42}K is found in the half of the bundle not exposed to radioactive potassium. Double tracer experiments indicate that the longitudinal movement of ^{82}Br, whose uptake by heart cells is quite small, has a shorter space constant than does the distribution of ^{42}K which was readily taken up. The exponential decay of radioactivity along the muscle has a length constant of 1.55 mm which clearly indicates that the longitudinal diffusion of ^{42}K is not hindered by the intercellular junctions (Weidmann, 1966). The quantitative analysis of these results lead to the conclusion that the permeability of the intercellular junctions is about 5.000 greater than that of the non-junctional cell membrane.

Cell-to-cell diffusion of Procion Yellow (mol. wt. 697 - Imanaga, 1974), tetraethylammonium (mol. wt. 130 - Weingart, 1974), ^{14}C-AMP (mol. wt. 328 - Tsien and Weingart, 1976) and fluorescein (mol. wt. 330 - Pollack, 1976; De Mello, 1979a) has been reported in cardiac tissues.

Recently, a new compound - Lucifer Yellow CH (mol. wt. 473) was introduced by Stewart (1978) as a fluorescent probe and proved extremely valuable in studies of cell-to-cell communication. This dye is a substituted four-amino naphthalimide with two sulfonate groups (see Bennett et al., 1978) and has the advantage of not diffusing through the non-junctional membrane.

We have carried out studies on the longitudinal movement of Lucifer Yellow along dog trabeculae after its introduction into the cell with the cut-end method (Imanaga, 1974). The results show that in myocardial fibers immersed in normal Tyrode solution at 37° C, an appreciable amount of the dye can be detected by spectrofluorometric methods 4 mm away from the rubber partition, 1 1/2 h later (see Fig. 4 - De Mello and Castillo, unpublished).

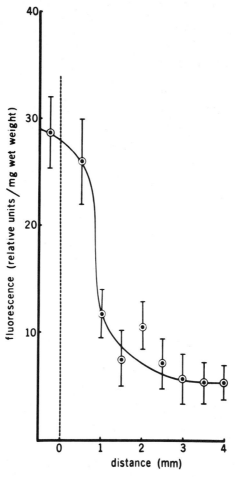

Fig. 4.   Longitudinal diffusion of Lucifer Yellow along dog
           trabeculae immersed in normal Tyrode solution. Diffusion
           period – 90 min. The vertical dotted line separates the
           loaded (left) from the unloaded area (Right). Average
           from 20 muscles. Vertical line at each point – S.D. of
           the mean. From De Mello and Castillo, unpublished.

The question remains if the longitudinal movement of Lucifer
Yellow is, indeed, due to intracellular diffusion. Washout studies
indicate that the dye leaves the extracellular space very quickly.
As is shown in Fig. 5 the washout curve consists of a first rapid
component ($t^{1/2}$ of 148 min.) which represents the loss of Lucifer
Yellow from the extracellular space and a second slow component
which correlates to the outward movement of the dye through the
surface cell membrane. The second component has an extremely large
$t^{1/2}$ (2×10^3 min. in some experiments), supporting the view that
the permeability of the non-junctional membrane to Lucifer Yellow
is negligible.

These results lead to the conclusion that the longitudinal
spread of Lucifer Yellow seen in myocardial fibers is, indeed, due
to transjunctional diffusion.

ON THE CONTROL OF JUNCTIONAL PERMEABILITY

Classical studies of Engelmann (1877) showed that in cardiac
muscle the injury potentials are quickly and spontaneously reversed
-a phenomenon called healing-over. The rapid disappearance of the
injury potentials is not due to depolarization of the non-damaged
cells because a new lesion produced near the previous one re-establish-
es the injury potential.

The healing-over process was initially interpreted as an
evidence of pre-established ionic barriers between the heart cells
(Rothschuh, 1951). This hypothesis was discarded because the core
resistivity in heart fibers was found to be quite low (105 Ωcm -
Weidmann, 1952). The formation of new membrane at the site of
injury (surface precipitation reaction - Heilbrunn, 1956) is
probably not involved in the healing process because in damaged
skeletal muscle fibers where a plug insulates the cytoplasm from
the external medium (Heilbrunn, 1956), the electrical sealing is
absent (see De Mello, 1973).

It seems then reasonable to think that new ionic barriers
established between damaged and non-damaged cells avoid the spread
of injury currents. The site of this barrier is probably the gap
junctions located near damage (see De Mello et al., 1969).

It is conceivable that a change in the internal ionic milieu
elicited by lesion would increase the junctional resistance
appreciably and promote healing-over. It is known, for instance,
that Ca ions are essential for the healing-over of cardiac muscle
(Déleze, 1965; De Mello et al. al., 1969, De Mello, 1972). These
findings led to the hypothesis that the junctional conductance
in heart might be modulated by variations in free $\{Ca^{++}\}_i$. In
order to check this possibility I injected Ca electrophoretically
inside a normal cardiac cell and searched for possible changes in

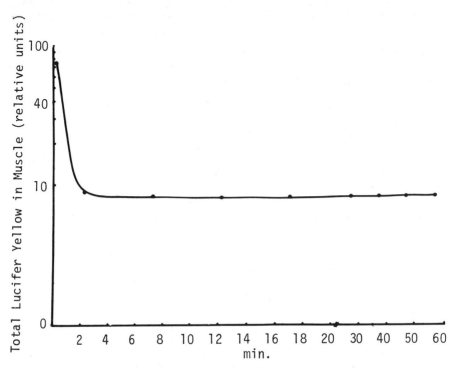

Fig. 5.   Loss of Lucifer Yellow from a dog trabecula. The wash-
               out curve shows a first rapid component ($t^{1/2}$ - 1^{48} min)
               and an extremely slow second component ($t^{1/2}$ about
               2×10^3 min). Temperature - 37°C (From De Mello and
               Castillo, unpublished).

cell-to-cell coupling. The results demonstrated that, indeed, cell
decoupling can be produced when the free $\{Ca^{2+}\}_i$ is increased above
a certain level (De Mello, 1972, 1975; - see Fig. 6). Interestingly,
the rate of healing is found to be greatly increased by stimulation
at a high rate (De Mello and Dexter, 1970) which is known to increase
the free $\{Ca^{++}\}_i$. Rose and Loewenstein (1975a) using aequorin,
demonstrated that the injection of Ca into salivary gland cells of
Chironomus produces a quick decrease of the electrical coupling
when the light emission is seen to spread all the way to the intercellular junctions.

The cell-to-cell decoupling produced by intracellular Ca
injection in heart fibers is accompanied by an increase in input
resistance of the injected cell (see Fig. 6). Both phenomena are
completely reversible. The re-establishment of cell-to-cell
communication is dependent upon homeosthatic mechanisms involved in
the maintenance of a low free $\{Ca^{2+}\}_i$ such as the active uptake of
the ion by mitochondria, sarcoplasmic reticulum or its extrusion
from the cell (see De Mello, 1975).

The mechanism by which Ca ions change the junctional conductance
is not known. Two hypotheses seem worth consideration: 1) Ca
activates enzyme reactions (through a Ca-ATPase?) which lead to
closure of the intercellular channels through a conformational
change in gap junction proteins. 2) Ca ions bind to negative polar
groups of gap junction phospholipids and abolish the permeability
of the hydrophilic channels. Phospholipids and proteins are normal
constituents of gap junctions (see Griepp and Revel, 1977).
Polyvalent cations such as La^{3+} cause cell decoupling in heart
fibers when injected into the cell (De Mello, 1979b). This finding
means that neutralization of negative charges at gap junctions
alter their conductance.

NA/CA EXCHANGE; ITS INFLUENCE ON CELL-TO-CELL COUPLING

It is known that in cardiac muscle as in nerve fibers the
extrusion of Ca is directly dependent on the energy provided by the
Na concentration gradient across the cell membrane (Reuter and
Seitz, 1968; Baker et al., 1969). The Na/K pump which depends on
ATP produces a sodium electrochemical gradient across the non-
junctional membrane which is used to energize the Ca extrusion. The
Na/Ca exchange can be reversed if the extracellular sodium
concentration is markedly reduced and if the $\{Na^+\}_i$ is enhanced.
Under these conditions, the Ca influx is large and the extrusion of
Ca small (see Blaustein and Hodgkin, 1969).

Evidence has been provided that the maintenance of a low intracellular Na concentration is essential for the preservation of cell-
to-cell coupling in heart cells (De Mello, 1974, 1976). When Na
ions are injected iontophoretically into the cytosol, r_i is

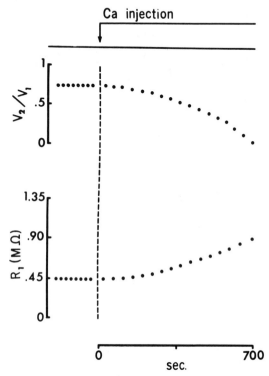

Fig. 6.   Typical effect of intracellular Ca injection on the
            input resistance (R_1) and coupling coefficient (V_2/V_1)
            of canine Purkinje cells (see also De Mello, 1975).

increased and cell decoupling is produced (see De Mello, 1976). The abolishment of the electrical coupling is dependent upon the extra-cellular Ca concentration. When $\{Ca^{++}\}_o$ is low the effect of Na injection on cell communication is negligible (De Mello, 1976). These findings strongly suggest that the decoupling action of Na injection was due to the activation of the Na/Ca exchange and consequent increase in free $\{Ca^{++}\}_i$. This idea is supported by the fact that the abolishment of the electrical coupling caused by high $\{Na^+\}_i$ is partially reversed by hyperpolarizing the non-junctional membrane (see De Mello, 1976). The recovery of cell-to-cell coupling is probably related to the fall in free $\{Ca^{++}\}_i$ produced by the increase in the Na electrochemical gradient across the non-junctional cell membrane (see Mullins and Brinley, 1975).

These observations indicate that the Na-pump is essential for the maintenance of the intercellular channels in an "open" state. Indeed, when the Na extrusion is inhibited by ouabain there is an increase in intracellular longitudinal resistance of heart fibers (Weingart, 1974) and cell-to-cell decoupling (De Mello, 1976). The drug also abolishes the cell-to-cell diffusion of Lucifer Yellow in cardiac fibers (De Mello, 1980a). The role of Ca in the decoupling action of ouabain is supported by the finding that the increase in r_i is accelerated by increasing the extracellular Ca concentration (Weingart, 1977) The exposure of heart fibers to K-free solution which is known to inhibit the Na-pump (Page et al., 1964) also caused cell decoupling (De Mello, 1980a).

As the inhibition of the Na-pump lead to electrical uncoupling the question arises whether activation of Na extrusion improves the cell-to-cell coupling. The evidence available is that this is the case. In cardiac Purkinje fibers partially depolarized by recent dissection the addition of nor-epinephrine which activates the Na-K pump in cardiac fibers (Vassalle and Barnabei, 1971), increases the resting potential and the cell-to-cell coupling (De Mello, 1977b).

The conclusion drawn from these results is that the Na pump contributes to the regulation of junctional permeability through the control of $\{Na^+\}_i$ and consequently of free $\{Ca^{++}\}_i$.

The intracellular free $\{Ca^{++}\}_i$ necessary to abolish the junctional permeability is difficult to estimate because the ion is taken up by the sarcoplasmic reticulum, mitochondria or even extruded from the cell. By comparing the increase in intracellular resistance and the time-course of the contractures produced by ouabain, Weingart (1977) reached the conclusion that the threshold concentration of free $\{Ca^{++}\}_i$ required to abolish the electrical coupling in myocardial fibers is larger than that necessary for the activation of the mechanical process. This means that a free $\{Ca^{++}\}_i$ larger than 1.8×10^{-7} M is necessary for the suppression of cell-to-cell coupling.

As the maintenance of a low intracellular free $\{Ca^{++}\}_i$ is dependent on metabolic energy it seems reasonable to think that metabolic inhibitors have an influence on intercellular communication in heart fibers. Evidence has been provided that 2-4-dinitrophenol, an uncoupler of oxydative phosphorylation, increases the intracellular resistance, abolishes the electrical coupling and the cell-to-cell diffusion of fluorescein in Purkinje fibers (see Fig. 7 and De Mello, 1979a). The suppression of intercellular communication is due to the release of Ca from intracellular stores since the contractures elicited by this compound are seen even in preparations exposed to Ca-free solution for 50 min. prior to the treatment with dinitrophenol. The depression of cell-to-cell coupling caused by the metabolic inhibitor is also found in preparations immersed in Ca-free solution. Cell communication, however, is re-established when EDTA is injected electrophoretically inside the cell (see De Mello, 1979a).

In Chironomus salivary gland the junctional permeability seems to be smoothly modulated by the free $\{Ca^{++}\}_i$ (Rose and Loewenstein, 1975b). It is not clear, however, if the modulation of junction permeability in heart is a smooth process in which all the intercellular channels are involved or if the number of active channels varies with the change in $\{Ca^{++}\}_i$.

JUNCTIONAL PERMEABILITY AND pH_i

In 1977, Turin and Warner showed that when embryonic cells of Xenopus are exposed to 100% CO_2 the pH_i falls, the cell depolarizes and the electrical coupling is abolished. More recently, an increase in r_i and cell decoupling of cardiac cells has been reported with intracellular injection of H ions (De Mello, 1980b), an effective way to reduce pH_i. In cardiac Purkinje fibers exposed to 100% CO_2, a similar increase in r_i has been found (Weingart and Reber, 1979). The question remains if the effect of intracellular acidosis on cell-to-cell coupling might be due to the increase in free $\{Ca^{++}\}_i$. In Chironomus salivary gland cells (Rose and Rick, 1978) or in barnacle muscle (Lea and Ashley, 1978) the fall in pH_i elicited by high pCO_2 is seen concurrently with a rise in free $\{Ca^{++}\}_i$. Hess and Weingart (1980) showed, however, that in sheep Purkinje fibers the exposure to high pCO_2 causes a fall in pH_i but the free $\{Ca^{++}\}_i$ is reduced.

These findings might indicate that H ions have a direct effect on junctional permeability in cardiac fibers. In embryonic cells of Fundulus acidification of the cytoplasm causes electrical decoupling -an effect due to a direct interaction of protons with gap junction macromolecules (Spray et al., 1981). However, as the buffer capacity of cardiac cells is quite high (Ellis and Thomas, 1976) it is not clear if pH_i plays a role in the modulation of junctional permeability under physiological conditions. During

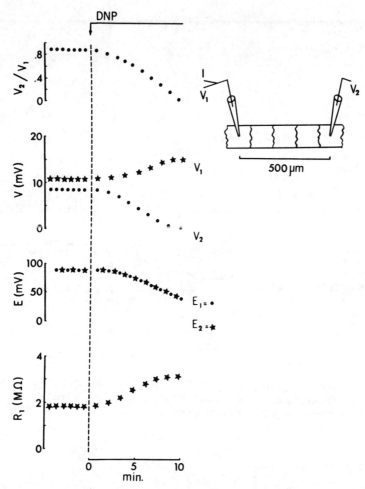

Fig. 7.   Effect of 2-4 dinitrophenol on the coupling coefficient
           (V_2/V_1), membrane potential (ε) and input resistance
           (R_1) of a canine Purkinje fiber (From De Mello, 1979a).

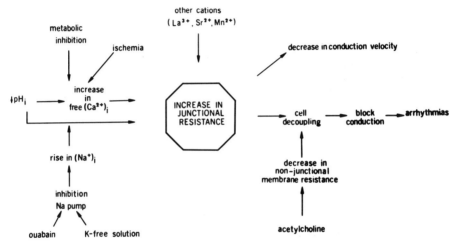

Fig. 8.   General diagram illustrating the influence of different
           factors on junctional conductance of cardiac fibers and
           their major consequences.

ischemia, however, when the pH_o and pH_i are reduced (Neely et al., 1975) the suppression of cell communication might be in part dependent on the fall in pH_i (De Mello, 1982).

Fig. 8 shows the influence of ionic and metabolic factors on junctional resistance and the major consequences of cell decoupling. As can be seen, a decrease in conduction velocity and cardiac arrhythmias can be ascribed to drastic changes in the electrical coupling.

IS CYCLIC AMP INVOLVED IN THE CONTROL OF JUNCTIONAL PERMEABILITY?

Cyclic nucleotides and Ca seem to be intimately related in the process of modulation of cell function induced by hormones (see Goldberg, 1975). In many systems, Ca ions seem to play a role as important as cyclic AMP as a second messenger (Rasmussen, 1975). The level of Ca in the cytosol seems to regulate the concentration of cyclic AMP. When the free $\{Ca^{++}\}_i$ rises the concentration of the nucleotide is reduced, in part due to inactivation of adenylate cyclase (see Rasmussen, 1975).

These observations lead to an important question - can cyclic AMP regulate the junctional permeability? In salivary glands of Drosophila cyclic-AMP increases cell-to-cell coupling (Hax et al., 1974). It has been suggested that in ovarian the oocyte receives cyclic AMP from the surrounding cummulus cells through gap junctions (Hertzberg et al., 1981) and that loss of the intercellular movement of the nucleotide might be important in the control of oocyte maturation.

Is cAMP involved in the control of junctional permeability in cardiac muscle? Preliminary studies performed on rat trabeculae show that theophylline, an inhibitor of phosphodiesterase, at low concentration (0.4 mM), increases the spread of electrotonic activity and the conduction velocity (Estapé and De Mello, 1982). As the time constant of the cell membrane is not changed by this compound it seems reasonable to conclude that the increment in space constant (59%) is not due to an increment in membrane resistance. Calculations of r_i on the basis of conduction velocity and the time constant of the "foot" of the action potential indicate that the intracellular longitudinal resistance (r_i) is reduced by theophylline (0.4 mM). Assuming that the myoplasmic resistivity is not changed these results indicate that the junctional conductance is increased by the phosphodiesterase inhibitor. The mechanism by which theophylline reduces r_i is not known.

The most plausible assumption is that the increment in intracellular concentration of cAMP produced by the drug may enhance the junctional conductance.

The effect of cAMP on cell-to-cell coupling is probably variable according to the concentration of the nucleotide. It is known, for

instance, that a substantial rise in concentration of cAMP leads to
an increase in membrane permeability to Ca ions (see Reuter, 1979;
Sperelakis, 1980). This means that small increments in concentration
of the nucleotide might reduce r_i while larger concentrations would
increase r_i through a rise in free $\{Ca^{++}\}_i$. Supporting this idea
is the finding that theophylline, at high concentration (4 mM) or
caffeine (6 mM) decreases the electrical coupling of heart cells
(De Mello, 1978).

It is known that receptor-hormone interaction at the surface
cell membrane leads to the production of cyclic AMP in the cell
interior. The increment in concentration of cAMP may change cell-
to-cell communication by varying the junctional conductance. This
mechanism probably plays a role in the long-term modulation of
junctional permeability.

Cell-to-cell coupling may be also influenced by hormonally
induced changes in membrane potential which activate voltage-
sensitive Ca channels.

In conclusion, the fine modulation of junctional permeability
seems to depend on intracellular and extracellular factors which
are intimately related to cell function.

Despite the fact that cardiac cells are in continuous
communication, cell privacy is preserved under circumstances in
which neighboring cells are inflicted by lesion or disease.

REFERENCES

Baker, P. F., Blaustein, M. P., Hodgkin, A. L., and Steinhardt, R.
    A., 1969, The influence of calcium on sodium efflux in
    squid axons. J. Physiol. (London), 200: 431.
Barr, L., Dewey, M. M., and Berger, W., 1965, Propagation of action
    potentials and the nexus in cardiac muscle. J. gen. Physiol.
    48: 797.
Bennett, M. V. L., 1977, Electrical transmission: a functional
    analysis and comparison to chemical transmission, in:
    "Cellular Biology of Neurons" (Handbook of Physiology,
    Section 1: The Nervous System, Vol. 1, E. R. Kandel, ed.,
    Williams and Wilkins, Baltimore. pp 357-416.
Bennett, M. V. L., Spira, M. E., and Spray, D. C., 1978,
    Permeability of gap junctions between embryonic cells of
    Fundulus; a reevaluation. Dev. Biol., 65: 114.
Blaustein, M. P., and Hodgkin, A. L., 1969, The effect of cyanide
    on the efflux of calcium from squid axons. J. Physiol.
    (London), 200: 497.

Clapham, D. E., Schrier, A., and De Haan, R. L., 1980, Junctional
    resistance and action potential delay between embryonic cell
    aggregates. J. gen. Physiol., 75: 633.
De Felice, L. J., and Challice, C. E. (1969), Anatomical and
    ultrastructural study of the electrophysiological atrio-
    ventricular node of the rabbit. Circulation Res., 24: 457.
De Haan, R. L., and Hirakow, R.,1972, Synchronization of pulsation
    rates in isolated cardiac myocytes. Exp. Cell Res., 70: 214.
Déleze, J., 1965, Calcium ions and the healing-over of heart fibres,
    in: "Electrophysiology of the Heart", B. Taccardi and G.
    Marchetti, eds., Pergamon Press, London. pp 147-148.
De Mello, W. C., 1972, The healing-over process in cardiac and
    other muscle fibers, in:"Electrical Phenomena in the Heart",
    W. C. De Mello, ed., Academic Press, New York. pp 323-351.
De Mello, W. C., 1973, Membrane sealing in frog skeletal muscle
    fibres. Proc. Natl. Acad. Sci. USA, 70: 4.
De Mello, W. C., 1974, Electrical uncoupling in heart fibres
    produced by intracellular injection of Na or Ca. Fedn.
    Proc., 17: 3.
De Mello, W. C., 1975, Effect of intracellular injection of
    calcium and strontium on cell communication in heart. J.
    Physiol. (London), 250: 231.
De Mello, W C.. 1976, Influence of the sodium pump on intracellular
    communication in heart fibres: Effect of intracellular
    injection of sodium ion on electrical coupling. J. Physiol.,
    (London), 263: 171.
De Mello, W. C., 1977a, Passive electrical properties of the atrio-
    ventricular node. Pflüg. Arch., 371: 135.
De Mello, W. C., 1977b, Factor involved on the control of
    junctional conductance in heart. Proc. Int. Union
    Physiol. Sci., 12: 319.
De Mello, W. C., 1978, Cell-to-cell diffusion of fluorescein in
    heart fibers. Fed. Proc., 37: 3.
De Mello, W. C., 1979a, Effect of 2-4-dinitrophenol on inter-
    cellular communication in mammalian cardiac fibres.
    Pflüg. Arch., 38: 267.
De Mello, W. C., 1979b, Effect of intracellular injection of La^{3+}
    and Mn^{2+} on electrical coupling of heart cells. Cell Biol.
    Intern. Rep., 3: 113.
De Mello, W. C., 1980a, Intercellular Communication and junctional
    permeability, in:"Membrane Structure and ·Function", E. E.
    Bittar, ed., John Wiley and Sons, Inc., New York, Vol. 3,
    pp 128-170.
De Mello, W. C., 1980b, Influence of intracellular injection of
    H$^+$ on the electrical coupling in cardiac Purkinje fibres.
    Cell Biol. Intern. Rep., 4: 51.
De Mello, W. C., 1981, Enhanced cell communication during diastolic
    depolarization in heart. The Physiologist, 24: 61.

De Mello, W. C., 1982, Intercellular communication in cardiac muscle. Circulation Res., 50: 2.

De Mello, W. C., and Dexter, D., 1970, Increased rate of sealing in beating heart muscle of the toad. Circulation Res., 26: 481.

De Mello, W. C., Motta, G., and Chapeau, M., 1969, A study on the healing-over of myocardial cells of toads. Circulation Res., 24: 475.

Dewey, M. M., and Barr, L., 1964, A study of structure and distribution of the nexus. J. Cell Biol., 23: 553.

Ellis, D., and Thomas, R. C., 1976, Direct measurement of the intracellular pH of mammalian cardiac muscle. J. Physiol. (London), 262: 755.

Engelmann, T. W., 1877, Vergleichende Untersuchungen zur Lehre von der Muskel-und Nervenelektricitat. Pflüg. Arch., 15: 116.

Estapé, E., and De Mello, W. C., 1982, Effect of theophylline on the spread of electrotonic activity in heart. Fed. Proc., 41: 1505.

Falk, G., and Fatt, P., 1964, Linear electrical properties of striated muscle fibres observed with intracellular electrodes. Proc. Roy. Soc. (London), Ser. B, Vol. 160, pp 69-123.

Fatt, P., and Katz, B., 1951, An analysis of the end-plate potential recorded with an intracellular microelectrode. J. Physiol., (London), 115: 320.

Gilula, N. B., 1978, Structure of intercellular junctions, in: "Intercellular Junctions and Synapses", J. Feldman, N. B. Gilula, and J. D. Pitts, eds, Chapman and Hall, London, pp 3-22.

Gilula, N. B., and Satir, P., 1971, Septate and gaps junctions in molluscan gill epithelium. J. Cell Biol., 51: 869.

Godlewsky, E., 1901, Ueber die Entwickelung des quergestreifen musculosen Gewebes. Bull. Inst. Acad. Sci. Krakaner Cracovie, 39: 45.

Godlewsky, E., 1902, Die Entwicklung des Skelet- und Herzmuskelgewebes der Säugethiere. Arch. fur Mikrosk. Anat., 60: 111.

Goldberg, N., 1975, Cyclic Nucleotides and Cell Function, in: "Cell Membranes; biochemistry, cell biology and pathology", G. Weismann and R. Claiborne, eds. H. P. Publishing Co., Inc. New York, pp 185.

Griepp, E. B., and Revel, J. P., 1977, Gap junctions in Development, in: "Intercellular Communication", W. C. De Mello, ed., Plenum Press, New York, pp 1-32.

Hax, Werner M. A., van Venrooij, Ger E. P. M., and Vossenberg, Joost B. J., 1974, Cell communication: A cyclic-AMP mediated phenomenon. J. Membrane Biol., 19: 253.

Heidenhain, M., 1901, Ueber die Structur des menschlichen Herzmuskels. Anat. Anz., 20: 33.

Heilbrunn, L. V., 1956, Dynamics of Living Protoplasm, L. V. Heilbrunn, ed., Academic Press, New York.

Hertzberg, E. L., Lawrence, T. S., and Gilula, N., 1981, Gap junctional communication. Ann. Rev. Physiol., 43: 479.

Hess, P., and Weingart, W., 1980, Intracellular free calcium
    modified by pHi in sheep Purkinje fibres. J. Physiol.
    (London), 307: 60.
Ikeda, N., Toyama, J., Shimizu, T., Kodama, I., and Yamada, K.,
    1980, The role of electrical uncoupling in the genesis of
    atrioventricular conduction disturbance. J. Mol. Cell
    Cardiol., 12: 809.
Imanaga, I., 1974, Cell-to-cell diffusion of Procion Yellow in
    sheeps and calf Purkinje fibres, J. Membrane Biol., 16: 381.
James, T. N., and Scherf, L., 1968, Ultrastructure of the atrio-
    ventricular node. Circulation, 37: 1049.
Kamiyama, A., and Matsuda, K., 1966, Electrophysiological properties
    of the canine ventricular fiber. Gap J. Physiol., 16: 407.
Kushmerick, M. J., and Podolsky, R. G., 1969, Ionic mobility in
    muscle cells. Science, N. Y., 166: 1297.
Lea, T. J., and Ashley, C. C., 1978, Increase in free Ca^{2+} in muscle
    after exposure to CO_2. Nature (London), 275: 236.
Maekawa, M., Nohara, Y., Kawamura, K., and Hayashi, K., 1967,
    Electron microscope study of the conduction system in
    mammalian hearts, in: "Electrophysiology and ultrastructure
    of the heart", T. Sano, V. Mizuhira, and K. Matsuda, eds.,
    Grune and Stratton, New York. pp 41 54.
Mark, G. E., and Strasser, F. F., 1966, Pacemaker activity and
    mitosis in cultures of newborn rat heart ventricle cells.
    Exp. Cell. Res., 44: 217.
Mullins, L. J., and Brinley, F. J., Jr., 1975, The sensitivity of
    calcium efflux from squid axons to changes in membrane
    potential. J. gen. Physiol., 65: 135.
McNutt, N. S., and Weinstein, R. S., 1970, Ultrastructure of the
    nexus. A correlated thin section and freezed cleave study,
    J. Cell Biol., 47: 666.
McNutt, N. S., and Weinstein, R. S., 1973, Membrane ultrastructure
    at mammalian intercellular junctions, in: "Progress in
    Biophysics and Molecular Biology", J. A. Butler and D.
    Noble, eds., Pergamon Press, London, Vol. 26, pp 45-101.
Neely, J. R., Whitmer, J. T., and Robetto, M. J., 1975, Effect of
    coronary flow on glycolitic flux and intracellular pH in
    isolated rat hearts. Circulation Res., 37: 733.
Noble, D., 1962, The voltage dependence of the cardiac membrane
    conductance. Biophys. J., 2: 381.
Page, E., Goerke, R. J., and Storm, S. R., 1964, Cat Heart Muscle
    In Vitro IV. Inhibition of transport in quiescent muscles.
    J. gen. Physiol., 47: 531.
Peracchia, C., 1980, Structural correlates of gap junction permeation
    Internat. Rev. Cytol., 66: 81-146.
Pöche, R., and Lindner, R., 1955, Untersuchungen zur Frage der
    Glanzstreifen des Herzmuskelgewebes bein Warmblüter and
    beim Kalbluter. Z. Zellforsch. Mikrosk. Anat., 43: 104.
Pollack, G. H., 1976, Intercellular coupling in the atrioventricular
    node and other tissues of the heart. J. Physiol. (London),

Rasmussen, H., 1975, Ions as "Second Messengers", in: "Cell
    Membranes, biochemistry, cell biology and pathology", G.
    Weismann and R. Claiborne, eds., H.P. Publishing Co., Inc.,
    New York. pp 203.
Reuter, H., 1979, Properties of two inward membrane currents in the
    heart. Ann. Rev. Physiol., 41: 413.
Reuter, H., and Seitz, N., 1968, The dependence of calcium efflux
    from cardiac muscle on temperature and external ion
    composition. J. Physio. (London), 195: 451.
Rose, B., and Loewenstein, W. R., 1975a, Calcium ion distribution
    in cytoplasm visualized by aequorin: diffusion in cytosol
    restricted by energized sequestering. Science, N. Y. 190:
    1204.
Rose, B., and Loewenstein, W. R., 1975b, Permeability of cell
    junction depends on local cytoplasmic reticulum activity.
    Nature (London), 254: 250.
Rose, B., and Rick, R., 1978, Intracellular pH, intracellular free
    Ca, and junctional cell-cell coupling. J. Membrane Biol.,
    44: 377.
Rothschuh, K. E., 1951, Ueber den funktionellen Aufbau des Herzens
    aus elektrophysiologischen Elementen and ueber den
    Mechanisms der Erregungsleitung in Herzen. Pflügers Arch.,
    253: 238.
Sakamoto, Y., 1969, Membrane characteristic of the canine papillary
    muscle fiber. J. gen. Physiol., 54: 765.
Sjöstrand, F. S., and Andersson, C. E., 1954, Electron microscopy
    of the intercalated discs of cardiac muscle tissue.
    Experientia, 10: 369.
Sperelakis, N., 1972, Electrical properties of embryonic heart
    cells, in: "Electrical Phenomena in the Heart", W. C. De
    Mello, ed., Academic Press, New York, pp 1.
Sperelakis, N., 1980, Changes in membrane electrical properties
    during development of the heart, in:"The Slow Inward
    Current and Cardiac Arrhythmias", D. P. Zipes, J. C. Bailey
    and V. Elharrar, eds., Martinus Nijhoff Publishers, The
    Hague, pp 221.
Spray, D. C., Harris, A. L., and Bennett, M. V. L., 1981, Gap
    junctional conductance is a simple and sensitive function
    of intracellular pH. Science, N. Y., 211: 712.
Stewart, W. C., 1978, Functional connections between cells as
    revealed by dye-coupling with a high fluorescent
    naphthalimide tracer. Cell, 14: 741.
Trautwein, W., Kuffler, S. W., and Edwards, C., 1956, Changes in
    membrane characteristics of heart muscle during inhibition.
    J. gen. Physiol., 40: 135.
Tsien, R., and Weingart, R., 1976, Inotropic effect of cyclic AMP
    in calf ventricular muscle studied by a cut end method. J.
    Physiol. (London), 260: 117.

Turin, L., and Warner, A. E., 1977, Carbon dioxide reversibly abolishes ionic communication between cells of early amphybian embryon. Nature (London), 27: 56.

Vassalle, M., and Barnabei, O., 1971, Nor-epinephrine and potassium fluxes in cardiac Purkinje fibres. Pflug. Arch., 322: 287.

Weidmann, S., 1952, The electrical constants of Purkinje fibres, J. Physiol. (London), 118: 348.

Weidmann, S., 1966, The diffusion of radiopotassium across intercalated discs of mammalian cardiac muscle. J. Physiol. (London), 187: 323.

Weidmann, S., 1970, Electrical constants of trabecular muscle from mammalian heart. J. Physiol. (London), 210: 1041.

Weingart, R., 1974, The permeability to tetraethylammonium ions of the surface membrane and the intercalated disks of the sheep and calf myocardium. J. Physiol. (London), 240: 741.

Weingart, R., 1977, The action of ouabain on intercellular coupling and conduction velocity in mammalian ventricular muscle. J. Physiol. (London), 264: 341.

Weingart, R., and Reber, W., 1979, Influence of internal pH on r_i of Purkinje fibres from mammalian heart. Experientia, 35: 929.

Woodbury, J. W., and Crill, W. E., 1961, On the problem of impulse conduction in the atrium, in: "Nervous Inhibition", E. Florey, ed., Pergamon Press, Oxford, pp 124-135.

THE ROLE OF CELL-TO-CELL COUPLING IN CARDIAC CONDUCTION DISTURBANCES

Madison S. Spach

Departments of Pediatrics and Physiology
Duke University Medical Center
Durham, North Carolina 27710, U.S.A.

INTRODUCTION

The propagation of electrical excitation in cardiac muscle has, since its identification more than a century ago, generally been treated as though it occurred in a continuous structure. While it has been well-appreciated that cardiac muscle is composed of individual cells connected together by low resistance connections, it has been considered that the electrical effects of the structural complexity produced by the connections between cells and between bundles are of minor importance, presumably to have the tissue fit a simple model for useful theoretical analysis. Because of this, most analyses of cardiac conduction have been based on the simplifying assumption that the structure has the electrical properties of continuously uniform geometry and intracellular resistivity in the direction of propagation.

It is well known that propagation in cardiac muscle exhibits a wide range of variations under both normal and abnormal conditions, such as preferential conduction, decremental conduction, slow propagation, conduction block, and reentry. Since all of these phenomena have been described in nonmyelinated nerves, it has been natural to account for the cardiac phenomena by the same mechanisms applied to nerves: differences in membrane properties and a branching structure. Thus, the analysis of the various forms of propagation in cardiac muscle have depended heavily on previous analyses for nerves (see recent review of Fozzard [8]).

Continuously Uniform Structures (Classical Concept)

Whenever a change in propagation has been observed or when

61

differences in propagation from region to region have been found in cardiac muscle, the traditional explanation has been a difference in membrane properties, just as in analyses of nerves. In such structures with passive electrical properties that approximate an ordinary continuous cable there is a positive correlation between the peak magnitude of the membrane sodium current (as expressed by $\dot{V}_{max}$) and the conduction velocity [11, 14, 24]. Thus, $\dot{V}_{max}$ and the velocity of propagation have long been closely associated in the analysis of action potentials that propagate in a continuous medium.

The association of $\dot{V}_{max}$ and the velocity of propagation in a continuous medium has profoundly affected the interpretation of the underlying mechanisms of conduction disturbances in cardiac muscle: altered membrane properties have been proposed as the basis of most all conduction phenomena necessary for cardiac arrhythmias caused by reentry. This is illustrated by several well-known analyses of cardiac impulse conduction. 1) Atrial fibers with higher $\dot{V}_{max}$ values have been thought to have special membrane properties producing large sodium currents and hence fast conduction [13, 23]. Many investigators believe there is clustering of such "specialized" fibers into a fixed-position narrow tract in some of the prominent atrial muscle bundles [15]. It is widely believed that each tract produces preferential fast and safe conduction in its muscle bundle. 2) Changes of the membrane properties along the fibers have long been considered a requirement for decremental conduction [12]. 3) A spatial difference in the refractory period is the basis for the classical model of Moe et al. [16] for reentry during atrial fibrillation and for the "leading circle" concept of Allessie et al. [1, 2]. 4) Slow conduction (<0.1 m/sec), which is routine in the AV node and in very depressed tissue [6, 17], has been attributed to slow response action potentials generated by a slow inward current rather than by the rapid sodium current. Cranefield [5] considers this mechanism necessary for reentry, noting that "It is all but certain that the slow conduction necessary for reentry can appear only in fibers that show slow response activity...."

Structural Discontinuities

The serious difficulty which the above ideas encounter when applied to the analysis of propagation of depolarization in cardiac muscle can be seen by examining recent experimental evidence and theoretical considerations that we have presented in detail elsewhere [19, 21, 22]. In essence, the evidence supports the theory that cardiac muscle is structured to propagate electrical activity in a discontinuous fashion owing to structural complexities related to the cell-to-cell couplings that produce discontinuities of effective axial (intracellular) resistivity, $\bar{R}_a$, that affect the membrane currents.

In this paper, I wish to discuss selected experiments we have done that demonstrate cardiac conduction disturbances in which the mechanisms of membrane alteration and discontinuities in axial resistance can be distinguished. The results provide a basis for explaining discontinuities of propagation at a microscopic and macroscopic size scale solely on the basis of discontinuities of axial resistance related to known structural complexities of cardiac muscle. A major implication is that the combination of discontinuities of effective axial resistivity at several size scales can produce a wide variety of complex abnormalities of propagation, including most currently known cardiac conduction disturbances that have been considered to require spatial nonuniformity of membrane properties.

METHODS

Propagation at a Microscopic Level

The in vitro methods have been described in detail previously [21, 22] and they will be summarized here. Preparations included pectinate muscles plus the crista terminalis and adjoining bundles for the atrium and papillary muscles from the right ventricle. All measurements were made at the constant temperature of 35°C. The concentration of the perfusate was 128 mM NaCl, 4.69 mM KCl, 1.18 mM $MgSO_4$, 0.41 mM NaH_2PO_4, 20.1 mM $NaHCO_3$, 2.23 mM $CaCl_2$, and 11.1 mM dextrose. The solutions were gased in a reservoir with a mixture of 95% O_2 and 5% CO_2 and perfused through the tissue bath through selective spouts at a rate of 100 ml/min to insure a high flow rate at the surface of the preparation.

The intracellular potentials were recorded with conventional glass microelectrodes. The extracellular electrodes were made of flexible tungsten wire, 50 μm in diameter, and insulated except at the tip. The separate reference electrodes for each extracellular or intracellular electrode were positioned 7 cm away from the recording site. Stimulation of the preparation was performed with extracellular electrodes using a stimulus of 0.5 to 1.0 msec in duration and 1.5 to 2.0 times threshold. A PDP-11/20 computer system [3] controlled the rate at one stimulus per second and synchronized the pacing with the data recording. A dissecting microscope equipped with a Nikon F250 35-mm camera was used to document the positions of all electrodes.

Changes in propagation velocity at one site were studied by analyzing the records (intracellular and extracellular) associated with the impalement of a single cell. Isochrone maps were constructed from the extracellular recordings, taking the time of the peak negative derivative (intrinsic deflection) as the instant of excitation. Conduction velocity then was calculated as the distance travelled normal to the isochrone per unit of time. The time constant of the

foot of the action potential (τ_{foot}) was calculated graphically by
plotting the first 8 mV of depolarization on semilogarithmic paper
and obtaining an appropriate straight line fit by eye. In the semi-
log plot of the initial 8 mV deviation from the resting potential,
there was some scattering of the points around a straight line that
resulted in a measurement error of about ± 35 µsec in τ_{foot}. The
signal-to-noise ratio of the data was not adequate to determine
whether or not the scatter was produced or increased by a non-expo-
nential component in the upstroke of the action potential.

Propagation at a Macroscopic Level

The same in vitro methods noted above were used to study propagation at a macroscopic level in the dog atrium. Macroscopic
anatomical discontinuities studied were those that could be identified easily by eye (Figure 1). They included sites of branching
where pectinate muscles arise from the crista terminalis and the
junction sites where two separate muscle bundles interconnect. Detailed isochrone maps were made from the extracellular waveforms
recorded at 30 to 100 sites within the area of conduction velocity
change; that is, in the muscle bundles forming the visible anatomical
discontinuity. It was impossible to detect and to analyze adequately
the velocity changes at these sites by means of intracellular
measurements. Therefore, the analysis was performed by using extracellular, rather than intracellular, potentials as suggested previously for detailed study of propagation in cardiac muscle [20].
They not only provided a means to detect the presence of the macroscopic discontinuities of propagation, but they provided a way to
study the mechanism associated with changes in axial resistance per
unit length at these sites.

Once an area of velocity change was identified in relation to an
anatomical discontinuity, 8 to 10 extracellular recording electrodes
were positioned along and across the muscle bundles that formed the
junctional area. Two to four stimulus electrodes were then positioned to produce propagation into the branch or junction site from
different directions. Propagation of normal action potentials was
measured while the stimulus site was varied randomly and the stimulus
rate remained constant at 1/sec. Action potentials that propagated
at different velocities were initiated at each stimulus site by the
following procedures: (1) The extracellular potassium concentration
was elevated by using a high-potassium solution that was identical
to the regular perfusing solution, except that the KCl concentration
was 15 mM. The KCl solution was introduced so that the concentration
increased gradually over 20 min. (2) Under conditions of normal
extracellular potassium concentrations (4.69 mM), a premature stimulus was injected after every 15th regular stimulus, which occurred
at a constant interstimulus interval of 800 to 1000 msec. The location of the stimulus was shifted randomly from one stimulus electrode
to another for each interval of delay between the prior normal

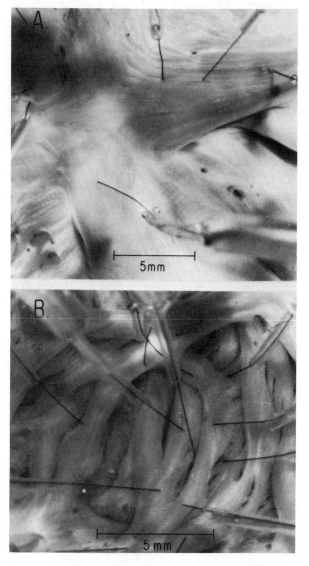

Figure 1: Structural Complexities That Result in Macroscopic Discontinuities of Axial Resistivity in the Adult Dog Atrium.
Panel A is a photograph of the junctional region of the
crista terminalis (vertical bundle) and the limbus of the
fossa ovalis (horizontal bundle) of the right atrium of a
dog. Note the abrupt directional change in the course of
the fibers in the junctional region of the two muscle
bundles. Panel B shows an endocardial view of the complex arrangement of the pectinate muscles and their
interconnections within a 1 cm^2 region. Multiple extracellular electrodes can be seen in both pictures.

stimulus and the premature stimulus. The refractory period of each
muscle bundle that formed the anatomical discontinuity was measured
in the usual way; that is, the time interval at which a 1-msec
additional delay just produced propagation to a distant recording
site located 2 to 3 cm from the stimulus electrode.

RESULTS

Anisotropic Propagation at a Microscopic Size Scale

Some of the electrical consequences of the structural anisotropy inherent in the parallel arrangement of elongated cells are
illustrated in Figure 2. The pattern of propagation is depicted on
the left side of the figure in the form of isochrones following point
stimulation by an extracellular electrode in the crista terminalis
of the right atrium of a newborn dog. The pattern is just what is
expected in a sheet with anisotropic internal resistance producing
fast propagation parallel to the long axis of the fibers and much
slower propagation in the transverse direction. The pattern shown
was reproduced when the stimulus site was moved to other positions
along the transverse axis of the bundle. Although the single pattern
shown in Figure 2 might be considered indicative of a specialized
tract that produces preferential conduction [15, 23], this cannot be
the case since the same pattern was repeatedly produced at multiple
stimulation sites across the bundle. This procedure confirms that
the pattern of propagation was related to the anisotropic properties
of the bundle, rather than to a specialized occult tract.

Evidence that the lower velocity in the transverse direction is
due to increased axial resistivity in that direction is provided by
the extracellular waveforms. Note that the largest amplitude occurred in the area of most rapid propagation (waveform d), and the
smallest amplitude of the extracellular potentials occurred when
propagation was slowest in the transverse direction (waveforms b and
c). At an intermediate velocity, the amplitude of the waveform was
intermediate in magnitude (waveform a). Thus, the amplitude of the
waveforms varied monotonically with the velocity and, in turn, the
velocity decreased monotonically as the direction of propagation
shifted from the longitudinal axis of the fibers to the transverse
axis. As shown previously [20], the extracellular potential decreases with the velocity as the intracellular current decreases
secondary to an increase in effective axial resistivity.

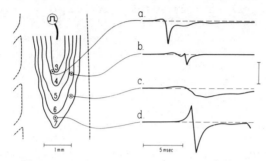

Figure 2:   Effects of Uniform Anisotropy on the Pattern of Excita-
            tion Spread and the Associated Extracellular Waveforms in
            An Atrial Muscle Bundle. Excitation was initiated at a
            point by an extracellular electrode (stimulus symbol).
            The sequence of excitation spread was derived from 30
            extracellular waveforms, four of which are shown along
            with their recording locations. The preparation was the
            crista terminalis of a newborn dog.   Vertical bar = 2 mV.

        According to continuous medium theory, the time course of the
upstroke of the transmembrane potential should not change when the
velocity is altered by changes in effective axial resistivity that
occurs when the direction of propagation is changed [4]. Figure
3 summarizes our recent results [21] which show that, contrary
to the predictions of continuous medium theory, the shape of
the action potential does change when the velocity is altered
by changing the direction of propagation with respect

to the fiber orientation. The schematic drawing shows the orientation of the individual cells with respect to the fastest and slowest
velocities θ_f and θ_s (panel 1). In atrial and ventricular muscle
bundles, high velocity is associated with a low $\dot{V}_{max}$ value and a
prolonged foot of the action potential while low velocity is associated with a high $\dot{V}_{max}$ value and a shortened foot of the action
potential. By comparing the transmembrane action potential shape
changes of Figure 3 with the extracellular waveforms of Figure 2, it
can be seen that the low velocities with high $\dot{V}_{max}$ in the transverse
direction are associated with small extracellular potentials and high
velocities with low $\dot{V}_{max}$ in the longitudinal direction are associated
with large extracellular potentials. These combined changes suggest
that the lower $\dot{V}_{max}$ is associated with low values of effective axial
resistivity in the longitudinal direction. Further, the variation in
$\dot{V}_{max}$ with changes in the direction of propagation is suggestive of a
varying load on the membrane. At low values of effective axial resistivity (longitudinal propagation), it is as though there were a
greater load on the membrane, as if more current were being drained
from a patch of membrane by a neighboring downstream patch, thus reducing the ionic current available for depolarizing itself.

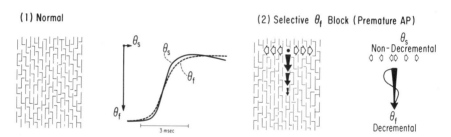

Figure 3: Directional Effects of Microscopic Discontinuities of
           Axial Resistance on (1) Normal Action Potentials (1)
           and Premature Action Potentials in Anisotropic Atrial
           Muscle (2).

As an explanation for these apparently anomalous changes in the
transmembrane action potential, we proposed that the decrease in
velocity in the transverse direction is due to the anisotropic
effects of the distribution of cell couplings, increasing the transverse coupling resistance and separating the excitable membrane into
loosely coupled units, thereby causing propagation to be discontinuous or saltatory -- jumping from unit to unit [21]. In the

longitudinal direction, the couplings make a contribution to the axial resistance comparable to that of the cytoplasmic resistivity so that little or no discrete effect is seen. In the transverse direction, however, the couplings represent the major axial resistance and produce recurrent discontinuities.

If we assume that at a microscopic level cardiac muscle is best described as a structure with recurrent discontinuities of axial resistivity, we can predict an unexpected kind of propagation that would not be possible in a continuous medium. Reduced $\dot{V}_{max}$ is generally associated with a decreased safety factor, which means a reduced capability for depolarizing downstream membrane. Thus, in spite of a higher velocity, longitudinal propagation with a low $\dot{V}_{max}$ should have a lower safety factor than transverse propagation with a higher $\dot{V}_{max}$. If the ability to supply depolarizating current is reduced by some independent means, propagation in an anisotropic sheet of cardiac muscle should fail first in the longitudinal direction -- the direction of low axial resistivity.

The right-hand panel of Figure 3 schematically represents the selective block along the longitudinal axis (θ_f) that occurred when we tested the above prediction [21]. A late premature stimulus produced steady propagation in all directions. However, when the premature stimulus interval was reduced to 155 msec, longitudinal propagation became decremental; that is, the amplitude and velocity continued to decrease with distance from the stimulus electrode until the impulse was extinguished. At the same time, however, stable propagation was still evident in the transverse direction (open arrows). We have been able to produce this type of selective directional block along the longitudinal axis of the fibers in repeated experiments, in atrial muscle bundles in which the anisotropic velocity ratios are large, and the selective block often has been associated with reentry [21, 22].

It should be emphasized that the predicted pattern of propagation for premature action potentials represented in the right-hand panel of Figure 3 depends on the presence of recurrent discontinuities in intracellular resistance. If the medium was continuous, propagation would have to fail simultaneously in both directions because, in that case, changes in effective axial resistivity scale only the spatial size of depolarization, but do not affect its time course.

Unidirectional block and decremental conduction usually have been attributed to nonuniform recovery of excitability where the action potential propagates into a region of cardiac muscle having a longer refractory period. In these experiments [21, 22] the refractory periods were measured in the region under study and, actually, there was a *decrease* in the refractory period with distance from the stimulus site along the longitudinal axis of the fibers --

the opposite of what is necessary to explain the propagation failure on the basis of different refractory periods.

Discontinuities of Propagation at a Macroscopic Size Scale

The above concept of discontinuous or saltatory propagation at a microscopic level was generalized to the premise that discontinuities of propagation also should occur at a macroscopic level when an action potential propagates into a region that represents an abrupt change in the distribution of the cell-to-cell connections; that is, when there is an abrupt change in the effective axial resistivity, $\overline{R}_a$, in the direction of propagation.

The photographs in Figure 1 of the endocardial surface of the right atrium of the dog show regions where one might expect to find abrupt changes in fiber orientation. Panel A shows the junction of the crista terminalis and limbus of the right atrium of the dog. Note the longitudinal striations in the limbus (the bundle with three electrodes orientated along the horizontal axis). These striations are produced by interrupted connective tissue septa which produce a nonuniform anisotropic type of propagation -- there is localized dissociation of excitation in adjacent fascicles during transverse propagation [22]. In the region where the crista (vertically orient-ed bundle) joins the limbus, marked changes in fiber orientation are evident. In panel B, the endocardial surface of the right atrial appendage is shown. This demonstrates the complex arrangement of the pectinate muscles as they branch and join one another.

Figure 4 summarizes the results of propagation changes at sites where muscle bundles branch or join with other bundles [22]. We found a directional dependence of the conduction velocity and the extracellular potential at branch sites (Panel 1). When the distal branch formed an acute angle with the parent branch, there was slow-ing of the wavefront as it changed direction to enter the distal branch. However, there was little or no change in the velocity or the extracellular waveforms when the wavefront entered branches that maintained the same fiber orientation as the parent branch, or de-viated from it at an obtuse angle. That is, the variation in velo-city at branches was related to the angle between the direction of propagation and the fiber orientation at the branch site. When the wavefront entered a branch that formed an acute angle with a parent branch, the direction of propagation was altered from the longitu-dinal to the transverse axis of the fibers. This was associated with a decrease in the velocity of propagation and a decrease in the extracellular waveform. Contrariwise, when there was no change in the fiber orientation as the wavefront entered a distal branch, there was no change in conduction velocity or in the amplitude of the extracellular waveforms. From these findings, we concluded that the cause of the abrupt slowing of propagation at branch sites is an abrupt increase in the effective axial resistivity in the

direction of propagation (a macroscopic discontinuity of $\bar{R}_a$). That
is, in one direction propagation into the branch proceeds along the
axis of the cells whereas, in the other direction, propagation must
change direction (with respect to the long cell axis).

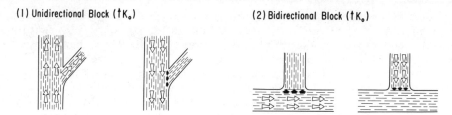

Figure 4:   Effects of High Extracellular Potassium Concentration
             (9 mM) at an Atrial Muscle Branch Site (1) and at the
             Junction of Two Separate Muscle Bundles (2).

        Figure 4 (Panel 1) shows a schematic representation of the re-
sult of a test of the mechanism of a velocity change that occurred
when the maximum membrane current was decreased by slowly elevating
the outside potassium concentration. The drawing shows a branch
formed by a small pectinate muscle arising from the considerably
larger crista terminalis (the fiber orientation is represented by
the parallel lines within the muscle bundles). At a normal extracellular potassium concentration (4.6 mM) action potentials propagated
into the smaller branch without block when the excitation wavefront
approached from either direction. When the extracellular potassium
concentration was elevated to 9 mM, there was unidirectional block
at the branch site. Propagation into the distal branch was still
successful from below, a direction that represented no change in
fiber orientation at the branch site. However, when propagation
occurred into the branch site from above, necessitating an abrupt
change in the direction of propagation and in the distribution of
the cellular connections encountered, block occurred at the branch.

        The question naturally arises as to whether the unidirectional
block at the branch site could be due to inexcitability of the membrane of some of the fibers; that is, differences in membrane properties along the course of the fibers within the branch. The
reversibility of the change shows that this mechanism cannot account
for the unidirectional block, since propagation was successful in
the same fibers in which conduction failed, depending upon the angle

from which the excitation wavefront entered the fibers.

The idea that propagation failure should occur at sites that
represent an abrupt change in the distribution of the cellular
couplings was tested further by studying propagation across the
junction of two separate muscle bundles [19]. A typical result is
illustrated schematically in Panel 2 of Figure 4.

Normal action potentials propagated across the junction from
one bundle to the other with only slight delay in either direction.
When the potassium concentration was elevated to 9 mM, however,
propagation ceased to occur into the distal bundle from either
direction. Bidirectional block at the junction site of two mutually
perpendicular muscle bundles was commonly encountered throughout
the atria when the extracellular potassium concentration was elevated.
It is interesting that the conduction block occurred at these localized sites, resulting in the disappearance of action potentials
distally. However, uniform propagation still occurred in the distal
bundle if it were stimulated directly.

Events During Reentry

Allessie et al. [1] demonstrated circus movement of the impulse
within a small segment of rabbit left atrium by applying an appropriately located and properly timed stimulus. The premature action
potential conducted in one direction and failed in another. They
considered the unidirectional block, which set the stage for circus
movement, to be caused solely by spatial nonuniformity of the recovery of excitability, which was consistent with their refractory
period measurements. They proposed the "leading circle" concept [2]
to emphasize that no insulated barrier is required to provide an
anatomical loop around which the impulse has to propagate to produce reentry. Our results, however, suggest that in addition to the
classical requirement of nonuniform recovery of excitability [1, 9],
the anatomical arrangement of the muscle bundles and the distribution of the muscle junctions also should be important determinants
of reentrant propagation within these small regions. That is, within a small region there are localized sites that represent abrupt
changes in the distribution of the cellular connections that produce macroscopic discontinuities of effective axial resistivity.
These sites should produce conduction block as an independent
mechanism.

We attempted to mimic the conditions of Allessie et al. [1] in
their atrial experiments by studying the propagation of premature
action potentials on the endocardial surface of the right atrial
appendage of the dog. It was easy to produce reentrant propagation
when the stimulus electrode was positioned at selected positions, a
finding similar to that of Allessie et al. Due to the arrangement
of the small bundles, the patterns of propagation were so complex

that we have not been able to successfully map a complete sequence
of excitation in all of the bundles within a region as small as
1 cm^2 during reentrant beats. However, we have confirmed the general
reentrant circuit within this small area and have found evidence that
several mechanisms can occur simultaneously to produce the "unidirectional" block during the initial beat that sets the stage for reentry. These mechanisms include: (1) spatially different refractory
periods, (2) decremental conduction due to anisotropic cellular
coupling at a microscopic level, and (3) macroscopic discontinuities
of effective axial resistivity that occur at the pectinate muscle
junctions [19, 22].

DISCUSSION

Discontinuous Propagation

     The term *saltatory* propagation in cardiac muscle is used to
indicate that propagation at a microscopic level would be "jumping"
or proceeding by steps (i.e., discontinuous) with slight hesitations
at recurrent sites of reduced conductivity which are due to the
cellular connections. The "low" resistance of the interconnections
between cells is not equivalent to complete cytoplasmic continuity,
although excitation propagates from excitable unit to excitable unit
through the significant electrical conductivity of the junctions. The
contribution of the interconnections to propagation will, in fact,
be determined by their location and frequency in relation to the cell
shape and packing. The defining characteristic of a discontinuous
spatial derivative of the transmembrane potential, originally described for myelinated nerve by FitzHugh [7], would also apply to
cardiac muscle [10]. We have found the term saltatory a useful
descriptor to emphasize the electrical representation of cardiac
muscle as recurrent discontinuities of axial resistivity, rather than
as geometric discontinuities in the form of changing core conductor
geometry.

     The features of myelinated nerve fibers that cause saltatory
propagation are not analogous, however, to those responsible for such
propagation in cardiac muscle. The discontinuities in the two tissues
are physically and electrically quite different. In myelinated nerve,
the node length is usually considered constant when the internode
distance is varied; patches of active membrane of fixed area are
coupled by different lengths of passive cable. In cardiac muscle,
the discontinuities consist of local reductions in the intracellular
conductivity where the cells are coupled. Future work will be necessary to distinguish the effects of discontinuities produced by the
cell-to-cell connections versus the side-to-side connections of the
unit bundles described by Sommer and Dolber [18].

     The directional difference in propagation velocity in cardiac

muscle is reasonable because the distribution of the cell junctions
should vary with direction. The reduced velocity in the transverse
direction then would be caused by increased intracellular (effective
axial) resistivity in that direction. When this explanation for
directional-velocity differences is combined with the presence of recurrent discontinuities of axial resistivity, an unexpected corollary
results. When there is the same change in membrane properties
throughout the sheet of muscle, propagation at a microscopic level
in the longitudinal and transverse directions responds differently.
Propagation can become decremental and stop in the longitudinal
direction while it continues as uniform propagation in the transverse direction. As the membrane activity is depressed, uniform
propagation ceases and becomes decremental first in the direction
having the highest velocity. Thus, the "safety factor" is lower
when the velocity is high and vice versa. The terms "optimal" and
"preferential" have been applied to regions of fast conduction, implying that conditions are advantageous and that propagation is
safer there. However, the introduction of recurrent discontinuities
of axial resistivity and modification of the propagation velocity by
changing the intracellular resistance reverse the relationship of
velocity and safety factor. For these conditions during premature
beats, slow propagation in the transverse direction is safer than
fast propagation along the axis of the fibers.

When the above electrical representation of cardiac muscle at
a microscopic level is generalized to a macroscopic size scale, it
is not surprising that we found additional discontinuities of propagation that are not accounted for by most current theories of
conduction disturbances. The macroscopic discontinuities of propagation occurred at locations where there were associated anatomic
(geometrical) discontinuities; such as branch sites and the junctions
of separate muscle bundles. Although these anatomical discontinuities represented easily visible changes in the gross geometry of
the muscular structures involved, the associated discontinuities of
propagation could not be accounted for by representing these sites
electrically as changes in core conductor geometry with continuous
properties of axial resistivity. The changes in velocity, as well
as the associated changes in the extracellular potentials, were
accounted for at these sites by macroscopic discontinuities of
effective axial resistivity due to abrupt changes in the distribution of the cellular couplings in the direction of propagation.

Reentry

The primary requirement for producing reentry in cardiac muscle
has been considered to be spatially nonuniform membrane properties;
i.e., nonuniform recovery of excitability [1]. Our results show
that reentry can occur within a small area having uniform membrane
properties [19, 21, 22]. Directional block can be produced at a
microscopic size scale by directional differences in cell-to-cell

coupling, so the pattern of propagation during reentry is related to
the cell orientation, not to regional differences in membrane properties. The effects on propagation produced by directional differences
in cellular couplings at a microscopic size scale are recapitulated
at a macroscopic level owing to resultant discontinuities of effective
axial resistivity at branch sites and junctions of separate muscle
bundles, locations at which the fiber orientation changes in the
direction of propagation. The safety factor of propagation is low
at these locations, as shown by the localized failure of propagation
at these sites during premature beats and during elevation of the
extracellular potassium concentration.

     In proposing the "leading circle" concept, Allessie et al. [2]
indicated that the reentrant propagation in the left atrium they
measured within a 1 cm^2 area was due to spatial differences in refractory periods without a gross obstacle for the impulse to circu-
late around; i.e., there was no inexcitable central obstacle. Our
results indicate that although the electrical discontinuities at
branch sites and the junction of two muscles present no significant
barrier to the propagation of normal or moderately depressed action
potentials, they can be the sole basis for propagation failure during early premature beats and depressed states. On the endocardial
surface of the pectinate muscle regions (Figure 1,B) the anatomical
arrangement of the small interconnecting muscle bundles provide
multiple discrete and separate "pathways" for propagation within a
very small area (1 cm^2), and the muscle junctions represent sites of
conduction block leading to reentrant propagation. Further, it was
interesting that block due to differences in refractory periods also
quite frequently was localized to the muscle junctions -- the differences in refractory periods along the course of the muscle bundles
was very small, and at the junction of two separate muscle bundles the
refractory periods changed up to 40 msec over a distance as small
as 100 μm [19]. Thus, the junction sites of two separate muscle
bundles provide a localized region of high resistance that can
maintain large intracellular potential gradients across a very small
distance during repolarization, resulting in markedly abrupt spatial
changes in the duration of action potentials.

     The results at a microscopic and macroscopic size scale suggest
that the occurrence of reentry in a given region of the heart depends on a combination of mechanisms related to both spatial differences in membrane properties and to anatomical complexities that
produce discontinuities in effective axial resistivity. The anatomical complexities include (1) anisotropic cellular coupling at a
microscopic level (producing saltatory or discontinuous propagation),
(2) macroscopic discontinuities of effective axial resistivity represented by branch sites and the junctions of muscle bundles, and
(3) the geometric arrangement of the muscle bundles and the locations
of their connection sites. In summary, reentry is a function of the
specific combination of several mechanisms, any one of which can

act independently or in combination with the others depending on
the state of the membrane properties and the anatomical complexities
involved within the area comprised by the reentrant pathway.

REFERENCES

1.   Allessie, M.A., Bonke, F.I.M, & Schopman, F.J.G. Circus move-
     ment in rabbit atrial muscle as a mechanism of tachycardia. II.
     The role of nonuniform recovery of excitability in the occur-
     rence of unidirectional block, as studied with multiple micro-
     electrodes. *Circulation Research* 39, 168-177 (1976).
2.   Allessie, M.A., Bonke, F.I.M. & Schopman, F.J.G. Circus move-
     ment in rabbit atrial muscle as a mechanism of tachycardia.
     III. The "leading circle" concept: A model of circus movement
     in cardiac tissue without the involvement of an anatomical
     obstacle. *Circulation Research* 41, 9-18 (1977).
3.   Barr, R.C., Herman-Giddens, G.S., Spach, M.S., Warren, R.B. &
     Gallie, T.M. The design of a real-time computer system for
     examining the electrical activity of the heart. *Computers and
     Biomedical Research* 9, 445-469 (1976).
4.   Clerc, L. Directional differences of impulse spread in trabe-
     cular muscle from mammalian heart. *Journal of Physiology
     London* 255, 335-346 (1976).
5.   Cranefield, P.F. *The Conduction of the Cardiac Impulse. The
     Slow Response and Cardiac Arrhythmias.* Mt. Kisco, New York:
     Futura Publishing Company (1975).
6.   Cranefield, P.F., Klein, H.O. & Hoffman, B.F. Conduction of
     the cardiac impulse. I. Delay, block, and one-way block in
     depressed Purkinje fibers. *Circulation Research* 28, 199-219
     (1971).
7.   FitzHugh, R. Computation of impulse initiation and saltatory
     conduction in a myelinated nerve fiber. *Biophysical Journal*
     2, 11-21 (1962).
8.   Fozzard, H.A. Conduction of the action potential. In *Handbook
     of Physiology*, Section 2, Volume I. The Heart, R.M. Berne,
     N. Sperelakis & S.R. Geiger, Eds, pp. 335-356. Bethesda:
     American Physiological Society (1979).
9.   Han, J. & Moe, G.K. Nonuniform recovery of excitability in
     ventricular muscle. *Circulation Research* 14, 44-60 (1964).
10. Heppner, D.B. & Plonsey, R. Simulation of electrical inter-
     action of cardiac cells. *Biophysical Journal* 10, 1057-1075
     (1970).
11. Hodgkin, A.L. & Katz, B. The effect of sodium ions on the
     electrical activity of the giant axon of the squid. *Journal
     of Physiology London* 108, 37-77 (1949).
12. Hoffman, B.F. & Cranefield, P.F. *Electrophysiology of the
     Heart.* New York: McGraw-Hill (1960).

13. Hogan, P.M. & Davis, L.D. Evidence for specialized fibers in the canine right atrium. *Circulation Research* 23, 387-396 (1968).
14. Hunter, P.J. McNaughton, P.A. & Noble, D. Analytical models of propagation in excitable cells. *Progress in Biophysics and Modecular Biology* 30, 99-144 (1975).
15. James, T.N. & Sherf, L. Specialized tissues and preferential conduction in the atria of the heart. *American Journal of Cardiology* 28, 414-427 (1971).
16. Moe, G.K. Rheinboldt, W.C. & Abildskov, J.A. A computer model of atrial fibrillation. *American Heart Journal* 67, 200-220 (1964).
17. Paes de Carvalho, A., Hoffman, B.F. & De Paula Carvalho, M. Two components of the cardiac action potential. I. Voltage-time course and the effect of acetylcholine on atrial and nodal cells of the rabbit heart. *Journal of General Physiology* 54, 607-635 (1969).
18. Sommer, J.R. & Dolber, P.C. Cardiac Muscle: The ultrastructure of its cells and bundles. In: *Normal and Abnormal Conduction of the Heart Beat*, A. Paes de Carvalho, B.F. Hoffman & M. Leiberman, Eds, Mt. Kisco, New York: Futura Publishing Company (1982) (To be published).
19. Spach, M.S. The electrical representation of cardiac muscle based on discontinuities of axial resistivity at a microscopic and macroscopic level. A basis for saltatory propagation in cardiac muscle. In *Normal and Abnormal Conduction of the Heart Beat*, A. Paes de Carvalho, B.F. Hoffman, & M. Lieberman, Eds. Mt. Kisco, New York, Futura Publishing Company (1982) (To be published).
20. Spach, M.S., Miller, W.T., III, Miller-Jones, E., Warren, R.B. & Barr, R.C. Extracellular potentials related to intracellular action potentials during impulse conduction in anisotropic canine cardiac muscle. *Circulation Research* 45, 188-204 (1979).
21. Spach, M.S., Miller, W.T.,III, Geselowitz, D.B., Barr, R.C., Kootsey, J.M. & Johnson, E.A. The discontinuous nature of propagation in normal canine cardiac muscle. Evidence for re-current discontinuities of intracellular resistance that affect the membrane currents. *Circulation Research* 48,39-54 (1981).
22. Spach, M.S., Miller, W.T., III, Dolber, P.C., Kootsey, J.M., Sommer, J.R. & Mosher, C.E., Jr. The functional role of structural complexities in the propagation of depolarization in the atrium of the dog. Cardiac conduction disturbances due to discontinuities of effective axial resistivity. *Circulation Research* 50, 175-191 (1982).
23. Wagner, M.L., Lazzara, R., Weiss, R.M. & Hoffman, B.F. Special-ized conducting fibers in the interatrial band. *Circulation Research* 18, 502-518 (1966).
24. Weidmann, S. The effect of the cardiac membrane potential on the rapid availability of the sodium-carrying system. *Journal of Physiology London* 127, 213-224 (1955).

"A MODEL STUDY OF THE EFFECT OF THE INTERCALATED DISCS ON

DISCONTINUOUS PROPAGATION IN CARDIAC MUSCLE"

Pedro J. Diaz, Yoram Rudy and Robert Plonsey
Case Western Reserve University
Department of Biomedical Engineering
Cleveland, Ohio 44106

There is considerable evidence (1,13,14,22,23) to support the existence of low resistance end to end junctions (gap junctions or connexons (10,12,17) which lie in the intercalated discs that make up the associated end-to-end plasma membranes of cardiac muscle cells. Even though these gap junctions are low resistance, they represent a significant discontinuity in the conductive medium. Indeed, while these low resistance contacts are low in the sense of permitting an adequate current to flow and excite the post-junctional cell, an often quoted value for the intercalated disc resistance, 1 ohm-cm^2 , would be an impediment to axial current flow comparable to the entire myoplasm of the cell. In order to study the effects of these discontinuities due to the intercalated discs on propagation in cardiac muscle a "microscopic" discontinuous cable model which includes the intercalated discs was developed.

Most of the work utilizing cable models to simulate the propagation of electrical activity in excitable tissue have dealt with conduction in nerve, for which the continuous cable model is applicable. Simulation of conduction in cardiac muscle has had to wait for the development of adequate action potential models, a task made difficult by the complexity of membrane ionic currents in cardiac muscle as well as uncertainty in the interpretation of voltage clamp results. However, recent models by McAllister and coworkers (9) for Purkinje action potentials and Beeler and Reuter (2) for ventricular action potentials have successfully extended the Hodgkin-Huxley (7) type model to cardiac tissue, and appear to faithfully reproduce many of the electrical phenomena of the cardiac membrane. Models of propagation in continuous cables have been developed using these

79

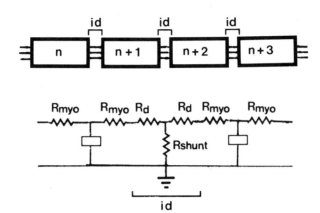

Figure 1.   Discontinuous cable model showing sequence of distinct
             cells connected by intercalated disc structure (id)
             (Top). Network representation of intercalated disc
             structure (Bottom).

membrane models (19). Recent models (11,16) take into account,
at least macroscopically, the experimentally observed (4, 20)
anisotropic nature of electrical propagation in cardiac muscle.
Since more intercalated discs per unit length area traversed by
an activation wavefront tarvelling perpendicular to the fiber
axis than by a wave travelling along the axis, it is reasonable
to assume that the anisotropy is due, at least to some extent,
to the discrete structure of the myocardium. In order to study
these effects we have developed a dimensionally correct "microscopic" model which includes the intercalated discs.

     The model shown in Figure 1 consists of a one dimensional
fiber made up of 35 to 50 cells, each 100μ long by 15μ in diameter. An intercalated disc, modeled as a T-resistance network
comprised of two axial resistances (Rd), and a radial leakage
resistance to the extracellular space (Rshunt). The intercalated
disc structure separates all neighboring cells in our model. The
individual cells are discretized and represented by ten membrane
patches 10μ in length with an axial myoplasm resistance,Rmyo,
connecting adjacent membrane patches as in a continuous cable.
The properties of each membrane patch are described by the
ventricular action potential model of Beeler and Reuter (2).
The cable equations for this discontinuous model were developed
and solved numerically on a digital computer using the method
of Crank and Nicolson (5). The equations describing the membrane properties were solved using the procedure proposed by Rush
and Larsen (18). Previous models involving the intercalated disc
in cardiac muscle have usually consisted of only two cells

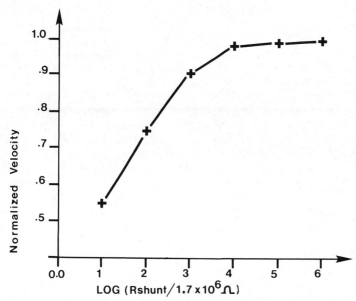

Figure 2.   The effects of Rshunt on conduction velocity. Values of Rshunt were varied from 1.7 x 10^6 ohms to 1.7 x 10^{12} ohms.

separated by a single intercalated disc (6). However, since the propagating action potential wavefront encompasses many cells, these models fail to adequately reflect the entire range of cell-to-cell interaction and the effect of the intercalated disc on propagation. These effects can only be examined using a multi-cell model such as the one described here.

Results

Variations in conduction velocity due to changes in the leakage resistance (Rshunt) are shown in Figure 2. A value for Rshunt (1.7 x 10^6 ohms) given by Heppner and Plonsey (6) for a specific disc resistivity of 1 ohm-cm^2 in their model is represented as 0.0 on the abcissa. In simulations utilizing this value of Rshunt, propagation was not sustained beyond three cells from the point of stimulus. A strong dependence of velocity on Rshunt is seen for Rshunt values of less than 1.7 x 10^9 ohms. These results suggest that structural changes at the intercalated disc which reduce the leakage resistance to the extracellular space may be a factor in slow conduction and possibly even complete conduction block.

In Figure 3 we show the effect of the periodic disc structure of our model on conduction velocity. The effective axial resistivity of the fiber, which is the sum of the contributions of the disc and myoplasm resistivities was varied in two ways. In the first case, the disc resistivity was kept constant at 1 ohm-cm^2, a typical value given in various experimental and theoretical studies (3,8,13,14,21), while the resistivity of the myoplasm was varied from 110 to 250 ohm-cm. The resulting decrease in conduction velocity is shown as curve 1. In the second case, the effective axial resistivity is increased by allowing the disc specific resistivity to vary from .1 ohm-cm^2 to 2.4 ohm-cm^2 while the myoplasm resistivity is kept constant at 200 ohm-cm. The resulting decrease in conduction velocity is shown as curve 2. For comparison the inverse square root relationship between conduction velocity and fiber resistivity, obtained from classical continuous cable theory, was utilized to compute expected changes in conduction velocity for the change in fiber resistivity. The result of this computation is shown as curve 3. Note that increasing the effective axial resisitivity by increasing the resistivity of the intercalated discs reduces conduction velocity to a greater extent than that predicted from the inverse square root relationship of continuous cable theory. In contrast, increasing the myoplasm resistivity while the resistivity of the intercalated discs is kept constant affects conduction velocity less than predicted by the inverse square root relationship.

The maximum velocity (normalized to 1 in Figure 3) is obtained in both cases for the same (210 ohm-cm) effective axial resistivity. The actual maximum velocity is 14.5 cm/sec in curve 1 and 22 cm/sec in curve 2. The reason for the lower velocity of curve 1 is the greater contribution from the discs to the total effective axial resisitivity in this case. In contrast, a higher velocity observed in curve 2 for the same effective axial resistivity results in this case due to the greater contribution of the myoplasm to the total resistivity.

These results demonstrate that the discrete disc structure has a much greater effect on conduction velocity than the diffuse myoplasm, and reflect the importance of the intercalated disc properties in determining conduction velocity in cardiac muscle.

Another departure from classical continuous cable theory is shown in Figure 4. The maximum rate of change of the temporal action potential ($\dot{V}$max),computed at the center of a cell in the midpoint of the fiber, and the conduction velocity in the fiber are plotted as functions of the fiber axial resistivity.

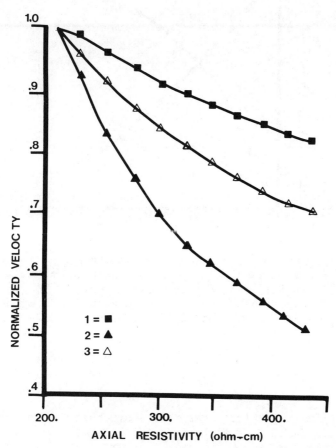

Figure 3.   Velocity changes due to variation in fiber
                   axial resistivity by changing the resistivity
                   of the myoplasm alone (Curve 1) or by changing
                   the resistivity of the discs alone (Curve 2).
                   Change predicted by inverse square root relation-
                   ship of continuous cable theory is shown for
                   comparison (Curve 3) .

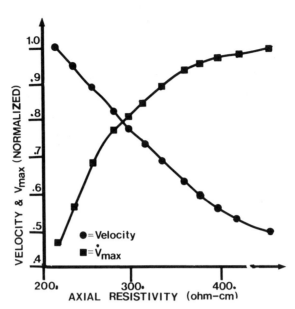

Figure 4.   Changes in conduction velocity and
                 V̇max obtained by increasing the disc resistivity
                 while keeping the myoplasm resistivity constant.
                 Note that direction of V̇max change is opposite
                 from that predicted by continuous cable theory.

The fiber axial resistivity was varied by changing the disc
resistivity from .1 to 2.4 $ohm-cm^2$ while the myoplasm resistivity
was kept constant at 200 ohm-cm. In contrast to the direct relation
between V̇max and conduction velocity of continuous cable theory,
our model shows an increase in V̇max with a decrease in conduction velocity. This type of behaviour was observed experimentally
by Spach and co-workers (20) in an isolated ventricular tissue
preparation.

    The effect of the periodic intercalated disc structure on
the nature of propagation and on the equivalent electrical source
configuration was also examined using our model. Figure 5 shows
the rising phase of a typical spatial action potential wavefront
obtained from our discontinuous model. . In contrast to the
smooth wavefront one observes in a continuous cable model, sharp
discontinuities are introduced at each disc location lying in the

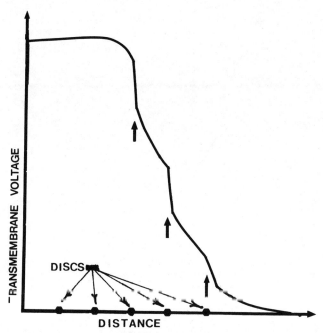

Figure 5.   Spatial transmembrane potential wavefront
                 computed from discontinuous model. Arrows
                 to abcissa point to intercalated disc locations.
                 Arrows to leading edge of wavefront point to
                 discontinuities in potential due to the inter-
                 calated discs.

leading edge. Since the equivalent dipole source density along
the fiber is proportional to the spatial derivative of the transmembrane potential along the fiber axis (15) one can immediately appreciate the effect of the periodic disc structure on the
electrical source distribution. A representation of the source
configuration obtained from the model is shown in Figure 6.
Large dipole sources are present at each intercalated disc, with
much weaker sources distributed throughout the cell volume (the
source density at the disc is 10^4 times the source density within
the cell). Computation of conduction velocity showed that the
propagation velocity within the cell (between the end-to-end
intercalated discs) was ten times higher than the average propagation velocity computed over many cells. The difference in the

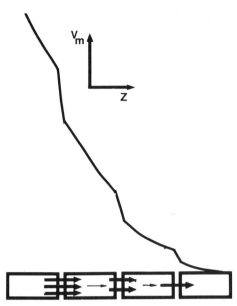

Figure 6.   Representation of equivalent dipole sources
                   obtained from the discontinuous model. Note the
                   large dipoles (arrows) present at the intercalated
                   discs and the weaker dipoles present within the
                   cell.

conduction velocity is due to a delay (.45 msec. for 1 ohm-cm^2
disc resistivity) encountered by the propagating wavefront
in crossing the intercalated disc. The picture that one obtains
is that there are strong persistent sources present at the intercalated discs with faster,much weaker sources travelling between
the discs during the passage of the activation wavefront. Propagation can be described, therefore, as discontinuous and saltatory in nature, with strong dipolar source "jumping" from disc to
disc.

        The strong persistent sources at the intercalated discs give
rise to sharp discontinuities in the extracellular potential
field generated by the fiber. In Figure 7 we show the spatial
extracellular field computed at the surface of the fiber from
the equivalent dipole sources. The sharp discontinuities reflect

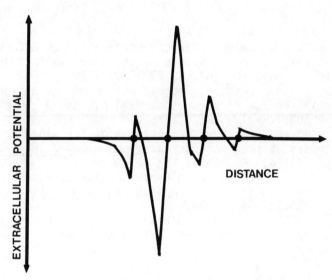

Figure 7.   Spatial extracellular potential field computed at
                   the surface of the fiber. Circles on the abcissa
                   indicate the location of the intercalated discs
                   which contribute to the field shown.

the distribution of equally spaced string disc sources. The potential field is smoothed out as one moves away from the fiber, reflecting both a diminished and more equal contribution form all the
disc sources.

   In summary, we have shown that the inclusion of a periodic
intercalated disc structure in a core conductor model of cardiac
muscle has allowed the examination of electrical propagation on
a microscopic cellular level. The results indicate that classical
continuous cable theory fails to adequately describe propagation
in cardiac muscle. In particular, $\dot{V}max$ can not always be utilized
as a measure of conduction velocity, and the classical inverse
square root relationship between conduction velocity and fiber
axial resistivity does not hold . The presence of the intercalated discs also influences the electrical source strength and
the nature of electrical propagation. As a result of the discrete periodic dis structure, the propagation in discontinuous with
large sources jumping from disc to disc in a saltatory fashion.
Based on these one dimensional results, it is clear that models
of cardiac muscle propagation must take into account the discontinuous nature of cardiac muscle.

REFERENCES

1. Barr,L., M.M. Dewey and W. Berger. Propagation of action
   potentials and the structure of the nexus in cardiac
   muscle. J. Gen. Physiol. 48:797-823, 1965.
2. Beeler, G.W. and H. Reuter. Reconstruction of the action
   potential of ventricular myocardial fibres. J. Physiol.
   London 286:177-210, 1977.
3. Chapman, R.A. and C.H. Fry. An analysis of the cable
   properties of frog ventricular myocardium. J. Physiol.
   London 283:263-281, 1978.
4. Clerc, L. Directional differences of impulse spread in
   trabecular muscle from mammalian heart. J. Physiol.
   London 255:335-346, 1976.
5. Crank, J. and P. Nicolson. A practical method for numerical
   evaluation of solutions of partial differential equations
   of the heat conduction type. Proc. Cambridge Phil. Soc.
   43:50-77, 1947.
6. Heppner, D.B. and R. Plonsey. Simulation of electrical
   interaction of cardiac cells. Biophys J. 10:1057-1075,
   1970.
7. Hodgkin,A.L. and Huxley, A.F. A quantitative description of
   membrane current and its application to conduction and
   excitation in nerve. J. Physiol. London 117:500-544, 1952.
8. Lowenstein, W.R. Junctional intercellular communication: The
   cell-to-cell membrane channel. Physiol. Rev. 61:829-913,
   1981.
9. McAllister,R.E., D. Noble and R.W. Tsien. Reconstruction of
   the electrical activity of cardiac Purkinje fibers. J.
   Physiol. London 251:1-59, 1975.
10. McNutt, N.S. and R.S. Weinstein. Membrane ultrastructure at
    mammalian intercellular junctions. Prog. Biophys. Mol.
    Biol. 26:45-101, 1973.
11. Miller, W.T. III and D.B. Geselowitz. Simulation studies of
    the electrocardiogram: I.The normal heart. Circ. Res.
    43:301-323, 1978.
12. Page, E. and L.P. McAllister. Studies on the intercalated
    discs of rat ventricular myocardial cells. J.
    Ultrastruct. Res. 43:388-411, 1973.
13. Page,E. and Y. Shibata. Permeable junctions between cardiac
    cells. Ann. Rev. Physiol. 43:431-442, 1981.
14. Pollack, G.H. Intercellular coupling in the atrioventricular
    node and other tissues of the rabbit heart. J. Physiol.
    London 255: 275-298, 1976.
15. Plonsey, R. Action potential sources and their volume
    conductor fields. Proc. IEEE 65:601-611, 1976.
16. Plonsey, R. and Y. Rudy. Electrocardiogram sources in a two
    dimensional anisotropic activation model. Med. Biol.
    Engr. Comput. 18:87-95, 1980.

17. Revel, J.P. and M.J. Karnovsky. Hexagonal arrays of subunits
    in intercellular junctions of the mouse heart and liver.
    J. Cell Biol. 12:571-588, 1962.
18. Rush, S. and H. Larsen . A practical algorithm for solving
    dynamic membrane equations. IEEE BME-25:389-392, 1978.
19. Sharp, G. and Joyner, R.W. Simulated propagation of cardiac
    action potentials. Biophysical J. 31:403-424, 1980.
20. Spach, M.S., W.T. MIller III, D.B. Geselowitz, R.C. Barr,
    J.M. Kootsey and E.A. Johnson. The discontinuous nature
    of propagation in normal cardiac muscle: Evidence for
    recurrent discontinuities of intra-cellular resistance
    that affect the membrane currents. Circulation Res.
    48:39-56, 1981.
21. Spira, A.W. The nexus in the intercalated disc of the canine
    heart: Quantitative data for the estimation of its
    resistance. J. Ultrastruct. Res. 34:409-425, 1971.
22. Weidmann, S. The diffusion of radiopotassium across
    intercalated disks of mammalian cardiac muscle. J.
    Physiol. London 187:323-342, 1966.
23. Woodbury, J.W. and W.E. Crill. On the problem of impulse
    conduction in the atrium. In: Nervous Inhibition ,edited
    by L. Florey. New York: Plenum , 1961, pp. 24-35.

BETA-ADRENERGIC STIMULATION OF ADENYLATE CYCLASE AND ALPHA-ADRENERGIC INHIBITION OF ADENYLATE CYCLASE: GTP-BINDING PROTEINS AS MACROMOLECULAR MESSENGERS

Lee E. Limbird

Dept. of Pharmacology
Nashville, TN

This review, which is a summary of an oral presentation made at the International Study Group for Research in Cardiac Metabolism, is a brief synopsis of work in our laboratory concerning the mechanism of hormonal regulation of adenylate cyclase. By its very nature, it refers almost entirely to our own work. However, since a number of laboratories have contributed to the field in ways at least as significant as our own, I recommend reading the reviews cited as references 4, 7 and 11 for a more comprehensive summary of the literature. The emphasis of this review is the role of GTP-binding proteins as important communicators between hormone-occupied receptors and the catalytic subunit of adenylate cyclase. The experimental work summarized emphasizes the extent to which one can determine the "intactness" receptor-effector coupling by focusing on receptor-agonist interactions, and modulation of these interactions by guanine nucleotides.

The adenylate cyclase system which responds to stimulation by hormones and drugs is now known to be composed of at least three distinct molecular components: the receptor (R), the catalytic subunit (C), and the multisubunit GTP-binding regulatory protein (G) that mediates the multiple regulatory effects of guanine nucleotides on the adenylate cyclase system. Data from a number of laboratories suggest that the flow of information from the receptor to the catalytic subunit proceeds from R → G → C. An important role of agonists appears to be the stabilization of the interaction between the receptor and the GTP-binding protein. Considerable experimental evidence suggests that the extent to which an agonist can stabilize R-G interactions correlates with the extent to which an agonist can stimulate adenylate cyclase activity.

This review will focus on agonist interactions with receptors coupled to adenylate cyclase and the so-called "R-G communication" stabilized by agonist occupancy of the receptor. Some of the methods used for evaluating putative R-G communication are listed below.

1) COMPETITION BINDING STUDIES. The observation is that guanine nucleotides decrease receptor affinity for agonists at receptors coupled to activation of adenylate cyclase. Thus, one way in which one can evaluate possible R-G communication is to determine the ability of GTP to decrease receptor affinity for agonists using competition binding studies. In these studies, the binding of radiolabeled antagonists is competed for by increasing concentrations of unlabeled agonists. Agonist competition for binding to the receptor is of greater potency in the absence of guanine nucleotides. In the presence of added guanine nucleotides, the agonist competition curve is "shifted to the right", consistent with the conclusion that guanine nucleotides decrease receptor affinity for agonists.

2) DISSOCIATION OF RADIOLABELED AGONIST BINDING. Since guanine nucleotides are able to decrease receptor affinity for agonist agents, another manifestation of R-G communication is the ability of GTP to facilitate agonist dissociation from prelabeled receptors. This observation follows directly from the equation K_D = k_{off}/k_{on}. Since a decrease in receptor affinity is paralleled by an increase in the value of the dissociation constant, K_D, then it follows that an increase in K_D might likely be accompanied by an increase in the rate of dissocation, k_{off}. The ability of guanine nucleotides to facilitate radiolabeled agonist dissociation from beta-adrenergic receptors coupled to activation of adenylate cyclase has often been used as a monitor of intact R-G communication [9, 16].

3) INCREASE IN APPARENT MOLECULAR SIZE OF THE RECEPTOR. We have tended to exploit a more molecular approach to evaluate the existence or not of agonist-stabilized R-G interactions. Since adenylate cyclase-coupled receptors appear to be particularly sensitive to guanine nucleotides when occupied by agonists, then one might predict that agonist occupancy of the receptor might stabilize the putative R-G interaction so that this interaction might not be disrupted upon detergent solubilization of the target membrane. Subsequent to detergent solubilization, the agonist-stabilized R-G complexes, if they exist, should be resolvable from unoccupied receptors using traditional biochemical techniques for resolving proteins based on their apparent molecular size, i.e. sucrose gradient centrifugation or gel exclusion chromatography.

We have exploited the third, more biochemical, approach noted
above in evaluating the beta-adrenergic receptor-adenylate cyclase
system of the frog erythrocyte [8] and rat reticulocyte [9, 10]. In
both target membranes, the adenylate cyclase is extremely sensitive to
catecholamines, and furthermore, a plasma membrane preparation of
reasonable purity can be simply prepared. The radiolabeled agonist
utilized for identification of the beta-receptor was [^{3}H]
hydroxybenzylisoproterenol (HBl).   Occupancy of beta-adrenergic
receptors with [^{3}H] HBl prior to solubilization of either target
membrane with the detergent, digitonin, resulted in an agonist-stabilized
increase in receptor size.

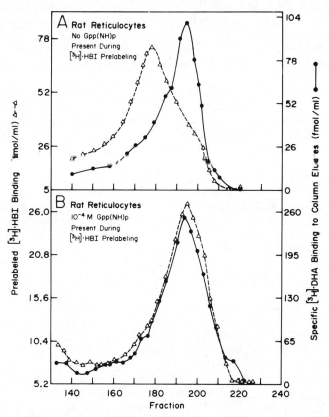

Figure 1:   Elution profile of prelabeled [^{3}H] HBl agonist- β -receptor
            complex and [^{3}H]DHA antagonist binding to column eluates
            from an AcA34 ultragel column.   A. Rat reticulocyte men-
            branes were preincubated with 16nM [^{3}H] HBl prior to
            digitonin solubilization and column chromatography.   [^{3}H]
            DHA binding to receptors unoccupied at the time of solu-
            bilization was assayed in the column eluates.   B. Rat
            reticulocytes were preincubated with 16nM [^{3}H] HBl in the
            presence of the GTP analog, Gpp(NH)p.   Details for ex-
            perimental procedures are provided in [9].

In the experiment shown in Figure 1, the target membrane employed is the rat reticulocyte. The elution of the prelabeled agonist-receptor complex earlier than unoccupied receptors, assayed in the column fractions using binding of the radiolabeled antagonist [^{3}H] dihydroalprenolol, is consistent with an agonist-stabilized increase in receptor size. The lower panel in Fig. 1 indicates that when radiolabeled agonist prelabeling of the membranes is carried out in the presence of the hydrolysis-resistant guanine nucleotide analog, Gpp(NH)p, the agonist-stabilized increase in apparent receptor size is no longer observed. Under these circumstances, the agonist-receptor complex elutes from the AcA34 column with a profile superimposable on that observed for unoccupied receptors in the same preparations. Thus, these data suggest that radiolabeled agonist and antagonist bind to the same protein, but that in the absence of guanine nucleotides the agonist can stabilize a receptor complex of larger size (Fig 1A) which appears to be reversed or prevented by the addition of guanine nucleotides (Fig 1B).

To determine more directly whether or not the agonist-stabilized complex of larger size indeed contained the GTP-binding protein of the adenylate cyclase system, we exploited a then recently developed technique for identifying the GTP-binding protein associated with activation of adenylate cyclase [10] . This technique involves the use of the A_1 subunit of cholera toxin (an enzyme) to transfer the ADP-ribose moiety from NAD^+ to the 42,000 Mr subunit of the GTP-binding protein associated with activation of adenylate cyclase. In cooperation with Dr. Michael Gill, one of the pioneers in establishing the catalytic activity of cholera toxin [6], we demonstrated that, in fact, the agonist-stabilized complex of larger size did include the [^{32}P] ADP-ribosylated 42,000 Mr subunit of the GTP-binding protein. These data are shown in Figure 2. In the upper panel, it can be seen that a large fraction of the ADP-ribosylated 42,000 Mr subunits elute from the AcA-34 Ultragel column with the prelabeled agonist-receptor complexes. However, as shown in the lower panel, the ADP-ribosylated proteins no longer demonstrate a peak in the region characteristic of the agonist-receptor complex of larger size, but distribute elsewhere throughout the column, when the receptors are unoccupied at the time of solubilization (or when they are occupied by antagonist, not shown here). These and subsequent reconstitution data led us to draw several conclusions. First, it appears that the agonist-stabilized β-adrenergic receptor complex of larger molecular size indeed contains the GTP-binding protein involved in activation of adenylate cyclase. Secondly, since the extent of covalent incorporation of ADP-ribose into this GTP-binding protein correlates directly with cholera toxin catalyzed enhancement of GTP-sensitive adenylate cyclase activity, these data also suggest that the same GTP binding protein that associates with the catalytic subunit and modulates adenylate cyclase activity also associates with the agonist-occupied receptor and modulates receptor-agonist interactions. This latter conclusion is strengthened by the experiments of Stadel et. al.

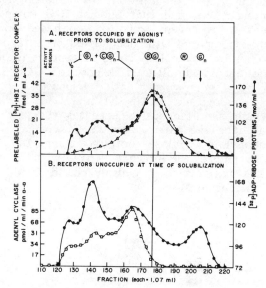

Figure 2: Gel filtration of digitonin-solubilized [^{32}p] ADP-ribosylated membrane proteins, β -adrenergic receptors and
adenylate cyclase. Rat reticulocyte membranes were exposed to cholera toxin and [^{32}p] NAD$^+$ under conditions
that covalently labeled the 42,000 Mr subunits of the
GTP-binding protein. The membranes were washed and pre-
incubated in presence (Fig. 2A) or absence (Fig. 2B) of
16nM [^{3}H] HB1, solubilized with digitonin and fractionated using AcA34 chromatography. Experimental details are
provided in [10].

[15] which demonstrated, using reconstitution studies, that the GTP-
binding protein isolated by virtue of its association with the agonist-
stabilized receptor complex can, upon interaction with catalytic subunit
of the turkey erythrocyte system, convey guanine nucleotide-sensitive
adenylate cyclase activity.

The preceding data as well as data from a number of laboratories
suggest that a reasonable model for hormonal activation of adenylate
cyclase is one such as is shown in Fig. [3]. Studies of catecholamine-
sensitive adenylate cyclase systems have suggested that the interaction
among the R,G, and C components appear to be dictated by the
catecholamine and nucleotide effectors themselves. As shown above, we

learned that the occupancy of the beta-adrenergic receptor by an agonist stabilizes R-G interactions, and that agonist R-G complexes can be isolated subsequent to detergent solubilization based on their larger molecular size when compared with unoccupied or antagonist-occupied beta-adrenergic receptors. The R-G complex appears to be responsible for promoting the agonist facilitated release of GDP from G [3]. Occupancy of G by a guanine nucleotide triphosphate, e.g. GTP or hydrolysis-resistant analogs such as Gpp(NH)p or GTPγS, dissociates the R-G complex, which simultaneously decreases receptor affinity for agonists, and stabilizes the interaction of G with C [5, 9, 12]. Expression of adenylate cyclase activity using the physiological substrate, ATP-Mg, requires the interaction of G with C, and activation of cyclase persists until GTP is hydrolyzed to GDP [1, 2], thus destabilizing G-C interactions.

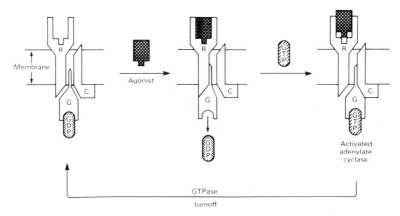

Figure 3: Postulated molecular interactions that accompany hormone-stimulated and guanine nucleotide-stimulated adenylate cyclase activity. R, receptor for hormones and drugs; G, multisubunit GTP-binding protein; C, catalytic subunit. From Reference 11.

The association of R with G has important consequences for the interaction of R with agonist agents, and these consequences are manifested in studies of radioligand binding to the beta-adrenergic receptor. The R-G complex possesses a higher affinity for agonist than the isolated moiety. Consequently, the effect of GTP occupancy of G to dissociate the R-G complex is paralleled by a GTP-promoted decrease in R affinity for agonist and the formation of the homogeneous population of beta-adrenergic receptors in the dissociated R form. R and RG possess an identical affinity for beta-adrenergic antagonists. In competition binding studies for radiolabeled antagonists, agonist competition profiles are observed to be of higher potency and of "shallow" shape (pseudo-Hill coefficient < 1) when the incubation of well-washed membranes is performed in the absence of exogenous guanine nucleotides. The addition of GTP or Gpp(NH)p to the incubation simultaneously decreases the affinity of the receptor for the agonist (shifts the competition curve to the right) and changes the shape of the competition curve to one of normal steepness i.e. that expected for an agent interacting via a simple bimolecular reaction with a homogeneous population of receptors. Computer modeling studies [5] as well as the biochemical studies mentioned above have suggested the interpretation that the shallow competition curve of overall higher potency ("to the left") represents the interaction of agonist with RG complexes ("the high affinity state" of the receptor for agonist) and R (the "low affinity state" of the receptor for agonist), thus accounting for the higher overall potency of the competition curve as well as the apparent receptor heterogeneity suggested by the shallowness of the competition curve for preparations evaluated in the absence of guanine nucleotides. The dissociation of R-G complexes promoted by the addition of GTP to the competition binding incubation results in formation of a homogeneous population of R moieties (accounting for the normal steepness of the agonist competition curve) possessing a lower affinity for agonists (accounting for the shift of the curve to the right). Thus, the important role of guanine nucleotides and the GTP-binding protein in receptor-cyclase coupling is manifested in both the requirement for guanine nucleotides for stimulation of adenylate cyclase and in the ability of guanine nucleotides to modulate receptor affinity for agonist agents.

Figure 3 implies that the extent to which an agonist can stabilize the interaction between R and G should correlate with the extent to which an agonist can amplify catalytic activity of adenylate cyclase. To test this hypothesis, we compared the biochemical properties of the beta-adrenergic adenylate cyclase system of the rat reticulocyte with those of the rat erythrocyte [9] . As the immature rat red cell, i.e. reticulocyte, matures to the erythrocyte, the catecholamine sensitivity of the adenylate cyclase system wanes. Thus, as shown in Figure 4, isoproterenol-stimulated adenylate cyclase activity is much lower in rat reticulocyte membranes, as is cyclase activity stimulated by exogenous guanine nucleotides or by GTP following exposure to cholera toxin. The data in Table I indicate that some quantitative differences do exist when comparing the density of R and G components in the rat reticulocyte and rat erythrocyte. However, in addition to the parallel decline in R and G density, a fundamental qualitative change occurs upon maturation of the rat reticyocyte, and that is the loss of R-G communication. Thus, as shown in Figure 5, the ability of the agonist isoproterenol to compete for [^{3}H] DHA antagonist binding to the beta-adrenergic receptors of the rat reticulocyte is of higher potency than observed in the erythrocyte. Furthermore, the ability of guanine nucleotides to decrease receptor affinity for agonists characteristic of rat reticulocyte membranes is almost entirely absent in rat erythrocyte membranes. Thus, one of the

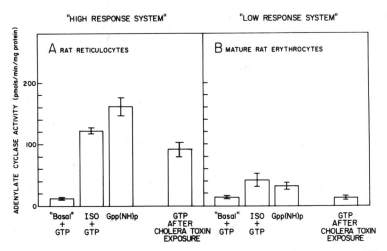

Figure 4. Adenylate cyclase activity in rat reticulocyte (A) and
rat erythrocyte (b) membrane preparations. Experimental
details are provided in [9].

TABLE I

Maturation of the Rat Erythrocyte: Changes in the Quantity of β-
Adrenergic Receptors and GTP Binding Proteins

	β-Adrenergic Receptors fmol/mg	42,000 Mr ^{32}P-ADP-Ribosylated GTP-binding proteins fmol/mg
RETICULOCYTES	680 ± 40	∿ 465 - 620
ERYTHROCYTES	220 ± 30	∿ 150 - 200

important parameters of monitoring R-G communication, namely the
responsiveness of receptor affinity for agonists to guanine nucleotides, is
lost upon maturation of the rat reticulocyte.

Figure 6 indicates that the "molecular monitor" of R-G
communication is also lost upon maturation of the rat reticulocyte.
Thus, the ability of agonist occupancy of the rat reticulocyte beta-
receptor to increase apparent beta-adrenergic receptor size is not
observed in rat erythrocyte membranes, as shown in Figure 6C.

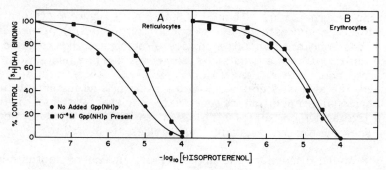

Figure 5: Competition of (-) isoproterenol for [³H] DHA antagonist binding to rat reticulocyte (A) and erythrocyte membranes (B). Experimental details are provided in [9].

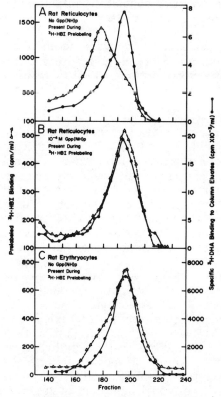

Figure 6: Comparison of prelabeled [³H] HBl-agonist- β-receptor complexes obtained in rat reticulocyte (A,B) and rat erythrocyte (C) preparations. Fig. 6A,B are identical to Fig. 1A,B and are provided for comparison. In Fig. 6C, rat erythrocyte preparations are treated identically to the rat reticulocyte preparations shown in Fig. 6A. Further experimental details are provided in [9].

Thus, if one returns to the schematic diagram in Figure 3, it can be observed that the decrease in the frequency (or quantity) of agonist-stabilized R-G encounters in rat erythrocyte membranes has resulted in decreased ability of both agonists and exogenous guanine nucleotides to stimulate the adenylate cyclase catalytic subunit. These data suggest that, indeed, the agonist-stabilized R-G interaction is an important first step in hormonal stimulation of adenylate cyclase, and loss of this important interaction correlates with loss in sensitivity of the enzyme to both hormones and exogenous guanine nucleotides.

In the above discussion, the dual role of guanine nucleotides has been emphasized, i.e. the ability of guanine nucleotides to enhance adenylate cyclase activity and decrease receptor affinity for agonists. It is now realized that hormones and drugs are not only capable of stimulating adenylate cyclase, but also a number of hormones, acting via receptors distinct from those coupled to activation of adenylate cyclase, are capable of inhibiting catalytic activity. These receptor populations include muscarinic receptors in the heart, opiate receptors in neuroblastoma-glioma cells, and alpha-adrenergic receptors of the alpha$_2$ subtype in adipose, pancreas and platelets. Little is known about the molecular basis for hormonal inhibition of adenylate cyclase. However, there are some interesting phenomenological similarities between systems coupled to activation of adenylate cyclase and those coupled to inhibition of adenylate cyclase. The most prominent similarity is the important role of guanine nucleotides in systems coupled to inhibition of adenylate cyclase. Thus, in much the same way that guanine nucleotides are required for hormonal stimulation of adenylate cyclase, GTP also appears to be absolutely required for inhibition of adenylate cyclase. In addition, guanine nucleotides are able to decrease receptor affinity for agonists at receptors coupled to inhibition of cyclase. Thus, one is provoked to ask whether or not the same GTP-binding protein, or population of GTP-binding proteins, is involved in mediating both activation and inhibition of adenylate cyclase.

A great deal of indirect experimental evidence has been accumulated to suggest that distinct GTP-binding proteins are involved in stimulation and inhibition of adenylate cyclase (cf Ref 4 for review), including the observation that approximately ten-fold higher concentrations of GTP are needed for inhibition than for stimulation of adenylate cyclase. In addition, although hydrolysis-resistant analogs result in persistent activation of adenylate cyclase, hormonal inhibition of adenylate cyclase requires GTP, and hydrolysis-resistant analogs of GTP will not support hormonal inhibition of the enzyme. Furthermore, differential sensitivity of guanine nucleotide-mediated stimulation and inhibition of cyclase to proteases, Mn^{++}, sulfhydryl-directed reagents and radiation inactivation have also suggested that separate GTP-binding proteins are involved in activation and attenuation of catalytic

activity [4].   However, a limitation of indirect data is that these
findings might simply indicate that discrete domains of a single GTP-
binding protein, responsible for communicating opposing signals to the
catalytic moiety, are differentially sensitive to the above preturbants.
Consequently, we chose to take a more direct look at the question of
whether or not the same GTP-binding protein might be involved in
activation and inhibition of adenylate cyclase.

We used the human platelet as our model system for exploring
hormonal inhibition of adenylate cyclase. This choice was predicated on
several factors. First, alpha-adrenergic receptors of the human platelet
are of a single pharmacological subtype, the $alpha_2$ subtype. In addition,
these α_2-adrenergic receptors can be identified directly using both a
radiolabeled agonist ([^{3}H] epinephrine) and a radiolabeled antagonist
([^{3}H] yohimbine) in membranes derived from human platelets. Thus,
we can focus on those molecular interactions uniquely promoted by
agonist occupancy of the receptor and not mimicked by antagonist
occupancy, thus giving us a handle on those molecular interactions
probably involved in receptor-cyclase coupling and transmembrane
signaling. In addition, the human platelet provides a homogenous, single
cell system in which particulate preparations possessing reasonable
specific activity of the functions that we are evaluating can easily be
obtained. Again, our studies on the α_2-adrenergic system of the human
platelet focus on R-G communication and the possibility that agonist
occupancy of the alpha-adrenergic receptor stabilizes a complex
between the α-receptor and a GTP-binding protein in a manner
analogous to observations for the β -adrenergic receptor coupled to
stimulation of cyclase.

As shown in Figure 7A, agonist competition for antagonist binding
to human platelet membranes is indeed sensitive to guanine
nucleotides [13] . Thus, epinephrine competition for [^{3}H] yohimbine
binding is of higher potency in washed platelet lysates than following the
addition of the GTP analog, Gpp(NH)p, which decreases receptor affinity
for the agonist. However, as shown in Figure 7B, when the alpha-
adrenergic receptor of the human platelet membrane has been
solubilized using the detergent digitonin, agonist competition is no longer
of such high potency, and guanine nucleotides fail to modulate receptor
affinity for agonist. This loss of agonist potency in competing for the
receptor is not a function of the receptor recognition site having been
altered by detergent solubilization.   This conclusion is based on the
observation that antagonist potency is unchanged in competing for
 [^{3}H] yohimbine binding to detergent-solubilized receptors when
compared with binding to receptors in the intact platelet
membrane [13]. Thus, this loss of agonist potency in human platelet
solubilized preparations is unique to agonist agents.   These data
suggested to us that detergent solubilization of unoccupied alpha-

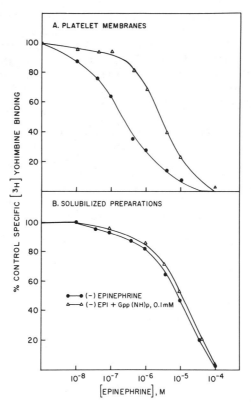

Figure 7. Effect of guanine nucleotides on agonist competition for
[3H] yohimbine binding to α2-adrenergic receptors in human
platelet membrane (A) and digitonin-solubilized (B) preparations. The specificity for the effect of guanine
nucleotides to decrease α -receptor affinity for agonist
is Gpp(NH)p>GTP=GDP>>GMP; App (NH)p is without effect at
0.1mM. Additonal experimental details are in [13].

adrenergic receptors from the human platelet membrane may result in
destabilization of receptor-effector interactions characteristic of the
intact membrane and responsible for higher receptor affinity for agonists
as well as sensitivity to guanine nucleotides. Consequently, we
postulated that digitonin solubilization of the human platelet membrane
had, in fact, disrupted R-G communication. Thus, we determined the
effect of prelabeling human platelet membranes with the radiolabeled
agonist, [3H] epinephrine prior to detergent solubilization. As shown
in Figure 8, agonist occupancy of receptors does stabilize R-G
communication to solubilization, as is demonstrated by the ability of
guanine nucleotides to facilitate [3H] epinephrine dissociation from
prelabeled, agonist-occupied alpha-adrenergic receptors. The data in

Figure 8B simply demonstrate that antagonist occupancy of the receptor at the time of solubilization does not yield an antagonist-occupied receptor that is sensitive to guanine nucleotides. This lack of sensitivity of antagonist-receptor complexes to guanine nucleotides is characteristic of that observed in the native human platelet membrane. However, the ability of agonist occupancy of the receptor to stabilize putative R-G interactions and hence sensitivity to guanine nucleotides is in distinct contrast to the lack of sensitivity of solubilized receptors to guanine nucleotides when the receptor is solubilized unoccupied (c.f. Figure 7B).

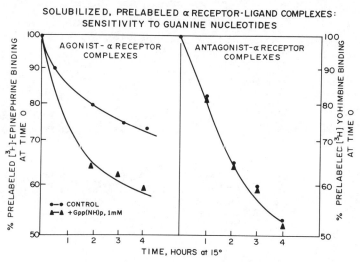

Figure 8. Dissociation of [3H] epinephrine (A) and [3H] yohimbine from α -adrenegic receptors in human platelets with radio-ligand prior to digitonin solubilization.

The guanine nucleotide-sensitive, [3H]epinephrine-alpha receptor complex that is solubilized from human platelet membranes is of larger molecular size than unoccupied or antagonist-occupied receptors. This conclusion is derived from the data shown in Figure 9. Prelabeled human platelet membranes were solubilized with digitonin and then fractionated using sucrose gradient centrifugation. As shown in the upper panel of Figure 9, the [3H] epinephrine-alpha receptor complex sediments more rapidly than unoccupied receptors in the same preparation, assayed using [3H] yohimbine binding to sucrose gradient fractions subsequent to centrifugation. The lower panel indicates that antagonist occupancy of the receptor does not promote the faster sedimenting form of the alpha-adrenergic receptor, since [3H] yohimbine prelabeled alpha-receptors sediment in a gradient position identical to that of unoccupied receptors, shown in the upper panel. Thus, in a manner completely analogous with beta-receptors coupled to activation of adenylate cyclase, alpha-adrenergic receptors of the human platelet coupled to inhibition of adenylate cyclase appear to interact with a GTP-binding protein upon agonist occupancy of the receptor. This agonist-stabilized R-G interaction is manifested by both the guanine nucleotide sensitivity of the prelabeled complex (Fig. 8) and the larger molecular size of the agonist stabilized complex (Fig. 9).

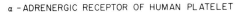

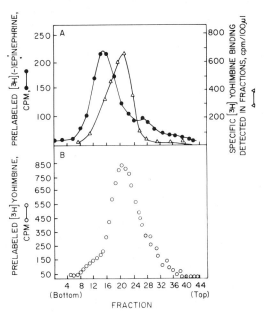

Figure 9. Comparison of the sedimentation characteristics of [3H] epinephine (AGONIST)-prelabeled α-receptors (A), [3H] yohimbine (ANTAGONIST)- prelabeled α-receptors (B) and unoccupied receptors (A), measured subsequent to sedimentation using [3H] yohimbine binding to the gradient fractions. Experimental details are provided in [13].

In order to determine more directly whether or not the guanine nucleotide-sensitive agonist-receptor complex of larger molecular size contained a GTP-binding protein, we developed a procedure for isolating the agonist-alpha-receptor complex (putative R-G complex) from the vast majority of GTP-binding proteins in the human platelet membrane. We utilized lectin chromatography to resolve GTP-binding proteins in association with cell surface moieties, e.g. the alpha-adrenergic receptor, from those on the inner lamella of the membrane. Using wheat germ agglutinin-Sepharose 6MB, we were able to adsorb 70% of the solubilized alpha-receptor preparation to the resin, while removing greater than 95% of the GTP-binding proteins from the solubilized material. Elution of the alpha-adrenergic receptor from the wheat germ agglutinin-Sepharose column was effected with N-acetyl-D-glucosamine, a preferred sugar for interaction with this lectin. The eluted material contained less than 5% of the original GTP-binding proteins in the total solubilized separation, but contained 60% of the starting alpha-adrenergic receptor material. In addition, the [^{3}H] epinephrine-alpha receptor complexes that were eluted by N-acetyl-D-glucosamine from the wheat germ agglutinin-Sepharose resin retained the properties uniquely conferred on the receptor by agonist occupancy, namely sensitivity to guanine nucleotides and a faster sedimentation in sucrose gradients [14].

The biological preparation eluted from wheat germ agglutinin-Sepharose appeared to be the appropriate starting material for determining whether or not the GTP-binding protein in association with the agonist-occupied alpha-adrenergic receptor was the GTP-binding protein that was able to associate with the catalytic subunit of adenylate cyclase and effect activation of the enzyme. To answer this question, we again exploited cholera toxin as a tool for identifying the GTP-binding protein responsible for activation of adenylate cyclase.

Figure 10 indicates that increasing concentrations of ^{32}P-NAD, the co-substrate for cholera toxin, can, in the presence of cholera toxin, cause an enhancement of GTP-sensitive adenylate cyclase activity in the human platelet. This enhancement of GTP-sensitive activity is paralleled by labeling of a 42,000 Mr peptide in human platelet membranes. In contrast to the dose-related effects of ^{32}P-NAD$^+$ on ^{32}P-ADP-ribosylation of the membranes and enhancement of GTP-sensitive adenylate cyclase activity, cholera toxin-catalyzed modification of human platelet membranes did not alter the ability of epinephrine to attenuate PGE$_1$-stimulated adenylate cyclase activity. These data provide indirect evidence that the cholera toxin substrate in these membranes is not the GTP-binding protein mediating inhibition adenylate cyclase. However, like all indirect data, another interpretation of the findings shown in Figure 10 is that the covalent modification of the GTP-binding protein by cholera toxin does not alter the function of the inhibitory domain of this protein.

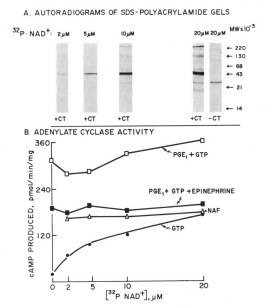

Figure 10. Effects of cholera toxin on ^{32}p-ADP-ribosylation and adenylate cyclase activities in human platelet membranes. Membranes incubated with 90 µg/ml cholera toxin and increasing concentrations of ^{32}p-NAD$^+$ for 20mm at 25° were washed and assayed for adenylate cyclase activity (B) or solubilized in SDS and applied to 10% SDS-polyacrylamide gels (A). Experimental details are provided in [14].

Thus, we continued our experiments to determine whether or not the guanine nucleotide sensitive [^{3}H] epinephrine-alpha receptor complex of larger molecular size indeed contains the cholera toxin-catalyzed ADP-ribosylated subunit of the stimulatory GTP-binding protein. For these experiments, human platelet membranes were first modified by cholera toxin under conditions that labeled all and nearly all of the 42,000 Mr subunits coupled to activation of cyclase [14]. These membranes were then thoroughly washed and exposed to the radiolabeled agonist, [^{3}H] epinephrine, prior to solubilization. The solubilized preparations were purified using wheat germ agglutinin-Sepharose 6MB chromatography, as described above. The material eluted from lectin using N-acetyl-D-glucosamine was concentrated and applied to sucrose gradients for fractionation. Identical treatment of preparations was carried out for [^{3}H] yohimbine-prelabeled alpha-receptor complexes.

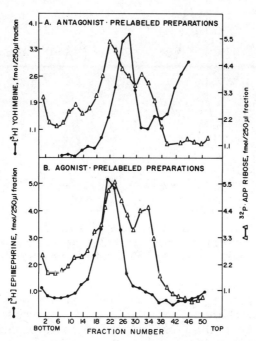

Figure 11. Sucrose gradient sedimentation profiles of ^{32}P-ADP-ribo-sylated proteins solubilized form human platelet membranes prelabeled with the antagonist [H] yohimbine (A) or the agonist [^{3}H] epinephrine (B). Membranes were preincubated with cholera toxin and ^{32}P-NAD$^+$, washed, prelabeled with [^{3}H]epinephine or [^{3}H] yohimbine, solubilized, exposed to wheat germ agglutinin-Sepharose 6MB, desorbed by N-acetyl-D-glucosamine, concentrated and applied to 7.5-20% sucrose gradients, as described [14].

The data shown in Figure 11 demonstrate the sedimentation profiles for ^{32}P-ADP-ribosylated proteins and compare them with the sedimentation position of agonist-receptor and antagonist-receptor complexes. As shown in Figure 11, a similar sedimentation profile was observed for ^{32}P-ADP-ribosylated proteins derived from membranes exposed to either alpha-adrenergic agonists (Figure 11B) or antagonists (Figure 11A). However, the possibility existed that a small fraction of the ^{32}P-ADP-ribosylated material might indeed have been associated with the agonist-occupied receptor but obscured in the heterogenous ^{32}P-ADP-ribose sedimentation observed profile in Figure 11. Therefore, to make rigorous quantitative comparisons between agonist- and antagonist-liganded preparations, gradient fractions corresponding to a portion of the peak region of the agonist-alpha-receptor complex were pooled from

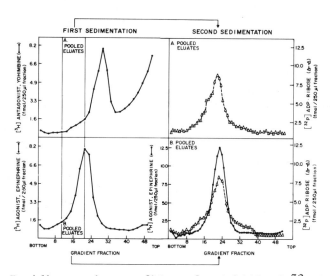

Figure 12. Residimentation profiles of solubilized ^{32}p-ADP-ribosylate
        proteins from human platelet membranes prelabeled with
        [^{3}H] epinephine or [^{5}H] yohimbine. Solubilized receptor-
        ligand complexes, prepared as in Fig. 10, were applied to
        7.5-20% sucrose gradients containing 0.1% digitonin buffer
        and centriguged for 15 hours at 100,000xg. In this experi-
        ment, cholera toxin incubation enhanced GTP-sensitive ac-
        tivity to 100% of 10mM NaF-stimulated activity; ^{32}p-ADP-
        ribose is 44cpm/fmol. SDS-autoradiograms documented that
        the cpm of ^{32}p sedimenting in the gradients are solely due
        to the 42,000 Mr peptide. The left hand panels demonstrate
        the sedimentation profile of [^{3}H] epinephine- and [^{3}H]
        ipinephine- and [^{3}H] yohimbine-receptor complexes. Frac-
        tions 10-20 of the gradients shown and of two additional
        gradients each for agonist- and antagonist-receptor pre-
        parations were pooled, concentrated and applied to a sec-
        ond sucrose gradient for recentrifugation. Additional ex-
        perimental details are provided in [14].

three separate gradients (Figure 12, left hand panel) and applied to a
second sucrose gradient for resedimentation (Fig. 12, right hand panels).
The peak height and sedimentation position of ^{32}P-ADP-ribosylated
proteins were virtually identical regardless of whether or not the
fractions for resedimentation were obtained from gradients containing
agonist-or antagonist-alpha-receptor complexes.   This is in distinct
contrast to what would have been anticipated if agonist occupancy of the
alpha-receptor resulted in a unique association of the alpha-receptor
with the ^{32}P-ADP-ribosylated GTP-binding protein, thus accounting for
the guanine nucleotide sensitivity and larger molecular size of the
agonist-receptor complex when compared with the antagonist-receptor
complex.   Since cholera toxin had increased GTP-sensitive adenylate
cyclase activity to 100% of NaF-stimulated activity in the starting

material for the experiment shown in Figure 12, it is not unreasonable to assume that a major fraction of the 42,000 Mr subunits coupled to activation of adenylate cyclase had incorporated ^{32}P-ADP-ribose. Hence, if the agonist-alpha-receptor complex had included the 42,000 Mr ^{32}P-ADP-ribosylated subunit in a 1:1 ratio with the receptor, then the height of the ^{32}P-ADP-ribose-containing peak obtained by resedimentation of agonist-receptor complexes should have been approximately 12 fmol greater than that obtained by resedimenting the corresponding fractions from antagonist-receptor-containing gradients. The absence of any quanititative change in ^{32}P-ADP-ribose-containing peaks from agonist-receptor vs. antagonist-receptor gradients suggests that the faster-sedimenting, [^{3}H] epinephrine-receptor complex does not uniquely contain ^{32}P-ADP-ribosylated 42,000 Mr proteins and, thus, that the ^{32}P-ADP-ribose migrating in similar fractions upon resedimentation is likely associated with distinct and independently sedimenting detergent-protein complexes [14] .

TABLE II

Characteristics of Hormone and Drug Effector
Systems which Regulate Adenyl Cyclase Actibity

ACTIVATING SYSTEMS	ATTENUATING SYSTEMS
↑ cAMP REQUIRES GTP $K_D \sim 10^{-7}$M	↓ cAMP REQUIRES GTP $K_D \sim 10^{-6}$M
GTP ↓ RECEPTOR AFFINITY FOR AGONISTS	GTP ↓ RECEPTOR AFFINITY FOR AGONISTS
AGONIST STABLIZES R-G INTERACTIONS (↑ MOLECULAR "SIZE")	AGONIST STABLIZES R-G INTERACTIONS (↑ MOLECULAR "SIZE")
AGONIST-R-G COMPLEX CONTAINS 42,000 Mr SUBUNIT ^{32}P-ADP-RIBOSYL-ATED BY CHOLERA TOXIN	AGONIST-R-G COMPLEX DOES NOT CONTAIN THE ^{32}P-ADP-RIBOSYLATED 42,000 Mr SUBUNIT

Table II compares the phenomenology for hormone receptor systems coupled to activation versus inhibition of adenylate cyclase. Both activation and inhibition of adenylate cyclase require GTP. GTP also modulates receptor affinity for agonists at receptors coupled to both activation and inhibition of adenylate cyclase. Furthermore, agonist occupancy of receptors coupled to activation as well as inhibition of cyclase appears to stabilize receptor interactions with effector components, presumably GTP-binding proteins. This conclusion is based on the ability of agonist occupancy of the receptor prior to detergent solubilization to yield a solubilized receptor-ligand complex which is sensitive to guanine nucleotides and which possesses a larger molecular size. However, an important difference between the systems coupled to activation versus inhibition of cyclase is the observation that the agonist-stabilized receptor complex of larger molecular size does not contain the ^{32}P-ADP-ribosylated 42,000 Mr subunit in systems coupled to inhibition of adenylate cyclase. This is in distinct contrast to beta-adrenergic receptors coupled to activation of adenylate cyclase. As shown in Figure 2, the agonist-beta receptor complex of larger molecular size is uniquely associated with the cholera toxin-catalyzed ^{32}P-ADP-ribosylated protein responsible for adenylate cyclase stimulation. Thus, it appears that at least two distinct GTP-binding proteins are involved in regulation of adenylate cyclase by receptors coupled to activation and inhibition of adenylate cyclase. In the case of activation of adenylate cyclase, however, it appears that the same GTP-binding protein both modulates receptor affinity for agonists and conveys regulatory information to the catalytic subunit of cyclase. Future studies will hopefully elucidate the biochemical nature of the GTP-binding protein that modulates affinity for agonists at receptors coupled to inhibition of adenylate cyclase as well as determine the relationship, if any, between this protein and the GTP-binding protein that conveys inhibitory signals to the catalytic moiety of the adenylate cyclase system.

REFERENCES

1.   Cassel, D. and Selinger, Z. Catecholamine-Stimulated GTPase Activity in Turkey Erythrocyte Membranes. Biochim. Biophys Acta 452, 538-551 (1976).

2.   Cassel, D., Levkovitz, H. and Selinger, S. The Regulatory GTPase Cycle of Turkey Erythrocyte Adenylate Cyclase. J. Cycl. Nucl. Res. 3, 393-406, 1977.

3.   Cassel, D. and Selinger, Z. Mechanism of Adenylate Cyclase Activation Through the β-Adrenergic Receptor: Catecholamine-induced Displacement of Bound GDP by GTP. Proc. Natl. Acad. Sci. USA 75, 4155-4159, 1978.

4.   Cooper, D.M.F. Bimodal Regulation of Adenylate Cyclase. FEBS Lett. 138, 157-163, 1982.

5.   DeLean, A., Stadel, J.M. and Lefkowitz, R.J. A Ternary Complex Explains the Agonist-specific Binding Properties of the Adenylate Cyclase-coupled β-Adrenergic Receptor. J. Biol. Chem. 255, 7108-7117, 1980.

6.   Gill, D.M. and Meren, R. ADP-ribosylation of Membrane Proteins Catalyzed by Cholera Toxin: Basis of the Activation of Adenylate Cyclase. Proc. Natl. Acad. Sci. USA 75, 3050-3054, 1978.

7.   Gilman, A.G. and Ross, E.M. Biochemical Properties of Hormone-sensitive Adenylate Cyclase. Ann. Rev. Biochem. 49, 533-564, 1980.

8.   Limbird, L.E. and Lefkowitz, R.J. Agonist-induced Increase in Apparent β-Adrenergic Receptor Size. Proc. Natl. Acad. Sci. USA 75, 228-232, 1978.

9.   Limbird, L.E., Gill, D.M. Stadel, J.M., Hickey, A.R. and Lefkowitz, R.J.   Loss of β-Adrenergic Receptor-Guanine Nucleotide Regulatory Protein Interactions Accompanies Decline in Catecholamine Responsiveness of Adenylate Cyclase in Maturing Rat Erythrocytes. J. Biol. Chem. 255, 1854-1861, 1980.

10.   Limbird, L.E., Gill, D.M. and Lefkowitz, R.J. Agonist-promoted Coupling of the β-Adrenergic Receptor with the Guanine Nucleotide Regulatory Protein of the Adenylate Cyclase System. Proc. Natl. Acad. Sci. 77, 775-779, 1980.

11.   Limbird, L.E. Activation and Attenuation of Adenylate Cyclase (Review Article) Biochem. J. 195, 1-13, 1981.

12.   Pfeuffer, T. Guanine-nucleotide-controlled Interactions Between Components of Adenylate Cyclase. FEBS Lett. 101, 85-89, 1979.

13.   Smith, S.K. and Limbird, L.E. Solubilization of Human Platelet α - Adrenergic Receptors: Evidence that Agonist Occupancy of the Receptor Stabilizes Receptor-Effector Interactions. Proc. Natl. Acad. Sci. 78, 4026-4030, 1981.

14.   Smith, S.K. and Limbird, L.E. Evidence That Human Platelet α - Adrenergic Receptors Coupled to Inhibition of Adenylate Cyclase are not Associated with the Subunit of Adenylate Cyclase ADP-ribosylated by Cholera Toxin. J. Biol. Chem. In Press, Sept./Oct., 1982.

15.   Stadel, J.M., Schorr, R.G.L., Limbird, L.E. and Lefkowitz, R.J. Evidence That a β-Adrenergic Receptor-associated Guanine Nucleotide Regulatory Protein Conveys Guanosine 5'-0-(3-thiotriphosphate)-dependent Adenylate Cyclase Activity. J. Biol. Chem. 256, 8718-8723, 1981.

16.   Williams, L.T. and Lefkowitz, R.J. Slowly Reversible Binding of Catecholamine to a Nucleotide-Sensitive State of the β - Adrenergic Receptor. J. Biol. Chem. 252, 7207-7213, 1977.

AGONIST REGULATION OF THE MUSCARINIC CHOLINERGIC RECEPTOR

IN EMBRYONIC CHICK HEART

Jonas B. Galper, Louise C. Dziekan and Thomas W. Smith

Brigham and Women's Hospital
Harvard Medical School
Boston, Massachusetts 02115

J. B. Galper, L. C. Dziekan and T. W. Smith. The correlation between number of muscarinic cholinergic receptor sites as measured by binding of the muscarinic agonist (^{3}H)methyl-scopolamine ((^{3}H)MS) and the ability of muscarinic agonists to mediate a physiologic response was determined in intact heart cells cultured from chick embryos 10 days in ovo. The increase in K^+ permeability and the decrease in beating rate mediated by the muscarinic agonist carbamylcholine were the responses studied. In cells labelled to equilibrium with $^{42}K^+$, exposure to 10^{-3}M carbamycholine caused a 33% increase in the rate of $^{42}K^+$ efflux from the cell with a half-maximal effect at a carbamylcholine concentration of 8×10^{-5}M. Steady state intracellular K^+ content remained at control levels. A 15% decrease in beating rate occurred in cells exposed to 10^{-3}M carbamylcholine.. Since muscarinic receptors on the surface of the intact cell are presumed to mediate the physiologic response to the agonist, an assay for binding of (^{3}H)MS to intact cells was developed. (^{3}H)MS bound specifically to intact heart cells (185fmol/mg protein) with a K_d of 0.48 nM. Exposure of cells for various times to 10^{-3}M carbamylcholine followed by washing and binding of (^{3}H)MS to intact cells demonstrated that following a brief lag period (12 min), a gradual loss of 70% of (^{3}H)MS binding sites took place over the next 6 h. Half of the receptor sites were lost during the initial 30 min. A decrease in the ability of carbamylcholine to stimulate K^+ efflux and to decrease beating rate was observed after pre-exposure of cells to muscarinic agonists. When half of the 70% receptor loss mediated by agonist pre-exposure was complete, both the K^+ permeability and beating rate responses decreased by 50%. These findings establish a close correlation between changes in the subclass of muscarinic receptors subject to agonist control and physiologic responsiveness following agonist exposure of cultured chick embryo heart cells and suggest the absence of significant numbers of "spare" receptors within this group.

Changes in the muscarinic receptor following agonist exposure were studied by comparing the binding of two muscarinic antagonists of markedly differing hydrophobicity. The binding of the more hydrophobic antagonist Quinuclidinyl benzilate ((^{3}H)QNB) was quite similar in extent to binding of the more hydrophilic antagonist ((^{3}H)MS), with K_d values of 0.11 nM and 0.47 nM respectively. However, following prolonged agonist exposure two subclasses of receptors were present, a form (A) that bound both (^{3}H)MS and (^{3}H)QNB and a form (B) which bound only (^{3}H)QNB. Binding of (^{3}H)MS and (^{3}H)QNB to cells following incubation for various times with agonist demonstrated a sequential interconversion of sites from form A to form B. The relationship of such a sequential mechanism to agonist-induced changes in the relationship of the receptor with the cell membrane and agonist-induced endocytosis of the receptor is discussed.

INTRODUCTION

The ability of hormone-sensitive cells to respond to changes in hormonal concentration by regulating the number and/or affinity of their cell surface receptors has been demonstrated in cells regulated by neurotransmitters, peptide and protein hormones, and factors such as lectins and immunoglobulins (1). The effect of such changes in receptor number and affinity on the physiologic response of the cell to hormone or neurotransmitter stimulation has been a subject of considerable interest (2). Even in the presence of "spare" receptors not obviously coupled to a physiologic response, reduction in membrane receptor number below a critical level would be expected to decrease the sensitivity of the cell to the effector. In luteal cells from rat ovaries in which hormone action mediates changes in adenylate cyclase activity, a close correlation has been demonstrated between luteinizing hormone (LH) induced decrease in LH receptors and a decrease in the ability of LH to stimulate the synthesis of cyclic AMP and progesterone (3).

Recently, experiments using the potent muscarinic antagonist (^{3}H)QNB for the measurement of muscarinic binding sites have demonstrated that prior exposure of neuroblastoma cells (4) or cultures of embryonic chick heart cells (5) to muscarinic cholinergic agonists decreased the number of muscarinic binding sites to as low as 30% of control levels. The response of embryonic chick heart cell cultures to muscarinic agonists revealed 3 subclasses of receptor sites: (^{3}H)QNB binding sites which are lost during the first minute of agonist exposure, 26% of total, accompanied by a decrease in apparent affinity of all remaining receptors for agonist; (^{3}H)QNB binding sites which are lost over 2.5 h of agonist exposure, 43% of total; and receptors which continued to bind (^{3}H)QNB after 3 h of agonist exposure, 30% of total (5). Whether any of these changes in receptor number are coupled to a decrease in physiologic response to muscarinic agonist has not been determined.

Muscarinic cholinergic stimulation of the heart causes a decrease in the rate and force of contraction. In atrial and nodal tissue vagal stimulation or application of exogenous acetylcholine have been associated with hyperpolarization of the resting membrane potential (6) and a shortening of the action potential duration. Both of these effects have been considered to be the consequence of the development of an outward K^+ current (7) whose magnitude is determined by the frequency of vagal stimulation. Harris and Hutter (8) were the earliest to demonstrate a vagally mediated increase in efflux of $^{42}K^+$ from tortoise and frog sinus venosus. However, more recently Giles and Nobel (9) and others have presented evidence that in atrial tissue the negative inotropic effect could also be mediated by a direct inhibitory effect of acetylcholine on the slow inward current.

In the present investigation we studied the relationship between changes in the properties and number of muscarinic receptors and the beating rate and K^+ permeability responses to muscarinic agonists in cultured heart cells. Specifically, we determined the ability of muscarinic agonists to elicit these responses before and after receptor number was altered by prior exposure to muscarinic agonists. We also examined the relationship between changes in a particular subclass of receptors (5) and altered K^+ permeability and beating rate responses.

Agonist-induced endocytosis of cell surface receptors has been demonstrated for several types of hormone binding sites (1). In one of the most extensively studied cases, epidermal growth factor interaction with the human fibroblast has been shown to involve endocytosis of the receptor-growth factor complex with probable subsequent lysosomal degradation of both the hormone and receptor within the cell (10). The slow loss of 43% of muscarinic receptors during a 3h exposure to agonist was only reversible after a twelve hour incubation in the absence of agonist, and required protein synthesis (5). Inhibitors of microtubule function inhibited 43% of total agonist-induced receptor loss. These data suggested that the subclass of 43% of receptors that disappear slowly during agonist exposure of cultured heart cells might be subject to endocytosis and degradation.

In order to study the changes in the state of the receptor following agonist exposure we compared the binding to intact cultured heart cells of two muscarinic antagonists with markedly differing hydrophobicities, $(^3H)QNB$ and (^3H)methylscopolamine. Our findings support the view that properties of binding of these radioligands to intact cells are capable of differentiating between two states of the receptor: the control state (before agonist binding) which bound both $(^3H)MS$ and $(^3H)QNB$ and a state present during the late phase of agonist exposure which bound only $(^3H)QNB$ and which may be an intermediate state in the process of receptor endocytosis.

METHODS

Heart Cell Cultures

Heart cell cultures were prepared by a modification of the method of DeHaan (11) as described (5). The heart cells were plated at a density of 1.3×10^5 cells per cm^2 on collagen-coated 100 mm Petri dishes or at a density of 2.0×10^5 cells/cm^2 in 16 mm multiwell dishes (CoStar) containing 24 wells per unit. On the third day of incubation, the medium was changed. Unless otherwise indicated cells were used for experiments on culture day 4.

Measurement of $(^3H)MS$ or $(^3H)QNB$ binding to intact cells

On the third culture day cells were fed with fresh medium containing leucine $(^{14}C(U))$, 0.01 mCi/ml, and incubation was continued for 24 hours. To study the binding of $(^3H)MS$ or $(^3H)QNB$, 0.5 ml of 4-(2-hydroxyethyl)-1-piperazine ethane sulfonic acid (HEPES) buffered medium M-199 2nM in $(^3H)MS$ or 1nM in $(^3H)QNB$ was added to each well and incubated at 37^oC for 1 hour.

Wells were rinsed rapidly 3 times with wash medium (120 mM NaCl, 5.4 mM KCl, 0.8 mM $MgSO_4$, 1.8 mM $CaCl_2$, 50 mM HEPES, 1.0 mM NaH_2PO_4 adjusted to pH 7.4 with NaOH). Solubilization of cell protein was as described previously (5). The mean protein content per 1,000 ^{14}C-counts was calculated. This factor permitted calculation of protein content in each well. All $(^3H)MS$ and $(^3H)QNB$ binding was normalized to specific binding per mg of cell protein. Total washing time was 10 seconds. $(^3H)MS$ and $(^3H)QNB$ binding was found to be constant during this period. Specific binding was defined as binding inhibited by a saturating concentration (0.1mM) of oxotremorine or 1.0 μM methyl-scopolamine. Nonspecific binding was determined in quadruplicate for each experimental point. Sixty percent of $(^3H)MS$ and 50% of $(^3H)QNB$ binding was specific under these conditions. Under the conditions described, specific binding at 2nM $(^3H)MS$ and 1nM $(^3H)QNB$ proceeded without a lag and reached equilibrium by 40 min. The relative potency of cholinergic ligands to inhibit $(^3H)MS$ or $(^3H)QNB$ binding was consistent with the relative pharmacologic potency of muscarinic agonists and antagonists.

Ion Flux Measurements: $^{42}K^+$ Uptake

Cells grown on coverslips for 3 days were labelled for 24 hrs with leucine $(4,5-^3H)$, 0.2 uCi/ml. As described previously (12) coverslips were placed in an uptake chamber containing fresh medium at 37°C in an atmosphere of 95% air 5% CO_2, transferred to a second chamber with medium containing $^{42}K^+$ (5 uCi/ml, total $K^+ = 4.5$) and incubated for the appropriate times. Coverslips were rinsed three times by dipping into Earle's saline solution, cells were then solubilized and $^{42}K^+$ determined as described (12). A zero time value was subtracted from each determination in order to correct for nonspecific binding of $^{42}K^+$. This value was usually less than 15 nmol/mg protein.

$^{42}K^+$ Efflux

Cells grown on glass coverslips were incubated for 24 h with leucine $(4,5-^3H)$, labelled to equilibrium (3h, $t_{1/2}$ of 14 min) with $^{42}K^+$ (5 mCi/ml, total K = 4.5 mM), rinsed once in fresh growth medium containing unlabelled K^+, transferred to a perfusion chamber and perfused with unlabelled growth medium at 0.98 ml/min at 37°C. The effluent was collected at 30 sec intervals for 5 min, 10 ml scintillation fluid added and $^{42}K^+$ determined. Uptake $^{42}K^+$ was maximum at 980 ± 15 (SEM, n=3) nmol/mg cell protein.

Measurement of Changes in Beating Rate

Cells grown on glass coverslips were placed in a Sykes-Moore chamber (Bellco Glass Inc., Vineland, N. J.) which could be continuously perfused via inlet and outlet ports. The chamber was placed on the stage of an inverted phase contrast microscope enclosed in a lucite box maintained at 37°C. Perfusion at 0.98 ml per min did not disturb cell adhesion to the coverslips. A stable baseline beating rate of 140 ± 10 (SEM, n=20) beats per min was observed for cultures of hearts 10 days in ovo. Beating was determined visually or by monitoring the movement of the border of a single cardiac cell with a video-motion detector and recording the output on a Hewlett-Packard physiological recorder as previously described (12). Cells were perfused with growth medium or medium containing $10^{-3}M$ carbamylcholine.

Computer Analysis

Data were fitted to equations describing a given binding model using a derivative free non-linear regression analysis described by W. J. Dixon and M. B. Brown (13).

RESULTS

Alterations in K^+ Permeability in Heart Cell Cultures
in Response to Muscarinic Agonists

In order to correlate agonist-mediated decreases in muscarinic receptor number in embryonic heart cell cultures with the ability of muscarinic agonists to alter beating rate and K^+ permeability, it was first necessary to determine the kinetics and concentration dependence of the effects of muscarinic agonists on these responses in cells not subjected to prior agonist exposure. Changes in the rate of efflux of $^{42}K^+$ following exposure of cells to muscarinic agonists were determined as a measure of change in permeability of the cell to K^+. To study K^+ efflux the intracellular K^+ pool was first labelled to equilibrium with $^{42}K^+$ (See Methods).

Efflux of $^{42}K^+$ from control cells equilibriated with $^{42}K^+$ was found to follow an exponential time course for up to 30 min during which $^{42}K^+$ remaining in the cells decreased from 960 ± 10 (n=3) nmol/mg protein to 285 ± 15 nmol/mg protein (data not shown). The half time of efflux was 14 min. However, in order to avoid simultaneous agonist mediated decreases in the ability of further exposure to agonist to increase $^{42}K^+$ efflux rate, during measurement of efflux, $^{42}K^+$ efflux was studied during a brief 5 min exposure to the agonist.

The effect of the cholinergic agonist carbamylcholine on the rate of efflux of K^+ from cultured cells is shown in Fig. 1. Each plot in Fig. 1 represents the least squares fit of a semilogarithmic plot of the data to a straight line. These data indicate that during the times studied, the efflux of $^{42}K^+$ follows an exponential time course and increases with increasing concentrations of carbamylcholine. The half times for efflux derived from the slopes of the curves in Fig. 1 are plotted in the insert. The half time for efflux of $^{42}K^+$ decreased 32% from 13.2 ± 0.3 (SEM, n=14) min to 9.0 ± 0.2 (n=14) min as the concentration of carbamylcholine varied from 0 to $10^{-3}M$. The increase in the rate of efflux of $^{42}K^+$ from the cells over this concentration range was half-maximal at a carbamylcholine concentration of $8 \times 10^{-5}M$. Incubation of cells with $10^{-3}M$ carbamylcholine in the presence of $10^{-6}M$ atropine completely inhibited the increase in the K^+ efflux rate (Fig. 1) indicating that these effects on K^+ movement were specific for interaction with muscarinic receptors.

Dishes containing heart cells cultured from chicken embryos 10 days in ovo and grown on glass coverslips were labelled overnight with 0.2uCi/ml leucine (4,5-3H), incubated for 3 hrs in growth medium 5 mCi/ml in $^{42}K^+$ = 4.5 nM), rinsed, and placed in an efflux chamber as described in Methods. Cells were perfused with growth medium con-

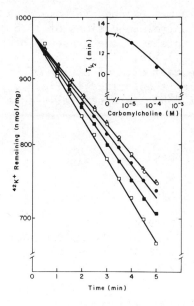

Figure 1
Effect of carbamylcholine on
$^{42}K^+$ efflux from cultured
heart cells.

taining unlabelled K^+ and the indicated concentrations of carbamylcholine o, no carbamylcholine; ●, $10^{-5}M$; ■,$10^{-4}M$; □, $10^{-3}M$; Δ, $10^{-3}M$
carbamylcholine plus $10^{-6}M$ atropine. $^{42}K^+$ efflux was determined at
the times indicated as described in Methods and plotted as $^{42}K^+$ remaining in the cells at time t, calculated by subtracting total
efflux of $^{42}K^+$ from the cell during time, t, from the initial $^{42}K^+$
content of the cell at time zero. $^{42}K^+$ at time zero was determined
as the mean K^+ content/mg protein of 14 coverslips exposed to 5
mCi/ml $^{42}K^+$ for 3 h, rinsed and $^{42}K^+$ determined as described in
Methods. Each curve is the mean of 2 sets of 7 reliate determinations each. The lines are the least squares fit of the $\log_{10}$ of
$^{42}K^+$ remaining at time t to a straight line and plotted on a logarithmic scale versus time. Correlation coefficients were at
least 0.99 for all plots. Insert: The effect of increasing carbamylcholine concentration on the half time of $^{42}K^+$ efflux. The half
time of efflux is calculated from the relationship $T_{1/2} = \ln 2/k_1$,
where k_1 is the slope of the curve at each carbamylcholine concentration in Figure 1 and equals the rate constant for the movement
of $^{42}K^+$ out of the cell.

Uptake of $^{42}K^+$ into Cultured Heart Cells in the Presence of Muscarinic Agonists

The effect of carbamylcholine on the rate of uptake of $^{42}K^+$
into cultured heart cells is shown in Fig. 2. The data are report-
ed as $^{42}K^+_{eq} - ^{42}K^+_t$ where $^{42}K^+_{eq}$ is the $^{42}K^+$ content of the cell
after a 3 h equilibriation with $^{42}K^+$-containing medium and $^{42}K^+_t$
is $^{42}K^+$ uptake at time t. Data are plotted on a logarithmic scale.
This analysis allows comparison of the data from efflux and uptake

studies. The time course of $^{42}K^+$ uptake was exponential over the
times studied, with a half time under control conditions of 13.8 ±
0.5 (SEM, n=21) min. The half time of uptake in the presence of
$10^{-3}M$ carbamylcholine was 8.8 ± 0.4 (n=21) min, similar to the
value of 9.0 ± 0.2 min obtained for the half time of efflux of $^{42}K^+$
at $10^{-3}M$ carbamylcholine in the experiments described in Fig. 1.
Hence the rates of efflux and uptake of $^{42}K^+$ are essentially equal.

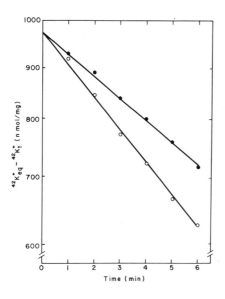

Figure 2
Effect of carbamylcholine on
uptake of $^{42}K^+$ by cultured
heart cells.

Cells were labelled with ^{14}C as described in Fig. 1. Discs were
incubated for the times indicated in medium containing 5m Ci/ml
$^{42}K^+$. Discs were rinsed and uptake of $^{42}K^+$ determined as described
in Methods. Data were plotted as $^{42}K^+_{eq} - ^{42}K^+_{t}$, $^{42}K^+_{eq}$, determined
from the mean of 14 determinations of $^{42}K^+$ uptake after a 3 h
incubation in medium containing 5 mCi/ml $^{42}K^+$, was 970 ± 15 nmol/
mg. Each curve represents the least squares fit of the $\log_{10}$ of
the mean of 21 determinations. Correlation coefficients were 0.99
for both regression lines. Half time of uptake was derived from
the data as described in Figure 1. open circles: $^{42}K^+$ uptake in the
presence of $10^{-3}M$ carbamylcholine; filled circles: control $^{42}K^+$
uptake.

K^+ Content of Cultured Heart Cells During Incubation
with Carbamylcholine

The efflux rate of K^+ is a function of membrane potential
(Em), K^+ gradient across the cell membrane, and permeability of the

membrane to K^+. The concentration gradient of K^+ across the cell
membrane is a major driving force in the movement of K^+ in response
to changes in membrane permeability. If muscarinic agonists increase the permeability of the cell membrane to K^+, prolonged exposure to muscarinic agonists might result in depletion of intracellular K^+ if changes in membrane potential and pump mechanisms were
unable to balance the accelerated K^+ loss. If the intracellular
K^+ concentration varied with time of exposure to muscarinic agonist,
the driving force for K^+ efflux would vary and the comparison of
relative efflux rates could not be used as an indicator of changes
in K^+ permeability in cells exposed to agonists for various times.
Therefore the effect of muscarinic agonists on steady state K^+
 ontent was measured in cells in which the intracellular K^+ pool
had been equilibriated with $^{42}K^+$, 5 uCi/ml, followed by incubation
for various times in $^{42}K^+$ plus $10^{-3}M$ carbamylcholine. A mean value
of 980 ± 20 (SEM, n=21) nmol/mg protein was obtained for control
cells and values of 960 ± 30 (n=14), 973 ± 15 (n=14), 975 ± 25
(n=14) and 980 ± 15 (n=14) nmol/mg protein were obtained for cells
incubated in $10^{-3}M$ carbamylcholine for 15, 45, 90 min and 3 h respectively. These values were not significantly different from
control. Hence changes in K^+ influx and efflux rates after incubation with carbamylcholine cannot be explained by alterations in
intracellular K^+ content and are consistent with changes in K^+
permeability.

Binding of Muscarinic Antagonist to Intact Cultured Heart Cells

The effects of muscarinic agonists on K^+ permeability and
beating rate require the interaction of agonist with receptors on
the surface of the intact cell. Since receptor number measured in
heart cell homogenates may not reflect the subset of receptors in
the intact cell available for agonist binding, correlations between changes in receptor number and functional response to the
agonist might be studied with greater validity using measurements
of receptor number in the intact cell. We chose the more hydrophilic muscarinic antagonist (^{3}H)MS for measurement of receptor
number in the intact cell. We felt that the more hydrophobic antagonist (^{3}H)QNB used in previous studies of ligand binding to
whole cell homogenates (5, 14), might diffuse readily through the
cell membrane and bind to receptors that were not available for interaction with the agonist at the cell surface. The specific binding of (^{3}H)MS was saturable at 195 ± 8 (SEM, n=6) fmol/mg protein,
with a K_d of 0.43 ± 0.05 nM (Fig. 3). Sixty percent of bound counts
were specific as measured by displacement by $10^{-4}M$ oxotremorine, a
potent muscarinic agonist.

Agonist-Induced Loss of (^{3}H)MS Binding Sites Assayed in Intact Cells: Dependence on Agonist Concentration During Pre-exposure

We have demonstrated previously that a 3 h incubation of heart cell cultures with muscarinic agonists caused a 70% decrease in the binding of (^{3}H)QNB to heart cell homogenates with a half-maximal effect of 35% for carbamylcholine at 0.8×10^{-5}M (5). When the effect of prior exposure of cells to various concentrations of agonist on receptor number was determined by binding (^{3}H)MS directly to intact cells (Fig. 4), exposure to carbamylcholine caused a maximum decrease of 67% in specific (^{3}H)MS binding with a half maximal effect of 34% at 3×10^{-5}M. Hence total receptor loss was the same as that assayed in homogenates.

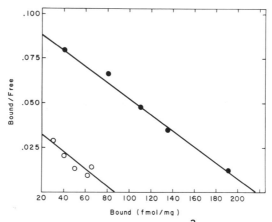

Figure 3 Scatchard plot of binding of (^{3}H)MS to chick heart cell homogenates at various (^{3}H)MS concentrations.

Replicate cultures in multiwell dishes were incubated overnight in medium containing 0.01u Ci/ml leucine (^{14}C (U)). Growth medium was replaced by fresh medium with and without 10^{-3}M caramylcholine, incubated for 3 h at 37º and washed twice with 3 ml each of HEPES buffered M199 and incubated for 2 h in the presence of the indicated concentrations of (^{3}H)MS. Cells were washed 3 times with 3 ml of ice cold wash solution and specific (^{3}H)MS binding determined as described in Methods. Each point represents the mean of 4 replicate determinations repeated n times and is corrected for nonspecific binding; ●, control cells (n=6); 0, cells incubated prior to (^{3}H)MS binding for 3 h with 10^{-3}M carbamylcholine (n=3).

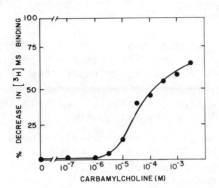

Figure 4 Effect of prior exposure of cells to graded concentrations of agonist on (^{3}H)MS binding to intact cells.

Replicate cultures in multiwell dishes were incubated overnight in
medium containing 0.01 µCi/ml leucine (^{14}C (U)). Growth medium
was replaced by fresh medium containing the indicated concentration
of carbamylcholine, incubated of 3 h at 37°C, washed twice with 3
ml each of HEPES buffered M-199 and incubated for 1 h in HEPES
buffered M-199 in the presence of 2 nM (^{3}H)MS. Cells were washed
3 times with 3 ml of ice cold wash solution and specific binding
of (^{3}H)MS determined as described in Methods. Each point represents the mean of 4 replicate determinations and is corrected for
nonspecific binding.

     One alternative explanation for the loss of (^{3}H)MS binding
sites following incubation with agonist is that agonist exposure
mediates a decrease in the affinity of the receptor for antagonist
and hence an apparent decrease of (^{3}H)MS binding. To rule out this
possibility an experiment comparing the concentration dependence of
the binding of (^{3}H)MS to control cells with binding to cells after
prior agonist exposure is illustrated in Fig. 3 . Scatchard analysis of the data gave two nearly parallel straight lines for car-
bamylcholine-treated and control cells, corresponding to K_d values
of 0.45 ± 0.07 (SEM n=6) and 0.43 ± 0.05 (n=3) respectively, and
intersecting the x-axis at 68 fmol/mg of protein for carbamylcholine treated cells and 195 fmol/mg of protein for control cells.
Hence these data are consistent with a 65% carbamylcholine-mediated
decrease in (^{3}H)MS binding with no significant effect on affinity
for (^{3}H)MS. Because of the low level of binding of (^{3}H)MS to
agonist treated-cells, these data were subject to somewhat more
scatter than in control cells.

Time Course of Agonist-Induced Loss of (^{3}H)MS Binding
Sites Assayed in Intact Cells

 We have determined previously that incubation of heart cell
cultures with muscarinic agonists caused a biphasic decrease in
(^{3}H)QNB binding sites with an early rapid loss of 26% of binding
sites followed by a lag phase and the gradual loss of another 43%
of receptors over 2.5 h.   The half time of this second phase of
loss of (^{3}H)QNB binding sites was 30 min.

 Fig. 5 summarizes data from an experiment in which we studied
the number of specific (^{3}H)MS binding sites in the intact cell
following exposure to carbamylcholine for various times. Following
a brief lag phase, the loss of 72% of (^{3}H)MS binding sites in the
intact cell took place during a 6 h exposure to agonists. The loss
of approximately half these receptors took place over the initial
30 min.   Hence the time course of agonist-induced receptor loss as
measured in the intact cell bears substantial similarity to the
slow phase of receptor loss seen in assays carried out in homogenates (5).   However, the rapid loss of 26% of receptors following
brief exposure of cells to agonists did not occur in the intact
cell.

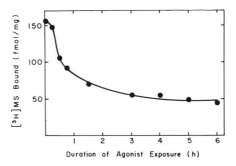

Figure 5   Time dependence of agonist-induced receptor loss measured
by the binding of (^{3}H)MS to intact cells.

Replicate cultures in multiwell dishes were incubated overnight in
medium containing 0.01uCi/ml leucine (^{14}C(U)).   Growth medium was
replaced by fresh medium containing 10^{-3}M carbamylcholine incubated
for the times indicated, rinsed and incubated for 1 h with 2 nM
(^{3}H)MS and washed as described in Fig. 4.   Each point represents
the mean of 4 replicate determinations repeated 6 times and is
corrected for nonspecific binding.

Effect of Prior Exposure to Agonist on the Ability of Muscarinic Agonists to Alter K^+ Permeability and Beating Rate

We compared the effect of carbamylcholine on K^+ permeability and beating rate in control cells and in cells exposed for various times to 10^{-3}M carbamylcholine (Fig. 6; Table 1). The results shown in Fig. 6 demonstrate that in cells not previously exposed to agonist, carbamylcholine decreased the half time for efflux of $^{42}K^+$ from 13.4 ± 0.2 (n=21) min to 8.8 ± 0.2 (n=21) min, a decrease of 4.6 min or 33% below control. However, after a 3 h exposure to 10^{-3}M carbamylcholine subsequent exposure to carbamylcholine had no significant effect on rate of $^{42}K^+$ efflux.

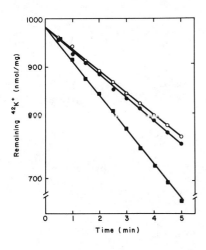

Figure 6
The effect of prior exposure to agonist on the ability of muscarinic agonist to increase K^+ permeability.

Efflux was measured as described in Fig. 1 except that cells were incubated for 3 h in growth medium 5mCi/ml in $^{42}K^+$ (total K^+=4.6 mM), with and without 10^{-3}M carbamylcholine prior to measurement of efflux. $^{42}K^+$ at time zero was determined for two sets of 14 coverslips each incubated for 3 h in medium 5mCi/ml in $^{42}K^+$ with or without 10^{-3} carbamylcholine as described in Methods. Total K^+ in control cells was 960 ± 20 nmol/mg protein while K^+ in cells exposed 3 h to agonist was 968 ± 15 nmol/mg protein. The lines are the least squares fit of a semilogarithmic plot of the data to a straight line. Correlation coefficients were at least 0.99 for all plots. (o), control; (■), 10^{-3}M carbamylcholine; (●), 10^{-3}M carbamylcholine following 3 h at 10^{-3} carbamylcholine.

Analysis of the time course over which carbamylcholine exposure decreased the response of K^+ efflux to muscarinic agonists is shown in Table 1. During the first 15 min of agonist exposure, no significant effect on the muscarinic response could be detected;

carbamylcholine decreased the half time for efflux by 4.4 min from
13.2 min to 9.0 min compared to a 4.6 min decrease for control
cells. However, after a 30 min agonist exposure, carbamylcholine
decreased efflux half time by only 2.3 min from 13.2 to 10.9 min,
a loss of 52% of the effect seen in control cells. After a 45 min
agonist exposure, carbamylcholine decreased efflux half time by
only 1.3 min from 13.3 min to 12.0, a loss of 74% of the effect
seen in control cells. After a 90 min exposure to agonist, carbamylcholine had no measureable effect on efflux rate. Since the
recovery of binding sites following agonist mediated receptor loss
takes place during a 12 h incubation in fresh medium, studies were

Table 1

Efflux rate of $^{42}K^+$ in cells previously exposed to carbamylcholine*

Duration of pre-exposure to agonist (min)	$T_{\frac{1}{2}}$ of $^{42}K^+$ efflux (min) (+ SEM, n=7)	
	Control	Carbamylcholine (10-3M)
0	13.4 ± 0.2	8.8 ± 0.2
15	13.2 ± 0.2	9.1 ± 0.5
30	13.2 ± 0.3	10.9 ± 0.3
45	13.3 ± 0.2	12.0 ± 0.1
90	13.7 ± 0.4	13.5 ± 0.1
180	13.0 ± 0.3	13.8 ± 0.2
180 + 12 hr recovery	13.8 ± 0.2	9.0 ± 0.2

*Experiments were carried out as described in Figure 6. After
labelling for 3 h with $^{42}K^+$, cells were incubated for the indicated
times in 5mCi/ml $^{42}K^+$ with or without $10^{-3}M$ carbamylcholine. $^{42}K^+$
efflux was measured as described in Figure 1.

Differences between $T_{1/2}$ of efflux in control cells and cells
exposed to carbamylcholine at 0, 15, 30 and 45 min are significant
within 99% confidence limits as demonstrated by the method of
covariance analysis (15). Differences between $T_{1/2}$ of efflux in
cells exposed to carbamylcholine for 0 and 30 min, 30 and 45 min
and 45 and 90 min are significant at 99% confidence limits by
similar criteria.

carried out to determine the ability of agonist to mediate an increase in K^+ efflux in cells subjected to agonist pre-exposure
followed by recovery in fresh medium. In the experiments summarized in Table 1, such a 12 h recovery period was accompanied by
full restoration of the K^+ permeability response.

We also determined the effect of prior exposure to carbamylcholine on the ability of muscarinic agonists to slow beating rate
in cultured heart cells. As summarized in Table II, in control
cells $10^{-3}M$ carbamylcholine decreased beating rate by 15% from 140
$\pm$ 3 (SEM, n=20) beats/min to 119 $\pm$ 3 beats/min. A 15 min prior
exposure to agonist had no effect on the beating rate response to
carbamylcholine. However, after a 30 min prior exposure to agonist, carbamylcholine decreased beating rate by only 8% to 129 $\pm$ 2
beats/min, a response only 47% of that in control cells. A 45 min
prior exposure to agonist decreased the response of beating rate
to 4% (136 $\pm$ 1.4 beats/min), which did not represent a statistically significant difference from the control rate of 140 $\pm$ 3
beats/min. Finally, after a 180 min prior exposure to agonist
no response in beating rate to carbamylcholine could be detected.
However, if these cells are washed and incubated for 12 h in fresh
medium, beating rate in these cells became fully responsive to
carbamylcholine.

Correlation Between Agonist-Induced Changes in Receptor Number and the Ability of Muscarinic Agonists to Alter K^+ Permeability and Beating Rate

Analysis of the time dependence of agonist-induced decrease
in receptor number (Fig. 5) demonstrated two subclasses of $(^3H)MS$
binding sites: a subclass of 70% of receptors which were lost with
a half time of 30 min and a subclass of 30% of receptors whose
binding of $(^3H)MS$ was unaffected by up to 6 h of exposure to agonist. Following a 90 or 180 min pre-exposure to agonist, no K^+
efflux rate or beating rate responses to agonist could be demonstrated (Table I and II). However, 30% of receptor sites were
still available for antagonist binding (Fig. 5). One explanation
of these data is that this 30% of sites alone is not sufficient to
elicit a cellular response and that the fraction of receptors subject to agonist control may play a critical role in mediating K^+
permeability and beating rate responses. The correlation between
the time course of the agonist mediated decrease in the binding of
$(^3H)MS$ to the subclass of receptors subject to agonist control and
the time course of the decrease in K^+ permeability and beating
rate response is shown in Fig. 7. A close correlation between the
decrease in the response in K^+ permeability and beating rate was
observed. Such a correlation is consistent with the view that the
increase in K^+ permeability occurs in parallel with and is related
to the decrease in beating rate. Agonist-mediated changes in

Table II

Effect of prior exposure to carbamylcholine on the decrease in
beating rate in response to muscarinic agonist exposure*

Duration of pre-exposure to agonist (min)	% decrease in beating rate (+ SEM, n=20) +
0	15 ± 2
15	15 ± 1
30	8 ± 1
45	4 ± 1
180	0 ± 2
180 + 12 hr recovery	15 ± 1

*Cells grown on glass coverslips were perfused in Sykes-Moore
chambers and beating rate determined as described in Methods.
Difference in the decrease in beating rate between 15 and 30 min
of agonist pre-exposure was significant with $p < 0.001$; the difference
between 30 and 45 min of pre-exposure was significant at $p < 0.01$,
while the difference between 45 min and 180 min of pre-exposure was
not statistically significant.

receptor number also closely approximated decreases in functional
response. A 15 min lag period was followed by a decrease in all 3
parameters which was maximal after 6 h with a half-maximal effect
at 30 min.

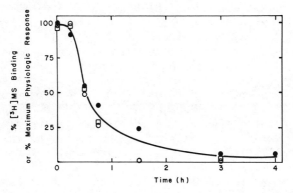

Figure 7 Correlation between the time course of agonist-mediated receptor loss and agonist-mediated decrease in K^+ permeability and beating rate response to muscarinic agonists. The fraction of (^{3}H)MS binding sites subject to agonist control remaining at each time (●) was derived from the data in Figure 5 by subtracting the subclass of receptors not subject to agonist control (46 ± 6 fmol/mg protein) from total (^{3}H)MS bound for each point and determining the % of maximum (^{3}H)MS binding remaining at each time point. Data for the % of maximum K^+ efflux response (□) and % maximal beating rate response (○) at each time was derived from the data in Tables I and II respectively.

Agonist-Mediated Changes in the Binding of (^{3}H)QNB and (^{3}H)MS to Intact Cells

Previously reported data support the hypothesis that the slow phase of agonist-induced receptor loss involves endocytosis of cell surface receptors (5). If this were the case, agonist-induced receptor loss might involve an agonist-mediated configurational change in the receptor followed by movement of the receptor into or across the cell membrane. We considered the possibility that although the (^{3}H)MS might bind only to receptors on the cell surface, a more hydrophobic ligand might diffuse through the intact cell membrane and bind to receptors that were not available for interaction with agonist at the cell surface. Hence, differences in binding of these two agonists might offer a probe of agonist-induced changes in the configuration and/or localization of receptors in the cell membrane. Although at pH 7.4 both (^{3}H)MS and (^{3}H)QNB are predominantly positively charged, we determined that (^{3}H)QNB is markedly more hydrophobic than (^{3}H)MS. A comparison of the partition of (^{3}H)QNB and (^{3}H)MS between an aqueous phase consisting of the wash solution described in Methods for ligand binding studies (pH 7.4, physiologic ionic strength) and an organic phase consisting of ether or chloroform revealed that the ether: aqueous phase partition coefficient for (^{3}H)QNB was 10 times greater than that for (^{3}H)MS and the chloroform: aqueous partition coefficient for (^{3}H)QNB was 30 times greater than the corresponding values for (^{3}H)MS.

An experiment comparing the binding of $(^3H)MS$ and $(^3H)QNB$ to intact cells after a 2h incubation with various concentrations of either $(^3H)MS$ or $(^3H)QNB$ is shown in Fig. 8. The specific binding of both ligands was saturable, and demonstrated a single apparent receptor affinity class for each antagonist ligand. The mean of 6 determinations such as that in Fig. 8 gave a K_d of 0.47 ± 0.12 nM with a maximum receptor number of 178 ± 14 fmol/mg protein for $(^3H)MS$ and a K_d of 0.11 ± 0.02 nM with a maximum receptor number of 183 ± 13 fmol/mg protein for $(^3H)QNB$ binding. The difference between the number of receptor sites measured by the two methods was not statistically significant, suggesting that all receptors are similarly accessible to both ligands and presumably available for agonist binding at the cell surface. Data from an experiment in which $(^3H)QNB$ and $(^3H)MS$ binding were compared in cells following a 6 h exposure to various concentrations of carbamylcholine is shown in Fig. 9. No difference could be detected between binding of the two ligands. Sixty-eight percent of radioligand binding sites were lost with a half-maximal effect at $3 \times 10^{-5}M$ carbamylcholine. A similar IC_{50} for carbamylcholine-induced receptor loss was noted previously for cell homogenates (5).

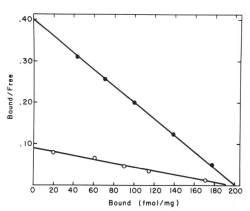

Figure 8 Scatchard plot of binding of $(^3H)QNB$ and $(^3H)MS$ to intact chick heart cells at various concentrations of the labelled antagonist. Replicate cultures in multiwell dishes were incubated overnight in medium containing 0.01 μCi/ml leucine $(^{14}C(U))$. Growth medium was replaced by HEPES buffered M-199 containing the indicated concentrations of $(^3H)MS$ or $(^3H)QNB$, incubated for 2 h at 37°C, washed three times with 3 ml each of wash solution, and specific (^3H) antagonist binding determined as described in "Methods". Each point represents the mean of 4 replicate determinations repeated six times and is corrected for nonspecific binding. Each curve represents the least squares fit of the data to a straight line. Correlation coefficients were at least 0.99. ●,$(^3H)QNB$: o, $(^3H)MS$.

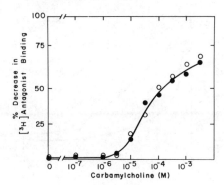

Figure 9   Effect of exposure of intact cultured heart cells to various concentrations of carbamylcholine on the binding of (^{3}H)MS and (^{3}H)QNB.

Cells from replicate cultures grown in multiwell dishes were grown overnight in medium containing 0.10µ Ci/ml leucine (^{14}C (U)). Cells were washed and incubated for 6 h at 37°C in HEPES-buffered M-199 containing the indicated concentrations of carbamylcholine, rinsed with 3 ml of fresh medium, and incubated with medium 1 nM in (^{3}H) QNB or 2 nM in (^{3}H)MS for 1 h at 37°C. The cells were then washed three times with 3 ml each of wash solution and specific (^{3}H) - antagonist bound determined as described in "Methods". Each point represents the mean of 4 replicate determinations repeated 4 times. Nonspecific binding was determined independently as the mean of 4 replicate determinations at each concentration. (●), (^{3}H)MS; (o), (^{3}H)QNB.
        An experiment comparing the time course of agonist-induced re- ceptor loss in intact cells as measured by the binding of (^{3}H)MS or (^{3}H)QNB is shown in Fig. 10, upper panel. The binding of (^{3}H)MS to intact cells (●) was unaffected by a 10-12 min prior exposure to muscarinic agonists similar to that shown in Fig. 5. Following this lag period nearly 80% of (^{3}H)MS binding sites were lost over the next 6 h of agonist exposure. Half of these receptors were lost during the first 30 min of agonist exposure following the lag phase (Fig. 10, upper panel). The time course of agonist-mediated receptor loss as measured by the binding of (^{3}H)QNB (o) was signi- ficantly slower than that measured with (^{3}H)MS. Following a 35-37 min lag period, 76% of (^{3}H)QNB binding sites were lost over the next 5½ h (Fig. 10, upper panel). Half of the receptor sites were lost approximately 107 min after the end of the lag phase. Hence, although a 6 h exposure to carbamylcholine caused a nearly identical decrease in total receptor number as measured by either (^{3}H)MS or (^{3}H)QNB binding (Fig. 9), the loss of (^{3}H)QNB binding sites takes place following a longer lag period and at a slower rate than does the loss of (^{3}H)MS binding sites.

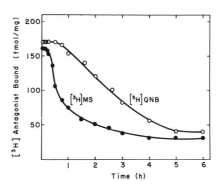

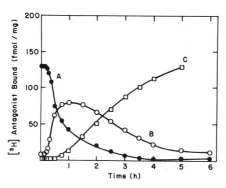

Figure 10   Time course of agonist-induced receptor loss in intact
             cells measured by the binding of (^{3}H)MS or (^{3}H)QNB.

Upper panel: Cells from replicate cultures gown in multiwell dishes
              were incubated with ^{14}C in the presence and absence of
              10^{-3}M carbamylcholine for the indicated times and (^{3}H)
              QNB and (^{3}H)MS binding determined as in Fig. 9. Each
              point represents the mean of 6 sets of 4 replicate
              determinations each. (o), (^{3}H)QNB bound; (•),
              (^{3}H)MS bound.
Lower panel: Derived From Fig. 10, upper panel. A (•), residual
              (^{3}H)MS binding sites plotted as a function of duration
              of agonist exposure; B (o), the number of receptors at
              a given time t that bind (^{3}H)QNB but not (^{3}H)MS, derived
              by subtracting A, the residual (^{3}H)MS binding sites at
              times t, from the total sites that bind (^{3}H)QNB at the
              same time; C (□), the number of receptor sties that no
              longer bind (^{3}H)QNB, derived by subtracting the total
              number of (^{3}H)QNB binding sites at time t (Fig. 10,
              upper panel) from total (^{3}H)QNB binding sites present
              at time zero. The residual ligand binding after a 6 h
              exposure to agonist has been subtracted from each curve.

Altered States of the Receptor Following Agonist Exposure

Since the loss of the ability of the receptor to bind $(^3H)MS$ precedes the loss of binding sites for $(^3H)QNB$, these data suggest the possibility of an agonist-mediated sequential conversion of the receptor to different forms. Such a conversion might be represented by a series of consecutive irreversible first order reactions:

$$A \xrightarrow{k_I} B \xrightarrow{k_{II}} C \qquad (1)$$

Here A can be viewed as a control state of the receptor which binds both $(^3H)MS$ and $(^3H)QNB$. In this model exposure to agonist would mediate conversion from from A to form B which binds only $(^3H)QNB$. More prolonged agonist exposure may result in conversion to a form C which binds neither $(^3H)MS$ nor $(^3H)QNB$. Here k_I and k_{II} are first order rate constants. The reactions can be considered irreversible during the time course of these studies since agonist-mediated loss of the ability to bind $(^3H)MS$ or $(^3H)QNB$ was not reversed for up to 3 h following removal of agonist and recovered fully only 9 to 12 h after agonist removal (data now shown). Three differential equations describe the time course of changes to A, B and C according to classical precursor-product considerations (16):

$$\frac{dA}{dt} = k_I A \qquad (2a)$$

$$\frac{dB}{dt} = k_I A - k_{II} B \qquad (2b)$$

$$\frac{dC}{dt} = k_{II} B \qquad (2c)$$

The predicted concentrations of A, B and C at any time may be derived from the data in Fig. 10. Computer analysis of these data by non-linear regression for two sequential irreversible reactions described by equations 2a-c demonstrated that k_I and k_{II} were approximately equal. Consequently the data were fit to a model in which k_I was set equal to k_{II}. The solutions of equations 3a-c when $k_I = k_{II}$ are:

$$A = e^{-kt} \qquad (3a)$$

$$B = kt \, A_o e^{-kt} \qquad (3b)$$

$$C = A_o - A - B \qquad (3c)$$

where A_o is the number of receptor sites at time zero.

A fit of the data in Fig. 10, to equations 3a-c gave $A_o = 157 \pm 4$ fmol/mg protein (n=10), $k = 0.0117 \pm 0.0006$ min^{-1}, and total receptor number remaining at 6 h = 30 ± 4 fmol/mg or about 20% of receptor sites. The equivalence of k_I and k_{II} suggests either that loss of both $(^3H)MS$ and $(^3H)QNB$ binding sites are part of a continuous time-dependent process rather than two independent

processes, or that k_I and k_{II} describe the rates of two independent
processes which happen to be similar in rate. In any event, these
data show that after a 10-12 min lag period (^{3}H)MS binding sites
began to decrease ($\bullet$) with the conversion of sites to a form which
binds only (^{3}H)QNB. Sites that bind only (^{3}H)QNB (o) reach a maximum at 1 hr and disappear over the next 5 h. At 30 min (^{3}H)QNB
binding sites begin to decrease slowly, reaching a minimum by 6 h
($\square$). These data strongly suggest that (^{3}H)MS and (^{3}H)QNB binding
data are capable of delineating two distinct states of the receptor.

DISCUSSION

Factors Acting to Maintain the Level of Intracellular K^+

     In the present studies the rate of K^+ efflux was increased by
33% in the presence of 10^{-3}M carbamylcholine. In the absence of
other compensatory mechanisms, the increase in K^+ flow down its
concentration gradient would tend to deplete intracellular K^+
((K^+)$_i$). Under these conditions the interpretation of changes in
the rate of K^+ efflux would be complicated because they would represent an increase in permeability to K^+ at the same time that the
driving force for movement of K^+ out of the cell was decreasing.
However, in the studies reported here, the undirectional rates of
efflux and uptake of $^{42}K^+$ are equal from 30 sec until 5 min after
exposure to agonist. Furthermore, exposure of cells to agonist for
time periods from 15 min to 6 h had no effect on (K^+)$_i$. The absence of any effect of prolonged agonist exposure on (K^+)$_i$ could
potentially be explained by the absence of an effect of muscarinic
agonists on K^+ permeability in cells following agonist exposures
of 90 min or longer (Table 1). However, agonist exposures of 15
min to 45 min are associated with a significant increase of K^+ permeability (Table I) and in these cells a compensatory mechanism for
maintenance of (K^+)$_i$ at control levels must exist. Hence, the passive
movement of K^+ down its concentration gradient is presumably bal-
anced by an increase in the passive movement of K^+ into the cell
due to the muscarinic agonist-induced hyperpolarization of the cell
membrane, by an increase in active transport of K^+ into the cell
via NaK-ATPase (which would also tend to cause hyperpolarization)
or by a combination of the two. Since efflux and influx rates for
K^+ are equal 30 seconds after addition of agonist, any compensatory
mechanism must respond within the first several seconds of agonist
exposure in order to maintain steady state levels of (K^+)$_i$. Experiments to delineate these phenomena are planned.

Relative Insensitivity of Cultured Cells to Carbamylcholine

     The relative insensitivity of these cells to carbamylcholine
is of concern. Comparison of the sensitivity of heart cell cultures and intact hearts to muscarinic agonists in prior studies

has demonstrated a marked decrease in sensitivity of beating rate
of cultured cells to muscarinic agonists. The half-maximal concentration of carbamylcholine for inhibition of beating in intact chick
embryo hearts removed from the embryos 7-10 days in ovo was 10 nM
(17). In the present study a 15% decrease in beating rate was seen
within 10-15 seconds after exposure of cultures of hearts taken from
embryos 10 days in ovo to 10^{-3} carbamylcholine. Speralakis and
Lehmkuhl (18) reported that heart cell cultures were insensitive
to muscarinic agonists; Ertel et al. (19) observed a response only
after a 15 min exposure to agonist, with a decrease in beating rate
which was independent of agonist concentration. A third group reported a response to as little as 1 nM acetylcholine using a rapid
flow technique (20).

     The limited sensitivity of our cultures to muscarinic agonists
may be related to several aspects peculiar to cultured systems. One
factor is the predominance in our cultures of ventricular cells,
which are relatively insensitive to muscarinic stimulation.

     Josephson and Speralakis (21) demonstrated that acetylcholine
produced a decrease in the slow inward current (I_{si}) in aggregates
of embryonic chick heart only in the presence of β-adrenergic stimulation. Watanabe et al. (22) and Jakobs et al. (23) demonstrated
that muscarinic agonists inhibit β-adrenergic agonist-stimulated
adenylate cyclase activity. The resulting decrease in cyclic AMP
levels could contribute to the effect of muscarinic agonists on the
intact heart. Although intact hearts are subject to some degree of
endogenous   β-adrenergic stimulation, the cultures of chick embryo
heart cells studied here are devoid of such effects. Hence muscarinic agonists could only affect adenylate cyclase activity by lowering basal adenylate cyclase activity. Biegon and Pappano (24)
observed that in embryonic chick ventricles studied prior to hatch-
ing, carbamylcholine decreased β-adrenergic agonist-stimulated
cyclic AMP levels, but had little effect on basal cyclic AMP levels.
Although other mechanisms probably account in part for the modest
muscarinic effects in these cultures, the absence of significant
β-adrenergic stimulation in cultured cells would be expected to contribute to the limited responsiveness of these cells to muscarinic
agonists.

"Spare" Muscarinic Receptors

     The availability of techniques for the measurement of changes
in K^+ permeability and beating rate, together with the ability to
quantify alterations in receptor number during pre-exposure to agonist, afforded us the opportunity to study the relationship of receptor number to the ability of agonist to effect a muscarinic response and to determine whether a particular subclass of receptors
was critical to the mediation of such a muscarinic response. Human
chorionic gonadotropin (hCG) binding to interstitial cells of the
rat testis, for example, has been shown to stimulate the synthesis

of testosterone and to increase levels of cyclic AMP. Low levels
of ^{125}I-hCG sufficient to bind to only 1% of receptor sites stimulated testosterone production, and a maximum cyclic AMP response was
seen at concentrations of ^{125}I-hCG capable of occupying only 50% of
sites. Hency, for the testosterone response, 99% of receptors are
not required to elicit an appreciable increase in synthesis while
50% of ^{125}I-hCG binding sites might be classified as "spare" receptors for the cyclic AMP response (25).

In the present studies of the agonist-induced decrease in muscarinic receptor number, a subclass of 30% of receptors appeard to
be unaffected by up to 6 h of agonist exposure. Cells exposed to
agonist for 90 min or 180 min, in which (^{3}H)MS binding demonstrated
the presence of only this subclass of 30% of receptors, did not respond to carbamylcholine as measured by an effect on either beating
rate or rate of K$^+$ efflux. Whether this subclass of 30% of receptors might mediate some as yet undefined muscarinic response, whether their presence is necessary for muscarinic activity but not
sufficient to mediate a response, or whether they represent a subclass of spare receptors cannot be determined from the available
data. What is clear is that the 70% of receptors subject to agonist
control is critical for mediation of the muscarinic responses studied, and that there are few if any spare receptors in this subclass.
Thus, agonist-induced changes in receptor number appear to modulate
responsiveness to muscarinic cholinergic stimuli in cultured heart
cells.

The absence of a more complete correlation of functional response and receptor number within the 70% subset could be due to the
fact that binding of (^{3}H)MS, an antagonist, may over-estimate the
number of physiologically active receptor sites and may not correspond on a one to one basis to those sites that form an active receptor complex with agonist. Comparison of the binding of radio-
labelled β-adrenergic agonist and antagonists in frog erythrocyte
membranes following pre-exposure to isoproterenol demonstrated that
antagonist binding over-estimated those receptor sites available for
agonist binding (26).

In addition to changes in the muscarinic receptor population
per se, the lack of responsiveness of cultured heart cells to muscarinic stimulation following agonist pre-exposure might be due, at
least in part, to uncoupling of the formation of an agonist-receptor
complex from an intermediate step critical to the mediation of a
functional response. A number of cellular events have been associated with the binding of muscarinic agonists including inhibition of
β-adrenergic agonist stimulated adenylate cyclase activity (22),
increased cyclic GMP levels (27), phosphorylation of specific cellular proteins by an activated protein kinase (28) and changes in
phosphatidyl inositol turnover (29). Uncoupling of any of these
events from agonist binding may prevent the expression of a muscarinic response.

Loss of Physiologic Response Parallels Loss of $(^3H)MS$ Binding Sites

We have demonstrated that prior exposure of cultured heart cells to agonist results in the loss of the ability of muscarinic agonist to decrease beating rate and to increase K^+ permeability as measured by altered efflux of $^{42}K^+$ from the cells. The time course of this agonist-mediated loss of physiologic response to muscarinic agonists corresponds closely to the agonist-mediated loss of $(^3H)MS$ binding sites shown in Fig. 10, with a 15 min lag period followed by loss of half the physiologic response after a 30 minute agonist exposure. Recently Halvorsen and Nathanson reported that agonist exposure of 6 h duration markedly decreased the ability of muscarinic agonist to mediate a decrease in beating rate in intact embryonic chick hearts 8 days in ovo. This effect was associated with the loss of high affinity receptors in heart homogenates (30). The close coupling between the loss of $(^3H)MS$ binding sites and the loss of physiologic response demonstrates that a modest change in receptor number is related to a comparable change in physiologic response. Such sensitivity of physiologic response to agonist exposure suggests that agonist-mediated receptor loss could be a sensitive mechanism for modulating the level of responsiveness of the heart to muscarinic stimuli. Prior studies demonstrated that a large fraction of agonist-mediated receptor loss (46% of total receptor sites) was inhibited by agents that interfered with microtubule function (5), suggesting that disappearance of this subclass of receptors involved endocytosis. Furthermore, the slow loss of receptors could only be demonstrated in intact cells or in homogenates of intact cells that had been exposed to agonist prior to homogenization (data not shown). This was also consistent with the view that the slow phase of agonist-induced receptor loss involves endocytosis of receptors and hence requires functions which take place in the intact cell.

To pursue this issue further, we postulated that following agonist exposure, but prior to irreversible degradation of the receptor, receptors might assume an altered configuration involving a more intimate association with membrane lipids. Such a change in configuration might prevent subsequent agonist binding or interfere with the ability of agonists to mediate a physiologic response. Although an agonist-receptor complex capable of mediating a physiologic response might not form in cells pre-exposed to agonist, we further postulated that a muscarinic ligand which was sufficiently hydrophobic might bind to such an altered form of the receptor. Hence comparison of the binding of radio-labelled ligands with markedly differing hydrophobicities might provide a means for studying the agonist-mediated transition in the state of the receptor.

Since $(^3H)MS$ contains one less phenyl group than $(^3H)QNB$ as well as an ether linkage, $(^3H)MS$ should be less capable of interacting with the lipid bilayer. The relative solubility of substances in the lipid bilayer of the cell membrane may be approximated by comparison of partition coefficients between an aqueous

phase at physiologic pH and ionic strength and immiscible organic
solvents such as ether and chloroform. We have demonstrated the
relative preference of (^{3}H)QNB over (^{3}H)MS for the organic phase in
terms of partition with an aqueous phase. By these criteria, one
might expect (^{3}H)QNB to be substantially more soluble (and permeant)
in the lipid bilayer of the cell membrane than (^{3}H)MS.

We compared the binding of (^{3}H)MS and (^{3}H)QNB to cells which
had been subject to prior exposure to high concentrations of agonists for various times. Prolonged exposure to agonist mediated
conversion of the receptor from a form (designated A, equation 1)
which binds (^{3}H)MS and (^{3}H)QNB to a form (designated B, equation 1)
which binds (^{3}H)QNB but which does not bind (^{3}H)MS, suggesting that
the configuration of the receptor and/or relationship of the receptor to the plasmalemma is altered. We observed a close temporal
correlation between loss of (^{3}H)MS binding sites in intact cells and
loss of physiologic response to agonist. This finding is consistent
with the hypothesis that accessibility of the receptor in the intact
cell to (^{3}H)MS is correlated with accessibility of the receptor to
agonist. Alternatively, (^{3}H)MS may bind preferentially to a func-
tioning state of the receptor. Hence, the receptors in form B do
not appear to mediate a physiologic response. More prolonged agonist exposure resulted in conversion to a form C, presumably a degraded form of the receptor that binds neither (^{3}H)MS nor (^{3}H)QNB.
Hence, form B of the receptor may constitute an intermediate state
of the receptor formed during the process of endocytosis. It
should be noted that the experiments described cannot distinguish
between differences in (^{3}H)QNB and (^{3}H)MS binding to an altered configuration of the receptor within the membrane (i.e. plasmalemma)
and differences in access to receptor sites that have been endocy-
tosed but not yet degraded.

In conclusion, binding of muscarinic agonist to a critical number of sites in a specific subclass of receptors was closely correlated with agonist-induced changes in unidirectional K^+ flux and
beating rate. Although the relatively high concentrations of muscarinic agonist required to produce changes in K^+ efflux and beating
rate leave uncertain the relevance of these findings to the physiologic muscarinic response, analogous mechanisms may operate in more
highly sensitive intact preparations (30). Our data also demonstrate the presence of a subclass of receptors that appears not to be
involved in a measurable physiologic response, but there is no evidence for the existence of a large fraction of "spare" receptors.
These findings support the concept that the cardiac cell is capable
of modulating the level of muscarinic responsiveness through agonist
induced changes in receptor number.

Figures 2,3,6, and 7 were reprinted with the permission of the
Journal of General Physiology. Figure 10 was reprinted with the
permission of the Journal of Biological Chemistry.

REFERENCES

1. Raff, M. Self regulation of membrane receptors. Nature $\underline{259}$, 265-266 (1976).

2. Catt, K.J., Harwood, J.P., Aguilera, G., and Dufau, M.L. Hormonal regulation of peptide receptors and target cell responses. Nature $\underline{280}$, 109-116 (1979). Cohen, I. and Kline, R. 1982. K^+ fluctuations in the extracellular spaces of cardiac muscle - evidence from voltage clamp and extracellular K^+ selective microelectrodes. Circ. Res. $\underline{50}$: 1-17.

3. Conti, M., Harwood, J.P., Dufau, M.L. and Catt, K.J. Effect of gonadotropin-induced receptor regulation on biological responses of isolated rat luteal cells. J. Biol. Chem. $\underline{252}$, 8869-8874 (1977).

4. Siman, R.G. and Klein, W.L. Cholinergic activity regulates muscarinic receptors in central nervous system cultures. Proc. Nat'l Acad. Sci. USA $\underline{76}$, 4141-4145 (1979).

5. Galper, J.B. and Smith, T.W. Agonist and guanine nucleotide modulation of muscarinic cholinergic receptors in cultured heart cells. J. Biol. Chem. $\underline{255}$, 9571-9579 (1980).

6. Glitsch, H.G., and Pott, L. Effects of acetylcholine and parasympathetic nerve stimulation on membrane potential in quiescent guinea-pig atria. J. Physiol. $\underline{279}$,655-668 (1978).

7. Antoni, H. and Rotman, M. Zum mechanisms der negative inotropen acetylcholine Wirkung auf das isolierte Froschmyocard. Pfluger's Arch. $\underline{300}$, 67-86 (1968).

8. Harris, E.J. and Hutter, O.F. The action of acetylcholine on the movements of potassium ions in the sinus venosus of the frog. J. Physiol. $\underline{133}$, 58-59. (1956).

9. Giles, W., and Noble, S.J. Changes in membrane currents in bullfrog atrium produced by acetylcholine. J. Physiol. $\underline{261}$, 103-123 (1976).

10. Carpenter, G., and Cohen, S. ^{125}I-Labeled Human Epidermal

Growth Factor. J. Cell Bid. 71, 159-71 (1976).

11. DeHaan, R.L. Regulation of spontaneous activity and growth of embryonic chick heart cells in tissue culture. Dev. Biol. 16, 216-249 (1967).

12. Biedert, S., Barry, W.H. and Smith, T.W. Inotropic effects and changes in sodium and calcium contents associated with inhibition of monovalent cation active transport by ouabain in cultured myocardial cells. J. Gen. Physiol. 74,479-494 (1979).

13. Dixon, W.J. and Brown, M.B. In: Biomedical Data Program (BMDP) 77, Biomedical Computer Programs P-Series. Derivative-Free Nonlinear Regression Analysis, University of California Press Berkley, California (1977).

14. Galper, J.B. and Smith, T.W. Properties of muscarinic acetyl-choline receptors in heart cell cultures. Proc. Natl. Acad. Sci. USA 75, 5831-5835 (1978).

15. Dixon, W.J. and Massey, F.J. Introduction to Statistical Analysis, New York, McGraw-Hill (1957).

16. Frost, A.A. and Pearson, R.G. in Kinetics and Mechanism. John Wiley & Sons, N.Y., 166-171 (1961).

17. Galper, J.B., Klein, W. and Catterall, W.A. Muscarinic acetyl-choline receptors in developing chick heart. J. Biol. Chem. 252, 8692-8699 (1977).

18. Sperelakis, N. and Lehmkihl, D. Insensitivity of cultured chick heart cells to autonomic agents and tetrodotoxin. Am. J. Physiol. 209, 693-698 (1965)

19. Ertel, R.J., Clarke, D.E., Chao, J.C. and Franke, F.R. Autonomic receptor mechanisms in embryonic chick myocardial cell cultures. J. Pharmacol. Exp. Ther. 178, 73-80 (1971).

20. Hermsmeyer, K. and Robinson, R. High sensitivity of cultured cardiac muscle cells to autonomic agents. Am. J. Physiol. 233, C172-C179 (1977).

21. Josephson, I. and Sperelakis, N. On the ionic mechanism under-lying adrenergic-cholinergic antagonism in ventricular muscle.

J. Gen. Physiol. 79, 69-86 (1982).

22.   Watanabe, A.M., McConnaughey, M.M., Strawbridge, R.A.,
      Fleming, J.W., Jones, L.R. and Besh, H.R., Jr. Muscarinic
      Cholinergic Receptor Modulation of β-Adrenergic Receptor
      Affinity for Catecholamines. J. Biol. Chem. 253, 4833-4836
      (1978).

23.   Jakobs, K.H., Aktories, K. and Schultz, G. GTP-dependent
      inhibition of cardiac adenylate cyclase by muscarinic
      cholinergic agonists. Naunyn Schmiedberg's Arch. 310,
      113-119 (1979).

24.   Biegon, R.L. and Pappano, A.J. Dual mechanisms for inhibi-
      tion of calcium dependent action potential by acetylcholine
      in avian ventricular muscle - relationship to cyclic AMP.
      Cir. Res. 46, 353-362 (1980).

25.   Mendelson, C., Dufau, M. and Catt, K. Gonadotropin binding
      and stimulation of cyclic adenosine 3':5'-monophosphate and
      testosterone production in isolated Leydig cells. J. Biol.
      Chem. 250, 8818-8823 (1975).

26.   Wessels, R., Mullikin, D. and Lefkowitz, R.J. Differences
      between agonist and antagonist binding following beta-
      adrenergic receptor desensitization. J. Biol. Chem.
      253, 3371-3373 (1978).

27.   George, W.J., Polson, J.B., O'Toole, A.G., and Goldberg, N.D.
      Elevation of guanosine 3', 5' - cyclic phosphate in rat
      heart after perfusion with acetylcholine. Proc. Nat'l.
      Acad. Sci. USA 66, 398-403 (1970).

28.   Greenguard, P. Possible Role for Cyclic Nucleotides and
      Phosphorylated Membrane Proteins in Postsynaptic Actions of
      Neurotransmitters. Nat. 260, 101-108 (1976).

29.   Michell, R.H., Jefferji, S.S. and Jones, L.M.   In: <u>Advances</u>
      <u>in Experimental Medicine and Biology</u>, Vol. 83 (Bazan, H.,
      Brenner, R., Giusto, H., ed.), Plenum Press, New York and
      London, pp. 447-464 (1976).

30.   Halvorsen, G.W. and Nathanson, N.M.   <u>In Vivo</u> regulation of
      muscarinic acetylcholine receptor number and function in
      embryonic chick heart.
      J. Biol. Chem. <u>256</u>, 7941-7948 (1981).

DEVELOPMENT AND REGULATION OF CARDIAC MUSCARINIC ACETYLCHOLINE RECEPTOR NUMBER, FUNCTION AND GYANYL NUCLEOTIDE SENSITIVITY

Stan W. Halvorsen, Bronia Engel, Dale D. Hunter, and
Neil M. Nathanson

Department of Pharmacology
University of Washington
Seattle, Washington 98195

INTRODUCTION

Acetylcholine is released from parasympathetic nerve terminals and binds to muscarinic acetylcholine (mACh) receptors to elicit negative chronotropic and inotropic effects on the heart. The molecular mechanisms for these cardiac effects are not well understood. Investigation of the mACh receptor has been greatly facilitated by the development of the potent cholinergic antagonist [3H] quinuclidinyl benzilate (QNB) which binds specifically and with high affinity to the mACh receptor (1). [3H]QNB can be used to study the interaction of agonists and antagonists with the receptor and quantitate the number of receptors present in cells and tissues.

Persistent exposure of neuronal (2-4) and cardiac muscle cells (5) in culture to muscarinic agents led to a decrease in the mACh receptor number and function on these cells. Taylor et al. (6) have shown that the long-term decrease of mACh receptor number in neuronal cells is distinct from short-term desensitization of receptor activity. Agonist-induced decrease of receptor number on cells in culture has been postulated to represent a model for the regulation of receptors by synaptic activity in vivo. Prolonged exposure to muscarinic agonists in vivo of embryonic chick (7) or mouse (8) led to a decrease in mACh receptor number in brain.

The negative chronotropic response of the chick heart to muscarinic agonists increases between 3 and 9 days of embryonic development (9-11). Parasympathetic ganglia can be found in the embryonic chick heart by the 4th to 6th incubation day (see ref.

143

12). Functional parasympathetic neurotransmission has been demonstrated by day 10-12 (13). Therefore mACh receptors are present and become functional prior to functional innervation of cardiac muscle by the parasympathetic nervous system.

Muscarinic agonists inhibit hormone-stimulated adenylate cyclase in several systems, including the heart (3,14-16). Evidence suggests this inhibitory action of mACh receptor agonists on adenylate cyclase activity involves a coupling of the mACh receptor to adenylate cyclase via a guanyl nucleotide-sensitive inhibitory regulatory subunit (N_i) (17-19). Guanyl nucleotides lower the apparent affinity of the mACh receptor for agonists in rat (20-22) and chick (23, 24) heart. Beta-adrenergic stimulation of adenylate cyclase activity is GTP-dependent and requires a functional stimulatory guanyl nucleotide regulatory protein (N_s) (see ref 17). Northup et al. (25) have demonstrated that the guanyl nucleotide binding protein purified from rabbit liver plasma membranes functions as a mult-subunit complex of 2-3 polypeptides. The relationship of N_s and N_i to guanyl nucleotide regulation of mACh receptor agonist binding has not been demonstrated.

We have used the chick embryonic heart to study the regulation and development of the mACh receptor in vivo. Specific stages of development of the embryonic heart can provide models of the mACh receptor at various stages of physiological coupling. In the studies reported here we temporally dissociate and correlate specific regulatory events with particular receptor-mediated physiological responses.

MATERIALS AND METHODS

Materials

White leghorn chick embryos were obtained locally and maintained at 38° C as previously described (24). Embryos were staged according to Hamburger and Hamilton (26). Chemicals were obtained as described earlier (24, 27).

Methods

Drugs for administration to embryos in ovo were dissolved in phosphate buffered saline (PBS) and administered as described (24). Washed cardiac membranes were prepared from freshly removed hearts by homogenizing and washing in 50 mM $NaPO_4$ (pH 7.4) for [^{3}H]QNB binding assays or 50 mM Tris HCl (pH 7.4) with 1 mM dithiothreitol, 0.2 M sucrose, 1 mM EDTA and 0.1 mM sodium ascorbate for adenylate cyclase assays as described (24, 27).

Protein was determined either by the method of McKnight (28) or a modification of the method of Lowry et al. (29) as described

(24). Muscarinic receptor number was assayed by a modification of the filter binding method of Yamamura and Snyder (1) which utilized the specific muscarinic antagonist [^{3}H]QNB. Experiments were incubated at room temperature for 60-90 minutes in 50 mM NaPO$_4$ or in beating rate media (see below) for carbachol binding studies as previously described (24). Specific binding was determined as binding inhibited in the presence of atropine, 10^{-6} M.

Carbachol [^{3}H]QNB competition binding studies were analyzed with an iterative computer program using a 2-site model for agonist binding which has been previously described (24,27). The adenylate cyclase assay contained 0.25 mM [α^{32}P]ATP (16-20 Ci/mol), 10 mM creatine phosphate, 50 units/ml creatine phosphokinase, 1 mM 2-mercaptoethanol, 1mM EDTA, 5 mM theophylline, 0.1% bovine serum albumin, 5 mM MgCl$_2$, 2 mM [^{3}H] cyclic AMP (18 mCi/mol), 100 mM NaCl, 0.1 mM sodium ascorbate in 50 mM Tris·HCl (pH 7.4), with drugs added as described. Assays were carried out in triplicate at 30° C for 10 minutes and [^{32}P] cyclic AMP was determined by a modification of Salomon et al. (30) as previously described (27).

The negative chronotropic response of spontaneously beating isolated atria to carbachol was determined visually as previously described (24) in oxygenated beating rate media (149 mM NaCl, 2.7 mM KCl, 1.8 mM CaCl$_2$, 1.0 mM MgSO$_4$, 10.0 mM 4-(2-hydroxyethyl)-1-piperazineethanesulfonic acid, 5.5 mM glucose, and 0.4 mM NaPO$_4$, pH 7.4) at 37° C.

Cardiac muscle cultures were prepared from 9-10 day embryonic hearts essentially as described by Galper and Smith (5). For binding studies with intact cells, cells grown in 35 mm dishes were washed twice with assay medium (116 mM NaCl; 1.8 mM CaCl$_2$; 2.7 mM KCl; 0.81 mM MgSO$_4$; 1.0 mM NaHPO$_4$; 5.56 mM glucose; and 25 mM 4-(2-hydroxyethyl) 1-piperazineethanesulfonic acid, pH 7.4), and then preincubated at 37° C in culture medium for 15-45 minutes prior to addition of ligands for assay. Incubations were stopped by aspiration of the medium, followed by 3 washes with 1-2 ml ice-cold PBS. The total time for washing was 5-7 seconds. After addition of 0.5 ml 1% sodium dodecyl sulfate, cells were scraped into scintillation vials, 4 ml of scintillation fluid was added, and radioactivity was determined by liquid scintillation counting.

RESULTS AND DISCUSSION

Regulation of Cardiac mACh Receptor Number in 8-day Embryos

Administration in ovo to 8-day old embryos of 0.3, 1.0 or 10 µmoles of the stable muscarinic agonist carbachol resulted in a dose and time-dependent decrease in bound [^{3}H]QNB in the heart compared to controls of 28%, 61% or 83%, respectively, which was maximal by 6-10 hours (24). Kinetic analysis of the rate of turn-

over of the receptor in the presence of these doses of carbachol
reveals no difference in the rate constant for the disappearance of
activated receptor ($t_{1/2}$ =1.82-1.86 hours (Fig. 1).

The decreased binding of [^{3}H]QNB in membranes from carbachol-
treated hearts could be due to either a change in affinity of the
mACh receptor for [^{3}H]QNB or a decrease in total receptor number.
To differentiate between the two possibilities the dependence of
binding on [^{3}H]QNB concentration was studied. Embryos were
pretreated in ovo with PBS as a control or 1 μmole of carbachol for
6 hours. Scatchard analysis of the binding data revealed no
significant change in the apparent affinity of the mACh receptor
for [^{3}H]QNB (control K_D = 6.4 x 10^{-11} M and treated K_D = 5.3 x
10^{-11} M) and a 58% decrease in the number of specific [^{3}H]QNB binding
sites (24).

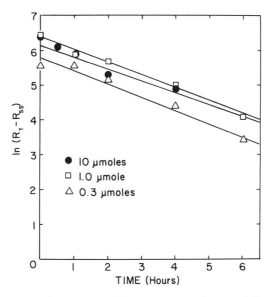

Figure 1.   Rate of mACh receptor loss with time

Kinetic analysis of rate of loss of mACh receptor number after 10
μmoles (●), 1.0 μmole (□) or 0.3 μmole (△) carbachol was performed
as described (24). R_T = receptor number at indicated time after
carbachol administration, R_{ss} = steady state receptor number at
t = 6-8 hours after carbachol. The slope is the negative
disappearance rate constant (0.37, 0.38 and 0.38, respectively).
The half-life for activated receptor is 0.69 ÷ disappearance rate
constant.

Table Ia

Specificity of carbachol action on the mACh receptor.

Treatment	Receptor Number (fmol/mg)	% of Control
Control (PBS)	1010	--
Carbachol (1 μmol)	530	52
Oxotremorine (0.1 μmol)	660	65
Oxotremorine (0.1 μmol) plus Atropine (0.1 μmol)	1010	100

Table 1b

Treatment	Receptor Number (fmol/mg)	% Inhibition of Receptor Loss
Control (PBS)	860	--
Carbachol (1 μmol)	450	--
Carbachol (1 μmol) plus Atropine (0.1 μmol)	830	93
or Scopolamine (0.1 μmol)	860	100
or d-Tubocurarine(0.1 μmol)	400	0
or Hexamethonium (0.1 μmol)	330	0

roups of 4 embryos were treated in ovo for 6.5 hours with each of the
rug combinations listed above. Hearts were harvested and assayed as
escribed in methods for specific [3H]QNB binding.

To determine whether this carbachol-induced decrease in receptor number was mediated by the mACh receptor, we investigated the dependence of down regulation on carbachol concentration. After pretreating embryos in ovo with increasing concentrations of carbachol, the cardiac mACh receptor number exhibited a dose-dependent decrease with an ED_{50} of 0.5 μmole (equivalent to 10^{-5} M if carbachol was uniformly distributed in a 50 ml egg volume) (24).

In ovo administration of the specific muscarinic agonist oxotremorine 0.1 μmole, led to a 35% decrease in mACh receptor number which was completely blocked by the muscarinic receptor antagonist atropine (Table Ia). We examined a number of other ACh receptor antagonists for their ability to prevent the decrease in mACh receptor number by carbachol administered in ovo. The specific mACh receptor antagonists scopolamine and atropine were both able to block greater than 90% of the effect of carbachol (Table Ib). The nicotinic acetylcholine receptor antagonists d-tubocurarine and hexamethonium were not able to block the carbachol-induced decrease in mACh receptor number (Table Ib). These results indicate that carbachol is specifically acting at the mACh receptor to cause a decrease in receptor number. In addition, these data are in agreement with earlier reports from cell culture experiments (2,3) that activation of the mACh receptor by an agonist is required to stimulate receptor decreases and that occupancy of the receptor by an antagonist is insufficient to cause receptor number to decrease.

The response to muscarinic agents on the spontaneous atrial beating rate was determined on atria isolated from control embryos and embryos treated in ovo with 1 μmole of carbachol. The EC_{50} for carbachol inhibition of beating was 2.7×10^{-6} M in control atria and 2.2×10^{-5} M in treated atria, an 8-fold increase at the EC_{50} (Fig. 2). The treated atria in these studies had a 52% reduction in mACh receptor number and yet all but 4 (out of 39) were capable of a complete inhibition of beating in response to carbachol indicating the presence of spare receptors. These results clearly demonstrate that the carbachol-induced decrease in mACh receptor number was accompanied by a decrease in the negative chronotropic response of the atria to subsequent mACh receptor stimulation.

The observed 8-fold shift in the carbachol dose response curve of treated atria could occur in part if receptors in treated atria have a lowered affinity for carbachol. Therefore we investigated the relative binding affinities of the mACh receptor for carbachol by competition binding experiments with [^{3}H]QNB. The binding of muscarinic agonists to the cardiac mACh receptor results in binding curves that are much flatter than expected from a simple mass action isotherm (10, 20-24, 27). In extensive studies of agonist binding the mACh receptor from rat cerebral cortex, Birdsall et al. (31) have shown that this deviation from simple mass action is due to a heterogeneity in the mACh receptor population which is most readily explained by the presence of at least two binding sites differing in affinity for agonists but not for antagonists. Studies of cardiac tissue from several species have shown that in physiological buffers guanyl nucleotides (e.g., GTP, GDP) lower the affinity of the mACh receptor for agonists with little or no effect on antagonist binding (20-22, 24). Since we expect endogenous GTP to be present in the intact atria these binding experiments were performed both in the absence and presence of the non-hydrolyzable GTP-analog guanyl-5'-yl-imidophosphate (GPP(NH)P), to more closely approximate in vivo conditions.

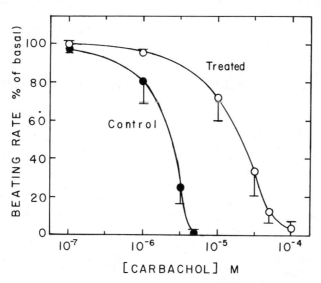

Figure 2.   Negative chronotropic dose-response curves of isolated atria.

The negative chronotropic response of isolated atria to carbachol was measured as described under "Methods." Curves show the response from 8-day control atria (●), and atria treated in ovo with carbachol, 1 μmole (O). Treated atria had 52% fewer mACh receptors than control. The response was measured as the minimum rate observed during carbachol exposure calculated as a percentage of the basal rate observed prior to carbachol exposure in the bath. Each point is the mean ($\pm$SEM) of 9-10 atria.

The curves for carbachol binding to cardiac mACh receptors in control and treated atria showed heterogeneity in agonist binding sites both in the absence and presence of guanyl nucleotides (24). The IC_{50} for carbachol inhibition of [^{3}H]QNB binding in the presence of GPP(NH)P was shifted 4-fold to the right in treated atria (24). The heterogeneity in the carbachol binding curves was computer-analyzed assuming a 2-site model for agonist binding as previously described (24, 27). Analysis showed that in the absence of GPP(NH)P there was an increase in the fraction of low affinity binding sites upon decreasing total receptor number with little change in the affinity of either site (Table II). However, analysis of binding in the presence of GPP(NH)P, 10^{-5} M, showed that the 48% decrease in receptor number was accompanied by a 3 to 4-fold decrease in the affinity of both receptor subtypes (Table II). This decrease in affinity of each receptor subtype accounted for the change in the IC_{50} seen in the carbachol binding curves but was not by itself sufficient to account for the 8-fold shift in the EC_{50} for inhibition of beating seen in treated atria. Therefore prolonged exposure to muscarinic agonists in vivo led to a loss of functional mACh receptors. GPP(NH)P altered carbachol binding in the 8-day embryonic chick heart by causing the ratio of the affinities for the low affinity site to the high affinity site to decrease from over 200 in the absence of GPP(NH)P to less than 50 when GPP(NH)P was present.

Recovery of Receptor Number and Function After in vivo Down-Regulation

We tested whether the carbachol-induced decrease in mACh receptor number was reversible by treating 7 to 8-day embryos in ovo with 1 µmole of carbachol for 6 hours and then blocking further carbachol-mACh receptor interaction with saturating doses of atropine. The administration of atropine with no prior exposure to carbachol gave no change in receptor number over a 28-hour period (24). Complete recovery of receptor number to control levels occurred between 6 and 16 hours after atropine administration (24). The long recovery time observed in our in vivo experiments agreed with studies on cells in culture that have shown the kinetics of agonist-induced receptor loss were consistent with an increase in receptor breakdown and that recovery of receptor number was dependent on de novo synthesis of protein (2,23).

Examination of the physiological activity of the mACh receptors which reappear after recovery from down-regulation may provide information on the kinetics of the coupling of the mACh receptors binding site to other components required for physiological activity (see below). Embryos were treated 8 hours in ovo with doses of carbachol (10-20 µmoles) sufficient to decrease receptor number by greater than 80%, then treated with atropine (0.1-0.5 µmole) for 16 hours, which allowed receptor number to

Table II

Agonist Binding Parameters of Atrial mAChR

			F_L	K_L (M)	K_H (M)	K_L/K_H
8-day:	Atria	-G	.32 (.27-.41)	6.8×10^{-6} (1.8-16.0)	3.2×10^{-8} (2.2-4.0)	213
		+G	.44 (.34-154)	1.2×10^{-5} (0.7-2.3)	2.8×10^{-7} 1.8-4.0)	43
	Treated Atria	-G	.44 (.38-.48)	9.5×10^{-6} (5.3-21.0)	2.7×10^{-8} (2.0-3.6)	352
		+G	.38 (.33-.41)	4.7×10^{-5} (3.9-7.2)	1.1×10^{-6} (1.0-1.3)	43
5-day:	Atria	-G	.54 (.51-.57)	3.9×10^{-6} (2.9-5.2)	2.4×10^{-8} (1.9-3.0)	163
		+G	.54 (.49-.60)	7.4×10^{-6} (5.7-9.4)	2.3×10^{-7} (1.7-2.9)	32
4-day:	Atria	-G	.24 (.22-.26)	1.4×10^{-5} (0.8-2.5)	2.5×10^{-8} (2.5-2.8)	560
		+G	.20 (.18-.21)	2.4×10^{-5} (1.4-4.6)	3.7×10^{-8} (3.4-4.2)	650

The mACh receptor binding parameters for atrial membranes from embryos of the indicated age were calculated from the carbachol/[^{3}H]QNB binding data as described in "Methods." The allowed variation is shown in parentheses and was determined as previously described (27). F_L is the fraction of mACh receptor with low affinity for agonists; K_L and K_H are the dissociation constants for agonist binding to the low and high affinity mACh receptor. 8-day treated atria had been exposed to 1 μmole of carbachol in ovo and had 58% of the 8-day control mACh receptor number. G = GPP(NH)P, 10^{-5} M.

return to 85–95% of the control level. Preliminary studies of the mAChR–mediated negative chronotropic response indicated that these recovered atria, with receptor levels close to that of controls, required at least 10-fold higher concentrations of carbachol than untreated atria in order to inhibit beating. After 27 hours of atropine treatment, the physiological sensitivity of the recovered atria had returned to control values. Thus these results suggest that receptors which initially reappear after agonist-induced down regulation may be physiologically less active than preexisting receptors.

Properties of Muscarinic Receptors on Intact Cells

Because guanyl nucleotides regulate agonist binding to the mACh receptor and endogenous GTP is present in the intact cell, it seems reasonable to expect the binding of agonist to receptors on intact cells would more closely resemble binding to mACh receptors in membrane homogenates in the presence rather than the absence of guanyl nucleotides. We have examined the properties of mACh receptors on living intact cardiac muscle cultures, using the membrane impermeable ligand [^{3}H]N-methyl scopolamine ([^{3}H]NMS). [^{3}H]NMS binds to a single class of sites on intact cultures, with a K_D of 0.12 nM, compared to a K_D of 0.20 nM for mACh receptors in membrane homogenates. In contrast to the heterogeneity of agonist binding sites in membranes prepared from either intact or cultured heart, [^{3}H]NMS/carbachol competition curves exhibit Hill coefficients of greater than 0.9, and are well described by the binding of carbachol to a single class of sites, with a K_D of 1.1 $\times 10^{-5}$ M. This is similar to the affinity of the low affinity agonist binding site as determined in membrane homogenates in the presence of guanyl nucleotides.

Competition curves between [^{3}H]QNB and carbachol are significantly different from those between [^{3}H]NMS and carbachol: the curves are much flatter with Hill coefficients of 0.3–0.5. In addition, 10^{-3} M carbachol can only block 50–60% of the [^{3}H]QNB. This difference between [^{3}H]NMS and [^{3}H]QNB may be due to agonist-promoted internalization of the receptor. [^{3}H]QNB is membrane-permeable and thus can still bind to internalized receptors, while [^{3}H]NMS and carbachol, being highly charged, could not interact with receptors after internalization.

Ontogenesis of mACh Receptor Regulation and Function

The onset of the negative chronotropic response to muscarinic agonists was investigated by determining the inhibition of the spontaneous beating of atria isolated from 4,5 and 8-day embryos to carbachol. Other workers have shown that atria isolated from 3-day embryos (9) and intact hearts from 4-day embryos (10) are much less responsive to the negative chronotropic effect of muscarinic agonists than are atria and hearts isolated from much older embryos. Our results showed that atria isolated from 4-day embryos were only minimally responsive to carbachol. 10^{-2} M carbachol inhibited the spontaneous beating rate only 30% in 4-day atria whereas in atria from 5-day embryos the spontaneous beating of 9 out of 12 atria was completely inhibited with only 3×10^{-5} M carbachol (27). Atria isolated from 5-day embryos exhibited a negative chronotropic response which closely resembled that seen in 8-day atria although a small number of individual atria were still less responsive.

Saturation binding experiments with [^{3}H]QNB revealed a similar density of mACh receptors and similar dissociation constants for [^{3}H]QNB binding in 4,5 and 8-day embryonic cardiac membranes (27). These results are consistent with those of Galper et al. (10) and Renaud et al. (11) which showed that unresponsive and responsive hearts have similar densities of mACh receptors and thus that 4-day embryonic atria possess physiologically inactive mACh receptors.

Administration in ovo of 1 or 2 μmoles of carbachol to 5 or 8-day embryos led to a similar decrease in cardiac mACh receptor number (Table III). However, 4-day embryos required a 5 to 10-fold greater dose of carbachol to achieve a similar degree of mACh receptor loss as 5 or 8-day embryos (Table III). These results suggest that not only must the receptor be occupied by agonist for receptor number to be decreased but the mACh receptor must be in a state that can be activated.

In order to compare the agonist binding properties of the mACh receptor from the less responsive 4-day atria to the older responsive 5 and 8-day atria, we performed competition binding experiments with [^{3}H]QNB and carbachol. In striking contrast to 8-day hearts, the agonist binding curves from 4-day atria were not significantly affected by the presence of GPP(NH)P. Computer analysis of binding to 4-day atrial membranes showed that GPP(NH)P had little or no effect on individual agonist binding parameters and that the fraction of low affinity agonist binding sites was much lower than in 5 or 8-day atria (Table II). This is consistent with our previous results (24, 27) which suggested that agonist binding to the low affinity form of the mACh receptor is necessary for the negative chronotropic response.

Carbachol binding curves from 5-day atria were shifted in the presence of GPP(NH)P 4-fold higher at the IC_{50} (27). The 4-fold shift in the binding curve was much less than in 8-day atria but GPP(NH)P altered the binding of carbachol by decreasing the affinity of the high affinity site 10-fold and the low affinity site 2-fold, similar to the effect seen in 8-day atria (Table II).

Table III

Developmental onset of agonist-induced decrease of receptor number

In vivo carbachol dose

Age	1 μmol	2 μmol	10 μmol
		(% loss of receptor number)	
4-day	13 ($^+_-$5) (n = 8)	n.d.	62 ($^+_-$1) (n = 4)
5-day	51 ($^+_-$7) (n = 6)	68 ($^+_-$4) (n = 2)	n.d.
8-day	54 ($^+_-$2) (n = 64)	70 ($^+_-$2) (n = 3)	86 ($^+_-$1) (n = 2)

Embryos were pretreated in ovo with PBS or the indicated amount of carbachol as described in "Methods". After 8h the hearts were removed and assayed for mACh receptor number with [^{3}H]QNB (0.67 nM) as described in "Methods." Table values indicate the mean percentage decrease ($^+_-$SEM) in mACh receptor number from control. The number of observations is n. (n.d. = not determined.)

In 3 to 4-day embryonic atria isoproterenol elicits a positive inotropic and chronotropic response (see ref. 12), suggesting the presence of N_s in these young atria. We found that in 4-day atria which did not exhibit guanyl nucleotide regulation of agonist binding to mACh receptors, isoproterenol plus GPP(NH)P or GTP stimulated enzyme activity (27). Thus, the adenylate cyclase in the atrial membranes of 4-day embryos can be stimulated via the N_s regulatory component.

We then tested the adenylate cyclase in 4-day atria for the expression of the inhibitory regulatory function, N_i, by studying the sensitivity to mACh receptor-mediated inhibition of activity. The carbachol concentration dependence for adenylate cyclase inhibition is shown in Table IV. Carbachol (10^{-4} M) inhibited GTP-dependent isoproterenol-stimulated adenylate cyclase activity to a similar degree in 8,5, and 4-day atria. The dose-response relationship for inhibition of adenylate cyclase activity in 4-day embryos was similar to 5-day embryos (Table IV). Thus at an age of development when mACh receptor activation elicited a much diminished negative chronotropic response, was less susceptible to agonist-induced decrease in receptor number and agonist binding was

Table IV

Inhibition of hormone stimulated adenylate cyclase

Carbachol	4-day	5-day	8-day
(M)	(% inhibition)		
10^{-4}	41 ($\pm$13)	40 ($\pm$3)	52 ($\pm$11)
10^{-5}	37 ($\pm$4)	36 ($\pm$8)	48 ($\pm$7)
10^{-6}	5 ($\pm$6)	7 ($\pm$9)	34 ($\pm$4)

Adenylate cyclase activity was measured in atrial membranes of
different ages as described in "Methods." The GTP concentration
was 10^{-5} M and isoproterenol 2 x 10^{-4} M. Values are %
inhibition of isoproterenol plus GTP activity compared to GTP alone
($\pm$SEM) for 2 to 4 experiments.

not regulated by guanyl nucleotides, mACh receptor stimulation
could significantly inhibit adenylate cyclase activity.

The physiological significance of the regulation of agonist
binding to the mACh receptor by guanyl nucleotides is not well
understood. Cardiac tissue from 4-day embryos displayed characteristics of possessing both stimulatory and inhibitory adenylate
cyclase regulatory components at a time when mACh receptors were
not coupled to guanyl nucleotide regulation of agonist binding.

The onset of mACh receptor-mediated negative chronotropic
response between 4 and 5 days was temporally correlated with an
increased fraction of low affinity agonist binding sites as well as
guanyl nucleotide regulation of agonist binding. However, it does
not seem likely that there are fewer active receptors in 4-day than
5-day atria, since there was no change in the dose-response curve
for inhibition of adenylate cyclase between 4 and 5-day atria
(Table IV). Alternatively, there may be a GTP-dependent regulatory
site separate from N_s and N_i which is required for guanyl
nucleotide regulation of agonist binding, and possibly the negative
chronotropic response, but is not expressed at 4 days and is at
5 days. Gross changes in the receptor do not appear to occur
between 4 and 5 days since neither [^{3}H]QNB binding nor agonist-
induced inhibition of adenylate cyclase changed appreciably.
Further investigation of this system should help to elucidate the
biochemical properties which are necessary for functional
activation and regulation of the mACh receptor.

REFERENCES

1. Yamamura, H.I. and Snyder, S.H. Muscarinic cholinergic binding
    in rat brain. Proceedings of the National Academy of Sciences
    USA 71, 1725-1729 (1974).
2. Klein, W.L., Nathanson, N.M., and Nirenberg, M. Muscarinic
    acetylcholine receptor regulation by accelerated rate of
    receptor loss. Biochemical and Biophysical Research
    Communications 90, 506-512 (1979).
3. Nathanson, N.M., Klein, W.L., and Nirenberg, M. Regulation of
    adenylate cyclase activity mediated by muscarinic acetylcholine
    receptors. Proceedings of the National Academy of Sciences USA
    75, 1788-1791 (1978).
4. Siman, R.G. and Klein, W.L. Specificity of muscarinic
    acetylcholine receptor regulation by receptor activity.
    Journal of Neurochemistry 37, 1099-1108 (1981).
5. Galper, J.B. and Smith, T.W. Properties of muscarinic
    acetylcholine receptors in heart cell cultures. Proceedings of
    the National Academy of Sciences USA 75, 5831-5835 (1978).
6. Taylor, J.E., El-Fakahany, E., and Richelson, E. Long-term
    regulation of muscarinic acetylcholine receptors on cultured
    nerve cells. Life Sciences 25, 2181-2187 (1979).
7. Meyer, M.R., Gainer, M.W., and Nathanson, N.M. In vivo
    regulation of muscarinic cholinergic receptors in embryonic
    chick brain. Molecular Pharmacology 21, 280-286 (1982).
8. Marks, M.J., Artman, L.D., Patinkin, D.M. and Collins, A.C.
    Cholinergic adaptations to chronic oxotremorine infusion.
    Journal of Pharmacology and Experimental Therapeutics 218,
    337-343 (1981).
9. Pappano, A.J. and Skowronek, C.A. Reactivity of chick embryo
    heart to cholinergic agonists during ontogenesis: decline in
    desensitization at the onset of cholinergic transmission. The
    Journal of Pharmacology and Experimental Therapeutics 191,
    109-118 (1974).
10. Galper, J.B., Klein, W., and Catterall, W.A. Muscarinic
    acetycholine receptors in developing chick heart. The Journal
    of Biological Chemistry 252, 8692-8699 (1977).
11. Renaud, J.F., Barhanin, J., Cavey, D., Fosset, M. and
    Lazdunski, M. Comparative Properties of the in ovo and in
    vitro differentiation of the muscarinic cholinergic receptor in
    embryonic heart cells. Developmental Biology 78, 184-200
    (1980).
12. Pappano, A.J. Ontogenetic development of autonomic
    neuroeffector transmission and transmitter reactivity in
    embryonic and fetal hearts. Pharmacological Reviews 29, 3-33
    (1977).
13. Pappano, A.J., Loffelholz, K. Ontogenesis of adrenergic and
    cholinergic neuroeffector transmission in chick embryo heart.
    The Journal of Pharmacology and Experimental Therapeutics 191,
    468-478 (1974).

14. Murad, F., Chi, Y.-M., Rall, T.W., and Sutherland, E.W. Adenyl cyclase. Journal of Biological Chemistry 237, 1233-1238 (1962).
15. Jakobs, K.H., Aktories, K. and Schultz, G. GTP-dependent inhibition of cardiac adenylate cyclase by muscarinic cholinergic agonists. Naunyn-Schmiedeberg's Archives Pharmacology 310, 113-119 (1979).
16. Watanabe, A.M., McConnaughey, M.M., Strawbridge, R.Z., Fleming, J.W., Jones, L.R., and Besch, H.R. Jr. Muscarinic cholinergic receptor modulation of α-adernergic receptor affinity for catecholamines. The Journal of Biological Chemistry 253, 4833-4836 (1978).
17. Rodbell, M. The role of hormone receptors and GTP-regulatory proteins in membrane transduction. Nature (London) 284, 17-22 (1980).
18. Hoffman, B.B., Yim, S., Tsai, B.S. and Lefkowitz, R.J. Preferential uncoupling by manganese of alpha adrenergic receptor mediated inhibition of adenylate cyclase in human platelets. Biochemical and Biophysical Research Communications 100, 724-731 (1981).
19. Koski, G. and Klee, W.A. Opiates inhibit adenylate cyclase by stimulating GTP hydrolysis. Proceedings of the National Academy of Sciences USA 78, 4185-4189 (1981).
20. Berrie, C.P. Birdsall, N.J.M., Burgen, A.S.V. and Hulme, E.C. Guanine nucleotides modulate muscarinic receptor binding in the heart. Biochemical and Biophysical Research Communications 87,1000-1005 (1979).
21. Rosenberger, L.B., Yamamura, H.I. and Roeske, W.R. Cardiac muscarinic cholinergic receptor binding is regulated by Na+ and guanyl nucleotides. The Journal of Biological Chemistry 255, 820-823 (1980).
22. Wei, J.-W. and Sulakhe, P.V. Requirement for sulfhydryl groups in the differential effects of magnesium ion and GTP on agonist binding of muscarinic cholinergic receptor sites in rat atrial membrane fraction. Naunynm-Schmiedeberg's Archves Pharmacology 314, 51-59 (1980).
23. Galper, J.B., and Smith, T.W. Agonist and guanine nucleotide modulation of muscarinic cholinergic receptors in cultured heart cells. The Journal of Biological Chemistry 255, 9571-9579 (1980).
24. Halvorsen, S.W. and Nathanson, N.M. In vivo regulation of muscarinic acetylcholine receptor number and function in embryonic chick heart. Journal of Biological Chemistry 256, 7941-7948 (1981).
25. Northup, J.K., Sternweis, P.C., Smigel, M.D., Schleiffer, L.S., Ross, E.M. and Gilman, A.G. Purification of the regulatory component of adenylate cyclase. Proceedings of the National Academy of Sciences USA 77, 6516-6520 (1980).
26. Hamburger, V. and Hamilton, H.L. A series of normal stages in the development of the chick embryo. Journal of Morphology 88,

49-92 (1951).
27. Halvorsen, S.W. and Nathanson, N.M. Ontogenesis of physiological responsiveness and guanyl nucleotide sensitivity of cardiac muscarinic receptors during chick embryonic development. Manuscript submitted for publication.
28. McKnight, G.S. A colorimetric method for the determination of submicrogram quantities of protein. Analytical Biochemistry 78, 86-92 (1977).
29. Lowry, O.H., Rosebrough, N.J., Farr, A.L., and Randall, R.J. Protein measurement with Folin phenol reagent. Journal of Biological Chemistry 193, 265-275 (1951).
30. Salomon, Y., Londos, C., and Rodbell, M. A highly sensitive adenylate cyclase assay. Analytical Biochemistry 58, 541-548 (1974).
31. Birdsall, N.J.M., Burgen, A.S.U. and Hulme, E.C. The binding of agonists to brain muscarinic receptors. Molecular Pharmacology 14, 723-736 (1978).

REGIONAL DISTRIBUTION OF CHOLINE ACETYLTRANSFERASE ACTIVITY

AND MULTIPLE AFFINITY FORMS OF THE MUSCARINIC RECEPTOR IN HEART

Robert Roskoski, Jr.

Department of Biochemistry
Louisiana State University Medical Center
New Orleans, Louisiana   70112 U.S.A.

INTRODUCTION

The autonomic nervous system plays an important role in the regulation of the heart. The parasympathetic division decreases heart rate and contractility while the sympathetic division mediates the opposite responses. The parasympathetic effect predominates at rest and provides tonic inhibitory influences. The parasympathetic system also predominates when both divisions are maximally stimulated (1). The preganglionic component of the parasympathetic system originates in the dorsal motor nucleus of the brain stem and courses to the heart through the vagus nerves. Postganglionic (intrinsic) neurons originate and terminate within the heart. Acetylcholine is the neurotransmitter of both the preganglionic and postganglionic divisions of the parasympathetic system. The response between the pre- and postganglionic neurons is mediated by the cholinergic nicotinic receptor. The postganglionic neurons interact with the myocardium and its specialized pacemaker tissue by means of the cholinergic muscarinic receptor. Choline acetyltransferase activity in heart is a neurochemical marker of both the pre- and postganglionic neurons of the parasympathetic system in unknown proportion.

The efferent sympathetic nerves originate in the upper thoracic spinal cord and travel to the stellate ganglia where they synapse with the postganglionic fibers extrinsic to the heart. The neurotransmitter of the preganglionic fibers is also acetylcholine and the receptor is nicotinic cholinergic

159

in nature. The postganglionic fibers course to the heart and
interact with the myocardium by means of the -adrenergic
receptor. The neurotransmitter is norepinephrine. Tyrosine
hydroxylase and dopamine -hydroxylase serve as neurochemical
markers of the postganglionic sympathetic neurons in heart.

Choline acetyltransferase catalyzes the following reaction:

$$\text{acetyl-CoA + choline} \rightleftharpoons \text{acetylcholine + CoA}$$

We developed a radiochemical assay for the enzyme in heart
homogenates based on the conversion of $[^{14}C]$ acetyl-CoA to
$[^{14}C]$acetylcholine (2). Low voltage paper electrophoresis was
used to resolve labelled acetylcholine from $[^{14}C]$acetyl-CoA,
$[^{14}C]$ acetylcarnitine and other metabolites. Heart contains
high activities of carnitine acetyltransferase and concentrations of endogenous carnitine sufficient to deplete
$[^{14}C]$acetyl-CoA. To eliminate the problem of $[^{14}C]$ acetyl-CoA
depletion, we first dialyzed the heart extracts (2) and later
made more dilute homogenates (1:20; w/v) to decrease adventitious utilization of labeled coenzyme. We also used 2 mM
choline to minimize conversion to acetylcholine by the greater
(1000-fold) endogenous carnitine acetyltransferase activity
(2). Although not saturating, this is well above the Km of
choline for choline acetyltransferase. Of all tissues in
which we have examined activity (brain, skeletal muscle,
heart, salivary gland, lung), the endogenous carnitine and
carnitine acetyltransferase activity of heart have made this
tissue the most difficult in which to measure choline acetyltransferase activity. The use of 1:20 homogenates or
dialyzing more concentrated extracts, the use of 2 mM choline,
and careful resolution of acetylcholine from acetylcarnitine
by paper electrophoresis provided the basis for a convenient,
reproducible and sensitive method for heart choline acetyltransferase activity determinations (2).

Neuroscientists readily accept the validity of using
tyrosine hydroxylase and dopamine -hydroxylase activity as
specific neurochemical markers of noradrenergic neurons (3).
On the other hand, there was considerable resistance to the
idea that choline acetyltransferase activity measurements in
heart represent a valid neurochemical marker for cholinergic
innervation. Primate placenta is one example of a non-inner-
vated tissue which contains substantial choline acetyltransferase activity (4). We performed a series of experiments to
test the validity of the hypothesis that choline acetyltransferase activity is neuronal and not myocardial in origin.

In collaborative studies with Dr. Kent Hermsmeyer and his co-workers, choline and carnitine acetyltransferase activities were compared in isolated cardiac muscle cells grown in culture and their tissue of origin (5). The specific activity of carnitine acetyltransferase activity in cells in culture was about half that found in the chick or rat heart from which the cultures were derived. Choline acetyltransferase activity, however, was undetectable (less than 1% of the activity of the starting tissue). Following trypsinization to disperse the myocardial cells, choline acetyltransferase activity was resolved from the myocardial cells by differential centrifugation. Moreover, extracts of cultured myocardial cells failed to inhibit enzyme activity in extracts of the embryonic heart of origin. This rules unlikely the presence of a diffusable inhibitor in the cultured cells. In collaboration with Drs. Marvin and Hermsmeyer, the ontogeny of choline acetyltransferase activity was determined in fetal rat (6). Carnitine acetyltransferase activity in heart was detected at day 15, the earliest time examined. Choline acetyltransferase activity, however, was first detected on day 19 (of the 21 day gestation). Similarly in chick, carnitine acetyltransferase activity was present well before the occurrence of choline acetyltransferase (which is first present at day 11 in ovo). Both studies support the notion that myocardial cells per se lack choline acetyltransferase activity. In our initial studies (2), we showed that the regional distribution of choline and carnitine acetyltransferase activities differed. The former was higher in the atria than in the ventricles; the latter was higher in the ventricles than atria.

In collaboration with Drs. Phillip Schmid and Donald Lund, the response of choline acetyltransferase activity to cardiac transplantation was determined.. During the transplantation, the preganglionic neurons are severed; the postganglionic intrinsic neurons remain intact (7). The donor hearts of isogenic rats were transplanted to the abdomen of recipients and enzyme activities were measured eight days later. This time allowed for the complete degeneration of the preganglionic fibers. Decreases of up to 95% activity occurred in the SA nodal region and the atria. Decreases in the ventricles ranged from 50%-80% (7). The wet weight, carnitine acetyltransferase and lactate dehydrogenase activities, however, were unchanged. We interpreted these results as arguing that choline acetyltransferase is a neuronal enzyme marker.

Another intervention to destroy preganglionic nerves, namely unilateral vagotomy, gave results which at first were surprising. Since the mortality of rats and guinea pigs with bilateral cervical vagotomy was 100%, we measured choline acetyltransferase activity following unilateral vagotomy in both rats and guinea pigs (8). Although this intervention abolished choline acetyltransferase activity distal to the lesion in the nerve, decreases were not seen in the heart after eight days. In some instances, there was an increase in the activity on the contralateral side of the heart. Decreases occurred in the SA nodal and AV nodal region one day post-operatively. The activities, however, returned to normal on the second post-operative day. We interpreted the increases in activity as indicating the occurrence of collateral sprouting. The growth of existing nerve fibers seems to parallel the disappearance of the severed fibers explaining the lack of change in total enzyme or the occassional increases seen contralaterally.

After establishing the validity of choline acetyltransferase activity in heart as a cholinergic neuronal marker, its regional distribution in heart will be reviewed. It will be compared with that of the total and multiple agonist affinity forms of the cholinergic muscarinic receptor. The agonist (methacholine) induced decreases of the receptor in perfused working rat heart will then be described.

METHODS

Choline acetyltransferase activity was determined by quantitating the formation of [^{14}C]acetylcholine from [^{14}C] acetyl-CoA as previously described (2). Tyrosine hydroxylase activity was determined by measuring the conversion of [^{3}H] tyrosine to [^{3}H]DOPA by the procedure of Coyle (9). Dopamine β-hydroxylase was measured by the procedure of Coyle and Axelrod (10). The specific protocols and modifications, if any, are given in the original papers. The dissections of heart utilized the landmarks specified by Anderson (11). The muscarinic receptor content was measured using [^{3}H](-)quinuclidinyl benzilate ([^{3}H]QNB) binding as previously described (12). The procedure for the methacholine displacement of the antagonist [^{3}H]QNB will be given in results.

RESULTS

Parasympathetic and Sympathetic Neuroenzyme Markers:

Regional Distribution in Guinea Pig Heart

Choline acetyltransferase activity was greatest in the SA node, the AV node, the proximal conduction bundles and the base of the right anterior papillary muscle and the moderator band of the right ventricle (Table 1). Enzyme activity is significantly lower in all other regions except the right

Table 1. Regional Distribution of Neurochemical Markers in Guinea Pig Heart

Region	Choline acetyltransferase[a] (nmol/h/g)	3H QNB binding (fmol/mg protein)	Tyrosine hydroxylase[b] (nmol/h/g)	Dopamine β-hydroxylase[b] (nmol/h/g)
Sinoatrial node	187 ± 37	184 ± 13	207 ± 15	1600 ± 170
Atrioventricular node	153 ± 26	162 ± 13	45 ± 16	620 ± 90
Atrioventricular bundle	133 ± 15	154 ± 17	47 ± 9	600 ± 74
Right ventricular moderator band	179 ± 19	N.D.	105 ± 10	890 ± 110
Right atrial appendage	137 ± 14	178 ± 14	234 ± 33	1800 ± 200
Left atrial appendage	64 ± 7	181 ± 14	130 ± 32	1100 ± 200
Interatrial septum	82 ± 11	183 ± 17	129 ± 9	950 ± 92
Interventricular septum				
anterior	N.D.	177 ± 21	33 ± 7	530 ± 67
posterior	N.D.	171 ± 13	28 ± 8	560 ± 110
Right ventricle				
anterior	108 ± 14	162 ± 14	74 ± 8	880 ± 130
posterior	94 ± 11	166 ± 17	67 ± 7	760 ± 160
Left ventricle				
anterior	55 ± 12	154 ± 15	39 ± 5	670 ± 120
posterior	49 ± 6	144 ± 10	33 ± 4	640 ± 140

Each value represent the mean ± S.E.M. of six animals. [a]From (13). [b]From (14). Activities are expressed per g wet weight; receptor content, per mg protein.

atrium. The right atrium, however, contains specialized internodal conduction pathways (15). The activity is similar in left atrium and right ventricle and lowest in the left ventricle. There is little variation in choline acetyltransferase activity in the different portions of the right ventricle, IV septum and left ventricle exclusive of those regions which are enriched in conduction tissue. There is a parallel distribution of acetylcholinesterase determined by histochemical procedures (16) and choline acetyltransferase activity in heart.

Based on these findings, we suggested that the para-sympathetic system plays a major role in the regulation of impulse initiation and conduction and a lesser role in the regulation of contractility. Priola and Fulton (17) demon-strated in canine heart that parasympathetic-mediated de-pression of contractility is greatest in right atrium (30%), followed by left atrium (12%), right ventricle (4-12%) and left ventricle (1-10%). Considering the different species (guinea pig vs dog), there is a very good correlation in these results. Although the absolute rates vary, we have obtained similar distributions for choline acetyltransferase in rat (8) and dog (18). Toscaro and Potter (19), moreover, report a similar regional distribution in human heart.

A parallel study on the regional distribution of the sympathetic markers (tyrosine hydroxylase and dopamine β-hydroxylase) was performed. The density of both enzymes is greatest in the SA node and right atrial appendage (Table 1). These values, which do not significantly differ from one another, are significantly higher ($p < .05$) than all other heart regions. The activities do not parallel those for choline acetyltransferase. There is no enrichment of activity in the AV node, AV bundle, or moderator band of the right papillary muscle. The activities in the AV node and bundle, for example, are only 25% that observed in the right atrium. In addition to regulation of heart rate, the sympathetic system increases cardiac contractility in both atria and ventricles (20) corresponding to the more uniform distribution of tyrosine hydroxylase and dopamine β-hydroxylase activities.

In general, the activities of tyrosine hydroxylase and dopamine β-hydroxylase are parallel. The activity of tyrosine hydroxylase is 5-15% that of dopamine β-hydroxylase. This is consistant with the notion that the former is the rate-deter-mining enzyme for norepinephrine biosynthesis. The effect of other components, however, may alter these activities observed in vitro. The role of feedback inhibitors and protein phos-phorylation may alter tyrosine hydroxylase activity (21).

Cu^{2+} added during the assay decreases the inhibition by an endogenous cofactor of dopamine β-hydroxylase (10).

Regional Distribution of the Cholinergic Muscarinic Receptor

Using the high affinity muscarinic cholinergic antagonist [^{3}H] quinuclidinyl benzilate ([^{3}H]QNB), the total receptor in the specified regions of the heart was quantitated by Scatchard analysis. The muscarinic receptor is uniformly distributed in guinea pig heart (Table 1). Using analysis of variance, none of the regions contained significantly different densities of receptor compared with the other regions. In contrast to the guinea pig heart, however, there are differences in the regional distribution in other species. In rat heart, for example, the right and left atria contain about four-fold more receptor (per mg protein) than in the ventricles or IV septum (Table 2). Rabbit (22) and human heart (19) have a pattern similar to that of rat (atria > ventricles = IV septum). Except for the higher absolute activity, the regional distribution of choline acetyltransferase in rat heart (Table 2) is similar to that of guinea pig heart. We guessed that the receptor distribution would parallel that of the parasympathetic system and still remain puzzled on why it does not. Perhaps like acetyl-cholinesterase, its distribution remains more widespread than choline acetyltransferase (which we believe is associated more specifically with cholinergic neurons).

Following the lead of Birdsall et al (23), we initiated an investigation of the multiple agonist affinity forms of the receptor. Whereas the muscarinic receptor (like other receptors) displays a single affinity state for antagonist, it displays multiple affinity states toward agonists. We performed displacement analysis of the antagonist [^{3}H]QNB by the agonist methacholine in order to quantitate these multiple affinity forms. We chose the latter since it has greater specificity for cardiovascular responses and because it is a muscarinic agent lacking nicotinic agonist activity. Oxotremorine and carbachol, for example, possess both nicotinic and muscarinic activity. With Dr. Paul Cook, we have developed the following displacement analysis for agonist binding. It can be more easily understood by comparing it with the equations of steady state enzyme kinetics.

$$v = \frac{V[A]}{K_A + [A]} \qquad\qquad \text{equation} \quad 1$$

Table 2. Regional Distribution of Cholinergic Markers in Rat Heart

Region	Choline Acetyltransferase (nmol/h/g)	3H QNB binding (fmol/mg/protein)
Right Atrial Appendage	1230 ± 108	533 ± 15
Sinoatrial node	1800 ± 300	N.D.
Left Atrial Appendage	324 ± 30	580 ± 14
Interventricular System	186 ± 24	119 ± 4
Right Ventricle	264 ± 24	181 ± 6
Left Ventricle	84 ± 12	154 ± 14

The values represent the mean ± S.E.M. of 4-6 animals. Choline acetyltransferase activity was measured as described in (2) and the total muscarinic receptor by Scatchard analysis as described in (12).

$$v = \frac{V[A]}{K_A(1 + I/K_I) + A} \qquad \text{equation} \quad 2$$

In the second equation, representing the competitive inhibition of an enzymatic reaction:

v = velocity
V = maximal velocity
A = substrate concentration
K_A = Michaelis constant
I = inhibitor concentration
K_I = K_d for the inhibitor

For displacement analysis, [^{3}H]-QNB binding corresponds to v and V_{max} and methacholine is the inhibitor whose affinity constants are to be determined. The equation for displacement can then be formulated in the following manner by analogy.

$$B_i = \frac{B_{max}[Q]}{K_Q(1 + [MeCh]/K_{MeCh}) + [Q]} \qquad \text{equation } 3$$

The equation can be recast in the following manner:

$$Bi(1 + K_Q/[Q]) = - Bi[MeCh]K_Q/[Q]K_{MeCh} + B_{max} \qquad \text{equation } 4$$

$K_Q = K_d$ for [^{3}H]-QNB determined by Scatchard analysis

[MeCh] = added methacholine concentration

B_{max} = [^{3}H-QNB] bound to receptor in the absence of the displacing agent MeCh (and not that determined by Scatchard analysis)

B_i = [[^{3}H]-QNB] bound to receptor in the presence of specified MeCh

[Q] = [Q]$_{added}$ - B_i or free [^{3}H]-QNB concentration

The quantity $Bi(1 + K_Q/[Q])$ is plotted on the y-axis and $B_i[MeCh]K_Q/[Q]$ is plotted on the x-axis. The slope of the lines generated in this manner is equal to $- 1/K_{MeCh}$. This is similar to a Scatchard analysis. The experiments are performed with added [^{3}H]-QNB (20-30 x 10^{-12}M) at a concentration sufficient to bind to only 10-15% of the receptor. It is assumed that only

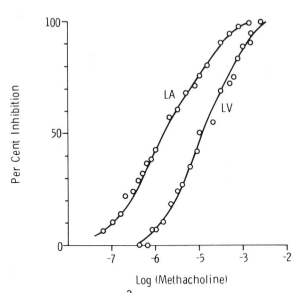

Figure 1.   Displacement of [^{3}H]-QNB by methacholine in guinea
            pig heart.   The total concentration of [^{3}H]-QNB
            was 20 pM in the atrial assays and 30 pM in the
            ventricular   assays.   The   protein   concentration
            was 1 mg/ml.   The values represent the mean of
            4 duplicate determinations.   The standard errors
            are less than 10% of the specified values.

a small fraction of added MeCh binds to receptor since
[MeCh] > > [R].   About 20-22 concentrations between 1 μM to
2 mM of MeCh are used.   The proportion of the multiple
affinity states are determined by extrapolation to the y axis.
Since subsaturating, constant additions of [^{3}H]-QNB are used,
it is not possible to determine the total receptor. This can
be independently measured by standard Scatchard analysis with
varying [^{3}H]-QNB.

     In left atrium and ventricle, the percent displacement
does not exhibit a characteristic sigmoidal curve with 9 to
91% displacement occurring over 2 log units as associated with
a single affinity binding site (Figure 1).   Both curves are

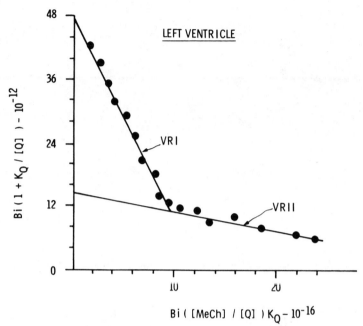

Figure 2. Demonstration of the multiple affinity states of
the muscarinic receptor for methacholine in guinea
pig left ventricle. The experimental data corresponding to those given in Figure 1 were plotted
as described in Results. The K_D is - 1/slope. The
percent of each affinity form is determined by extrapolation to the ordinate. The K_D's and percent determined by computer fitting of the equations are
5.3 ± 0.31 μM (62%) and 220 ± 14 μM (38%).

flattened and extend further than 2 log units. By non-linear
least squares regression, the proportion and K_D's of the
multiple agonist affinity states have been determined for
brain (23). Plotting the data in Figure 1 according to
equation 4 gives the results shown in Figures 2 and 3. The
left and right ventricle and IV septum exhibit two affinity
states. The right and left atrium and the SA node exhibit
three affinity states. Since the SA node is contaminated by
contiguous right atrium, this finding was anticipated. The AV
node, in the superior portion of the IV septum, is contaminated by septal tissue with the two affinity states.

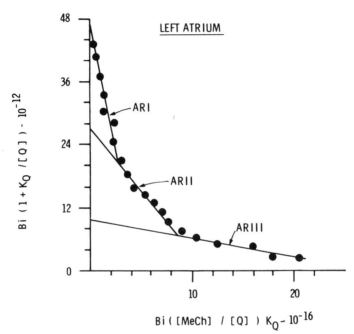

Figure 3. Demonstration of the multiple affinity states of
the muscarinic receptor for methacholine in the
guinea pig left atrium. The K_D's and percent
were determined as described in Figure 2 and
were 0.59 ± 0.11 µM (41%), 15 ± 2.5 µM (47%)
and 1100 ± 350 µM (12%).

Displacement analysis of homogenates containing the AV node,
however, reveals the three affinity states seen in the atrium.
This represents the first demonstration of three affinity sites
by agonist/antagonist displacement.

In summary, the specialized pacemaker tissue (SA node,
right atrium and AV node) contain three affinity states one of
which is of high affinity (0.57 µM). The left atrium also
contains these three forms. The contractile regions (right
and left ventricle and IV septum) contain two affinity sites.

Both the cholinergic muscarinic receptor and the
β-adrenergic receptors are associated with GTP-regulatory

proteins (24,25). The binding of GMPPNP, a non-hydrolyzable
GTP analogue, decreases the affinity of agonists to the receptor and converts them into a form of uniform affinity. In
collaboration with Dr. Enseleit, we performed dose-dependent
titrations with GMPPNP to determine its effect on the multiple
affinity states (26). In guinea pig and rat heart 0.1 µM
GMPPNP converted the two affinity forms to a single form with
intermediate K_d. In the atria, 300 µM GMPPNP abolished the
high affinity state and two states remained. Higher concentrations (1 mM) converted the receptor into a single
affinity form. There was no change in the total amount or
affinity of [^{3}H]-QNB binding as measured by Scatchard
analysis. We conclude that all forms of the receptor have the
potential to interact with the GTP-regulatory proteins. Two
novel findings will be more thoroughly characterized in future
experiments. First, the dose-response to GMPPNP differs in
atria and ventricles. Higher concentrations of GMPPNP (1 mM)
are required to convert the atrial receptor into a single
affinity state than in the ventricle (1 µM). Second, the
affinity state in both atria and ventricles and in both rat
and guinea pig resulting from GMPPNP is intermediate in
affinity. This is in contrast with other systems where the
affinity state reverts to a lower affinity form (24,25)

Methacholine Down Regulation of the Muscarinic Receptor in the Perfused Rat Heart

In an effort to determine the significance of the multiple affinity states, Rick Reinhardt studied the regulation of
receptor in the perfused working rat heart as described by
Morgan and co-workers (27). The heart is perfused with a
Krebs-Henseleit buffer containing glucose (10 mM), the twenty
amino acids required for protein synthesis, and bovine serum
albumin (to increase viscosity). The left ventricle beats
against a pressure of 160/100 mm Hg. The right side of the
heart is more passive. The purpose of the experiments was to
determine whether the agonist methacholine would bring about a
decrease in the amount of muscarinic receptor as has been seen
in heart and brain cells in culture (28,29). In the latter
case, down regulation was brought about with 1 mM concentrations of agonist. In the case of the perfused heart,
the highest concentration of methacholine that could be added
without producing asystole was 4 µM. Moreover, it had to be
added in increments until the final concentration was
obtained. This suggested that the high affinity form of the
receptor is the important one.

In the first series of experiments, the receptor content
in the five regions of the heart (atria, ventricles and IV

Table 3.   Reversibility of Down Regulation of the Muscarinic Receptor in Rat Heart

Region	Receptor Content (fmoles/mg protein)			
	2.5 h Control Perfusion	2.5 h Methacholine Perfusion	5 h Control Perfusion	2.5 h Methacholine Perfusion Followed by 2.5 h Control Perfusion
Left Atrium	570 ± 15	469 ± 14[a]	540 ± 20	531 ± 20
Right Atrium	524 ± 13	470 ± 12[a]	511 ± 19	504 ± 17
Left Ventricle	147 ± 5	118 ± 5[a]	139 ± 9	130 ± 8
Right Ventricle	179 ± 7	169 ± 8	166 ± 8	169 ± 9
IV Septum	111 ± 5	108 ± 5	110 ± 6	114 ± 7

Each value is the mean ± S.E.M. of determinations from four perfused rat hearts. Receptor content was determined by Scatchard analysis. [a]Significantly different from control ($p < 0.01$). From (30).

septum) was found to be stable during five hours of perfusion in the absence of added methacholine (not shown). In the presence of 4 μM methacholine, however, there was a significant decrease in receptor content (Table 3). Decreases occurred in the right and left atrium and left ventricle. The lack of decrease in the right ventricle may reflect the fact that it is only passively perfused in this preparation. To test for reversibility, the methacholine was removed after 2.5 hours and the perfusion was continued for an additional 2.5 hours. The receptor number returned to control levels. This indicates that the decreased receptor number was not due to non-specific toxic effects, but was related to the methacholine. To further substantiate this hypothesis scopolamine (1 μM), a muscarinic receptor antagonist, completely blocked the methacholine mediated down regulation (not shown). Scopolamine per se lacked any effect on receptor number. The proportion and K_D's of the multiple affinity states in response to methacholine perfusion was determined. After 2.5 hours, there was a conversion of the three agonist affinity states to two states in the left atrium (Table 4). There was a loss of the high affinity state and formation of two states with K_D's between those of the initial three states. These K_D's correspond in apparent affinity to the two states seen in the ventricles and IV septum. Following an additional 2.5 hour perfusion in the absence of methacholine, not only did the receptor content return, but the three affinity states reappeared. The multiple affinity states in the right atrium showed exactly the same pattern: conversion to two states after 2.5 hours and return to three states after an additional 2.5 hours in the absence of methacholine. In contrast, there was no change of the proportion or apparent affinity states of the muscarinic receptor in the left ventricle (Table 4).

DISCUSSION

In guinea pig, rat, dog and human heart, choline acetyltransferase activity parallels the distribution of specialized pacemaker and conduction tissue. This is in contrast to the regional distribution of tyrosine hydroxylase and dopamine β-hydroxylase activity in guinea pig heart where the AV node, proximal bundle and moderator band have the activity of the contiguous contractile tissue (Table 1). The density of cholinergic muscarinic receptor in rat heart is greater in the atria than in the ventricles or IV septum (Table 2). This is the pattern seen in human heart (19). In contrast, total receptor is more uniformly distributed in guinea pig heart. For both guinea pig and rat, the ratio of choline acetyltransferase activity to receptor density is greatest in right atrium and ventricle and lowest in left atrium and left

Table 4. Down Regulation of Muscarinic Receptors and Receptor Interconversion in Rat Heart

| Region | Apparent Receptor K_D, μM (% total) Time, hour | | | |
	0 h	2.5 h Meth	2.5 h Meth 2.5 h Control	5 h Control
Left Atrium				
ARI	16 (28)	46 (32)	15 (30)	13 (33)
ARII	140 (38)	230 (69)	132 (39)	152 (35)
ARIII	650 (32)		689 (30)	643 (33)
Left Ventricle				
VRI	34 (21)	35 (24)	39 (25)	41 (23)
VRII	246 (79)	250 (76)	229 (75)	213 (77)

The values represent the means of 4 determinations. The data were fitted by eye. Methacholine (4 μM) or control buffer was perfused through the working rat heart as described by Morgan et al (27) for the time indicated. The multiple agonist affinity states were determined as described in results.

ventricle. These do not necessarily correlate with the physiological situation since both indices are reflections of maximal possible responses and not activity in vivo. It is unlikely that choline acetyltransferase, for example, is performing at optimal substrate concentrations in vivo; the presence of spare or uncoupled receptors also makes the total receptor content only an approximation of functional receptor activity.

The distribution of the multiple affinity forms of the receptors is similar in guinea pig and rat even though the distribution of total receptor differs. The atria, SA node and AV node contain three affinity states for methacholine. The highest and lowest affinity states parallel the distribution of the specialized pacemaker and conducting tissue. The ventricles and IV septum contain only two affinity forms. Their apparent magnitude is intermediate between those of the three atrial affinity states. Whether the five affinity states are truly different will require additional experimentation.

We measured choline acetyltransferase activity and quantitated the total amount of muscarinic receptor in guinea pigs exposed to hypobaric hypoxia for one and two weeks (12). We observed major increases in choline acetyltransferase activity (54%) in only the SA nodal region. We interpreted this as representing an increase in neuronal mass or activity. There was a concomitant down regulation of receptor which was more widespread. After two weeks, for example, there were significant decreases in the right atrium and ventricle, and SA and AV node. It is our working hypothesis that muscarinic receptor number is a more sensitive, reciprocal index of parasympathetic nerve action than choline acetyltransferase activity. At the time that these studies were performed, we had not yet developed our procedures for determination of the multiple affinity forms. The presence of multiple affinity states for muscarinic receptor agonists prompts the question of their possible physiological significance. Birdsall et al have proposed that the low affinity state is the physio-logically important one (23). This is based in part on the observation that the high affinity state is uniformly dis-tributed in the rat brain but the low affinity state is non-uniform. Occupancy of the low affinity state is correlated with cGMP levels in neuroblastoma cells and in striated brain slices, modulation of neurotransmitter release in hippocampus and contraction in ileal smooth muscle.

Our studies with the heart, however, may not be in agreement with this notion. The high affinity state of the receptor parallels that of the pacemaker and conduction tissue and choline acetyltransferase. Futhermore, the highest dose of methacholine that can be perfused through the heart corresponds more closely with the high affinity form.

The molecular explanation for the multiple affinity states also requires clarification. Guanine nucleotides decrease the binding of many substances to their receptor (24). This appears to be related to coupling of the receptor to the specific responses. The multiple affinity forms of the atrial and ventricular receptors are all converted to an intermediate affinity state by GMPPNP. Higher concentrations of GMPPNP are required in atria than ventricles. These experiments support the notion that the apparent affinities for agonists are altered by the environment (GTP-regulatory proteins). There may be more than one type or conformation of GTP-regulatory protein which may also confer different apparent agonist affinities upon the receptor. Agonist affinity may also be altered by the receptor environment. This might include different subunits making up the receptor, multiple forms of the GTP-regulatory protein, other proteins (specific and unspecific) in the environment and membrane lipid interactions. Perhaps one of the observed forms represents receptor undergoing endocytosis and degradation or biosynthesis and translocation to a functional site.

The multiple affinity forms might represent coupling to different effector sites. Different receptor populations may govern, inter alia, the following: rate, contractility, inhibition of adenylate cyclase, activation of guanylate cyclase, or K^+ ion permeabability. The presence of the multiple affinity states has raised more questions than it has answered.

ACKNOWLEDGEMENTS

This research was supported by grant HL 24791 from the U.S. Public Health Service and by a grant from the American Heart Association and its Louisiana Affiliate. I thank Wanda Santa Marina for secretarial assistance.

REFERENCES

1. M.N. Levy, Parasympathetic control of the heart. In: Neural regulation of the heart. W.C. Randall, ed., pp. 95-129 New York: Oxford University Press (1977).
2. R. Roskoski, Jr., H.E. Mayer, and P.G. Schmid, Choline acetyltransferase activity in guinea pig heart in vitro. J. Neurochem. 23:1197 (1974).

3.   P.B. Molinoff, and J. Axelrod, Biochemistry of Catechola
     mines. Ann. Rev. Biochem. 40:465 (1971).
4.   Potter, L.T., Acetylcholine in Handbook of Neurochemistry.
     Vol IV, A. Lajtha ed., New York, Plenum Press, pp 263-284
     (1970).
5.   R. Roskoski, Jr., R. McDonald, L.M. Roskoski, W. Marvin,
     K. Hermsmayer, Choline acetyltransferase activity in
     Heart: Evidence for neuronal and not myocardial origin.
     Am. J. Physiol. 233:H642 (1977).
6.   W.J. Marvin, Jr., K. Hermsmeyer, R.I. McDonald, L.M.
     Roskoski, and R. Roskoski, Jr., Ontogenesis of
     cholinergic innervation in the rat heart. Circ. Res.
     46:690 (1980).
7.   D.D. Lund, P.G. Schmid, S.E. Kelly, R.J. Corry, and
     R. Roskoski, Jr., Choline acetyltransferase activity
     in rat heart after transplantation. Am. J. Physiol.
     235:H367 (1978).
8.   D.D. Lund, P.G. Schmid, and R. Roskoski, Jr., Choline
     acetyltransferase activity in rat and guinea pig heart
     following vagotomy. Am. J. Physiol. H620 (1974).
9.   J.T. Coyle, Tyrosine Hydroxylase in rat brain. Biochem.
     Pharmacol. 21:1935 (1972).
10. J.T. Coyle, and J. Axelrod, Dopamine -hydroxylase in
     the rat brain: Developmental characteristics. J.
     Neurochem. 19:449 (1972).
11. R.H. Anderson, The disposition, morphology and
     innervation of cardiac specialized tissue in the
     guinea pig. J. Anat. 111:453 (1972).
12. L.H. Crockatt, D.D. Lund, P.G. Schmid, and R.
     Roskoski, Jr., Hypoxia-induced changes in
     parasympathetic neurochemical markers in guinea
     pig heart. J. Appl. Physiol. 50:1017 (1981).
13. P.G. Schmid, B.J. Greif, D.D. Lund, and R. Roskoski, Jr.,
     Regional Choline Acetyltransferase Activity in the
     Guinea Pig Heart. Circ. Res. 42:657 (1978).
14. Dickson, D.W., Lund, D.D., Subieta, A.R., Prall, J.L.,
     Schmid, P.G., Roskoski, R. Jr., Regional Dis-
     tribution of Tyrosine Hydroxylase and Dopamine B-
     Hydroxylase Activities in Guinea Pig Heart, J. Autonomic
     Nervous System, 4:319-326 (1981).
15. T.N. James, The connecting pathways between the sinus node
     and the A-V node and between the right and left atrium in
     the human heart. Am. Heart J. 66:498 (1963).
16. T.N. James, Cardiac innervation: Anatomic and pharmacologic
     relations. Bull. N.Y. Acad. Med. 43:1041 (1967).
17. D.V. Priola, and R.L. Fulton, Positive and negative ino-
     tropic responses of the atria and ventricles to vagosym-
     pathetic stimulation in the isovolumic canine heart. Circ.
     Res. 25:265 (1969).

18. D.D. Lund, P.G. Schmid, U.J. Johannsen, and R. Roskoski,Jr., Biochemical indices of cholinergic and adrenergic autonomic innervation in chronic right heart failure. J. Mol. Cell Cardiol. in press.

19. P. Toscano, and L.T. Potter, Distribution of muscarinic receptors (MR) in relation to choline acetyltransferase in the human heart. Fed. Proc. 41:1327.

20. W.C. Randall, Sympathetic control of the heart. In: Neural regulation of the heart, W.C. Randall, ed., pp. 43–94. New York, Oxford University Press (1977).

21. W. Lovenberg, E.A. Bruckwick, and I. Hambauer, ATP, Cyclic AMP and magnesium increase the activity of rat striatal tyrosine hydroxylase for its cofactor. Proc. Natl. Acad. Sci. (U.S.A.). 72:2955 (1975).

22. J.Z. Fields, W.R. Roeske, E. Morkin and H.I. Yamamura, Cardiac Muscarinic Cholinergic Receptor., J. Biol. Chem. 253:3251 (1978).

23. N.J.M. Birdsall, A.S.V. Burgen, and E.C. Hulme, The binding of agonists to brain muscarinic receptors. Mol. Pharmacol. 14:723 (1978).

24. M. Rodbell, The role of hormone receptor and GTP-regulatory proteins in membrane transduction. Nature 284:17 (1980).

25. L.E. Limbird, Activation and attenuation of adenylate cyclase. Biochem. J. 195:1 (1981).

26. W.H. Enseleit, R.G. Bassett, Jr. and R. Roskoski, Jr., Modification of muscarinic receptor-ligand binding in the rat heart by 5'-guanylylimidodiphosphate, Fed. Proc. 41:1211 (1982).

27. H.E. Morgan, B.H.L. Chua, and E.O. Fuller, Regulation of protein synthesis and degradation during in vitro cardiac work. Am. J. Physiol. 238:E431 (1980).

28. J.B. Galper, and T.W. Smith, Properties of muscarinic acetylcholine receptors in heart cell cultures. Proc. Natl. Acad. Sci. (U.S.A.). 75:5831 (1978).

29. R.G. Simon, and W.L. Klein, Cholinergic activity regulates muscarinic receptors in central nervous system cultures. Proc. Natl. Acad. Sci. (U.S.A.) 76:4141 (1979).

30. R.R. Reinhardt, and R. Roskoski, Jr., Methacholine induced decrease of the cholinergic muscarinic receptor in the perfused working rat heart. Fed. Proc. 41:898 (1982).

NEUROCHEMICAL INDICES OF AUTONOMIC INNERVATION OF HEART IN

DIFFERENT EXPERIMENTAL MODELS OF HEART FAILURE

Donald D. Lund, Phillip G. Schmid, and Robert Roskoski, Jr.

VA Medical Center, The Cardiovascular Center, and
Departments of Internal Medicine and Biochemistry
The University of Iowa, Iowa City, Iowa   52242

ABSTRACT

Parasympathetic neural regulation of the failing heart is impaired. In order to investigate parasympathetic mechanisms in experimental heart failure, measurements were made of choline acetyltransferase (CAT) activity and [^{3}H]-quinuclidinyl benzilate (QNB) binding in hearts of 1) hamsters with skeletal and cardiac myopathy, 2) dogs with pulmonary artery constriction and tricuspid avulsion, and 3) guinea pigs with pulmonary artery constriction. Tyrosine hydroxylase (TH) and dopamine-beta-hydroxylase (DBH) activities and norepinephrine levels served as indices of sympathetic innervation. In myopathic hearts, total CAT activity decreased ($P<0.05$) compared to age-matched controls. In canine and guinea pig right heart failure, total CAT activity was normal in contractile and specialized tissues. Alterations in [^{3}H]-QNB binding paralleled CAT activity being decreased ($P<0.05$) only in myopathic hearts. In all three models, indices of sympathetic innervation were altered in ways qualitatively different from parasympathetic indices; TH and DBH activities were increased ($P<0.05$) in myopathic ventricles, decreased ($P<0.05$) in hypertrophied canine and guinea pig ventricles and non-hypertrophied canine ventricles, and normal in non-hypertrophied guinea pig ventricles. These results indicate that alterations in cardiac parasympathetic indices vary depending on the etiology of heart diseases and differ qualitatively from alterations in sympathetic indices. Selective determinants are necessary to explain the varied changes.

INTRODUCTION

Cardiac hypertrophy and failure are associated with catecholamine depletion (3,8,9,19,27-31). This gives rise to the concept
that sympathetic neural abnormalities occur in diseased hearts.
Further, there is recent evidence to suggest that sympathetic neural
changes vary in experimental models of heart diseases. Tyrosine
hydroxylase activity, which regulates norepinephrine synthesis, is
decreased in models with pressure- and volume-induced hypertrophy
(19) and increased in the cardiomyopathic hamster (28). Therefore,
depending on the specific intervention used to produce experimental
heart disease, heart failure may be associated with decreases or
increases in a biochemical index of sympathetic innervation.

Preliminary information suggests that the parasympathetic
innervation of diseased hearts may be affected differently than the
sympathetic innervation (18,21). The activity of choline acetyltransferase, which catalyzes synthesis of acetylcholine, is not
altered detectably (21) under circumstances associated with reduced
activity of tyrosine hydroxylase (18). There remains also, the
possibility that parasympathetic neural changes, like those of the
sympathetic system, vary in experimental models of heart disease.
To investigate these issues further, biochemical indices of parasympathetic and sympathetic innervation were determined in hearts
from three experimental preparations: 1)Syrian golden hamsters
with generalized skeletal myopathy and cardiac myopathy; 2) dogs
with tricuspid avulsion and pulmonary artery constriction; and 3)
guinea pigs with pulmonary artery constriction.

Cardiac innervation in contractile regions has been investigated in previous studies (21,24). There has been limited biochemical information about the innervation of pacemaking and conductive regions in diseased hearts despite suggestive evidence of
abnormalities based on studies of baroreflexes (13,15). Therefore,
a second goal was to investigate choline acetyltransferase activity
in the sino-atrial and atrioventricular nodal regions of the guinea
pig model and segments of the right atrium (including segments with
the sinus node and artery) in the canine model of right heart disease

In conjunction with these studies, measurements also were made
of specific binding of ligand, [^{3}H]-quinuclidinyl benzilate, to
muscarininc cholinergic receptors in homogenates of hearts from
the three models.

METHODS

Male and female Syrian golden hamsters (Bio 2.4) and their
counterparts with hereditary skeletal myopathy (Bio 14.6) (Bio-
Research Inst., Cambridge, Mass.) were obtained at age 20 days and

maintained three to a cage in the University of Iowa Animal Facility until sacrifice and study. The two groups were treated similarly and given a standard laboratory diet (Tecklab, Winfield, IA) and water ad libitum.

Male guinea pigs were obtained at a weight of 500-600 gm. Twenty-one were prepared surgically with pulmonary artery constriction as previously described (21,22,24,25). Fifteen additional guinea pigs from the same source were subjected to sham surgery at the same time with dissection around the pulmonary artery and encirclement with a string but without constriction of the vessel. All of the guinea pigs were caged individually and given standard pellet chow and water ad libitum for 30 days until sacrifice and study.

Seven male mongrel dogs weighing 19-22 kg were anesthetized and prepared using the technique of Barger et al. (6) to produce tricuspid avulsion and pulmonary artery constriction. Tricuspid insufficiency was produced by avulsing the chordae tendineae of the tricuspid leaflets via an incision of the right atrial appendage. Approximately one week later pulmonic stenosis was created by placing a Teflon constricting band around the main pulmonary artery. Seven male mongrel dogs of corresponding size had sham surgery. The dogs were maintained in runs and fed standard laboratory chow and water ad libitum until they were studied and sacrificed approximately three to five years after the initial surgical preparations. Dogs representing control and heart failure groups were monitored over the same period, but dogs entered and terminated the study at varying times so that the duration of heart failure is characterized as chronic without implying that it was exactly the same for all dogs.

Hamsters and guinea pigs were sacrificed by cervical dislocation. Dogs were anesthetized with chloralose (50 mg/kg) and urethane (500 mg/kg); central venous pressures were determined in the dogs before excising the hearts.

Sampling of tissues was accomplished as fast as possible. Pilot studies have demonstrated that muscarinic receptor binding properties and choline acetyltransferase activity are stable up to 45 minutes post-mortem and remain stable in liquid nitrogen for at least three months (12). Canine and hamster hearts were dissected over ice. In the hamster, samples were obtained from the contractile regions of the right and left atria and right and left ventricles. In the guinea pigs, samples were obtained from regions that Anderson previously identified as containing the sinus node (SA node), the atrio-ventricular node (AV node) and the proximal conduction bundles (Prox bund.) (2,23). In the dog, samples were obtained from the right and left atria and from multiple sites in the right and left ventricular free walls. The right atrium was dissected and sampled as described by White et al. (32) (Figs. 3 & 5). This standardized approach was intended to facilitate reproducible sampling of 16 atrial segments, some with predominantly specialized tissue and some with predominantly contractile tissue.

Biochemical Determinations

Total tissue norepinephrine was measured by modification of the alumina-trihydroxyindole procedure (24,25). This procedure allows 75% recovery of added catecholamine throughout the tissue analysis and is sensitive to the 50 pgm level. Frozen tissue samples were homogenized with a Tekmar Tissuemizer (Cincinnati, OH) in 50 volumes of iced 0.4N perchloric acid, absorbed onto alumina at a pH of 8.6, and eluted with 3-5 ml of 0.05N perchloric acid. Samples were then analyzed for catecholamine determination using a high performance liquid chromatography unit (Waters) with electrochemical detection (Bioanalytical Systems) (25).

Other tissue samples were homogenized (20 volumes of ice-cold 5 mM potassium phosphate, 0.1 mM EDTA [pH 7.4] per g wet weight tissue) using four 10-sec bursts of the Tekmar Tissumizer at a setting of 70%. After removing aliquots for [^{3}H]-QNB binding, 10% Triton X-100, a non-ionic detergent, was added to the remaining homogenate to give a concentration of 0.2% (v/v). Choline acetyltransferase activity was measured as previously described using a 15-min incubation at 37°C (17,20,21,23). Tyrosine hydroxylase activity was measured by the procedure of Coyle using a 10-min incubation at 37°C (10,26). The final concentrations of tyrosine and 2-amino-4-hydroxy-6, 7-demethyl-tetrahydropteridine were 0.2 mM and 1.0 mM respectively. Dopamine-β-hydroxylase was measured by the procedure of Coyle and Axelrod using a 20-min incubation at 37°C (11,26).

The measurements of muscarinic cholinergic receptor density in heart was performed by a modification of the method of Galper and co-workers (12,14). Incubations were performed in Ringer's solution (10 mM Tris-HCl, pH 7.4, 10 mM glucose, 150 mM NaCl, 3.5 mM KCl, 1.2 mM MgSO$_4$, 1.2 mM Na$_2$HPO$_4$) containing a 2 nM [^{3}H]-quinuclidinyl benzilate ([^{3}H]-QNB, 13-17 Ci/mmol). Portions of tissue homogenate (0.25 mg tissue in 50 μl) were added to the Ringer's solution containing the [^{3}H]-QNB and incubated at 24°C for 45 minutes in duplicate. Nonspecific binding was determined in parallel assays in the presence of saturating concentrations of oxotremorine (0.2 mM). The reaction was terminated by filtration through a Whatman glass fiber filter (GF/A) positioned over a vacuum. Unbound ligand was then washed through a filter with saline (0.9M NaCl, 5 x 5 ml). Filters were dried for ten minutes at 100°C and radioactivity was measured by liquid scintillation spectrometry. Duplicate protein determinations were performed accoring to the method of Lowry et al. (16).

A two-factor analysis of variance was used to analyze differences between control and heart failure groups. All variables except norepinephrine, dopamine and CAT activity were transformed to a $\log_{10}$ scale to acheive homogeneity of variance among groups. Multiple comparisons among group means was accomplished using the multiple t method with an overall level of significance of 0.05 (1).

RESULTS

Heart Weights and Evidence of Heart Failure

Syrian golden hamsters with skeletal myopathy. Five different age groups of myopathic (Bio 14.6) and age-matched control (Bio 2.4) hamsters were studied. Younger hamsters from either source (30, 90, and 180 days old) had age related increases but no detectable differences in heart weight. Older myopathic hamsters (290-360 days old) had significantly greater (P<0.05) heart weights (515±17) than control hamsters (415±12) and some had evidence of heart failure such as ascites, hepatic congestion, and peripheral edema.

Dogs with tricuspid avulsion and pulmonary artery constriction. At the time of sacrifice and study, control dogs averaged 22.1±0.7 kg and heart failure dogs averaged 20.4±0.8 kg body weight ($\bar{x}$±SE). All of the latter animals had ascites (4.4±1.7 kg), and demonstrated gross pathological evidence of chronic hepatic congestion. The central venous pressure in dogs with right-sided congestive heart failure was significantly greater (8.5±2.2 mmHg) than the sham animals (3.1±0.4 mmHg) (P<0.05). The ratio of right ventricular weight to body weight was significantly elevated (P<0.05) in the chronic heart failure dogs compared with the sham surgery group (2.8±0.2 vs 1.9±0.2 g/kg respectively) but there was no difference (P>0.1) in the left ventricular weight to body weight ratio between the two groups (5.7±0.2 vs 6.0±0.3 g/kg).

Guinea pigs with pulmonary artery constriction. The right ventricular weight normalized for body weight (g/kg) was 0.58±0.03 ($\bar{x}$±SE) for seven sham-operated guinea pigs, 1.03±0.04 for 15 guinea pigs with mild to moderate hypertrophy (P<0.05 vs C) and 1.64±0.05 for five guinea pigs with severe hypertrophy (P<0.05 vs C and moderate hypertrophy groups). Those in the latter group with severe hypertrophy had histologic evidence of hepatic congestion and, therefore, heart failure. Two guinea pigs with loose constrictor bands around the pulmonary artery had minimal increases in right ventricular weight. The left ventricular weights normalized for body weight were similar in all of the groups.

Indices of Sympathetic Innervation

Syrian golden hamsters with skeletal myopathy. In adult

hamsters (290-360 days) tyrosine hydroxylase (TH) activity (nmol, mg prot^{-1}, hr^{-1}) was significantly increased in the stellate ganglia of myopathic (M) hamsters but not in control (C) hamsters (C=34±4; M=50±3). Increased TH activity also occurred in the adrenal gland of myopathic hamsters compared to control hamsters (C=26±4; M=54±9) but not in the superior cervical ganglia (C=36±3; M=33±5). In parallel with the enzyme activity in stellate ganglia, TH activity and dopamine-beta-hydroxylase (DBH) activity increased in myopathic hearts to greater levels than in control hearts (Fig. 1). When values were evaluated per unit weight, norepinephrine, but not dopamine concentration was markedly reduced only in failing myopathic hearts (Table 1) while tyrosine hydroxylase and dopamine hydroxylase activities were maintained. In terms of age-related changes, the increases in DBH activity in myopathic hearts were evident at all ages, and there was a trend for an increase in TH activity although it was only significantly increased at 180 days and older (Fig. 1). There was no appreciable difference between old hamsters with heart failure and those with myocardial hypertrophy alone with respect to these changes.

Table 1. Indices of Sympathetic Innervation in Control and Cardiomyopathic Hamster Hearts

Age (days)	Dopamine Concentration (ng/g)		Norepinephrine Concentration (ng/g)	
	Control	Myopathic	Control	Myopathic
30 (6)	70±10	80±3	970±7	1572±30*
90 (6)	130±10	90±20	1680±130	1850±110
180 (6)	120±10	100±10	1570±60	1730±30
290-360 (9) (Hypertrophy)	80±15	67±7	1298±88	1313±158
290-360 (6) (Failure)	94±19	87±24	1519±199	932±83*

All values represent mean±SEM. Numbers in parentheses denote the number in each group.

* Differs from Control, P<0.05.

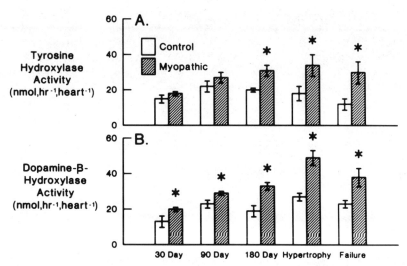

Fig. 1.   Total cardiac a) tyrosine hydroxylase activity and b)
dopamine-β-hydroxylase activity of control and cardiomyopathic hamsters at various ages. Hypertrophy and
failure groups were 290-360 days old. Each value is
the mean ± SEM for at least 6 animals, (* Significantly
different from Control; P<0.05)

Dogs with tricuspid avulsion and pulmonary artery constriction.
Unlike the myopathic heart in which TH activity increased and norepinephrine concentration decreased, the stressed canine heart exhibited marked reductions in both TH activity and norepinephrine.
Norepinephrine concentration in the right ventricles of stressed
hearts averaged 24±5 ng/g ($\bar{x}$±SE) vs 862±53 ng/g in control hearts
(P<0.01). Likewise, norepinephrine concentration in left ventricles
averaged 190±58 ng/g and 658±51 ng/g, respectively (P<0.01). Norepinephrine content (μg/ventricle) averaged 1.4±0.2 vs 38±3 and
22±5 vs 89±5 in the right and left ventricles, again clearly indicating norepinephrine depletion in both chambers of failing canine

hearts (P<0.01). Similar decreases were evident with regard to TH
and DBH activities in the right and left ventricles of stressed
canine hearts (Table 2). However, neither enzyme appeared to be
affected in the left atrium and total DBH activity appeared to be
maintained selectively in the right atrium (Table 2).

Guinea pigs with pulmonary artery constriction. Like the
canine model of heart failure, guinea pigs with pulmonary artery
constriction have a marked reduction in norepinephrine concentration
and tyrosine hydroxylase activity in the stressed right ventricle
(Table 3). However, unlike the canine model of heart failure,
the norepinephrine concentration and tyrosine hydroxylase activity
in the left ventricle of pulmonary banded animals were similar
to the control animals (Table 3).

Indices of Parasympathetic Innervation in Contractile Regions

Syrian golden hamsters with skeletal myopathy. The time
course of changes in choline acetyltransferase (CAT) activity in
myopathic hearts differed markedly from that of TH activity (Fig. 2).
Whereas TH activity (Fig. 1) increased progressively from 30 to 360
days of age in myopathic hearts, total CAT activity (Fig. 2) increased early (from 30-90 days of age) in parallel with CAT activity
in control hearts and then decreased progressively in the myopathic
heart so that heart failure was associated with markedly reduced
CAT activity compared to age-matched control hamsters' hearts.
The decrease in CAT activity was most pronounced in the failing
myopathic hearts.

Dogs with tricuspid avulsion and pulmonary artery constriction.
Unlike the myopathic heart in which CAT activity decreased, the
stressed canine heart had no detectable change in CAT activity in
either the right or the left ventricle (Table 4).

Guinea pigs with pulmonary artery constriction. Like the
canine model of right heart failure there was no detectable change
in choline acetyltransferase activity in either the right or left
ventricle (Table 3).

Indices of Parasympathetic Innervation in Specialized Pacemaking
and Conductive Regions

Dogs with tricuspid avulsion and pulmonary artery constriction.
The segments of the normal (control) right atrium near the point
where the sinus node artery enters the atrial myocardium (segments
9 and 13) had the highest choline acetyltransferase activity (Fig. 3)
and enzyme activity tended to decrease in segments away from these
two. When enzyme activity was expressed per unit weight of tissue,
values in most segments from heart failure dogs were significantly
lower (P<0.05) than corresponding sham (C) values. However, when

Table 2. Tyrosine Hydroxylase and Dopamine-β-Hydroxylase Activities in Hearts of Control and Heart Failure Dogs

	Right Atrium		Left Atrium		Right Ventricle		Left Ventricle	
	TH	DBH	TH	DBH	TH	DBH	TH	DBH
Control (nmol, g^{-1}, hr^{-1})	28.3 ±8.1	83 ±5	28.2 ±7.2	13 ±4	35.4 ±9.6	29 ±4	29.1 ±6.5	97 ±6
Heart Failure (nmol, g^{-1}, hr^{-1})	1.9*† ±1.1	43* ±8	26.6 ±2.6	19 ±4	5.2*† ±3.2	2*† ±1	3.1*† ±3	31* ±6
Control (nmol, chamber^{-1}, hr^{-1})	194 ±65	512 ±43	---	---	1677 ±312	1292 ±138	3972 ±928	13201 ±1644
Heart Failure (nmol, chamber^{-1}, hr^{-1})	23* ±13	429 ±94	---	---	307* ±158	9.7* ±9.2	411* ±409	3752* ±570

Each value is the mean ± SEM (n=7).

* Differs from Control, $P<0.05$.

† Estimate only; activity less than twice the blank lacking enzyme.

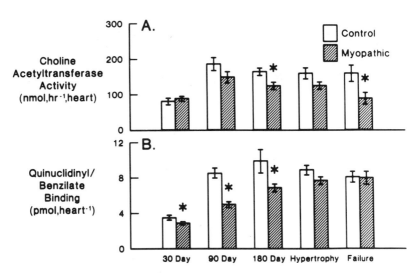

Fig. 2. Total cardiac a) choline acetyltransferase activity and
b) quinuclidinyl benzilate binding of control and cardiomyopathic hamsters at various ages. Hypertrophy and failure
groups were 290-360 days old. Each value represents the
mean ± SEM for at least 6 animals. (* Significantly different from control; P<0.05).

values were expressed per entire right atrium, choline acetyltransferase activity was similar (P>0.01) in sham and heart failure dogs
(1150±60 vs 1020±210 nmol, chamber^{-1}, hr^{-1}).

In order to assess the significance of reduced CAT activity per
unit weight of tissue, DBH activity in the same segments also was
measured (Fig. 4). Values of CAT and DBH activities in segments of
atria from heart failure dogs tended to be reduced to a similar
extent since the ratio of CAT activity to DBH activity decreased
slightly but not significantly in segments 2, 4, 5, 6, 7, 9, 11, and
13 of heart failure dogs when compared to control dogs; the ratio
increased slightly but not significantly in segments 3, 12, and 16
and increased markedly from 2.7 to 7.7 (P<0.05) only in segment 14,

Table 3. Norepinephrine Concentration, Tyrosine Hydroxylase Activity
and Choline Acetyltransferase Activity in Contractile Tissue
of Hearts of Guinea Pigs with Sham Surgery and Pulmonary
Artery Constriction (PAC)

	Right Ventricle		Left Ventricle	
	Sham (15)	PAC (16)	Sham (15)	PAC (16)
Norepinephrine (ng/g)	987 ±48	481* ±50	725 ±39	775 ±59
Tyrosine Hydroxylase Activity (nmol, vent^{-1}, hr^{-1})	73 ±8	29* ±3	97 ±6	100 ±12
Choline Acetyltransferase Activity (nmol, vent^{-1}, hr^{-1})	43 ±4	44 ±4	108 ±15	126 ±17

Values are means ± SEM.
Numbers in parentheses denote the number in each group.
* Differs from Control, $P < 0.05$.

which is clearly away from the SA node.

Guinea pigs with pulmonary artery constriction. Despite marked
right ventricular hypertrophy and evidence of hepatic congestion in
the animals with the most marked hypertrophy, CAT activity was maintained in samples from the regions of the SA node and the AV node
(Fig. 5). This was confirmed in a separate study (Table 5).

Muscarinic Cholinergic Receptors

Binding of [^{3}H]-quinuclidinyl benzilate (QNB) to homogenates
of hearts. Binding of [^{3}H]-QNB to myopathic hearts, like CAT
activity, was reduced compared to control hearts (Fig. 2) but the
time course of changes in [^{3}H]-QNB binding differed from the time
course of changes in CAT activity. When expressed in terms of whole
heart, the reductions in [^{3}H]-QNB binding were evident early (30, 90,
and 180 days) whereas, reductions in CAT activity were evident late
(180-360 days) (Fig. 2). Scatchard analysis of the binding data
suggested that the early reduction in [^{3}H]-QNB binding in myopathic
hearts was the result of a lower number of cholinergic muscarinic
receptors rather than an alteration in receptor affinity. The K_d
for QNB binding in myopathic and control hearts averaged 124±24 pmol
and 112±22 pmol, respectively, ($\bar{x}$±SE, $P > 0.1$, n=7).

In contrast to myopathic hearts where [^{3}H]-QNB binding appeared

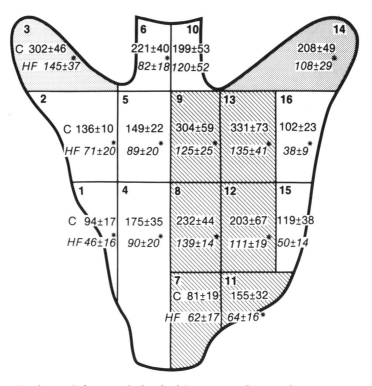

Fig. 3. Canine right atrial choline acetyltransferase activity
for Control (C) and Heart Failure (HF) dogs. Each value
represents the mean ± SEM for 7 animals.
* Significantly different from Control (P<0.05).
The atria were subdivided into segments as reported
previously (32).

reduced, the specialized regions of guinea pigs with pulmonary
artery constriction (Table 5) and the right and left ventricles of
dogs with tricuspid avulsion and pulmonary artery constriction
(Table 4) maintained similar levels of specific [^{3}H]-QNB binding
to those observed in the respective control groups.

Table 4.   Choline Acetyltransferase Activity and Quinuclidinyl Benzilate Binding in Hearts of Control and Heart Failure Dogs

	Right Ventricle		Left Ventricle	
	Control	Heart Failure	Control	Heart Failure
Choline Acetyltransferase Activity				
$(nmol, gm^{-1}, hr^{-1})$	83±7	61±5	51±5	47±5
$(nmol, chamber^{-1}, hr^{-1})$	3590±810	3557±745	6790±1019	5968±722
Quinuclidinyl Benzilate Binding				
$(fmol, mg\ prot^{-1})$	124±14	131±10	107±15	153±39
$(pmol, gm^{-1})$	16.8±1.8	15.9±1.9	14.6±1.7	17.3±31

Each value is the mean ± SEM.
There are no differences between control and heart failure dogs.

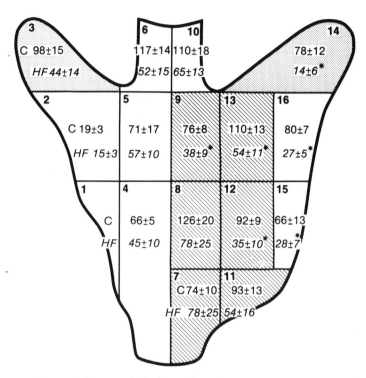

Fig. 4.   Canine right atrial dopamine-β-hydroxylase activity for
          Control (C) and Heart Failure (HF) dogs, Each value
          represents the mean ± SEM for 7 animals. (* Significantly
          different from Control; P<0,05).

DISCUSSION

    Syrian golden hamsters with cardiomyopathy and heart failure
had reductions in choline acetyltransferase activity, an index of
parasympathetic innervation, and reductions in [^{3}H]-QNB binding,
an index of cholinergic muscarinic receptors, The finding of

Table 5.   Choline Acetyltransferase Activity and Quinuclidinyl
            Benzilate Binding in Specialized Regions of the Hearts
            of Guinea Pigs with Sham Surgery and Pulmonary Artery
            Constriction (PAC)

	Choline Acetyltransferase Activity (nmol, gm^{-1}, hr^{-1})		Quinuclidinyl Benzilate Binding (pm, gm^{-1})	
	Sham (7)	PAC (7)	Sham (7)	PAC (7)
SA Node	114±19	114±12	16.9±2.9	12.7±2.8
AV Node	104±9	126±23	19.3±0.9	16.9±1.6
Prox Bundles	123±4	87±13	15.9±2.0	13.4±2.0

Values are means + SEM.
Numbers in parentheses denote the number in each group.
There are no differences between sham and PAC guinea pigs.

markedly impaired parasympathetic mechanisms in myopathic hearts is
distinctly different from the paucity of such changes in dogs with
pulmonary artery constriction and tricuspid avulsion and in guinea
pigs with pulmonary artery constriction. The results indicate,
therefore, that parasympathetic abnormalities, like sympathetic
abnormalities, vary with the experimental model of heart disease.

In all three models studied, the parasympathetic system was
affected differently than the sympathetic system. In the myopathic
heart, indices of sympathetic innervation increased, whereas those
of parasympathetic innervation decreased. In the stressed right
ventricles of dogs and guinea pigs, indices of sympathetic innervation decreased, whereas indices of parasympathetic innervation were
unchanged. The present results indicate first, that the response
of the parasympathetic nervous system in heart failure varies depending on the circumstances that cause the heart disease and second,
parasympathetic responses differ qualitatively from sympathetic
responses.

Since both adrenergic and cholinergic nerve terminals often
lie side by side in the same nerve separated only by their axonal
membranes (7), the selective decrease in only one of the neuronal
enzymes suggest that the reduction is due to damage of the individual
neurons and is not the result of generalized, chronic inshemia related to hypertrophy alone. In the hypertrophied heart of myopathic

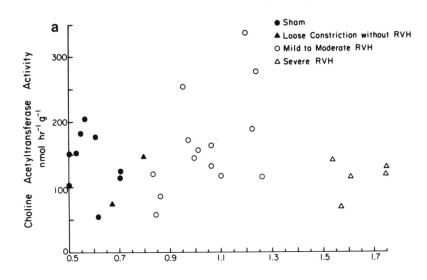

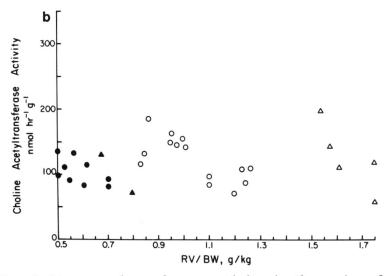

Fig. 5. Choline acetyltransferase activity in the region of the
        a) sinus node and b) atrio-ventricular node of guinea
        pigs. These values are expressed in terms of normalized
        right ventricular weights of the individual animal from
        which the samples were obtained.

hamsters where the adrenergic enzymes are increased, the changes
suggest that there is an adaptive augmentation of sympathetic
mechanisms. The factors responsible for these phenomena, however,
are as yet unknown.

The major reasons for evaluating indices of sympathetic innervation in this study were 1) to confirm that changes similar to those
previously reported (19,27-29) had occurred, and 2) to faciliate
a qualitative comparison between changes in sympathetic and parasympathetic innervation in each model. The major new information resulting from this study concerns the parasympathetic system and the
contrast between sympathetic and parasympathetic changes.

In myopathic hamsters, there were contrasts between the time
course of changes in indices of sympathetic innervation, DBH and
TH activities (Fig. 1), which seemed evident at all ages and indices
of parasympathetic innervation, CAT activity (Fig. 2), which seemed
to be reduced progressively in the myopathic hearts of older hamsters.
However, young myopathic hamsters had less than the normal complement
of cholinergic muscarinic receptors so that cholinergic and adrenergic
defects characterized the entire age range of myopathic hearts under
study (30-360 days).

Investigators have proposed that excessive sympathetic neural
activity damages the heart and leads to cardiomyopathy and heart
failure in the myopathic hamsters (3-5,27-31). Parasympathetic
defects (the early reductions in cholinergic muscarinic receptors and
the later reductions in choline acetyltransferase activity) might
contribute to a deleterious influence of sympathetic overactivity by
virtue of impaired cholinergic modulation of this influence. The
present data do not directly support this speculation, but they do
indicate a need to explore this possibility further since cardiac
disease is a common feature of muscular dystrophy.

Choline acetyltransferase activity and the binding of [^{3}H]-QNB
were maintained per unit weight in specialized pacemaking and conductive tissues of guinea pigs with pulmonary artery constriction
(Table 5). These variables also were maintained per mg protein,
and per unit weight, in the right and left ventricles of dogs with
tricuspid avulsion and pulmonary artery constriction (Table 4).
However, in various segments of the right atria of heart failure dogs,
the activity of CAT per unit weight was decreased significantly
compared to the values in control dogs. These reductions are consistent with an increase in the mean interval between nerve fibers
such as has been observed for sympathetic fibers in hypertrophied
heart chambers (7) and they suggest the possibility that there may
be important alterations in the relationship of parasympathetic
innervation to effector sites in the stressed right atria of some
pressure-and volume-induced heart failure preparations, as well as
in the myopathic hamster model of heart failure. This possibility
merits further investigation.

The major findings in this study are different heart failure models have disparate changes in cardiac sympathetic and parasympathetic innervation. The striking observation was that biochemical indices of parasympathetic innervation and cholinergic muscarinic receptors are both reduced significantly in the hearts of Syrian golden hamsters with skeletal myopathy and cardiomyopathy. The possibility that impaired parasympathetic mechanisms contribute to augmented sympathetic mechanisms and the pathogenesis of heart disease in this hamster model is raised by these results and should be investigated in the future.

ACKNOWLEDGMENTS

We thank Alberto Subieta, James Johannsen, Janine Davis, Robert Oda, and Carol Whiteis for technical assistance and Lisa Jo Lowenberg for secretarial assistance.

This work was supported by Grants HL-20768, HL-24246, and Program Project Grant HL-14388 from the U.S. Public Health Service and a Grant from the Veterans Administration.

REFERENCES

1.   Afifi, A.A., and Azen, S.P. Statistical Analysis: A Computer Oriented Approach. Academic Press, New York, p 75 (1972).
2.   Anderson, R.H. The disposition, morphology and innervation of cardiac specialized tissue in the guinea pig. Journal of Anatomy 111, 453 (1972).
3.   Angelakos, E.T., King, M.P., and Carballo, L. Cardiac adrenergic innervation in hamsters with hereditary myocardiopathy: chemical and histochemical studies. In Recent Advances in Studies on Cardiac Structure and Metabolism, vol. 2, edited by E. Bajusz, and G. Rona. Baltimore, University Park Press, pp 529-532 (1973).
4.   Bajusz, E., Homburger, F., Baker, J.R., and Opie, L.H. The heart muscle in muscular dystrophy with special reference to involvement of the cardiovascular system in the hereditary myopathy of the hamster. Annals of the New York Academy of Science 138, 213-231 (1966).
5.   Bajusz, E., Homburger, F., Baker, J.R., and Bogdonoff, P. Dissociation of factors influencing myocardial degeneration and generalized circulatory failure. Annals of New York Academy of Science 156, 396-420 (1969).
6.   Barger, A.C., Roc, B.B., and Richardson, G.S. Relations of valvular lesions and of exercise to auricular pressure, work tolerance, and to development of chronic congestive failure

in dogs. American Journal of Physiology 169, 384-399 (1952).

7.   Borchard, F. The adrenergic nerves of the normal and hyper-
     trophied heart. In Normal and Pathological Anatomy, Vol. 33,
     edited by W. Bargmann and W. Doerr, P.S.G. Publishing Company,
     Inc., Massachusetts, pp 1-68.

8.   Chidsey, C.A., Kaiser, G.A., Sonnenblick, E.H., Spann, J.F.
     Jr., and Braunwald, E. Cardiac norepinephrine stores in ex-
     perimental heart failure in dogs. Journal of Clinical Investi-
     gation 43, 2389-2393 (1964).

9.   Covell, J.W., Chidsey, C.A., and Braunwald, E. Reduction of
     cardiac response to postganglionic sympathetic nerve stimulation
     in experimental heart failure. Circulation Research 19, 51-56
     (1966).

10. Coyle, J.T. Tyrosine hydroxylase in rat brain. Cofactor
     requirments, regional and subcellular distribution. Biochemical
     Pharmacology 21, 1935-1944 (1972).

11. Coyle, J.T., and Axelrod, J. Dopamine-β-hydroxylase in the rat
     brain. Developmental characteristics.Journal of Neurochemistry
     19, 449-459 (1972).

12. Crockatt, L.H., Lund, D.D., Schmid, P.G., and Roskoski, R. Jr.
     Hypoxia-induced changes in parasympathetic neurochemical
     markers in guinea pig heart. Journal of Applied Physiology:
     Respiration Environmental Exercise Physiology 50, 1017-1021
     (1981).

13. Eckberg, D.L., Drabinsky, M., and Braunwald, E. Defective
     cardiac parasympathetic control in patients with heart disease.
     New England Journal of Medicine 285, 877-883 (1971).

14. Galper, J.G., Klein, W., and Catterall, W.A. Muscarinic acetyl-
     choline receptor in developing chick heart. Journal of Biologi-
     cal Chemistry 252, 8692-8699 (1977).

15. Higgins, C.B., Vatner, S.F., Eckberg, D.L., and Braunwald, E.
     Alterations in the baroreceptor reflex in conscious dogs with
     heart failure. Journal of Clinical Investigation 51, 715-724
     (1972).

16. Lowry, O.H., Rosebrough, N.J., Farr, A.L., and Randall, R.J.
     Protein measurement with folin phenol reagent. Journal of
     Biological Chemistry 193, 265-275 (1951).

17. Lund, D.D., Schmid, P.G., Kelley, S.E., Corry, R.J., and
     Roskoski, R. Jr. Choline acetyltransferase activity in rat
     heart after transplantation. American Journal of Physiology
     235, H367-H371 (1978).

18. Lund, D.D., Schmid, P.G., Johannsen, U.J., and Roskoski, R. Jr.
     Biochemical indices of cholinergic and adrenergic autonomic
     innervation in dog heart: Disparate alterations in chronic
     right heart failure. Journal of Molecular and Cellular
     Cardiology (In press).

19. Pool, P.E., Covell, J.W., Levitt, M., Gibb, J., and Braunwald,
     E. Reduction of cardiac tyrosine hydroxylase activity in ex-
     perimental congestive heart failure. Circulation Research
     20, 349-353 (1967).

20. Roskoski, R. Jr., Mayer, H.E., and Schmid, P.G. Choline acetyltransferase activity in guinea pig in vitro. Journal of Neurochemistry 23, 1197–1200, 1974.

21. Roskoski, R. Jr., Schmid, P.G., Mayer, H.E., and Abboud, F.M. In vitro acetylcholine biosynthesis in normal and failing guinea pig hearts. Circulation Research 36, 547–552 (1975).

22. Schmid, P.G., Mayer, H.E., Mark, A.L., Heistad, D.D., and Abboud, F.M. Differences in the regulation of vascular resistance in guinea pigs with right and left heart failure. Circulation Research 41, 85–93 (1977).

23. Schmid, P.G., Greif, B.J., Lund, D.D., and Roskoski, R. Jr. Regional choline acetyltransferase activity in guinea pig heart. Circulation Research 42, 657–660 (1978).

24. Schmid, P.G., Lund, D.D., and Roskoski, R. Jr. Efferent autonomic dysfunction in heart failure. In Disturbances in Neurogenic Control of Circulation. Edited by F.M. Abboud, H.A. Fozzard, J.P. Gilmore, and D.J. Reis, Bethesda: American Physiological Society, pp 33–49 (1981).

25. Schmid, P.G., Lund, D.D., Davis, J.A., Whiteis, C.A., Bhatnagar, R.K., and Roskoski, R. Jr. Selective sympathetic neural changes in hypertrophied right ventricle. American Journal of Physiology (In press).

26. Schmidt, R.H., and Bhatnagar, R.K. Regional development of norepinephrine, dopamine-β-hydroxylase, and tyrosine hydroxylase in the rat brain subsequent to neonatal treatment with subcutaneous 6-hydroxydopamine. Brain Research 166, 293–308 (1979).

27. Sole, M.J., Lo, C., Liard, C.W., Sonnenblick, E.H., and Wurtman, R.J. Norepinephrine turnover in the heart and spleen of the cardiomyopathic Syrian hamster. Circulation Research 37, 855–862 (1975).

28. Sole, M.J., Wurtman, R.J., Lo, C.M., Ramble, A.B., and Sonnenblick, E.H. Tyrosine hydroxylase activity in the heart of the cardiomyopathic Syrian hamster. Journal of Molecular and Cellular Cardiology 9, 225–233, (1977).

29. Sole, M.J., and Hussain, M.N. A possible change in the rate-limiting step for cardiac norepinephrine synthesis in the cardiomyopathic Syrian hamster. Circulation Research 41, 814–817 (1977).

30. Spann, J.F. Jr., Chidsey, C.A., Pool, P.E., and Braunwald, E. Mechanisms of norepinephrine depletion in experimental heart failure produced by aortic constriction in the guinea pig. Circulation Research 17, 312–321 (1965).

31. Strobeck, J.E., Factor, S.M., Ghan, A., Sole, M., Liew, C.C., Fein, F., and Sonnenblick, E.H. Hereditary and acquired cardiomyopathies in experimental animals: Mechanical, biochemical, and structural features. Annals of New York Academy of Science 317, 59–88 (1979).

32. White, C.W., Marcus, M.L., and Abboud, F.M. Distribution of coronary artery flow to the canine right atrium and sino-atrial node. Circulation Research 40, 342–347 (1977).

MECHANICAL AND CONTRACTILE PROPERTIES OF ISOLATED SINGLE INTACT

CARDIAC CELLS

Merrill Tarr

University of Kansas College of Health Sciences

Kansas City, KS 66103

INTRODUCTION

During the last 20 years a great deal of effort has been expended attempting to define cardiac muscle contractile performance in terms of the performance of the sarcomere within the cardiac muscle. The early studies of cardiac contractile performance assessed sarcomere performance indirectly due to the inherent difficulties of directly visualizing the sarcomeres in most intact cardiac preparations. In order to assign certain contractile properties (e.g., force and velocity) of the intact tissue to the so-called contractile element (i.e., sarcomere) within the tissue it was necessary to use mechanical equivalent models (the so-called Maxwell or Voigt models) composed of a contractile element and at least two elastic elements: parallel and series elastic. By the mid 1970's it was generally accepted that such attempts to deduce sarcomere performance from whole tissue performance would yield questionable results due to 1) the uncertainties in quantitating the physical properties of the intact tissue as represented by equivalent series and parallel elastic elements, 2) the inability of any unique mechanical model to represent both the static and dynamic contractile properties of heart muscle, and 3) the dramatic nonuniformities in the distribution of structures (elastic and contractile) within the intact muscle.

Clearly, one definitive way to assess cardiac sarcomere performance would be to measure directly the lengths of sarcomeres within intact preparations. Such measurements, however, necessitate the use of very thin preparations. Two laboratories

199

in the mid 1970's initiated the application of laser diffraction
techniques to thin intact bundles of frog [17] or rat [15] cardiac
tissue to directly assess the average sarcomere length within
relatively large groups of sarcomeres. These experiments gave
both interesting and somewhat unexpected results. First, they
demonstrated that the performance of the observed sarcomeres
within the tissue can bear little relation to overall muscle
performance. For example, when the intact tissue undergoes a so-
called isometric contraction (i.e., overall tissue length does
not change) the sarcomeres in the central region shorten by as
much as 10-15% and extend those in other regions of the tissue.
Thus, the central sarcomeres are actually developing force auxotonically rather than isometrically. Second, they demonstrated
that the sarcomeres in the central region shorten at a rather
constant velocity even though force is increasing dramatically.
In discussing these results, Manring et al. [16] emphasized that
some uncertainty will always exist in defining the force-length
and force-velocity relationships of sarcomeres within intact
multicellular preparations simply due to uncertainties regarding
the distribution of the total external force among the cells,
connective tissue, and elastic tissue which comprise the tissue.
Manring et al. [16] emphasized that "the ultimate solution to the
problem can lie only in the simplification of the experimental
preparation".

The simplest intact preparation, of course, is the single
intact isolated cardiac cell. My laboratory as well as several
other laboratories have been involved over the last 5-7 years in
developing the technology by which the mechanical and contractile
properties of the single cardiac cell and the sarcomeres within
the cell can be investigated. The purpose of this paper is to
summarize the progress that has been made in this endeavor as well
as to summarize what the single cell studies have shown concerning the mechanical and contractile properties of the cardiac
sarcomere. The literature cited in this paper is not meant to be
exhaustive, but rather it is intended to direct the reader to
representative papers dealing with the topics discussed.

METHODS

A variety of enzymatic dispersion techniques using various
combinations of trypsin, collagenase and hyaluronidase have been
used to prepare isolated single cardiac cells. Early attempts to
prepare single mammalian heart cells generally produced cells
that were spontaneously active and which went into contracture
when exposed to physiological calcium concentrations [1,2,28].
Fabiato and Fabiato [8] showed that the spontaneous beating cells

did not have intact cell membranes and stated that one criterion of a healthy intact cardiac cell should be that it is quiescent in the presence of low calcium. The cells should also, of course, be relaxed and quiescent at physiological extracellular calcium concentrations. Mammalian cardiac cells can now be prepared which satisfy these criteria [3,7,14], although the yield of such cells is relatively low (10-50%). Fabiato [7] indicates that one major factor for increasing the cells tolerance to calcium is to increase the extracellular calcium concentration gradually so as to favor a decrease in membrane permeability and a healing over of the intercalated discs. In contrast to mammalian cells, isolated frog atrial cells can be obtained in high yields (~70% or greater) relatively simply by digesting minced atrial tissue with either trypsin alone [25] or a combination of trypsin and collagenase [11,22].

The isolated mammalian cardiac cell and frog atrial cell are dimensionally different. The mammalian cell has a length on the order of 100 μm and is somewhat rectangular in cross-section being approximately 20 μm wide and 12 μm deep [7,14]. In contrast, the single frog atrial cell [11,22] is quite long (300-500 μm) and thin (3-5 μm dia). Thus, the mammalian cell contains many more myofibrils (~16-20) than the frog atrial cell (~1-2). The limited number of myofibrils in the frog atrial cell is advantageous, since the total external force is distributed between a very limited number of parallel myofibrillar elements. We have observed that the sarcomere performance is uniform across the width of the frog atrial cell indicating that the total force is distributed equally between the parallel myofibrils. Thus, the force at the sarcomere level is relatively well defined in the single frog atrial cell. In contrast to the frog cardiac cell, the force is distributed between approximately 20 parallel myofibrils in the mammalian cell and the force at the sarcomere level is defined only if the force is uniformly distributed between the myofibrils.

Both the mammalian and frog cells have some common instrumentation requirements regarding the investigation of the contractile and mechanical properties of these cells and the sarcomere performance within the cell. First, it must be possible to attach to the cell in order to measure force. Second, it must be possible to measure the relatively small forces developed by the cell. Third, it must be possible to directly measure sarcomere lengths within the cell.

Attachment to the single cell poses the problem that it must be nondestructive; thus, clamping to the cell's ends is precluded. Attachment to the single frog atrial cell can be accomplished simply by contacting the cell surface with a poly-L-lysine coated glass beam [26]. Such an attachment does not appear to damage the cell and is strong enough to withstand the maximum forces developed by the frog cell provided the cell is secured to the beam by wrapping the cell once or twice around the beam. The polylysine method does not appear to work for the mammalian cell presumably because the attachment is not strong enough to withstand the large forces developed by the mammalian cell. At present two other attachment techniques have been used and neither is entirely satisfactory. Brady et al. [3] have used suction pipettes to hold on to single rat heart cells but can do so only when the force generated by the cell is reduced by low extracellular calcium. Fabiato [7] has attached to mammalian cells by forcing microtools into damaged cells which are attached to each end of a healthy cell which is electrically but not mechanically uncoupled from the damaged cells. The success rate of this procedure is extremely low (<10%), but it does allow the investigation of the contractile performance of the cell at normal extracellular calcium concentrations.

Several techniques have been developed for the measurement of force from the single cardiac cells. Fabiato [9] uses a photodiode force transducer in which the deflection of the force member is sensed by a change in light intensity on a pair of photodiodes. The lever arm of the transducer is attached to the cell via a glass microtool. This tranducer system has a compliance on the order of 2 μm/mg and is useful in resolving forces in excess of 10 μg (~100 nN). Since the maximum tension which can be developed by the mammalian cardiac cell is on the order of 2.5 mg [7], the force developed by a 100 μm long cell can be measured under relatively isometric conditions (<10% cell shortening). Brady et al. [3] also use a photodiode system to detect motion of the force beam but attach the cell to the force beam by suction pipettes which add considerable mass and therefore inertia to the transducer system. The frequency response of these photodiode transducer systems can be quite low (~5 Hz) making them unsuitable for investigating rapid changes in force. It would be expected that a frog atrial cell would develop only about 5% of the force developed by the mammalian cardiac cell due to the decreased amount of myofibrillar material. To measure these small forces Tarr et al. [26] have used a relatively compliant (0.1-0.5 μm/nN) glass beam as a cantilevered force beam. The displacement of this beam by the cell as it shortens and develops force is monitored microscopically and recorded by a closed circuit TV-videotape system. The frame-by-frame analysis of the videotape allows the determination of force at time intervals of 16.67 msec. One advantage of this system is that the relatively light glass beam does not introduce any significant acceleration components into the force measurement as indicated by the observation that when the end of a typical force beam is deflected by as much as 50 μm and released the beam returns to its unloaded position and is stable within 16.67 msec (unpublished observation). Thus, the force beam when driven by its own restoring force has a free velocity in excess of 3000 μm/sec which is significantly greater than the force beam velocities of 500 μm/sec or less which occur during a typical contraction. Thus, the force supported by the cell is primarily determined by the force beam compliance and deflection and not by acceleration force or viscous drag. However, one disadvantage of using a very compliant force measuring device is that considerable shortening (10-30%) of the cell can occur during contraction, and the simultaneous changes in force and length can complicate the interpretation of the data.

The determination of sarcomere lengths within the single cell can be accomplished using either laser diffraction techniques or direct imaging techniques. The laser diffraction technique has been successfully applied to single rat heart cells [14], but whether or not it can be successfully applied to the frog atrial cell containing limited myofibrillar material remains to be determined. Direct imaging of the sarcomere pattern can be accomplished by projecting the sarcomere pattern on to some form of a photosensitive device be it a television camera tube [26], a linear array of photosensitive charge coupled devices, [21] or film. Each of these techniques has advantages and disadvantages. The laser diffraction technique has the advantage that computation of sarcomere length can be done rapidly with appropriate electronic circuitry thereby producing an electronic signal which is related to sarcomere length. This allows essentially on-line analysis during the course of the experiment. In contrast direct imaging techniques generally require off-line analysis following the experiment by techniques which can be extremely time consuming. For example, the frame-by-frame analysis of either video taped or filmed data is extremely tedious and time consuming. Computerized analysis of direct imaged data is possible [21] but can be expensive to implement as it requires not only high speed computing capabilities but also requires the development of extensive software for the management of data acquisition, storage, retrival and analysis. One distinct advantage of the direct imaging technique, however, is that it allows the analysis of the performance of relatively small groups of sarcomeres within the cell and therefore a fairly detailed analysis of contractile homogeneity within the cell. In contrast, the laser diffraction technique determines the average length of the sarcomeres in the entire length of the cell although the dispersion of the diffraction pattern can be used to gain some information concerning sarcomere length homogeneity.

One concern that has been raised regarding direct imaging techniques is that the time intervals between successive measurements during the contraction may be relatively long. For example, a conventional TV-videotape system such as that used by Tarr et al. [26] has a time resolution of 16.67 msec. This time resolution, however, is not excessive when considered in light of the time required for an accurately detectable change in sarcomere length to occur as measured over the length occupied by a small population (6-10) of sarcomeres. This detectable length change is in effect equal to the resolving power (R.P.) of the optical system which in this case is primarily determined by the resolving power of the light microscrope optics used to view the sarcomeres. The resolving power expresses the ability of the optical system to discriminate between two objects and gives the minimum separation at which two objects can be seen as separate entities. Similarly, a single object or the distance between two objects (e.g., the total length occupied by a group of sarcomeres) must change by this minimum separation for this change in distance to be accurately measured. The time (t) required for this minimum length change to occur is given simply by the equation $t = R.P./nV$ where n = the number of sarcomeres over which the length change occurs and V = the average sarcomere velocity. If R.P. = 0.5 μm (a typical value for a light microscope at relatively high magnification), n = 10, and V = 2.5 μm/sec then t = 20 msec which is on the same order as the 16.67 msec time resolution.

RESULTS

Excitability Properties

There is now a variety of experimental evidence which indicates that the enzymatic dispersion techniques used to prepare single cardiac cells can produce isolated single cells having an intact excitable membrane. Tarr et al. [25] assessed the excitability properties of their isolated frog atrial cells by determining the characteristics of the contractile response of the cells to electrical stimulation. They found that the cells responded to a short duration (1-10 msec) electrical stimulus with an all-or-none contractile response. The threshold stimulus strength-stimulus duration relationship for the frog atrial cell was described by the Lapicque-Hill equation (an equation that adequately described the strength-duration relationship of a variety of excitable tissue) having a time constant of 15 msec.

Also, tetrodotoxin shifted the strength-duration relationship as expected if the excitatory response of the single frog atrial cell depended on the fast inward sodium current. The conclusion drawn by Tarr et al. [25] that the isolated frog atrial cell has normal excitability properties has been confirmed recently by direct measurements of transmembrane potentials from single frog atrial cells by Hume and Giles [11]. These investigators found that these cells had normal resting potentials (-88 mv) and produced normal long duration (~720 msec) action potentials in response to electrical stimulation. Furthermore, the upstroke velocity of the action potential was significantly tetrodotoxin sensitive. The membrane time constant of 20±7 msec found by Hume and Giles was also similar to that predicted from the strength-duration relationship reported by Tarr et al. [25]. Intra-cellular potential measurements have also been obtained on single mammalian cardiac cells which demonstrate that these isolated cells can also have normal resting potentials and normal action potentials [19].

Unloaded velocity of sarcomere shortening and lengthening

The single cardiac cell provides an opportunity to investigate sarcomere shortening and lengthing during contraction and relaxation at essentially zero external force. Such an investigation is of interest in light of the question of whether or not the ability of muscle to shorten at zero external force is independent of its ability to generate force. To answer this question one generally determines if sarcomere shortening velocity at zero external force (V_o) depends on sarcomere length or the level of contractile activation. In this regard, Edman [5] has recently demonstrated in intact skeletal muscle that V_o is independent of sarcomere length over a range of 1.7 μm to about 2.8 μm. Also Edman found that depression of the force generating capacity of the muscle by the drug dantrolene (a drug which apparently reduces calcium release from the sarcoplasmic reticulum) did not alter V_o. These results suggest that V_o in intact skeletal muscle is neither activation-dependent nor sarcomere length-dependent. In contrast, other investigators [12] have presented evidence indicating that V_o in skinned skeletel muscle is calcium dependent and would, therefore, be activation-dependent.

Tarr et al. [25] investigated the characteristics of sarcomere shortening in single frog atrial cells and found that under very lightly loaded conditions (external forces < 10 nN) the cardiac sarcomere shortened with relatively constant velocity down to sarcomere lengths as short as 1.6-1.7 μm. Typical examples of sarcomere shortening and lengthening at light loads (< 10 nN) are shown in Figure 1. We have recently confirmed the

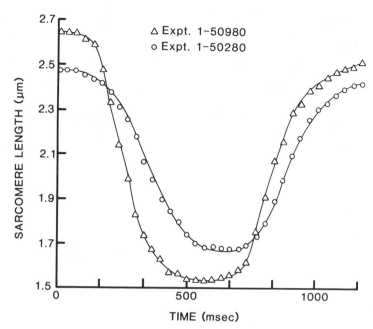

Fig. 1.   Sarcomere   length-time   relationships   during   lightly
           loaded twitch contractions in two cells.   The perfor-
           mance of a group of ten sarcomeres was analyzed in each
           experiment.   The   maximum   velocities   of   sarcomere
           shortening were 4.2 μm/sec (Expt. 1-50980) and 2.2
           μm/sec (Expt. 1-50280). Maximum lengthening velocities
           were 4.1 μm/sec and 2.7 μm/sec.

finding of a constant velocity of sarcomere shortening down to
sarcomere lengths as short as 1.6-1.7 μm under truely unloaded
conditions by allowing the frog atrial cell to take up various
amounts of slack (unpublished observation). Krueger et al. [14]
have also reported similar results in isolated rat cardiac cells
in which the cells were unattached and therefore the external
forces on the cell were essentially zero.   The finding of a
constant sarcomere velocity down to sarcomere lengths as short as
1.6-1.7 μm is different than that observed in rat papillary
muscle where Pollack and Krueger [18] found that the velocity of
sarcomere shortening under very lightly loaded conditions
decreased markedly at sarcomere lengths below 2.0 μm.   For
example, they found that the velocity at a sarcomere length of 1.8
μm was only 30% that at a sarcomere length of 2.2 μm.

However, the finding of a constant V_o over a wide range of sarcomere lengths does not necessarily mean that V_o is independent of either length or the level of activation. In fact, it can easily be demonstrated that a constant V_o can occur under conditions where V_o is highly length- and time- dependent. An example of this is shown in Figure 2 which gives a simulated unloaded contraction in which the sarcomere velocity (V) is defined at all times by the equation $V=bP_o/a$. The b-variable and a-variable are time- and length-independent in this simulation and, therefore the unloaded velocity has the same length and time dependency as the force generating capacity (P_o) of the sarcomere. The figure gives the sarcomere length-time relationship (left half) and isochronal V_o-sarcomere length relationships at 16.67 msec time intervals (right half). The point of interest is that for a considerable period of time the sarcomere shortens at relatively constant velocity (7 ± 1 μm/sec) even though at any instant V_o is highly length-dependent. Thus a constant velocity phase for V_o could result from offsetting length-and time- dependent alterations in P_o.

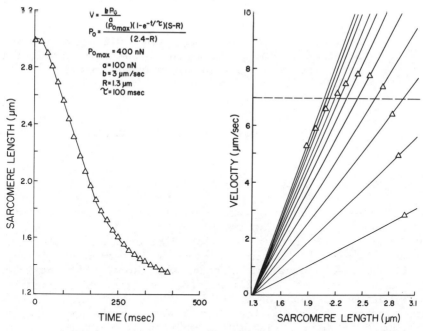

Fig. 2   Time course of sarcomere shortening (left) and length dependency of sarcomere velocity at time intervals of 16.67 msec (right) during a simulated contraction at zero external force. The computations were done by computer using Euler's iterative method.

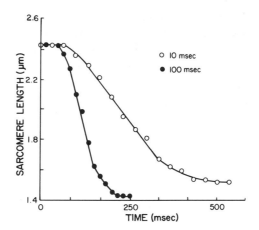

Fig. 3   Sarcomere length-time relationships in one cell during
          lightly loaded twitch contractions elicited by constant
          current   stimulation   at   two   different   stimulus
          durations.   The performance of the same group of ten
          sarcomeres was analyzed in each experiment.

A time-dependent V_o would occur if V_o were activation-
dependent provided the activation effect on V_o developed slowly
during the twitch contraction. Both Tarr et al. [25] and Krueger
et al. [14] found that the velocity of sarcomere shortening at
small   or   zero   external   forces   was   apparently   activation
dependent. Tarr et al. [25] altered the level of activation by
using different duration stimuli.   Short duration stimuli (10
msec) produced lightly loaded sarcomere shortening velocities
ranging from about 1-5 μm/sec, whereas long duration stimuli
produced velocities as high as 12 μm/sec. A typical example of
the stimulus effect on the time course of sarcomere shortening
under lightly loaded conditions is shown in Figure 3.   In this
example, the constant velocity for the 10 msec duration stimulus
was 3.1 μm/sec compared to a velocity of 9.7 μm/sec for the 100
msec stimulus. Krueger et al. [14] reported unloaded velocities

on the order of 9 μm/sec when the rat cardiac cells were exposed to 1 mM $CaCl_2$ and of about 3.7 μm/sec when they were exposed to 0.5 mM $CaCl_2$. These data strongly suggest that V_o in cardiac muscle is activation-dependent. However, these findings do not force the conclusion that V_o is also length-dependent, since it is possible that the activation time course of V_o (a reflection of myosin ATPase activity) is different than that for the force-generating capacity (a reflection of the number of attached cross-bridges) of the sarcomere. A definitive conclusion requires more information concerning the time-dependency of V_o. Regardless of interpretation, the data of Tarr et al. [25] and Krueger et al. [14] indicate that the V_o of the enzymatically prepared single cardiac cell ranging from about 1-4 initial muscle lengths/sec is not impaired relative to what would be predicted from studies on nonenzymatically treated intact muscle.

Figure 1 also demonstrates an interesting and consistent finding concerning sarcomere extension during relaxation. That is, sarcomere extension during relaxation occurs at high velocity even when external forces are negligible. Krueger et al. [14] reported a similar finding in isolated rat heart cells which were unattached. The finding that sarcomere length returns during relaxation to its rest length in the absence of significant external force indicates that an intracellular restoring force must be present. This internal force may also help explain a constant velocity phase of unloaded shortening which is activation-dependent. If we assume that sarcomere velocity is defined by Hill's force-velocity equation then in the presence of an internal force (P_i) the unloaded sarcomere velocity (V_o) would be given by the equation $V_o = b(P_o - P_i)/(P_i + a)$. In this case a constant V_o could occur if the time-dependent increase in P_o were offset by a length dependent increase in P_i which occurs with sarcomere shortening below rest length. Computer simulations (unpublished) indicate that this could be the case.

Force Generating Capacity

At present there have been only a few measurements of the force generating capacity of single mammalian cardiac cells. Brady et al. [3] reported peak twitch forces in rat heart cells on the order of 9 μN. Fabiato [7] reported a value on the order of 17 μN for single rat heart cells and 5 μN for single rabbit heart cells. The fully activated skinned heart cell (both rat and rabbit) developed a force on the order of 25 μN. The cross-sectional area of the mammalian cell is on the order of 200 $μm^2$. Thus, the maximum force generating capacity of the fully activated mammalian cardiac cell is on the order of 125 $nN/μm^2$; a value typical of striated muscle (1 kg/cm^2 = 98 $nN/μm^2$). Twitch forces would appear to be on the order of 20% (in rabbit) to 70% (in rat) of the fully activated force. A twitch stress of 88

$nN/\mu m^2$ (i.e., 70% of 125 $nN/\mu m^2$) would be similar to the 75 $nN/\mu m^2$ value reported by Julian and Sollins [13] for maximum twitch force from intact rat papillary muscle.

Figure 4 shows typical sarcomere length vs. time and force vs. time relationships obtained on a single frog atrial cell during an auxotonic twitch. This cell developed a peak force of about 185 nN. Typical values of peak auxotonic force range from as low as 100 nN to as high as 800 nN depending to some extent on the compliance of the force beam to which the cell is attached. At a typical peak force of 300 nN, the frog atrial cell would be developing a stress of about 24 $nN/\mu m^2$. This value is similar to the values of about 10-30 $nN/\mu m^2$ which can be computed from data obtained on intact frog atrial tissue as presented by Manring et al. [16]. Thus, it would appear that single cardiac cells (both frog atrial and mammalian) prepared by enzymatic dispersion of intact tissue are capable of generating typical stresses characteristic of striated muscle and thus the force generating capacity of these cells appears to be normal.

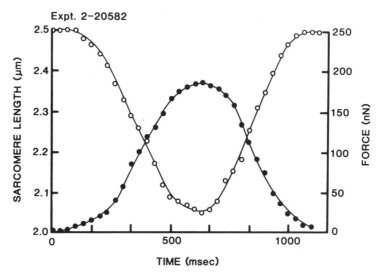

Fig. 4   Sarcomere length-time and force-time relationships during an auxotonic contraction. The performance of a group of ten sarcomeres was analyzed in this experiment. The maximum shortening velocity was 1.3 $\mu m/sec$ and the maximum lengthening velocity was 1.4 $\mu m/sec$.

Figure 4 also demonstrates that the time course of the change in the average sarcomere length as computed for a population of sarcomeres (in this case 10) within the tissue is quite similar to the time course of auxotonic force change. Since in this type of experiment there is a direct relationship between the rate of change of force and the average sarcomere velocity within the region of cell between the points of attachment to the beams, the finding of similar time courses for sarcomere length changes and auxotonic force suggest that sarcomere performance is homogeneous over the length of the cell. This figure also demonstrates the consistent finding that sarcomere shortening during auxotonic contraction can occur at constant velocity even though force is increasing dramatically. This result is similar to that found by Nassar et al. [17] and Krueger and Pollack [15] on intact cardiac tissue. Computer simulations by Tarr et al. [27] demonstrated that a constant sarcomere shortening velocity in the face of increasing force can occur if the cardiac sarcomere has a time-dependent Hill type force-velocity relationship. In this case the constant velocity phase results from the time-dependent increase in P_o being offset by the decrease in P_o which occurs with sarcomere shortening. The experimental results of Tarr et al. [27] clearly demonstrated that sarcomere shortening velocity in the single cardiac cell is force-dependent as evidenced by the observations that 1) the velocity of sarcomere shortening in a given cell was greater during a very lightly loaded contraction than during an auxotonic contraction in which the cell developed significant force, 2) during auxotonic contractions in which a given cell contracted against an adjustable compliance force beam the sarcomere velocity decreased as the compliance of the beam decreased, and 3) quick release of a cell to a very light load during an auxotonic contraction resulted in an immediate increase in sarcomere velocity. These observations clearly indicate that the cardiac sarcomere has some type of a force-velocity relationship.

Force-Sarcomere Length Relationships

The single cardiac cell can provide an opportunity to determine the active and resting force-length relationships over a wide range of sarcomere lengths. Figure 5 gives typical examples of total force (open symbols) and resting force (closed symbols) obtained from three frog atrial cells.

The resting force-sarcomere length relationship of the single frog atrial cell has two important features: 1) the resting sarcomere length of the single frog atrial cell is on the order of 2.2-2.4 μm even when external force is zero, and 2) the resting cell is very compliant and can be extended to sarcomere lengths in excess of 3.0 μm with very little force. As discussed

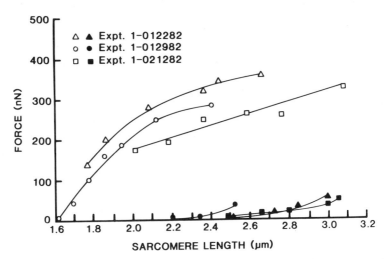

Fig. 5   Sarcomere length-force relations obtained on three
          cells: resting force (filled symbols), peak total force
          (unfilled symbols).   The performance of a group of
          seven sarcomeres was analyzed in each experiment.

by Tarr et al. [26], the resting stress in the single frog atrial
cell at a sarcomere length of 2.6 μm is generally on the order of
1 nN/μm^2 which is approximately thirty-fold less than that found
in intact frog atrial tissue [29].   Thus, in the case of frog
atrial tissue, it appears that the individual cardiac cells are
responsible for very little of the resting stiffness characteristic of the intact tissue.

     The relationship between peak total force developed
auxotonically and the sarcomere length at peak force can be
obtained over a range of sarcomere lengths by a combination of
initiating the contraction from different sarcomere lengths above
the normal rest length and by allowing the cell to take up various
amounts of slack prior to auxotonic force development.   The
typical results presented in Figure 5 obtained from three cells
demonstrate that the total force-sarcomere length relationship
increases up to sarcomere lengths of at least 2.8-3 μm: see also
Tarr et al. [24].   This finding indicates that the single frog
atrial cell operates during a twitch on the ascending limb of an
isometric force (P_o)-sarcomere length relationship up to
sarcomere lengths on the order of 3 μm. This result is similar to
that which has been reported for 1) twitch contractions in
skeletal muscle [4,20], and 2) for partially activated skinned

cardiac [10] and skinned skeletal muscle cells [6]. The finding of such an ascending P_o-sarcomere length relationship indicates that contractile activation in cardiac muscle is sarcomere length dependent and supports the concept that length-dependent changes in contractile activation may play a major role in the improved contractile performance which accompanies increased ventricular filling (i.e., Starling's Law of the Heart).

At present there is very little available information concerning the force-sarcomere length relationships of intact single mammalian cardiac cells. The quiescent single rat heart cell [3,14] does, however, have a significantly shorter resting sarcomere length (~1.9 μm) than the frog atrial cell (~2.4 μm). The resting rat heart cell also appears to be considerably stiffer than the resting frog atrial cell. Brady et al. [3] reported a value of 3 nN/μm^2 for the resting stress of the rat cell at a sarcomere length of 1.9 μm. Fabiato and Fabiato [10] reported that the resting tension in skinned rat cardiac cells increased considerably more steeply with increasing sarcomere length than that in skinned frog cardiac cells. The data presented by Fabiato and Fabiato [10] indicates that the resting tension of the rat cell at a sarcomere length of 2.2 μm is about 5% of the maximum active tension. If we assume a maximum active stress of 125 nN/μm^2, then the resting stress would be on the order of 6 nN/μm^2. At a sarcomere length of 2.6 μm this value would increase to approximately 41 nN/μm^2 (30% of maximum active tension) which is about 40-fold greater than that of the single frog atrial cell at this length. The resting stress of intact rat papillary muscle at sarcomere lengths in the range 2.2-2.3 μm has been reported to be in the range of 13 nN/μm^2 [13] to 24 nN/μm^2 [15].

Chemical Activation of Single Cells

In addition to investigating the characteristics of sarcomere performance in the single frog atrial cells, Tarr and Trank [23] reported a totally unexpected result obtained while attempting to record intracellular potentials from these cells. I would like to direct the reader to this result in the hopes that it might generate some interest and suggestions for future work. These investigators found that a dying frog atrial cell (killed by impalement with an unfilled microelectrode) liberates some unknown substance which diffuses away from the cell and activates contractile activity in other cells within the vicinity of the dying cell. From the time-distance squared relation it was possible to calculate a diffusion coefficient for the substance of 8.8 X 10^{-6} cm^2/sec which indicates that the substance has a fairly small molecular weight (60-300). Also, the substance must

be able to activate the cardiac cell at relatively small concentrations (μmolar or less). At present we have no idea what this
substance is, but the possibility that some potent cardioactive
agent is contained within the single cardiac cell is certainly
exciting.

SUMMARY

In light of the demonstrated contractile and mechanical nonuniformities which exist in many of the commonly used intact
cardiac preparations, there is now a recognized need to evaluate
cardiac sarcomere performance directly in relatively simple
cardiac preparations. The single cardiac cell represents the
simplest intact cardiac preparation and it can provide the opportunity for relatively definitive studies of cardiac sarcomere
performance, since the force at the sarcomere level is fairly
well defined compared to the situation in more complex intact
cardiac preparations and sarcomere lengths can be measured
directly. Considerable progress has been made within the last
five years in developing the methodology for preparing intact
isolated single cardiac cells and for investigating the
mechanical and contractile properties of these cells. There is
now sufficient information available to warrant the conclusion
that the isolated cardiac cell can have normal force generating
and sarcomere shortening capacity as well as normal electrical
activity. Studies on single cardiac cells have already given
insight into the characteristics of 1) sarcomere shortening and
extension at essentially zero external force, 2) sarcomere
shortening during auxotonic force development, 3) the contribution which the cell makes to the resting tension-sarcomere length
relationship of intact cardiac tissue, and 4) the sarcomere
length-dependency of the force generating capacity of cardiac
muscle during twitch contractions. These studies have also
clearly demonstrated that the cardiac sarcomere has some type of
a force-velocity relationship although the exact nature of this
relationship remains to be determined.

ACKNOWLEDGMENTS

Dr. Tarr's research work on single heart cells has been
supported by U.S. Public Health Service Grant HL 18943.

REFERENCES

1. Berry, M. N., Friend, D. S. & Scheuer, J. Morphology and
    metabolism of intact muscle cells isolated from adult rat
    heart. Circulation Research 26:679-687 (1970).

2. Bloom, S. Spontaneous rhythmic contraction of separated heart muscle cells. Science 167:1727-1729 (1970).
3. Brady, A. J., Tan, S. T. & Ricchiuti, N. V. Contractile force measured in unskinned isolated adult rat heart fibres. Nature 282:728-729 (1979).
4. Close, R. I. The relations between sarcomere length and characteristics of isometric twitch contractions of frog sartorius muscle. Journal of Physiology 220:745-762 (1972).
5. Edman, K. A. P. The velocity of unloaded shortening and its relation to sarcomere length and isometric force in vertebrate muscle fibres. Journal of Physiology 291:143-159 (1979).
6. Endo, M. Length dependence of activation of skinned muscle fibers by calcium. Cold Spring Harbor Symposium of Quantitative Biology 37:505-510 (1973).
7. Fabiato, A. Myoplasmic free calcium concentration reached during the twitch of an intact isolated cardiac cell and during calcium-induced release of calcium from the sarcoplasmic reticulum of a skinned cardiac cell from the adult rat or rabbit ventricle. Journal of Physiology 78:457-497 (1981).
8. Fabiato, A. & Fabiato, F. Excitation-contraction coupling of isolated cardiac fibers with disrupted or closed sarcolemmas. Calcium-dependent cyclic and tonic contractions. Circulation Research 31:293-307 (1972).
9. Fabiato, A. & Fabiato, F. Techniques of skinned cardiac cells and of isolated cardiac fibers with disrupted sarcolemmas with reference to the effects of catecholamines and of caffeine, in: "Recent Advances in Studies of Cardiac Structure and Metabolism", Vol. 9, P. E. Roy and N. S. Dhalla, Eds., pp. 71-94, University Park Press, Baltimore (1976).
10. Fabiato, A. & Fabiato, F. Myofilament-generated tension oscillations during partial calcium activation and activation dependence of sarcomere length-tension relation of skinned cardiac cells. Journal of General Physiology 72:667-699 (1978).
11. Hume, J. R. & Giles, W. Active and passive electrical properties of single bullfrog atrial cell. Journal of General Physiology 78:19-42 (1981).
12. Julian, F. J. & Moss, R. L. Effects of calcium and ionic strength on shortening velocity and tension development in frog skinned muscle fibres. Journal of Physiology 311:179-199 (1981).
13. Julian, F. J. & Sollins, M. R. Sarcomere length-tension relations in living rat papillary muscle. Circulation Research 37:299-308 (1975).
14. Krueger, J. W., Forletti, D. & Wittenberg, B. A. Uniform sarcomere shortening behavior in isolated cardiac muscle cells. Journal of General Physiology 76:587-607 (1980).

15. Krueger, J. W. & Pollack, G. H. Myocardial sarcomere dynamics during isometric contraction. Journal of Physiology 251:627-643 (1975).

16. Manring, A., Nassar, R. & Johnson, E. A. Light diffraction of cardiac muscle: An analysis of sarcomere shortening and muscle tension. Journal of Molecular and Cellular Cardiology 9:441-459 (1977).

17. Nassar, R., Manring, A. & Johnson, E. A. Light diffraction of cardiac muscle: Sarcomere motion during contraction. Ciba Foundation Symposium 24:57-82 (1974).

18. Pollack, G. H. & Krueger, J. W. Sarcomere dynamics in intact cardiac muscle. European Journal of Cardiology 4(Suppl):53-65 (1976).

19. Powell, T., Terrar, D. A. & Twist, V. W. Electrical properties of individual cells isolated from adult rat ventricular myocardium. Journal of Physiology 302:131-153 (1980).

20. Rack, P. M. H. & Westbury, D. R. The effects of length and stimulus rate on tension in the isometric cat soleus muscle. Journal of Physiology 204:443-460 (1969).

21. Roos, K. P., Brady, A. J. & Tan, S. T. Direct measurement of sarcomere length from isolated cardiac cells. American Journal of Physiology 242:H68-H78 (1972).

22. Tarr, M. & Trank, J. W. Preparation of isolated single cardiac cells from adult frog atrial tissue. Experientia 32:338-339 (1976).

23. Tarr, M. & Trank, J. W. Chemically mediated cell-to-cell contractile activation in isolated frog atrial cardiac cells. Experientia 34:1472-1474 (1978).

24. Tarr, M., Trank, J. W., Goertz, K. K. & Leiffer, P. Effect of initial sarcomere length on sarcomere kinetics and force development in single frog atrial cells. Circulation Research 49:767-774 (1981).

25. Tarr, M., Trank, J. W. & Leiffer, P. Characteristics of sarcomere shortening in single frog atrial cardiac cells during lightly loaded contractions. Circulation Research 48:189-200 (1981).

26. Tarr, M., Trank, J. W., Leiffer, P. & Shepherd, N. Sarcomere length-resting tension relation in single frog atrial cardiac cells. Circulation Research 45:554-559 (1979).

27. Tarr, M., Trank, J. W., Leiffer, P. & Shepherd, N. Evidence that the velocity of sarcomere shortening in single frog atrial cardiac cells is load dependent. Circulation Research 48:200-206 (1981).

28. Vahouny, G. V., Wei, R., Starkweather, R. & Davis, C. Preparation of beating heart cells from adult rats. Science 167:1616-1618 (1970).

29. Winegrad, S. Resting sarcomere length-tension relation in living frog heart. Journal of General Physiology 64:343-355 (1974).

STUDIES OF SUBSTRATE METABOLISM IN ISOLATED MYOCYTES

John J. Spitzer

Department of Physiology
Louisiana State University Medical Center
New Orleans, LA 70112

INTRODUCTION

Although techniques of isolating heart myocytes from adult animals have been available for over a decade, the often encountered low yield, poor viability, contamination by non-muscle cells and extreme sensitivity to the presence of calcium ions have limited the use of such preparations. During the last two to three years several laboratories have reported techniques of isolating adult myocardial cells with good yield, good viability, minimal contamination by non-muscle cells, as well as calcium-tolerance (1,2,3,4). Thus, the use of freshly isolated adult heart myocytes in myocardial biology has become more widespread (5) primarily, because of the following advantages of the preparation: a) Homogeneous population of myocytes is obtained which is virtually free of other cellular elements, whereas in the rat heart, myocytes comprise only about 25 percent of the total cell population (6). b) A cell population, free of neuronal and hormonal influences is obtained. c) During an experiment the isolated myocyte preparation can be divided into several aliquots and thus, internal controls for each preparation can be employed. d) Cells can be exposed to environmental changes without the necessity to consider capillary and extracellular barriers.

This review will summarize some of the available data concerning the metabolic behavior of the freshly isolated myocardial cells and compare them to the metabolic characteristics of isolated perfused heart preparations. The brief overview will consist of four parts: 1) a short description of the method of isolation and characterization of the cell preparation, 2) substrate utilization and oxygen consumption by myocytes from control animals, 3) substrate metabolism

217

and oxygen consumption by myocytes isolated from diabetic rats, and
4) a few selected examples of the use of isolated myocytes in different aspects of myocardial research. It should be noted that the
data obtained from freshly isolated myocytes were derived from
"calcium resistant" cells; i.e. from cells that were not hypersensitive to physiological Ca^{2+} concentration.

METHOD OF CELL ISOLATION

     Cells were prepared by using the method of Montini et al.
(7,8). Hearts were mounted to a recirculating perfusion apparatus
and retrogradely perfused with Joklik's minimal essential medium
(MEM) supplemented with 8 mM glutamate and 1.2 mM $MgSO_4$. The perfusion fluid was further supplemented with 0.1% collagenase and
0.1% FFA-free bovine serum albumin (BSA). The ventricle was then
diced and placed in siliconized Erlemeyer flasks containing the
enzyme medium. After sieving and resuspending the cells, the cells
were washed three times and allowed to settle in substrate-free
Joklik's MEM supplemented with 1.2 mM $MgSO_4$ and 1% BSA. Prior to
the last washing, cells were resuspended in 0.5 mM $CaCl_2$ containing
buffer. As indicated in previous publications (7,8), this preparation resulted in cells that maintained high viability in a medium
containing 1.5 mM Ca^{2+} as indexed by elongated cell morphology and
trypan blue exclusion. The cells contained physiologic concentrations of ATP and creatine phosphate (CP) during the incubation
period, and met their energy requirement through the uptake and
oxidation of exogenously provided substrates (8). Finally, the
preparation was virtually free of non-myocytic elements, as indicated in Table 1. Few, if any, nuclei of non-myocytic elements
could be stained in the preparation. Also, connective tissue,
cholinergic or adrenergic elements were barely or non-detectable
in the preparation. This method of preparation however, was not
optimal when hearts from diabetic rats were used, as it resulted
in relatively low yield and viability. The less-than-optimal cell
preparation obtained from diabetic rats was presumably due to the
fact that these cells have an impaired rate of glucose utilization
and thus, we modified the method of preparation by adding 0.2 mM
palmitate to the perfusate during the initial perfusion (and also
reduced the perfusion rate from 8 to 6 ml/min).

SUBSTRATE UTILIZATION AND OXYGEN CONSUMPTION BY MYOCYTES
AND PERFUSED HEARTS

     The presence or absence of Ca^{2+} exerted a major effect on the
rate of glucose or lactate oxidation by myocytes (Table 2). Complete removal of Ca^{2+} from a nominally calcium-free medium resulted
in a 28% decrease in glucose oxidation and a 14% decrease in lactate
oxidation. Adding 1.5 mM Ca^{2+} to the calcium-free incubation medium increased glucose oxidation by 49% and lactate oxidation by 30%
No significant effect of the presence of Ca^{2+} was noted on palmitate

TABLE 1
PURITY OF FRESHLY ISOLATED
RAT HEART MYOCYTE PREPARATION

EVALUATION	CONTAMINATION
GIEMSA TOLUIDENE BLUE STAINING	< 1.5% NON-MYOCYTIC ELEMENTS STAINED
HYDROXYPROLINE	< 4% OF THAT FOUND IN INTACT HEART
TYROSINE HYDROXYLASE ACTIVITY[a]	NOT DETECTABLE
ACETYLCHOLINE TRANSFERASE ACTIVITY[a]	NOT DETECTABLE

a. Courtesy of Dr. Robert Roskoski, Jr.

TABLE 2
GLUCOSE OR LACTATE OXIDATION IN THE PRESENCE OR ABSENCE OF Ca^{2+}

| | PERCENT CHANGE IN | |
	GLUCOSE OXIDATION	LACTATE OXIDATION
+0.1 mM EGTA	−28%	−14%
+0.1 mM EGTA +1.6 mM Ca	+49%	+30%

Myocytes (2.5 mg protein) were incubated (37°C, 60 min) with either $[U^{14}C]$ glucose (5 mM), or $[U^{14}C]$ lactate (7.5 mM).

oxidation (7). Cellular ATP content was also better preserved following incubation in the presence of Ca^{2+} (7).

ATP and CP concentrations in the isolated myocytes and in perfused hearts are shown in Table 3. Both ATP and CP concentrations of the myocytes are well preserved and are within the range found in perfused hearts.

The rate of oxygen consumption by isolated myocytes when either glucose or palmitate served as substrate, is indicated in Table 4. These values are essentially identical to those obtained in

TABLE 3

ATP AND CP CONCENTRATION IN ISOLATED MYOCYTES
AND IN PERFUSED HEARTS

	MYOCYTES[a]	PERFUSED HEARTS[b,c]
VIABILITY (percent)	72-79	--
ATP (nmoles/mg protein)	22-24	15-26
CP (nmoles/mg protein)	28-32	19-37

a. Incubated with 5.5 mM glucose (Chen, V., Bagby, G.J. &
    Spitzer, J.J.: unpublished data)
b. Langendorff preparation with 5.5 or 11.0 mM glucose, at 65 cm
    H_2O perfusion pressure
c. From references 9, 10, 11.

Langendorff non-working heart perfusion experiments. The exact
cause of the striking increase in O_2 consumption in the presence of
palmitate (as compared to O_2 consumption in the presence of glucose)
is not known. The decreased efficiency of ATP yield from O_2 when
palmitate is being oxidized as compared to glucose could not fully
account for the marked difference. Other factors, e.g. futile cycling (lipolysis followed by reesterification), alteration in ion
transport, etc. are also likely to contribute to the observed increase.

TABLE 4

O_2 CONSUMPTION BY ISOLATED MYOCYTES AND PERFUSED HEARTS
(nmoles/hr/mg protein)

	IN THE PRESENCE OF	
	GLUCOSE	PALMITATE
ISOLATED MYOCYTES[a]	1140	1860
PERFUSED HEARTS[b,c]	1080	1860

a. Incubated with 5.5 mM glucose or 0.4 mM plamitate (Chen, V.,
    Bagby, G.J. & Spitzer J.J.: unpublished data)
b. Langendorff preparation with 5.5 mM glucose or 1.7 mM plamitate,
    at 65 cm H_2O perfusion pressure
c. From references 9, 12.

The rate of oxidation of the three major substrates, fatty acids, lactate and glucose, is shown in Table 5. The first line of this table represents oxidation rates in the presence of one of the three major substrates, whereas the second line contains oxidation rates when all three substrates were presented simultaneously. From the information included on the second line of this Table, one can calculate the total ATP production and also the percent contribution of the individual substrates to ATP production under conditions of incubating the cells in the presence of 5 mM glucose, 1 mM lactate and nmoles/hr/mg 0.4 mM palmitate. Of the 6,600 nmoles/hr/mg of ATP production, 18% was attributable to glucose, 21% to lactate and 60% of palmitate oxidation (Table 6). Thus, palmitate was by far the most important energy yielding substrate for the myocytes. These results, as well as substrate competition data (18) show that fatty acids are the preferred substrates for the isolated myocytes, just as they are for the myocardium in the isolated perfused heart, or under _in vivo_ conditions.

TABLE 5

RATE OF SUBSTRATE OXIDATION BY ISOLATED MYOCYTES
AND PERFUSED HEARTS
(nmoles/hr/mg protein)

	GLUCOSE	LACTATE	PALMITATE OXIDATION
ISOLATED MYOCYTES[a]			
in the presence of a single exogenous substrate	150	298	61
in the presence of all three exogenous substrates	34	81	35
PERFUSED HEARTS[b,c]	77		50

a. Incubated with 5.5 mM glucose, 1.0 mM lactate, or 0.4 cm M palmitate (Chen, V., Bagby, G.J. & Spitzer, J.J.: unpublished data)
b. Langendorff preparation with 5 mM glucose, or 0.4 MM palmitate at 60 cm H_2O perfusion pressure
c. From references 13, 14.

SUBSTRATE METABOLISM OF MYOCYTES ISOLATED FROM DIABETIC RATS

Myocytes used in these experiments were prepared from hearts

222

J. J. SPITZER

TABLE 6
CALCULATED RATE OF ATP PRODUCTION IN MYOCYTES
FROM EXOGENOUS SUBSTRATES[a]

| | ATP PRODUCTION | PERCENT CONTRIBUTION BY INDIVIDUAL SUBSTRATES | | |
		GLUCOSE	LACTATE	PALMITATE
CONTROL	$6,600 \pm 360$[b]	18	21	60
DIABETIC	$6,420 \pm 660$	6	11	83
INSULIN-TREATED DIABETIC	$7,420 \pm 540$	23	25	52

a. In the presence of 5 mM glucose, 1.0 mM lactate and 0.4 mM palmitate
b. Mean $\pm$ SEM; nmoles/hr/mg protein (N = 7), (Chen, V., Bagby, G.J. & Spitzer, J.J.: unpublished data)

of rats given 70 mg/kg streptozotocin 4 weeks prior to the experiment The viability of cell preparations and ATP and CP concentrations are shown in Table 7. All values are similar to those obtained in myocytes from control rats (Table 3). Also, ATP and CP concentration are within, or above the range reported in perfused hearts.

TABLE 7
ATP AND CP CONCENTRATION IN ISOLATED MYOCYTES
AND IN PERFUSED HEARTS OF DIABETIC RATS

	MYOCYTES[a]	PERFUSED HEARTS
VIABILITY (percent)	69-78	---
ATP (nmoles/mg protein)	20-23	15-22
CP (nmoles/mg protein)	26-30	16-17

a. Incubated with 25 mM glucose (Chen, V., Bagby, G.J. & Spitzer, J.J.: unpublished data)
b. Working heart perfusion with 5.5 or 11.0 mM glucose, at 20 cm H_2O hydrostatic pressure
c. From references 9, 11, 15.

The rates of oxidation of glucose, lactate and palmitate in the presence of all three substrates are indicated in Figure 1. The oxidation of both glucose and lactate is markedly decreased in cells prepared from diabetic animals. These changes are completely reversed in cells obtained from animals treated twice daily with insulin (5U NPH-insulin per kg administered subcutaneously).

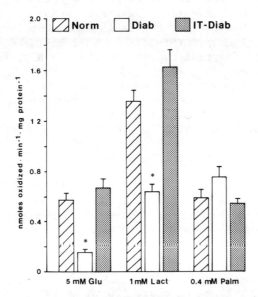

Figure 1. Rates of oxidation of glucose, lactate
and palmitate in myocytes prepared from control,
diabetic, or insulin-treated diabetic (IT-Diab)
rats. The three substrates were present simultaneously in the incubation medium at the concentrations indicated in the figure. From Chen, V.,
Bagby, G.J. and Spitzer, J.J.: unpublished data.

Calculated ATP production in myocytes from diabetic rats was
6,420 nmoles/hr/mg (Table 6). This value is comparable to the one
obtained in myocytes from control rats. However, the contribution
of glucose and lactate to total ATP production was much less (6 and
11 percent respectively) and the contribution of palmitate was considerably more (83%) than in myocytes from control rats. Insulin
treatment eliminated these changes.

In the presence of glucose, or lactate oxygen consumption by

myocytes obtained from diabetic rats was markedly different from
that measured in myocytes from control animals (Table 8). However,
oxygen consumption in the presence of palmitate was substantially
lower when cells from diabetic rats were used as compared to values
contained in cells from control rats. The reason for this difference remains to be elucidated. Oxygen consumption of the perfused
heart is higher than that of the isolated myocyte, especially in
the presence of glucose. This discrepancy may be due to the relatively high aortic perfusion pressure (100 cm H_2O) employed in
those investigations.

TABLE 8

O_2 CONSUMPTION BY ISOLATED MYOCYTES AND PERFUSED HEARTS
FROM DIABETIC RATS
(nmoles/hr/mg protein)

	IN THE PRESENCE OF		
	GLUCOSE	LACTATE	PALMITATE
ISOLATED MYOCYTES[a]	960	1020	1260
PERFUSED HEARTS	2160[b,c]	1440[d]	

a. Incubated with 25 mM glucose, 1.0 mM lactate, or 1.0 mM palmi-
    tate (Chen, V., Bagby, G.J. and Spitzer, J.J.: unpublished data)
b. Langendorff preparation with 11.0 mM glucose, at 100 cm H_2O
    perfusion pressure
c. From reference 9
d. Burns, A.H.: unpublished data.

SELECTED EXAMPLES OF THE USE OF ISOLATED MYOCYTES IN MYOCARDIAL
RESEARCH

There are numerous examples of the use of isolated myocytes in
different areas of research. Three examples have been arbitrarily
selected:

1. In earlier experiments Bagby et al. had demonstrated the
presence of lipoprotein lipase (LPL) activity in freshly isolated
rat myocytes (16). In subsequent investigations, Bagby demonstrated
a positive correlation between heparin-nonreleaseable LPL activity
(intracellular LPL) in the heart and myocytic LPL activity. This
correlation was established by experimentally manipulating intracellular LPL activity via the administration of E. coli endotoxin
(an agent known to decrease activity), or colchicine (an agent
known to increase activity). Myocytes appear to be the major intracellular compartment of LPL in the heart. These studies are

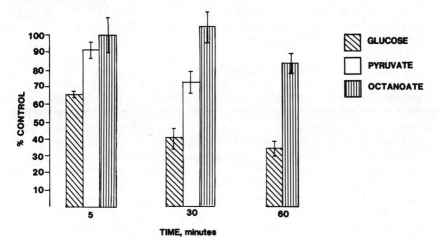

Figure 2.   Changes in glucose, pyruvate octanoate oxidation by isola-
            ted myocardial cells following exposure (for 5, 30 or 60
            minutes) to nitorogen atmosphere and reoxygenation. Sub-
            strate concentration in the medium was 5 mM glucose, 1 mM
            pyruvate or 1 mM octanoate. From McDonough, K.H. and
            Spitzer, J.J.: unpublished data.

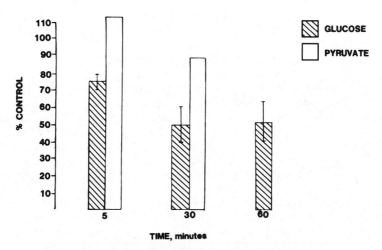

Figure 3.   Changes in lactate production by isolated myocardial cells
            following exposure (for 5, 30 or 60 minutes) to nitrogen
            atmosphere and reoxygenation. Incubation medium contained
            5 mM glucose or 1 mN pyruvate. Drom McDonough, K.H. and
            Spitzer, J.J.: unpublished data.

consistent with the view that the LPL pool in myocytes serves as
precursor to the functional extracellular enzyme located on capillary endothelial surfaces (17).

2.   Hypoxic insult and subsequent reoxygenation have been
known to cause marked metabolic changes in the myocardium. Since
contractile activity and metabolism are functionally related,
alterations in mechanical activity can obscure some of the effects
of oxygen deprivation upon cell metabolism. For this reason
in vitro exposure of isolated quiescent adult rat heart cells to
hypoxia and reoxygenation is a useful experimental model to assess
the effects of an hypoxic episode on myocardial metabolism. In
order to determine the rate of oxidation of the different substrates,
McDonough and Spitzer (18) exposed freshly isolated heart myocytes
to nitrogen atmosphere for 5, 30 or 60 minutes which was followed
by reoxygenation and incubation (for 30 min) in glucose, pyruvate
or octanoate containing buffer. Five minutes of exposure to hypoxia
followed by reoxygenation produced a significant depression of
glucose oxidation (Figure 2) and lactate production (Figure 3).
The oxidation of pyruvate, or octanoate was unaltered. Thirty
minutes of oxygen deprivation resulted in more marked changes in
glucose oxidation and slight alterations of pyruvate utilization.
Octanoate oxidation was slightly depressed after sixty minutes of
hypoxia followed by reoxygenation. These results indicated that
changes in cytosolic metabolism were detectable after short periods
of hypoxia followed by reoxygenation, whereas mitochondrial function
was more resistant to the insult.

3.   A highly potent fast-acting natriuretic factor has been
recently described and found to reside in atrial, but not in ventricular heart tissue (19, 20). Extracts of rat atria when injected
into assay rats produced an 30 fold increase in urinary sodium excretion with 10 minutes. The substance, now referred to as atrial
natriuretic factor (ANF), has been found in the atria of several
species of mammals, including man (21). ANF may have important
regulatory influence on urinary sodium excretion. The isolated
adult myocardial heart cell preparation lends itself well for the
further study of the properties of ANF (22), as this preparation is
virtually free of non-myocytic elements. Isolated atrial myocytes
were prepared from adult Sprague Dawley rats according to a previous
technique used for isolated ventricular myocytes (7). Extracts of
isolated atrial myocytes, as well as of ventricular myocytes were
prepared and assayed for natriuretic activity using the same rat
bioassay method that was employed in the earlier experiments on extracts of whole atria (20). The natriuretic response elicited by
injection of atrial myocyte extract was similar to that previously
demonstrated by extracts of whole atria. The rapid increase in
urinary sodium excretion and urine output reached peaks within 10

minutes (Figure 4). Only a moderate increase in urinary potassium
excretion was noticed. This time course of action is one of the
characteristics that distinguishes the ANF from other natriuretic
factors. No such elevations in water and electrolyte excretion
were found following injection of ventricular myocyte extract
(Figure 4).

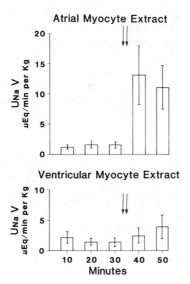

Figure 4. Urinary sodium excretion in rats (N=8)
receiving atrial myocyte extract, and in animals
(N-7) receiving ventricular myocyte extract. Injections (arrows) were made intravenously (4 mg/kg)
using phosphate buffered saline (pH 7.4) as the
vehicle. Mean ± SE are given. From Trippodo, N.C.,
MacPhee, A.A. and Cole, F.E.: unpublished data.

Acknowledgement: The investigations reported in this review
were supported by NIH Grant HL 23157.

REFERENCES

1. Frangakis, C.J., Bahl, J.J., McDaniel, H. and Bressler, R.
    Tolerance to physiological calcium by isolated myocytes
    from the adult rat heart; an improved cellular preparation.
    Life Sciences 27, 815-825 (1980).

2. Kao, R.L., Christmas, E.W., Luh, S.L., Kraubs, J.M.,
    Tylers, G.F. and Williams, E.H. The effect of insulin and
    anoxia on the metabolism of isolated mature rat cardiac
    myocytes. Archives of Biochemistry and Biophysics 203,
    587-599 (1980).

3. Haworth, R.A., Hunter, D.R. and Bekhoff, H.A. Contracture
    in isolated adult rat heart cells. Role of Ca^{2+}, ATP, and
    compartmentation. Circulation Research 49, 1119-1128 (1981).

4. Dow, J.W., Harding, N.G.L. and Powell, T. Review: Isolated
    cardiac myocytes: I Preparation of adult myocytes and their
    homology with intact tissue. Cardiovascular Research 15,
    483-514 (1981).

5. Dow, J.W., Harding, N.G.L. & Powell, T. Review: Isolated
    cardiac myocytes: II Functional aspects of mature cells.
    Cardiovascular Research 15, 549-579 (1981)

6. Morkin, E. and Ashford, T.P. Myocardial DNA synthesis in
    experimental cardiac hypertrophy. American Journal of
    Physiology, 215, 1409-1413 (1968).

7. Montini, J., Bagby, G.J., Burns, A.H. & Spitzer, J.J.
    Exogenous substrate utilization in Ca^{2+}-tolerant myocytes
    from adult rat hearts. American Journal of Physiology,
    240, H659-H663 (1981).

8. Montini, J., Bagby, G.J. & Spitzer, J.J., Importance of
    exogenous substrates for the energy production of adult
    rat heart myocytes. Journal of Molecular and Cellular
    Cardiology 13, 903-911 (1981).

9. Opie, L.H., Mansford, K.R.L. & Owen, P. Effects of in-
    creased heart work on glycolysis and adenine nucleotides
    in the perfused heart of normal and diabetic rats. Bio-
    chemical Journal 124, 475-590 (1971).

10. Neely, J.R., Denton, R.M., England, P.J. & Randle, P.J.
    The effects of increased heart work on the Tricarboxylate
    Cycle and its interactions with glycolysis in the perfused
    rat heart. Biochemical Journal 128, 147-159 (1972).

11. Opie, L.H., Tansey, M.J. & Kennelly, B.M. The heart
    in diabetes mellitus, I. Biochemical basis for myo-
    cardial dysfunction. South African Medical Journal
    56, 207-211 (1979).

12. Neely, J.R., Bowman, R.H. & Morgan, H.E. Effects of
    ventricular pressure development and palmitate on
    glucose transport. American Journal of Physiology,
    216, 804-811 (1969).

13. Crass, M.F., McCaskill, E.S. & Shipp, J.C. Effect of
    pressure development on glucose and palmitate metabolism
    in perfused heart. American Journal of Physiology,
    216, 1569-1576 (1969).

14. Evans, J.R., Opie, L.H. & Shipp, J.C. Metabolism of
    palmitic acid in perfused rat heart. American Journal
    of Physiology, 205, 766-770. (1963).

15. Miller, T.B. Cardiac performance of isolated perfused
    hearts from alloxan diabetic rats. American Journal of
    Physiology 236, H808-H812 (1979).

16. Bagby, G.J., Liu, M.S. & Spitzer, J.A. Lipoprotein
    lipase activity in rat heart myocytes. Life Sciences
    21, 467-474 (1977).

17. Bagby, G.J. & Corll, C.B. Importance of lipoprotein
    lipase activity to intracellular activity in the adult
    rat heart. Journal of Mollecular and Cellular Cardiology,
    14 Supplement 1, 24 (1982).

18. McDonough, K.H. & Spitzer, J.J. Effects of anoxia upon
    carbohydrate utilization by isolated rat heart cells.
    Federation Proceedings 40, 561, (1981).

19. de Bold, A.J., Borenstein, H.B., Veress, A.T. &
    Sonnenberg, H.: A rapid and potent natriuretic response
    to intravenous injection of atrial myocardial extract
    in rats. Life Sciences 28:89-94 (1981).

20. Trippodo, N.C., MacPhee, A.A., Cole, F.E. & Blakesley, H.L.:
    Partial chemical characterization of a natriuretic sub-
    stance in rat atrial heart tissue. Proc Soc Exp Biol
    Med (in press).

21. MacPhee, A.A., Trippodo, N.C. & Cole, F.E.: Natriuretic
    activity in extracts of the human atrium. Presented at
    the 1982 meeting of The Endocrine Society.

22. Trippodo, N.C., MacPhee, A.A. & Cole, F.E.: Natriuretic
     factor in isolated rat atrial myocytes. J Mol Cellul
     Cardiol 14 (Suppl 1): 65, 1982.

ION MOVEMENTS IN ADULT RAT HEART MYOCYTES

Gerald P. Brierley, Charlene Hohl, and Ruth A. Altschuld

Department of Physiological Chemistry
College of Medicine
Ohio State University
Columbus, Ohio 43210

INTRODUCTION

Recent improvements in methodology for the isolation of adult heart cells (6,9,10,18,22,25,31,36,46) yield myocytes that are more suitable for the study of cellular and intracellular ion movements than those previously available. For example, 92% of the cells in the myocyte preparations currently in use in our laboratory are viable by trypan blue exclusion, 85% show the elongated, rod-like configuration of heart cells in situ (Fig. 1A), and the rod cells show morphology in the electron microscope that is indistinguishable from cells in intact heart tissue (Fig. 2). These cells also contain enzyme profiles corresponding to those of heart cells in situ (34) and ATP, total adenine nucleotide, and creatine phosphate at levels quite comparable to those found in intact heart tissue (19,24, and 34 nmol·mg protein^{-1}, respectively; Ref. 22).

These cells show good viability when incubated aerobically with glucose in a Ca-free buffer (80% viable after 2 hours at 37°), and the majority of the cells are Ca-tolerant. When a population of these cells is exposed to 1 mM Ca, about 15% of the rod-shaped cells go into an irreversible hypercontracture and assume a round configuration (Fig. 1C) characterized by blebs of cytosol containing mitochondria (see 32,35,44 for micrographs of the round cells in hypercontracture). More than 60% of the cells remain in the rod-cell form when exposed to Ca, however, and 50% of all cells survive in this form after 2 hours at 37° in a buffer containing glucose and 1 mM Ca (22). As pointed out by Dow et al (9,10) the Ca-sensitivity of heart myoctyes is an issue of crucial

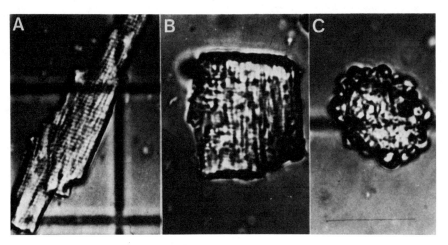

Figure 1 - Morphological forms of myocytes. A. Rod-shaped cell.
More than 85% of the cell population has this appearance when
first isolated. B. Contracted myocyte. These cells have
markedly decreased sarcomere length but retain the normal
alignment of contractile elements. C. Round cell in
hypercontracture. These cells are characterized by blebs of
cytoplasm containing mitochondria and extensive derangement of
contractile elements (see 32,35, and 44 for electron micrographs
of this cell form). The hemotcytometer grid is 50μ.

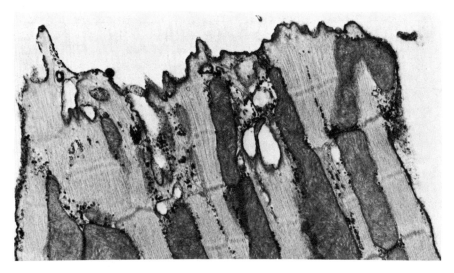

Figure 2 - Electron micrograph of a typical rod-shaped myocyte
(courtesy of Dr. J. R. Hostetler).

importance if the cells are to be used for ion transport or metabolic studies. We shall return to this point several times in the course of this discussion.

It should be noted that, although a number of laboratories now have satisfactory preparations of heart myocytes available, there is no consensus as to the best methodology for cell preparation. A systematic analysis of the factors that lead to acceptable cell preparations is clearly needed. The experience in our laboratory suggests that three factors can be controlled to improve cell quality. The first is an empirical screening of various batches of serum albumin to eliminate those that seem to promote cytotoxicity. The second is the addition of taurine, creatine, and the amino acid and vitamin additives specified in the procedure of Kao et al (25). A third consideration (to be discussed below) is the increase in intracellular Na (Na_i) and decrease in K_i seen when cells are washed or stored in the cold (2). To prevent this increase in cellular Na/K ratio these steps are now carried out at room temperature (22).

TRANSPORT AND ION CONDUCTANCE IN THE MYOCYTE SARCOLEMMA

The sarcolemma of heart cells contains pathways for the conductance of Na and Ca during the action potential, the so-called fast and slow channels (8,24). The permeability of this membrane to K is large compared to that of other ions and there are indications (8) that K conductance may be controlled by intracellular Ca (Ca_i). When heart cells are stimulated, inward Na current, inward Ca current, and outward K current all depend on membrane conductances and the existing electrochemical gradients. Restoration of these gradients is accomplished by the electrogenic Na-K pump (15), by Na/Ca exchange, (33) and by a Ca extruding pump (26). In the intact cell Ca_i is extensively compartmentalized (40). The Ca_i is bound to and released from endogenous chelators such as adenine nucleotides and Ca-receptor proteins (calmodulin and troponin), it is taken up by the sarcoplasmic reticulum (SR) as a result of the activity of the SR Ca-pump and released from SR during excitation, and under some circumstances Ca_i can be accumulated into and released from the mitochondrial fraction. Cellular K also appears to be distributed between cytosolic and mitochondrial matrix compartments (3) and Na_i may move into and out of the mitochondrion in conjunction with Ca uptake and release. Ion movements observed in a suspension of myocytes therefore reflect a net interplay between ion uptake and extrusion at the level of the sarcolemma and the available intracellular ion-distribution reactions.

The presence of these competing or opposing pathways for ion movement make the study of such reactions in myocyte suspensions complex. However, the adult heart myocyte preparation has certain experimental advantages over intact heart tissue for some types of transport studies. The isolated cells can be exposed to media of well-defined composition and the cell suspension can be sampled serially to establish the time-course of a reaction. If the suspension is gently agitated, the cells are exposed uniformly to the suspending media and questions as to cell orientation and solute diffusion can be largely eliminated. In addition, since there are virtually no cells other than myocytes present, complications introduced by the presence of fibroblasts, connective tissue, and of cells of vascular origin in other preparations are minimized.

The cells can be washed rapidly through solutions containing chelators to estimate surface binding of Ca and Mg and the sarcolemma can be lysed selectively with digitonin (3). Such digitonized myocytes retain an intact mitochondrial population so that matrix-cytosol compartmentation can be examined by this procedure.

Such advantages are offset by a number of drawbacks, including the difficulty of stimulating a population of myocytes uniformly, the rapid time frame of shifts in ion-conducting channels from "resting" to "open" to "inactive" states following stimulation (24), and heterogeneity of cell response. This latter problem comes into play in the assessment of even slow ion-distribution reactions in myocytes. As mentioned above, a portion of the cells appear predisposed to hypercontracture when exposed to Ca. These hypercontracted cells remain viable by all available criteria, but since the intracellular components have been extensively realigned, it is not certain that intracellular ion movements in such cells will be equivalent to those in normal myocytes. In addition, it is apparent that functional mitochondria are present to a varying extent in some of the so-called non-viable cells (those that have released cytosolic enzymes and stained with trypan blue) and that these mitochondria can contribute to ion movements under some conditions. An additional difficulty is the comparatively short life span of adult heart myocytes and the fragility of some cells, especially when magnetic stirring is employed. The cells also settle to the bottom of a cuvette rapidly and therefore present problems when direct spectrophotometric analysis is required.

However, it has been established that the completely dissociated myocyte retains the electrophysiological properties of cells in situ (10) as well as appropriate hormone receptor sites (10,12,25,36), and contractile properties (42). These properties, in addition to the maintenance of intracellular compartments in their native relationships, provide compelling reasons for attempting to address certain specific questions of ion transport to the myocyte model. It now seems apparent that alterations in myocyte Na and Ca distribution may account for(or at least make a major contribution to) the remarkable morphological transformations seen when myocytes hypercontract and that the process of hypercontracture may be of relevance to pathophysiological conditions seen in situ. The studies that led to these conclusions will be summarized in the following sections.

ROLE OF Na IN HYPERSENSITIVITY OF MYOCYTES TO Ca

Our initial attempts to prepare rat heart myocytes by collagenase pefusion yielded cells that were virtually all hypersensitive to Ca (2). These cells were routinly washed and stored in the cold. Analysis showed that the cells contained elevated Na_i and decreased K_i relative to intact heart tissue. When these myocytes were exposed to 1 mM Ca they were quantitatively converted to the bizarrely contorted, round hypercontracture forms (Fig. 1C). Since the cells were prepared using a nominally Ca-free buffer (containing an average of 25 μM Ca from adventitious and cellular sources), their hypersensitivity to Ca is formally equivalent to a "Ca-paradox" protocol in an intact heart (1,16,17,20,43). Re-introduction of Ca after a period of Ca-free perfusion in an intact heart results in massive cellular damage characterized by cell contracture and the release of creatine kinase and other soluble enzymes (20).

It should be emphasized that the bulk of the hypercontracted myocytes produced by exposure to Ca retain an intact sarcolemma. These cells exclude trypan blue, retain lactic dehydrogenase, creatine phosphokinase and other cytosol enzymes, and re-establish low Na/K ratios on continued incubation. These round cells deteriorate more rapidly than normal rod cells, however, especially if mechanical agitation is involved. This may explain the widely held view (9 for example) that hypercontracture is a symptom of disruption of the sarcolemma. Despite the metabolic competence of these round cells it is clear that hypercontracture produces morphological alterations that are irreversible and that an equivalent reaction in situ would result in the loss of contractile function in a heart cell. It seems likely that the process of rounding and hypercontracture of the isolated myocytes is equivalent to the formation of contracture bands in intact heart tissue (see 13, for example). In an unattached myocyte completely dissociated from its neighboring cells, the contracture process appears to occur with considerable distortion of intracellular structure but without rupture of the sarcolemma. The equivalent process occuring in partially or completely attached cells would result in mechanical rupture of the sarcolemma with a spilling out of cytosolic enzymes and metabolites (13). It is our contention that hypercontracture represents a form of heart cell death that can occur without obligatory loss of the integrity of the sarcolemma.

If Na-loaded myocytes are permitted to respire in a Ca-free medium for a short time, the activity of the Na-K-ATPase (15) results in restoration of a low Na/K ratio and cells subjected to this pre-incubation step become largely insensitive to Ca (2). The development of Ca-tolerance in these cells follows the same time course as the restoration of a normal Na/K ratio. The cells remain hypersensitive to Ca if the restoration of this ratio is prevented by addition of sufficient ouabain to block the Na-pump in rat heart cells (2). Cells prepared in a Na-free medium are not hypersensitive to Ca (2). These studies lead to the conclusion that the Ca-sensitivity of heart myocytes is related to elevated Na_i and that cells prepared (or treated) in such a way as to maintain (or establish) low Na/K ratios are Ca-tolerant. A similar conclusion has been reached by Goshima (16) in an elegant study using cultured myocytes.

It is also of interest that the Na-loaded myocytes contract spontaneously when first isolated and that these cells become quiescent when incubated in a Ca-free medium to restore a normal low Na/K ratio (2). Ventricular cells in situ do not contract unless stimulated and the spontaneous contractile activity of these myocyte preparations is probably an indication of high ionic permeability (11). Cells that have a low Na/K as isolated and cells in which low Na/K ratios are established by the activity of the Na-pump do not beat spontaneously.

Myocytes with elevated Na/K ratios take up ^{45}Ca much more rapidly than do cells from the same preparation pre-incubated to lower the Na/K ratio (2). This increased Ca uptake could result from inward exchange of Ca_o for Na_i on the Ca/Na exchanger of the sarcolemma (33), or alternatively it could merely reflect an elevated ionic permeability of cells with high Na/K ratios. This latter explanation would require that reactions that restore low ion permeability (membrane sealing) occur simultaneously with Na-pump activity. For this reason we feel that direct Ca/Na exchange provides a more straightfoward rationale for the observations.

Regardless of the mechanism of the increased Ca_i, it would seem that the rapid increase in this component in Na-loaded cells contributes to the observed hypercontracture. However, as we will develop below, the hypercontracture response appears complex and has several features that are not yet understood completely.

The hypercontracture reaction requires respiration since it is strongly inhibited by rotenone, antimycin, and other inhibitors of mitochondrial respiration (5). Rotenone also eliminates 35% of the net uptake of ^{45}Ca in these cell suspensions (5), a result that indicates that significant amounts of Ca are being deposited in the mitochondrial fraction. It is also of interest that the

myocytes do not go into hypercontracture when suspended at acid pH
(5). The production of viable, round cells is virtually
eliminated at pH 6.2 in both Na-loaded cells and cells
pre-incubated to restore a low Na/K ratio. The low pH also
inhibits net uptake of [45]Ca into these cells and largely
eliminates the burst of respiration seen at neutral pH when the
cells are exposed to Ca (5). It appears that less Ca is available
to the mitochondria at pH 6.4 than at neutral pH and it seems
likely that less Ca is able to cross the sarcolemma under the acid
conditions (5).

Table I - Effect of Ca on Na/K Ratio and Lactate Production of
          Anaerobic Myocytes

Incubation Conditions	ΔNa^+ (nmol.mg^{-1})	Na/K	ΔLactate (μmol.mg^{-1})	Ca (nmol.mg^{-1})
1. Anaerobic, no glucose				
no added Ca	193±21	8.0±0.9	0.11±0.01	-
+ Ca (1 mM)	109±14	2.2±0.1	0.10±0.01	-
2. Anaerobic + glucose				
+EGTA (1 mM)	48±3	1.4±0.1	1.03±0.11	-
+EGTA + ouabain	219±33	4.4±0.4	0.45±0.05	-
+Ca (1 mM)	53±14	1.2±0.1	0.45±0.05	10.6±0.6
+Ca + ouabain	141±43	2.4±0.3	0.51±0.06	9.1±1.2

Rat heart myocytes (22) were incubated at 2 mg protein.ml^{-1},
37°, under N_2 in Krebs-Ringer-phosphate (22) containing rotenone
(8 μg•ml^{-1}). In experiment number one, no glucose was added;
experiment number two contained 11mM glucose. When no Ca was
added, the Ca concentration (from cellular and adventitious
sources) was 25 μM. Where indicated Ca (1mM), EGTA (1mM), or
ouabain (0.5mM) were also present. After 30 minutes of incubation
the cells were centrifuged through a layer of bromododecane (29)
into perchloric acid and the Na and K content of the resulting
extracts determined by atomic absorption spectroscopy. Parallel
incubations were stopped with acid and lactate determined. Data
tabulated are the means ± S.E. for 5 experiments. Lactate
production was linear with time during these incubations. Cell
viability by trypan blue exclusion averaged 78% for EGTA-treated
cells in experiment number two and 65% for Ca-treated cells. The
viability of these preparations prior to incubation averaged 90%
for Ca-free cells and 84% in the presence of mM Ca. Ca uptake was
estimated using [45]Ca (2,5).

Since increased Ca_i due to Ca/Na exchange represents a possible vector for the production of hypercontracture (2,16), we have recently examined some of the factors contributing to the Na permeability of myocytes. Non-energized myocytes (i.e. cells incubated under N_2 in the absence of glucose) lose K and take up Na as expected (22). In the presence of Ca_0 both the increase in Na_i and loss of K_i are decreased (21), so that the Na/K ratio is only about one quarter of that found after a comparable incubation in the absence of added Ca (Table I). Under these conditions the myocyte Na/K ratio was found to be an inverse function of Ca_0 in the range from 25μM (nominally Ca-free) to 2 mM Ca (21). These studies suggest that Ca_0 acts to limit the permeability of non-energized myocytes to Na and K.

When heart cells are exposed to high concentrations of EDTA or EGTA their ionic permeability increases to the extent that the cells are referred to as "chemically skinned" (11,30,45). Such cells have low resting potentials consistent with free permeability to ions and respond to low concentrations of Ca_0 (45). Miller (30) has pointed out that the sarcolemma of frog heart cells is not disrupted by these conditions and that the results are more consistent with the operation of the Ca/Na exchange system whose activity has been modified by depolarization and by extracellular ATP. Our studies with rat heart myocytes treated with low levels (1mM) of EGTA are consistent with the presence of an intact sarcolemma but with increased permeability to Na and K (Table I). Anaerobic myocytes supplemented with glucose carry out glycolysis and maintain low Na/K ratios both when Ca_0 is set at 1mM and when Ca_0 is removed by chelation with 1mM EGTA. When the Na-pump of these cells is blocked with ouabain, Na/K increases under both incubation conditions, but the increase is much greater in the presence of EGTA (Table I). The lactate produced by Ca-treated myocytes is only half that produced in the presence of EGTA (Table I) and the additional lactate produced in the presence of the chelator is abolished by ouabain. The ouabain-sensitive production of lactate under these conditions can be taken as an indication of the energy demand of the Na-pump (Na-K ATPase activity). The EGTA-treated myocytes maintain a low Na/K ratio, but they appear to expend considerable energy in influx-efflux cycling of monovalent cations compared to cells treated with 1 mM Ca.

These results would be explained if Ca_0 inhibited passive monovalent cation permeability via the slow channel (28) or any other pathway that would permit monovalent cation conduction in de-energized myocytes. Removal of Ca would therefore result in increased Na_i and increased Na-pump activity which would be reflected in increased glycolysis. It should be noted that there are indications that Na and Ca may compete for binding sites on the sarcolemma (37,38) and that a similar role for Ca as an

inhibitor of monovalent cation permeability has been suggested in
a lymphocyte system (39). An alternative explanation would be
that Na-permeability is unchanged in the presence or absence of
Ca, but that Na_i extrusion in exchange for Ca_0 is no longer
possible in the presence of EGTA. The elevated Na_i would result
in increased Na-pump activity in this case, as well. This
explanation would require either a net accumulation of Ca_i or an
expenditure of energy for Ca extrusion. There is a net increase
in ^{45}Ca uptake equivalent to only 10 $nmol \cdot mg^{-1}$ under these
conditions (Table I). Of this amount 5 $nmol \cdot mg^{-1}$ is removed
by a rapid wash through EGTA and may be regarded as surface bound
(or otherwise readily released) and 2 $nmol \cdot mg^{-1}$ are sedimented
with digitonin-lysed cells. This latter fraction may be bound to
mitochondria and other intracellular membrane components. It
therefore appears that there is insufficient net uptake of Ca
under these conditions to account for the lower Na/K ratio seen in
the presence of Ca_0 (Table I) by Ca/Na exchange.

Regardless of the exact mechanisms involved, it is possible
to conclude from these studies that (a) Ca_0 minimizes the uptake
of Na and loss of K from non-energized myocytes, and (b) myocytes
with elevated Na/K ratios are hypersensitive to re-addition of Ca.
Both of these observations appear relevant to the phenomenon of
Ca-paradox (1,16,17,20,43).

RESPONSE OF HEART MYOCYTES TO HYPOXIA AND REAERATION

Heart myocytes deteriorate by two distinctive pathways when
incubated under conditions chosen to simulate various aspects of
ischemia (5,22). Cells incubated anaerobically in the absence of
glucose show a progressive loss of creatine phosphate and ATP and
a decline in the total adenine nucleotide pool after about 15
minutes at 37° (22). After 60 minutes under these conditions the
adenine nucleotide has decreased to less than 5 $nmol \cdot mg^{-1}$ and
ATP is virtually undetected. As anaerobic incubation is
continued, more and more rod-cells contract into nearly square
forms (Fig. 1B) that retain the structural features of rod-cells
but with decreased sarcomere length (18,22). These forms
eventually take up trypan blue and lose cytosolic enzymes but do
not round up or show the distorted morphology of the contracture
forms (Fig. 1C). The loss of sarcolemmal integrity in these
de-energized cells appears to be an all-or-none phenomenon, in
that the uptake of dye and the release of cytosolic lactic
dehydrogenase, creatine kinase, and aspartate aminotransferase all
appear to occur simultaneously and there is no indication of a
graded increase in permeability as a function of molecular size
(34). The permeable cells retain mitochondrial creatine kinase
and particulate aspartate aminotransferase, however. The factors
responsible for the loss of sarcolemma integrity with time in
de-energized myocytes have not been identified. This type of cell
death would appear analogous to that seen in hearts maintained in
global ischemia in vitro (23,41) and can be related to the lack of

high-energy phosphate compounds required to maintain structural
integrity.

When cells are incubated anaerobically in the absence of
glucose for 30 minutes or more and then re-aerated, large numbers
of round cells in hypercontracture (Fig. 1C) are produced. Nearly
40% of the cells assume this form when re-aerated after 30
minutes, for example (Table II). The round cell forms produced by
this protocol are indistinguishable from those produced by
addition of Ca to Na-loaded cells (see above). The
hypercontracted cells exclude trypan blue, restore high-energy
phosphate to the extent permitted by the adenine nucleotide level,
re-establish the creatine phosphate pool (73% of control) and
restore low ratios of intracellular Na to K (22).

Table II - Hypercontracture of Myocytes on Anaerobic to Aerobic
          Transition

Incubation Conditions	Viable Cells			AN	ATP
	Total	Rod	Round		
	(% Total Cells)			(nmol·mg^{-1})	
Control - no incubation	92±2	85±1	7±1	24±2	19±2
anaerobic 30 min; no glucose					
no reaeration-15 min	77±5	66±7	11±3	5±2	<1
re-aerated 15 min	75±4	38±7	37±3	8±2	5±1
re-aerated 15 min + rotenone	67±4	57±4	10±2	-	-
anaerobic 15 min + iodoacetate					
no re-aeration-15 min	78±1	67±2	12±2	4±1	<1
re-aerated 15 min.	70±4	3±1	67±5	4±1	2±1

The percentages of total cells maintaining rod-like configurations
(Fig. 1A and 1B) and viable cells rounded in hypercontracture
(Fig. 1C) were determined as previously described (5,22). The ATP
and total adenine nucleotide (AMP+ADP+ATP) content was estimated
by HPLC (22). Cells were maintained in Ca-free
Krebs-Ringer-phosphate (22) under N_2 for the indicated time at
37° and then either re-aerated for 15 min or anaerobic incubation
was continued for that time. Where indicated iodoacetate (5mM) or
rotenone (8μg/ml) were present throughout the incubation.

The hypercontracture of myocytes on anaerobic to aerobic
transition shares several features of the so-called
"oxygen-paradox" observed in intact hearts (13,14,19,20). In such
protocols hearts subjected to anoxic perfusion in the absence of

glucose show contracture of the cells and release of enzymes when
re-oxygenated. The oxygen-induced release of enzymes is prevented
by inclusion of glucose during hypoxic perfusion and inhibited by
cyanide or uncouplers of oxidative phosphorylation present during
re-oxygenation (13,14,19,20). The hypercontracture of myocytes on
anaerobic to aerobic transition shows an identical inhibitor
profile (22). The process is inhibited by rotenone (Table II) and
uncouplers and prevented by inclusion of glucose during the
anaerobic incubation (22). In addition, if glycolytic
ATP-formation is abolished by inclusion of iodoacetate (4), there
is a very rapid loss of high-energy phosphate and total adenine

nucleotide during anaerobic incubation, and re-aeration of such
cells produces a nearly complete conversion to the round
hypercontracture forms (Table II). This result suggests that a
portion of the cell population may maintain ATP levels by
glycogenolysis when incubated anaerobically in the absence of
glucose and that these cells can possibly account for the portion
of the cell population that does not go into hypercontracture when
re-aerated. Again, as with Ca-paradox discussed above, it would
appear that hypercontracture of myocytes with retention of
sarcolemmal integrity is equivalent to the cell contracture in
situ that leads to rupture of the sarcolemma and enzyme release
(13).

When cells are incubated under nitrogen in the absence of
glucose in buffer containing 1 mM Ca some round cells are produced
immediately (see above). The presence of Ca accelerates the loss
of myocyte viability during anaerobic incubation and increases the
number of cells that go into hypercontracture when re-aerated
(22). However, the presence of EGTA during anaerobic incubation
and re-aeration does not abolish the contracture. It appears that
large numbers of cells have sufficient Ca available from
intracellular sources to support the contracture process. It
should be noted that the anaerobic cells are contracted into
nearly square forms (Fig. 1B) and following aeration these forms
are seen to relax and contract for several cycles before rounding
up in hypercontracture (22). The restoration of ATP levels in
these cells occurs before the hypercontracture process is complete
(22) and the bulk of the mitochondria appear to remain competent
during and after hypercontracture (22). It appears therefore that
the production of ATP by mitochondrial oxidative phosphorylation
is contributing to the process of hypercontracture and that the
greatly diminished adenine nucleotide pool is probably the primary
lesion in this type of cellular deterioration. It also appears
likely that derangements of intracellular Ca metabolism that
develop under low-energy conditions contribute to
hypercontracture.

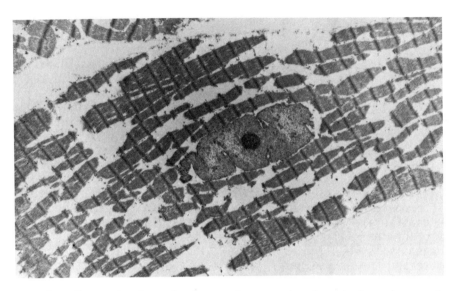

Figure 3 - Transmission electron micrograph of rod-shaped myocyte
extracted with Triton X-100 (2%) to remove mitochondria, SR, and
other detergent-soluble components. Note the maintenance of
overall cell configuration and the presence of fibrous components
of the sarcolemma (see 27). Micrograph courtesy of Owen Kindig.

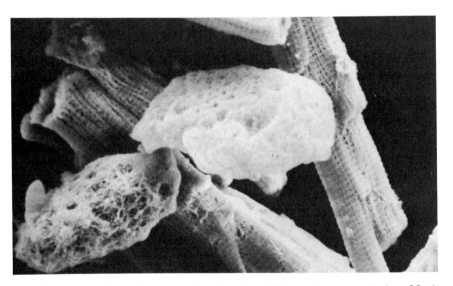

Figure 4 - Scanning micrograph of rod-cells and a rounded cell in
hypercontracture after Triton-extraction. The cytoskeleton
appears as a protein mesh after removal of detergent-soluble
components (see Figure 3; courtesy of Owen Kindig).

Studies using myocytes with a shunted sarcolemma indicate that the SR plays a primary role in the transient release of Ca during phasic contraction (7). In this preparation, elevation of free Ca above 10^{-6} M produces contracture and cell degeneration. In a recent study relating myoplasmic free Ca levels to the tension developed during a twitch of a myocyte, Fabiato (11) reported that a free Ca level of 4 µM is attained under optimal conditions of release from the SR and that this level of Ca corresponds to that which produces an optimal twitch in an intact cell. Full activation of myofibril contraction was not attained until 12 µM Ca was present. It would seem that either an over contraction due to elevated Ca or a failure of SR might be involved in the hypercontracture observed in our studies (2,5,22).

Two forms of lysed myocytes have proven useful in studies of the development of hypercontracture in myocytes. Cells lysed with digitonin (3) lose all soluble cytosolic components but retain intact mitochondria. These cells do not exhibit phasic contractions, so we assume that the SR is damaged. Digitonin lysis of respiring myocytes suspended in a nominally calcium-free buffer converts all cells to a round form stained by trypan blue. Addition of either rotenone or EGTA (1mM) prior to the digitonin yields a uniform population of elongated, dye-permeable cells (5). These results suggest that hypercontracture requires both Ca and ATP and that, in the absence of inhibitors, mitochondrial oxidative phosphorylation is able to satisfy the ATP requirement by continuous regeneration of high-energy phosphate (even in the presence of a markedly reduced total adenine nucleotide level in the lysed cells).

Cells lysed with Triton X-100 have been used to rule out a direct involvement of micochondria in hypercontracture. Triton-lysed cells (final concentration 1-5%) closely resemble intact elongated myocytes by light microscopy, but in the electron microscope it is clear that mitochondria and other membranous organelles (SR) are absent (Fig. 3). Triton extracted cells contain bundles of well-aligned contractile proteins and nuclei held together by filamentous structures continuous with the Z lines. Contracture of these cells is comparable to digitonin-lysed cells with regard to effects of ATP and chelators, but because there are no organelles to be extruded during hypercontracture, organization of contractile proteins is more easily visualized. Scanning electron microscopy of elongated Triton-extracted cells shows good preservation of cell shape and sarcomere organization, while hypercontracted cells are intact but grossly disorganized (Fig. 4).

The remarkable contribution of the filamentous cytoskeleton (27) to myocyte morphology is clearly evident in these preparations. This feature is even more striking when

triton-extracted cells are further treated with 0.6 M KCl to
remove the myofibrils (not shown). It seems clear, even after
these very preliminary studies, that the cytoskeleton is not
disaggregated during the contracture process but rather is twisted
and disorganized as the myofibrils contract.

ACKNOWLEDGEMENTS

These studies were supported in part by United States Public
Health Services Grant HL23166 and by a Grant-in-Aid from the
Central Ohio Heart Chapter. We thank Karla Lamka for expert
technical assistance and Owen Kindig for the electron micrographs.

REFERENCES

1. Alto, L.E. and Dhalla, N.S. Role of changes in microsomal
    calcium uptake in the effects of reperfusion of
    Ca^{2+}-deprived rat hearts. Circulation Research 48, 17-24
    (1981).

2. Altschuld, R., Gibb, L., Ansel, A., Hohl, C., Kruger, F.A.,
    and Brierley, G.P. Calcium tolerance of isolated rat heart
    cells. Journal of Molecular and Cellular Cardiology 12,
    1383-1395 (1980).

3. Altschuld, R., Hohl, C., Ansel, A., and Brierley, G.P.
    Compartmentation of K^+ in isolated rat heart cells.
    Archives of Biochemistry and Biophysics 209, 175-184 (1981).

4. Altschuld, R.A., Hohl, C. and Brierley, G.P. Role of
    anaerobic glycolysis in contracture of rat heart myocytes on
    anaerobic to aerobic transition. Federation Proceedings 41,
    447 (1982).

5. Altschuld, R.A., Hostetler, J.R., and Brierley, G.P.
    Response of isolated rat heart cells to hypoxia,
    re-oxygenation, and acidosis. Circulation Research 49,
    307-316 (1981).

6. Bahl, J., Navin, T., Manian, A.A., and Bressler, R.
    Carnitine transport in isolated adult rat heart myocytes and
    the effect of 7,8-diOH chlorpromazine. Circulation Research
    48, 378-385 (1981).

7. Chiesi, M., Ho, M.M., Inesi, G. Somlyo, A.V.A and Somlyo,
    A.P. Primary role of sarcoplasmic reticulium in phasic
    contractile activity of cardiac myocytes with shunted
    myolemma. The Journal of Cell Biology 91, 728-742 (1981).

8. Coraboeuf, E., Deroubaix, E., and Hoerter, J. Control of ionic permeabilities in normal and ischemic heart. Circulation Research Supplement I, 38 I-92-I-98 (1976).

9. Dow, J.W., Harding, N.G.L., and Powell, T. Isolated cardiac myocytes I. Preparation of adult myocytes and their homology with intact tissue. Cardiovascular Research 15, 483-514 (1981).

10. Dow, J.W., Harding, N.G.L., and Powell, T. Isolated cardiac myocytes II. Functional aspects of mature cells. Cardiovascular Research 15, 549-579 (1981).

11. Fabiato, A. Myoplasmic free calcuim concentration reached during the twitch of an intact isolated cardiac cell and during calcium-induced release of calcium from the sarcoplasmic retriculum of a skinned cardiac cell from the adult rat or rabbit ventricle. The Journal of General Physiology 78, 457-497 (1981).

12. Farmer, B.B., Harris, R.A., Jolly, W.W., Hathaway, D.E., Katzberg, A., Watanabe, A.M., Whitlow, D.R. and Besch Jr. H.R. Isolation and characterization of adult rat heart cells. Archives of Biochemistry and Biophysic 179, 545-558 (1977).

13. Ganote, C.E., and Kaltenbach, J.P. Oxygen-induced enzyme release: early events and a proposed mechanism. Journal of Molecular and Cellular Cardiology 11, 389-406 (1979).

14. Ganote, C. E., McGarr, J., Lui, S.Y. and Kaltenbach, J.P. Oxygen-induced enzyme release. Assessment of mitochondrial function in anoxic myocardial injury and effects of the mitochondrial uncoupling agent 2,4-dinitrophoenol (DNP). Journal of Molecular and Cellular Cardiology 12, 387-408 (1980).

15. Glitsch, H.G. Characteristics of active Na transport in intact cardiac cells. American Journal of Physiology 236, H189-H199 (1979).

16. Goshima, K., Wakaboyashi, S. and Masuda, A. Ionic mechanism of morphological changes of cultured myocardial cells on successive incubation in media without and with Ca^{2+}. Journal of Molecular and Cellular Cardiology 12, 1135-1157 (1980).

17. Grinwald, P.M. and Nayler, W.G. Calcium entry in the calcium paradox. Journal of Molecular and Cellular Cardiology 13, 867-880 (1981).

18. Haworth, R.A., Hunter, D.R. and Berkoff, H.A. Contracture in
     isolated adult rat heart cells. Role of Ca^{2+}, ATP, and
     compartmentation. Circulation Research 49, 1119-1128 (1981).

19. Hearse, D.J. and Chain. E.B. The role of glucose in the
     survival and recovery of the anoxic isolated perfused heart.
     The Biochemical Journal 128, 1125-1133 (1982).

20. Hearse, D.J., Humphrey, S.M. and Bullock, G.R. The oxygen
     paradox and the calcium paradox: two facets of the same
     problem. Journal of Molecular and Cellular Cardiology 10,
     641-668 (1978).

21. Hohl, C., Altschuld, R.A., and Brierley, G.P. Effects of
     calcium on the sodium and potassium content of adult rat
     heart myocytes. Federation Proceedings 41, 447 (1982).

22. Hohl, C., Ansel, A., Altschuld, R., and Brierley, G.P.
     Contracture of isolated rat heart cells on anaerobic to
     aerobic transition. American Journal of Physiology, 243, in
     press (1982).

23. Jennings, R.B., Reimer, K.A., Hill, M.L. and Mayer, S.E.
     Total ischemia in dog hearts in vitro. 1. Comparison of
     high energy phosphate production, utilization, and depletion,
     and of adenine nucleotide catabolism in total ischemia in
     vitro vs severe ischemia in vivo. Circulation Research 49,
     892-900 (1981).

24. Katz, A.M., Messineo, F.C., and Herbette, L. Ion Channels in
     membranes. Circulation 65 (supplement I) I-2-I-10 (1982).

25. Kao, R.L., Christman, E.W., Luh, S.L., Kraubs, J.M., Tylers,
     G.F.O. and Williams, E.H. The effects of insulin and anoxia
     on the metabolism of isolated mature rat cardiac myocytes.
     Archives of Biochemistry and Biophysics 203, 587-599 (1980).

26. Lamers, J.M.J. and Stinis, J.T. An electrogenic Na^{+}/Ca^{2+}
     antiporter in addition to the Ca^{2+} pump in cardiac
     sarcolemma. Biochimica et Biophysica Acta 640, 521-534
     (1981).

27. Lazarides, E. Intermediate filaments as mechanical
     integrators of cellular space. Nature 283, 249-256 (1980).

28. Linden, J. and Brooker, G. Properties of cardiac
     contractions in zero sodium solutions: intracellular free
     calcium controls slow channel conductance. Journal of
     Molecular and Cellular Cardiology 12, 457-478 (1980).

29. McCune, S.A. and Harris, R.A. Mechanism responsible for
     5-(tetradecyloxy)-2-furoic-acid inhibition of hepatic
     lipogenesis. The Journal of Biological Chemistry 254,
     10095-10101 (1979).

30. Miller, D.J. Are cardiac muscle cells "skinned" by EGTA or
     EDTA? Nature 277, 142-143 (1979).

31. Montini, J., Bagby, G.J., Burns, A.H. and Spitzer, J.J.
     Exogenous substrate utilization in Ca^{2+}-tolerant
     myocytes from adult rat hearts. American Journal of
     Physiology 240, H659-H663 (1981).

32. Moses, R.L. and Kasten, F.H. Ultrastructure of dissociated
     adult mammalian myocytes. Journal of Molecular and Cellular
     Cardiology 11, 161-162 (1979).

33. Mullins, L.J. The generation of electric currents in cardiac
     fibers by Na/Ca exchange. American Jounral of Physiology
     236, C103-C110 (1979).

34. Murphy, M., Altschuld, R.A. and Brierley, G.P. Patterns of
     enzyme release from adult rat heart myocytes. Federation
     proceedings 41, 381 (1982).

35. Nag, A.C., Fischman, D.A., Aumont, M.C. and Zak, R. Studies
     of isolated adult rat heart cells: the surface morphology
     and the influence of extracellular calcium ion concentration
     on cellular viability. Tissue and Cell 9, 419-436 (1977).

36. Onorato, J.J. and Rudolph, S.A. Regulation of protein
     phosphorylation by inotropic agents in isolated rat
     myocardial cells. The Journal of Biological Chemistry 256,
     10697-10703 (1981).

37. Philipson, K.D., Bers, D.M., Nishimoto, A.Y., and Langer,
     G.A. Binding of Ca^{2+} and Na^+ to sarcolemmal membranes:
     relation to control of myocardial contractility. American
     Journal of Physiology 238, H373-H378 (1980).

38. Philipson, K.D. and Nishimoto, A.Y. Efflux of Ca^{2+} from
     cardiac sarcolemmal vesicles. Influence of external Ca^{2+}
     and Na^+. The Journal of Biological Chemistry 256,
     3698-3702 (1981).

39. Quastel, M.R., Segal, G.B., and Lichtman, M.A. The effect of
     calcium chelation on lymphocyte monovalent cation
     permeability, trnasport, and concentration. The Journal of
     Cellular Physiology 107, 165-170 (1981).

40. Rasmussen, H. "Calcium and cAMP as synarchic messengers."
     John Wiley and Sons, New York, 1981.

41. Reimer, K.A., Jennings, R.B. and Hill, M.L. Total ischemia
     in dog hearts in vitro. 2. High energy phosphate depletion
     and associated defects in energy metabolism, cell volume
     regulation and sarcolemmal integrity. Circulation Research
     49, 901-911 (1981).

42. Roos, K.P., Brady, A.J., and Tan, S.T. Direct measurement of
     sarcomere length from isolated cardiac cells. American
     Journal of Physiology 242, H68-H78 (1982).

43. Ruigrok, T.J.C., Boink, A.B.T.J., Spies, F., Blok, F.J.,
     Maas, A.H.J. and Zimmerman, A.N.E. Energy dependence of the
     calcium pradox. Journal of Molecular and Cellular Cardiology
     10, 991-1002 (1978).

44. Russo, M.A., Cittadini, A., Dani, A.M., Inesi, G. and T.
     Terranova. An ultrastructural study of calcium induced
     degenerative changes in dissociated heart cells. Journal
     of Molecular and Cellular Cardiology 13, 265-279 (1981).

45. Winegrad, S. Studies of cardiac muscle with a high
     permeability to calcium produced by treatment with
     ethylenediaminetetraacetic acid. The Journal of General
     Physiology 58, 71-93 (1971).

46. Wittenberg, B.A. and Robinson, T.F. Oxygen requirements,
     morphology, cell coat and membrane permeability of
     calcium-tolerant myocytes from hearts of adult rats. Cell
     and Tissue Research 216, 231-251 (1981).

CARDIAC MUSCLE CELL PROLIFERATION AND

CELL DIFFERENTIATION IN VIVO AND IN VITRO

William C. Claycomb

Department of Biochemistry
Louisiana State University School of Medicine
New Orleans, Louisiana 70112 U.S.A.

INTRODUCTION

Terminal differentiation of the cardiac muscle cell can be viewed as a series of events. These events can be broadly separated into two divisions. One is the activation of specific genes and acquisition of cell specific functions such as the synthesis and assembly of the contractile proteins and the establishment of contractile force. The other division can be viewed as the inactivation of specific genes and the loss of specific functions such as the loss of enzymes and other proteins which are needed to replicate DNA and cessation of DNA replication and cell division. There are a multitude of changes which occur in the biochemistry, physiology, pharmacology and morphology of the cardiac muscle cell as it differentiates and in the intact heart in general, during early growth and development. This review will be confined to the ventricular cardiac muscle cell of the laboratory rat and will be concerned with selected aspects of cellular proliferation, differentiation, morphology and metabolism and will deal primarily with studies carried out in this laboratory. It will be divided into those events occurring in intact cardiac muscle in vivo during early neonatal development and with studies of cardiac muscle cells isolated from neonatal and adult animals and grown in primary cell culture. The reader is refered to several recent excellent reviews which have dealt extensively with many other aspects of growth and development of the heart (1-5).

249

DNA REPLICATION, CELL PROLIFERATION AND CELL HYPERTROPHY IN VIVO

In skeletal muscle, cytodifferentiation and cellular pro- liferation are mutually exclusive (6-8). In contrast, cardiac muscle cells containing actin, myosin, and highly organized contractile proteins continue to replicate their DNA and undergo mitosis (10-17). Autoradiographic studies have shown that in the rat, DNA synthesis occurs during the early stages of postnatal development (1,10-12) but not in the terminally differentiated adult cells (1,10,18-20). Autoradiographic and histologic data of Rumyantsev (10,11) demonstrate that the percentage of labeled nuclei and the percentage of those cells undergoing mitosis in cardiac muscle of the rat has reached nearly zero by about the 13th day of postnatal development. Semiconservative DNA replication in the intact rat heart and in purified individual cardiac muscle cells has been determined to essentially cease by the 17th day of postnatal development (21-23). When these studies were done it was widely believed that once semiconservative DNA replication stopped in these muscle cells it was irreversibly repressed for the remaining life of the animal. In a later section, recent work will be discussed which demonstrates that DNA replication is reactivated in the terminally differentiated adult ventricular cardiac muscle cell grown in culture.

An important aspect of the growth of the heart during early development should be emphasized here. Growth and the increase in the mass of the heart muscle during early development is primarily by cell division and proliferation or hyperplasia. After the third week of postnatal development of the rat, hyperplastic growth ceases because DNA replication and cell division cease. After this time period the increase in muscle mass is due to the enlargement or hypertrophy of these pre-existing cells. This is documented in Fig. 1 which shows how much the cardiac muscle cell enlarges from the period during growth when cell division ceases to the adult animal (Fig. 1 B-C). These cells acquire and assemble large quantities of contractile proteins and it has been estimated that they enlarge some 10 fold in size (24). Thus, at about 3 weeks of postnatal development growth of the heart essentially changes from one of cell hyperplasia to cell hypertrophy. As has been suggested and will be discussed in the next section this change in growth pattern may be brought about by an increase in the functional demand placed on the developing heart (22,25). An increase in functional demand exerted on the heart of the adult animal is known to result in hypertrophy of the cardiac muscle cells and enlargement of the heart (26-29). It was suggested previously (25) that the

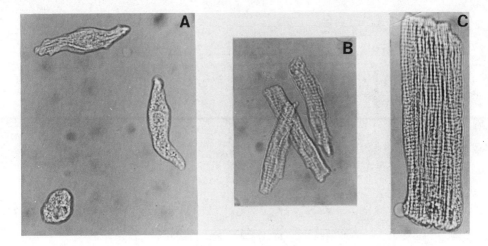

Figure 1. Cardiac muscle cells were prepared from (A) 1-day;
(B) 17-day; (C) adult rats (23). As the cells
differentiate they acquire and assemble the contractile proteins into sarcomeres (B). Since all of
these cells are at the same magnification (x500)
it can readily be appreciated how much they enlarge
during development.

developing animal may offer an excellent experimental system
which can be used to study cardiac muscle hypertrophy. The
model is always reproducible and it may very well be that the
molecular mechanism(s) which induces cellular hypertrophy in
the neonatal animal is similar to that which operates in the
adult animal when the heart enlarges.

POSSIBLE MECHANISMS RESPONSIBLE FOR CESSATION OF DNA
REPLICATION AND CELL DIVISION

Once the time period during development when DNA
replication is repressed in cardiac muscle cells was
established, the next obvious question was to ask how this
repression was achieved. It had previously been observed that
the concentration of cyclic AMP increases progressively as the
concentration of cyclic GMP decreases in cardiac muscle of the
rat during late fetal and early neonatal development (Fig. 2)
(30,31). The activity of adenylate cyclase is also higher in
the adult than in the newborn (32-34). Since cyclic AMP had
been implicated both in the regulation of cell proliferation
and cell differentiation in many cellular systems, it was

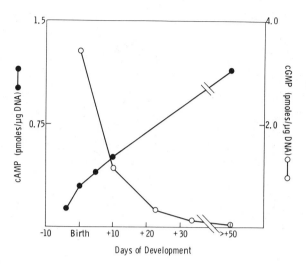

Figure 2. Concentrations of cyclic AMP and cyclic GMP in
cardiac muscle of the developing rat. Cyclic
AMP values are from (30) and are recalculated
on a per μg of DNA (per cell) basis. Cyclic GMP
values are from (31) and also are recalculated on
a per μg of DNA (per cell) basis.

decided to examine whether this cyclic nucleotide might be
involved with the regulation of cell proliferation and cell
differentiation in cardiac muscle (22). It was observed that
a single injection of either isoproterenol or dibutyryl cyclic
AMP results in an inhibition in the rate of [^{3}H] thymidine
incorporation into the DNA of differentiating cardiac muscle
of the neonatal rat (22) and that this inhibition could be
potentiated by theophylline. This inhibition was also
observed (22) in tissue slices of the heart prepared from
neonatal rats that had been injected with isoproterenol or
cyclic AMP 16 hours prior to preparing the slices.
Isoproterenol and cyclic AMP were also found to accelerate the
pattern of biochemical events which normally occurs in cardiac
muscle of the neonatal rat during the course of early
development. This pattern includes an increase in protein and
myosin synthesis, an increase in the activity of poly
(ADP-ribose) polymerase and decreases in the synthesis of DNA
and the activity of the replicative DNA polymerase (22,35).
A significant increase in the cellular concentration of NAD
was also observed (35). These experiments demonstrated that
cyclic AMP and agents which elevate intracellular
concentrations of cyclic AMP would accelerate the normal

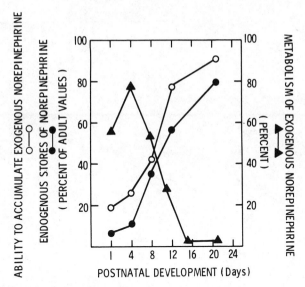

Figure 3. Uptake, metabolism and endogenous stores of norepinephrine in cardiac muscle of the rat during
development. Redrawn from data of Glowinski et al.
(36) and Iversen, et al. (37).

events which occur as the cardiac muscle cell terminally
differentiates. In reviewing the literature concerning the
adrenergic innervation of the heart during development it was
found that not only does the concentration of cyclic AMP
increase in the heart but that there also is a progressive
development-dependent increase in endogenous stores of
norepinephrine and in the ability to take up, accumulate, and
not catabolize exogenous norepinephrine (36,37) (Fig. 3).
These parameters are used to judge the functional maturation
of an adrenergic neuron (38,39). The tissue content of
norepinephrine is held to reflect the density of the
adrenergic neurons and it has been observed that the density
of the adrenergic neurons in the heart increases with
development (38-42). A few single axons are observed at
birth; innervation continually increases thereafter,
approximating the adult pattern by about the 22nd day of
postnatal development. Thus, in cardiac muscle of the rat the
cessation of DNA replication and cell proliferation, and the
degree of cellular differentiation and the rise in the
intracellular concentration of cyclic AMP, are correlated
temporally with the anatomical and physiological development
of the adrenergic nerves and innervation of the heart.
Because of these observations and the experiments
demonstrating that cyclic AMP and catecholamines could

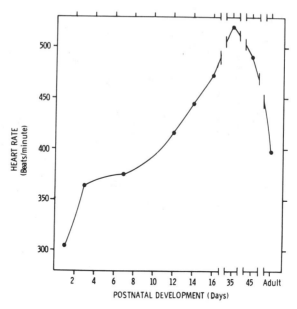

Figure 4. Development of the heart rate in the rat. Redrawn from (Adolph (52) and Wekstein (53)).

prematurely accelerate the normal developmental program of the
heart, it was proposed that DNA replication, cell proliferation
and differentiation in cardiac muscle is ultimately
controlled by adrenergic innervation with norepinephrine and
cyclic AMP serving as the chemical mediators and that the
elevation in the intracellular concentration of cyclic AMP
during development resulted from the stimulation of
adenylate cyclase by norepinephrine (22). It was also
proposed that one level of growth control (or at least the size
an organ attains) during growth and development may be mediated
by the autonomic nervous system's influence on cellular
proliferation (22).

Thus, it is hypothesized that the physiological signal
for the heart to change its growth pattern from hyperplasia to
hypertrophy is functional adrenergic innervation with
norepinephrine and cyclic AMP serving as chemical mediators.
Several studies of Slotkin and colleagues add support to this
concept (43-46). Cardiac hypertrophy in the adult is in
response to an increased functional demand placed on the
heart. The stimulus for the muscle cells to enlarge and
increase their synthesis of contractile proteins in the
neonatal animal could be the same, with the increase in
functional demand originating from an increase in adrenergic
nerve activity. The heart rate of the laboratory rat

Table 1. Heart weight/body weight ratio and heart rate of various animals. From Welty (54).

Animal	Heart Weight (% of Body Weight)	Heart Rate (Beats/Minute)
Frog	0.57	22
Man	0.42	72
Canary	1.68	514
Hummingbird	2.37	615

increases from approximately 300 beats/min to approximately 500 to 600 beats/min during the first 3 weeks after birth (Fig. 4) and this increase in heart rate is due exclusively to the adrenergic sympathetic nervous system (43,44). This increase stops apparently when the parasympathetic restraint counterbalances the sympathetic influence and thus a new steady state heart rate is reached. Apparently this increase in heart rate is a mechanism that is used by the autonomic nervous system to compensate the neonatal animal to the increased hemodynamic load encountered after birth. It was suggested (25) that as a response to this increased functional demand, the muscle cells cease dividing and increase their production of contractile elements. These contractile elements may act as a physical barrier to prevent cell division and therefore subsequent growth of the heart is by cell hypertrophy. The size of an organ is largely determined by the work it has to perform. The physiological mechanisms that regulate function apparently also control growth (see Table 1 which demonstrates a correlation between heart weight and heart rate). This biological concept would appear to be exemplified by the developing heart and hypertrophy of the cardiac muscle cell.

Cyclic AMP is known to influence many events which occur in the nucleus of the cell. At a molecular level the adrenergic nervous system may also be exerting a control on cell division by influencing the activity of genes which specify the synthesis of the enzymes and proteins needed to replicate DNA or which code for the synthesis of the contractile proteins. A cell that is actively synthesizing DNA has already made the decision to continue through the cell cycle, enter mitosis and divide. Thus, the control of the cell cycle and hence cell division resides in the factors which control the initiation and regulate the rate of DNA synthesis. The adrenergic nervous system may influence DNA synthesis and hence cell proliferation by a programmed and selective repression in the genes coding for the enzymes and proteins needed for DNA replication. Cyclic AMP could act via a specific cyclic AMP-dependent protein kinase to selectively repress or activate genes coding for DNA enzymes or the contractile proteins. This could occur by phosphorylation of certain chromosomal proteins.

It should be noted here that thyroid hormone is known to influence differentiation of the cardiac muscle cell. An excess or lack of this hormone can also influence other biochemical parameters in cardiac muscle of both neonatal and adult animals. Thyroid hormone may exert these effects on development of the heart and differentiation of the cardiac muscle cell by influencing maturation of sympathetic neurotransmission in the heart (47-51). This in turn could alter or help determine the developmental program.

CONTROL OF DNA REPLICATION BY DNA ENZYMES

Semiconservative DNA replication declines progressively in intact cardiac muscle of the rat and in isolated cardiac muscle cells and essentially ceases by the 17th day of postnatal development (21,23). Temporally correlated with the loss of this synthetic activity is the disappearance from these cells of measurable activities of at least 2 DNA enzymes, DNA polymerase α and thymidine kinase (21,23,55). DNA polymerase α is now felt by most investigators to be the replicative DNA polymerase in the eukaryotic cell. Thymidine kinase is a key enzyme providing nucleotide building blocks needed for DNA replication. A logical question to ask of this data is: does DNA synthesis cease in this tissue because the activities of these and other DNA enzymes are lost, or are the activities of these enzymes lost because DNA synthesis ceases? Which is the cause and which is the effect? What metabolic changes cause, and which are merely associated with, cessation of DNA synthesis and terminal cell differentiation? This was tested directly (56) by isolating nuclei and chromatin from cardiac muscle at various times during the developmental period in which DNA synthesis is being and has been restricted. To determine if the ability of DNA to serve as a template for DNA replication changes, both template availability (as determined by the amount of DNA in nuclei or chromatin which is accessible for DNA polymerase binding and that can be used as a template to catalyze incorporation of deoxyribonucleotides into DNA) and the number of 3'-OH termini in the DNA which can serve as primer termini for polymerization were measured. If either of these were restricted during the terminal differentiation of the muscle cell then no matter how much DNA polymerase was present in the cell, DNA synthesis would not occur. Three different DNA polymerases were used, DNA polymerase α, E. coli DNA polymerase I and M. luteus DNA polymerase. Density-shift experiments with bromodeoxyuridine triphosphate and isopynic analysis in cesium chloride equilibrium density gradients showed that DNA chains being replicated semiconservatively in vivo continued to be elongated by these exogenous DNA polymerases. DNA template availability and 3'-OH termini available to exogenously added DNA polymerases were found not to change as cardiac muscle differentiates and the rate of DNA synthesis decreases and ceases in vivo. Template availability and 3'-OH termini were also not changed in nuclei isolated from cardiac muscle in which DNA synthesis had been inhibited by administration of isoproterenol and theophylline to newborn rats. It was concluded from these studies (56) that DNA synthesis ceases in terminally differentiating cardiac muscle because the activity of the replicative DNA polymerase and other enzymes needed for DNA replication are lost from the cell, rather than the activity of these enzymes being lost because DNA synthesis ceases. The loss of the enzymes which are needed for DNA replication is probably due to a selective and programmed repression in the genes coding for them. Adrenergic innervation of the heart may ultimately be responsible for this developmental program with norepinephrine and cyclic AMP serving as the chemical mediators of the nerves.

A point that should be emphasized with all in vivo studies of cardiac muscle tissue is that this tissue is heterogeneous as to cell type. It has been estimated that only 55% of the total cell population of the ventricular muscle of the one-day-old rat are actually myocytes; the remaining 45% are fibroblasts, phagocytes, circulating erythrocytes and cells comprising nerve and vascular tissue (24). Myocytes comprise only 20-25% of the total cell population of cardiac muscle of the adult rat (19, 24). Therefore, studies carried out using whole tissue or organelles isolated from whole muscle tissue may not accurately reflect the metabolic state of the cardiac muscle cell. These studies do provide useful information but the results should be interpreted with this caveat in mind. For this reason further studies were extended to pure populations of cardiac muscle cells grown in culture (57-61).

IN VITRO STUDIES WITH CARDIAC MUSCLE CELLS IN CULTURE

Neonatal cells in serum-free media

Culture of cardiac muscle cells from neonatal rats has provided a system which can be used to study directly the proliferation, differentiation and growth of this cell. In

addition cultured cells are useful for studies of the
structure and function of the cardiac myocyte. One
disadvantage of the culture system is that the cultures
eventually become overgrown with fibroblasts and that crude
animal serum is needed for maintenance and growth of the
cells. These sera contain many undefined substances such as
hormones and growth factors. This makes it difficult to
determine precisely what factors are needed for
differentiation and growth of these cells and makes the
assessment of the effect of substances added to the cells complex and difficult. Recently, cardiac muscle cells from
neonatal rats have been cultured in completely defined
serum-free media (57). The most successful system consists of
precoating the bottom of the culture flask with fibronectin
and adding fetuin and either dibutyryl cyclic AMP, cholera
toxin, epidermal growth factor or insulin plus dexamethasone
to the medium. A serum- and a hormone or growth factor-free
medium was defined by growing the cells in the presence of
fibronectin, fetuin and dibutyryl cyclic AMP for the first 4
days of culture, after which time the dibutyryl cyclic AMP was
omitted from the medium. Under these conditions the cells
continue to maintain their differentiated state for at least 4
days thereafter. This system thus offers a means to study the
cardiac muscle cell in the absence of serum, hormones or
growth factors. These studies also add support to the
proposal that cyclic AMP is involved with the differentiation
of the cardiac muscle cell. Dibutyryl cyclic AMP and cholera
toxin (which is known to increase the activity of adenylate
cyclase and elevate the intracellular concentration of cyclic
AMP) both accelerated the rate of morphological
differentiation of these cells in serum containing (Fig. 5)
and serum-free medium (57). These agents also will prematurely increase the activity of creatine phosphokinase and
decrease the synthesis of DNA when added to cultures of
neonatal cells (unpublished observations). Another advantage
of the serum-free culture system is that fibroblast
contamination has almost been eliminated. Apparently cyclic
AMP and cholera toxin inhibit the proliferation of the
non-muscle cells and they die and do not overgrow the culture.
A disadvantage of using neonatal cells in culture is that they
differ in many respects biochemically, physiologically,
morphologically and pharmacologically from the cardiac muscle
cell of the adult animal (59,60,62-65). Therefore, what we
have learned or will learn from studies of neonatal cardiac
muscle cells in culture may not be directly applicable to the
fully differentiated adult cell.

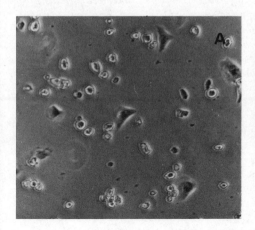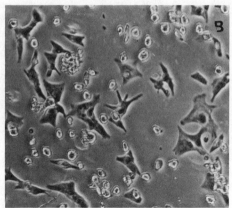

Figure 5. Effect of dibutyryl cyclic AMP on neonatal rat
cardiac muscle cells in culture. Cells were isolated
from 2-day old rats and were grown in the absence (A)
or presence (B) of dibutyryl cyclic AMP (10^{-3}M) for
the first 16 hours of culture. This nucleotide
greatly decreases the time needed for these cells
to attach and spread out and accelerates the differentiation of these cells in culture. These
cells have been in culture for 16 hrs.

Terminally differentiated adult ventricular cardiac muscle cells in culture

Recently the methodology to culture ventricular cardiac
muscle cells isolated from adult rats has been perfected (58,
66-68). We have been successful in maintaining spontaneously
contracting cells in culture for as long as 128 days. The
freshly isolated cells are striated and cylindrical in shape,
typical of intact ventricular cardiac muscle cells. When
placed in culture they shorten, round up and lose their cross
striations. They then attach to the surface of the culture
flask and extend pseudopod-like processes. With increased time
the cells spread out and become entirely flattened and
organized bands of myofibrils reappear (58). At the light and
scanning electron microscope level these cells appear to be
similar morphologically to cardiac muscle cells isolated from
neonatal rats and grown in culture, however, they are much
larger. Many of the cells continue to contract spontaneously

during the rounding and spreading out process and nearly all
of the completely flattened, spread-out cells are contracting
(58). We have recently completed an ultrastructural study of
this rounding and spreading out process and have fully
characterized the ultrastructure of the completely flattened,
spread-out cell, maintained in long term culture (59,60). The
cardiac muscle cell is fairly well organized immediately after
isolation but becomes disorganized with respect to sarcomeric
arrangement after 24 hours in culture (59). The cells are
damaged by the dissociation process and exhibit large surface
blebs which are full of mitochondria. The blebs are
eventually pinched off and produce mitochondria - filled
vesicles. Cellular damage is also exhibited as bloated
mitochondria, supercontracted myofilaments and breakdown of Z
lines. Although sarcomere organization was profoundly
disturbed, some minimal signs of prior filament interrelations
persisted. Non-junctional sarcoplasmic reticulum was no longer
recognizable. Some elements of the transverse tubular system
(T system) were observed in the tangled mass of disorganized
filaments. Myofilaments in the rounded cells were largely
disorganized, however, some elements of myofibrillar
organization were still apparent. Focal Z densities were
present among the disorganized filaments and some groups of
filaments ran in parallel, unregistered arrays. Former
intercalated disc regions could not be recognized. After 5
days in culture the cells begin to reconstruct their in vivo
ultrastructure (60). Fine structural evidence for protein
synthesis was abundant, and the cells appear to reorganize
their contractile apparatus using a mechanism similar to that
observed during normal mammalian cardiac muscle
differentiation. Other myocyte features which reappeared as
the myofilaments reorganized included intercalated discs,
sarcoplasmic reticulum and a fully formed T system.
Lipofuscin granules also were present and probably were of de
novo origin. It was concluded from this developmental study
(60) that the changes observed in these cells during the
initial culture period when they round up and then spread out
into spontaneously contracting cells, is due to both a simple
reorganization and to cellular dedifferentiation and
redifferentiation. This redifferentiation may be by a process
which is identical or similar to that which occurs during
embryonic and neonatal development when the premyoblasts
differentiate into cardiac muscle cells.

A detailed thin-section study of the fully established
flattened out adult cardiac muscle cell in culture revealed
that they more closely resemble the adult in vivo cardiac
muscle cell than does the cultured neonatal cardiac myocyte
(59). These cells contain typically distributed organelles
such as nuclei, mitochondria, Golgi apparatus, and elements of

the sarcoplasmic reticulum. Myofilaments are highly organized and sarcomeres are in register. Typical intercalated discs were observed between adjacent cells. Unlike cultured neonatal cardiac muscle cells, the adult cells contained a well developed transverse tubular system and numerous residual bodies. The T system is present only in rudimentary form in cultured neonatal myocytes. Therefore, at the ultrastructural level these cells look identical to the cardiac muscle cell in the intact heart except that they are flattened and spread out.

It has recently been observed that these terminally dif-fereintiated cells in culture acquire multiple nuclei (69). In one cultured myocyte as many as 10 nuclei have been counted. The number of nuclei seen thus far has ranged from one to ten. The nuclei generally occur in multiples of two and pairs usually had similar sizes, however, individual pairs within the same cell sometimes differed in their size and morphology. Cells containing multiple nuclei may be formed by DNA replication followed by karyokinesis; the cells then must fail to complete mitosis and divide. To investigate whether DNA synthesis was occuring they were cultured in the presence of [^{3}H]thymidine and then processed for autoradiography. Both binucleated and multinucleated cells were observed to incorporate [^{3}H] thymidine into DNA as evidenced by the high concentration of silver grains over their nuclei (69). Peak periods of incorporation were observed to occur at 10- to 20-day intervals. Maximum periods of incorporation occurred at 11-, 23- and 33-days after placing the cells in culture. If the cells were cultured continuously for 30 days in the presence of [^{3}H] thymidine, 56% of the cells incorporated [^{3}H] thymidine (61). Isopynic analysis of bromodeoxyuridine-labelled DNA in equilibrium density gradients demonstrated that this [^{3}H] thymidine incorporation is into DNA that is replicating semiconservatively and is not due to some type of DNA repair phenomenon (70). Recent studies have shown that these cells also reacquire activities of DNA enzymes which are needed to provide nucleotide building blocks and which polymerize these nucleotides into DNA (61). These studies demonstrate that the terminally differentiated mammalian ventricular cardiac muscle cell, previously thought to have permanently lost the capacity to synthesize DNA during early development, is able to reinitiate DNA replication when grown in culture.

The adult mammalian ventricular cardiac muscle cell grown for weeks or months in cell culture offers a new and unique system which can be used to study the heart muscle cell. These cultured adult cells offer advantages over neonatal cells grown in culture because they more closely resemble the

muscle cells in the adult intact heart and they are easier to
maintain for prolonged time periods. We are able to eliminate
fibroblast contamination by including cytosine arabinoside in
the medium during the first seven days of culture. They also
offer distinct advantages over freshly isolated adult cells
because they can be maintained for long time periods. The
freshly isolated cells clearly are damaged and leaky and what
is most likely being measured in short-term studies (1-2 hour
incubations) using these cells are changes or events due to
repair processes. In many instances studies using freshly
isolated cells most likely reflect measurements of processes
that are occurring in dying or in dead cells and do not
reflect the metabolism or transport processes of a normal
myocyte. Unlike freshly isolated cardiac muscle cells which
oxidize glucose preferentially, cultured adult cardiac muscle
cells more closely resemble metabolically the in vivo heart
muscle and the isolated perfused heart, in that their
preference for exogenous substrates is in the order of fatty
acid > lactate > glucose (71). What ever is damaged or
altered and accounts for the changed metabolic pattern in the
freshly isolated myocyte apparently is repaired or returned to
the in vivo normal situation in these cultured adult cardiac
muscle cells.

In conclusion, the cultured adult rat ventricular cardiac
muscle cell provides a unique in vitro model of the in vivo
terminally differentiated adult cardiac muscle cell.

REFERENCES

1.   Rumyantsev, P.P., 1977, Int. Rev. Cytol., Bourne G.H. and
     Danielli, J.F., eds., Academic Press, New York, 187-273.
2.   Harary, I., 1979, Handbook of Physiology Cardiovascular
     System I, Berns, R.M., Sperelakis, N. and Geiger, S.R.,
     eds., Am. Physiol. Soc. Bethesda, MD, 43-60.
3.   Bugaisky, and Zak, R., 1979, Texas Reports Biol. Med.
     39: 123-138.
4.   Dowell, R.T., 1980, Hearts and Heart-Like Organs, 2:
     419-433.
5.   Rakusan, K., 1980, Hearts and Heart-Like Organs, 2:
     301-348.
6.   Stockdale, F.E. and Holtzer, H., 1961, Exp. Cell Res.
     24: 508-520.
7.   Okazaki, K. and Holtzer, H., 1965, J. Histochem.
     Cytochem. 13: 726-739.
8.   Okazaki, K. and Holtzer, H., 1966, Proc. Natl. Acad.
     Sci. U.S.A. 56: 1484-1490.
9.   Manasek, F.J., 1968, J. Cell Biol. 37: 191-196.

10. Rumyantsev, P.P., 1963, Folia Histochem. Cytochem. 1: 463-471.
11. Rumyantsev, P.P., 1965, Fed. Proc. (Trans. Suppl.) 24: T899-T904.
12. Rumyantsev, P.P. and Snigirevskaya, E.S., 1968, Acta Morphol. Acad. Sci. Hong. 16: 271-283.
13. Weinstein, R.B. and Hay, E.D., 1970, J. Cell Biol. 47: 310-316.
14. Przybylski, R.J. and Chlebowski, J.S., 1972, J. Morphol. 137: 417-432.
15. Hay, D.A. and Low, F.N., 1972, Am. J. Anat. 134: 175-202.
16. Chacko, S., 1973, Folia Histochem. Cytochem. 1: 463-471.
17. Polinger, I.S., 1973, Exp. Cell Res. 76: 253-262.
18. Klinge, O. and Stocker, E., 1968, Experientia 24: 167-168.
19. Morkin, E. and Ashford, T.P., 1968, Am. J. Physiol. 215: 1409-1913.
20. Mandache, E., Unge, G., Appelgren, L.-E. and Ljungquist, A., 1973, Virchows Arch Abt. B Zellpath. 12: 112-122.
21. Claycomb, W.C., 1975, J. Biol. Chem. 250: 3229-3235.
22. Claycomb, W.C., 1976, J. Biol. Chem. 251: 6082-6089.
23. Claycomb, W.C., 1979, Exp. Cell Res. 118: 111-114.
24. Sasaki, R., Watanabe, Y., Morishita, T. and Yamagata, S., 1968, Tohoku J. Exp. Med. 95: 177-184.
25. Claycomb, W.C., 1976, Biochem. J. 168: 599-601.
26. Fanburg, B.L., 1970, N. Engl. J. Med. 282: 723-732.
27. Rabinowitz, M. and Zak, R., 1972, Ann. Rev. Med. 23: 245-261.
28. Rabinowitz, M., 1974, Circ. Res. 34: Suppl. 2, 3-11.
29. Morkin, E., 1974, Circ. Res. 34: Supl. 2, 37-48.
30. Novak, E., Drummond, G.I., Skala, J. and Hahn, P., 1972, Arch. Biochem. Biophys. 150: 511-518.
31. Kim, G. and Silverstein, E., 1975, Fed. Proc. 34:231.
32. Brus, R. and Hess, M.E., 1973, Endocrinol. 93: 982-985.
33. Brus, R., 1974, Pol. J. Pharmacol. 26: 337-340.
34. Yount, E.A. and Clark, C.M., Jr., 1976, Fed. Proc. 35: 423.
35. Claycomb, W.C., 1976, Biochem. J. 154: 387-393.
36. Glowinski, J., Axelrod, J., Kopin, I.J. and Wurtman, R.J., 1964, J. Pharmacol. Exp. Ther. 146: 48-53.
37. Inversen, L.L., DeChamplain, U., Glowinski, J. and Axelrod, J., 1967, J. Pharmacol. Exp. Ther. 157: 509-516.
38. Mirkin, B.L., 1972, Fed. Proc. 31: 65-73.
39. Burnstock, C. and Costa, M., 1975, Adrenergic Neurons. Their Organization, Function and Development in the Peripheral Nervous System. John Wiley and Sons, New York.
40. DeChamplain, J., Malmfors, T., Olson, L. and Sachs, C., 1970, Acta Physiol. Scand. 80: 276-288.

41. Schiebler, T.H. and Heene, R., 1968, Histochemie 14: 328-334.
42. Friedman, W.F., Pool, P.E., Jacobowitz, D., Seagren, S.C. and Braunwald, F., 1968, Cir. Res. 23: 25-32.
43. Bartolome, J. Lau, C. and Slotkin, T.A., 1977, J. Pharmacol. Exp. Ther. 202: 510-518.
44. Bareis, D.L. and Slotkin, T.A., 1978, J. Pharmacol. Exp. Ther. 205: 164-174.
45. Slotkin, T.A., Seidler, F.S. and Whitmore, W.L., 1980, Life Sci. 26: 1657-1663.
46. Bareis, D.L. and Slotkin, T.A., 1980, J. Pharmacol. Exp. Ther. 212: 120-125.
47. Deskin, R., Mills, E., Whitmore, W.L., Seidler, F.J. and Slotkin, T.A., 1980, J. Pharmacol. Exp. Ther. 215: 342-347.
48. Lau, C. and Slotkin, T.A., 1979, J. Pharmacol. Exp. Ther. 208: 485-490.
49. Lau, C. and Slotkin, T.A., 1980, Mol. Pharmacol. 18: 247-252.
50. Lau, C. and Slotkin, T.A., 1980, J. Pharmacol. Exp. Ther. 212: 126-130.
51. Lau, C. and Slotkin, T.A., 1982, J. Pharmacol. Exp. Ther. 220: 629-636.
52. Adolph, E.F., 1967, Am. J. Physiol. 212: 595-602.
53. Wekstein, D.R., 1965, Am. J. Physiol. 208: 1259-1262.
54. Welty, C., 1955, Sci. Am. 192: 88-96.
55. Gillette, P.C. and Claycomb, W.C., 1974, Biochem. J. 142: 685-690.
56. Claycomb, W.C., 1978, Biochem. J. 171: 289-298.
57. Claycomb, W.C., 1980, Exp. Cell Res. 131: 231-236.
58. Claycomb, W.C. and Palazzo, M.C., 1981, Develop. Biol. 80: 466-482.
59. Moses, R.L. and Claycomb, W.C., 1982, Am. J. Anat. 164: 113-131.
60. Moses, R.L. and Claycomb, W.C., 1982, In Press.
61. Claycomb, W.C. and Bradshaw, H.D., Jr., 1982, In Press.
62. Carmeliet, E., Horres, C.R., Lieberman, M. and Vereeck, J.S., 1975, Developmental and Physiological Correlates of Cardiac Muscle, Liberman, M. and Sano, T., eds., Raven Press, New York, 103-116.
63. Dehaan, R.L., McDonal, T.F. and Sachs, H.G., 1975, Developmental and Physiological Correlates of Cardiac Muscle, Liberman, M. and Sano, T., eds., Raven Press, New York, 155-168.
64. Sperelakis, N., Shiegenobu, K. and Mc Lean, M.J., 1975, Developmental and Physiological Correlates of Cardiac Muscle, Liberman, M. and Sano, T., eds., Raven Press, New York, New York, 169-184.

65. Langer, G.A., Brady, A.J., Tan, S.T. and Serens, S.D.,
     1975, Cir. Res. 36: 744-752.
66. Jacobson, S.L., 1977, Cell Struct. Func. 2: 1-9.
67. Schwarzfeld, T.A. and Jacobson, 1981, J. Mol. Cell
     Card., 13: 563-576.
68. Nag, A.C. and Cheng, M., 1981, Tiss. Cell 13:
     515-523.
69. Claycomb, W.C., 1981, J. Cell. Biol. 91: 342a.
70. Bradshaw, H.D., Jr. and Claycomb, W.C., 1981,
     Fed. Proc. 40: 1628.
71. Claycomb, W.C. and Burns, A.H., 1982, Fed. Proc. 41:
     1418.

RADIONUCLIDE VENTRICULOGRAPHY TO EVALUATE MYOCARDIAL FUNCTION

Robert L. Huxley, James R. Corbett,
Samuel E. Lewis, and James T. Willerson

Departments of Internal Medicine (Cardiovascular Division
and Radiology (Nuclear Medicine), The University of Texas
Health Science Center, 5323 Harry Hines Boulevard
Dallas, Texas 75235

INTRODUCTION

Over the past decade, radionuclide ventriculography has developed from being solely an investigational tool to one of wide spread use in the clinical assessment of myocardial function. Visualization of the cardiac chambers and qualitative and quantitative assessment of ventricular function provide the clinician with important diagnostic and prognostic information. In addition, radionuclide ventriculography is non-invasive, can be applied during stress including exercise, or during pharmacologic intervention, and provides a means of following patients serially.

METHODOLOGY

Ventricular images are obtained using two general methods: (1) the "first-pass" and (2) the equilibrium blood pool technique. The first-pass method follows the initial transit of radiotracer through the heart. The equilibrium blood pool method is performed after an intravascular radiotracer has reached equilibrium; data acquisition relies on synchronizing ("gating") data collection intervals to specified portions of the cardiac cycle. In this manner, end-diastolic and end-systolic images may be obtained. A popular approach is to acquire data using multiple frames obtained throughout a cardiac cycle ("MUGA" or multiple gated acquisition). Each of these methods is discussed below.

First-Pass Method

1. _Technique_. This technique is based on indicator-dilution principles and assumes that there is homogeneous mixing of the

267

radioactive tracer with blood as it passes through each of the cardiac chambers (5,13,14,75). Both right and left ventricular function can be evaluated from the same study because of temporal and anatomic separation of radioactivity within the cardiac chambers (Figures 1 and 2). First pass studies may be performed either upright or supine.

Injection of the radionuclide material may be made through an antecubital vein, an external jugular vein or directly into the pulmonary artery. However, the radionuclide tracer must be injected as a compact bolus into the circulation to provide subsequent homogenous mixing of the tracer so that changes in radiographic count rates correspond to changes in cardiac chamber volumes (38). The adequacy of the injection technique should be assessed visually in each study by analyzing the transit of activity through the superior vena cava as well as by analyzing the time activity curve over the subclavian vein and superior vena cava (118).

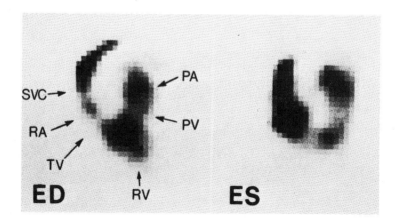

Figure 1.   End-diastolic and end-systolic frames recorded in multiple acquisition mode in the right anterior oblique projection during the right heart phase of the first-pass method.   SVC = superior vena cava; RA = right atrium; TV = tricuspid valve; RV = right ventricle; PV = pulmonic valve; PA = pulmonary artery.   Reproduced from SCHELBERT, H.R., WISENBERG, G. & MARSHALL, R.G.   Assessment of ventricular function by radionuclide techniques.   In Progress in Nuclear Medicine: Cardiovascular Nuclear Medicine, S. Karger, New York (1980) by permission of author and publisher.

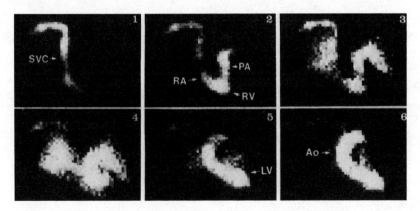

Figure 2. Radionuclide angiocardiogram (1 sec/frame) recorded in 30° right anterior oblique projection. Note anatomic and temporal separation of cardiac chambers. Abbreviations: See Figure 1. Reproduced as in Figure 1.

Any technetium-99m labeled radiopharmaceutical agent (except macroaggregated particles) can be used since they remain within the intravascular space long enough for recording first transit. When sequential studies are planned, different Tc-99m labeled compounds may be used. For example when two sequential studies are performed (such as rest and exercise), the first injection is often made with Tc-99m sulfur colloid, which is cleared rapidly from the blood pool by the reticuloendothelial system leaving no residual blood pool activity. The second injection may be made with technetium-99m pertechnetate (67). An alternative tracer for the first injection of a pair or when three injections are needed is Tc-99m-DPTA (diethylenetriamine pentaacetic acid), which is cleared rapidly by the kidneys.

The scintillation camera used for first pass studies must provide adequate temporal and spatial resolution with acceptable counting statistics. A multicrystal camera is often used because of their excellent performance at high count rates. Using a computer system, various framing intervals per second can be acquired, the optimal framing interval dependent upon heart rate. Time activity curve may be obtained for both ventricles using these images (Figure 3) (13). Data are acquired via a dedicated computer system in either "frame" or "list" mode for 30-60 seconds. In frame mode, data are acquired as a sequence of conventional images. The spatial resolution of the images is usually 32 X 32 or 64 X 64. The temporal resolution of the images varies from 10-50 msec per image. The optimal framing interval depends upon heart rate and the information sought. In "list" mode, acquisition data are not recorded as images. Instead, the position of each detected photon is recorded on magnetic disk memory. Also included in the data

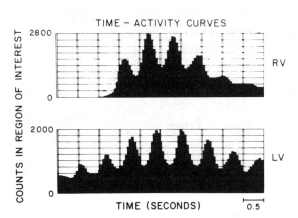

Figure 3.   Right ventricular (RV) and left ventricular (LV) time
    activity   curves   obtained   at   20   frames/sec   with   the
    computerized multicrystal scintillation camera.   Reproduced
    from Reference 14 by permission of author and publisher.

"list" are specially encoded time markers; and in some cases the
occurrence of the R-wave is also recorded.   After acquisition is
completed, the data list is converted to one or more series of
sequential images.   The advantage of list mode acquisition is that
the final images may be reformatted at different temporal
resolutions and with and without R-wave gating as required.

     An alternative to frame or list mode first-pass studies for
the evaluation of the right heart is the multigated first-pass
study performed as follows.   The patient is placed in the supine
position with the scintillation detector in a 30° right anterior
oblique projection.   The patient's electrodes are connected to a
dedicated computer system which is set to acquire 16 images per
cardiac cycle beginning with the R-wave.   The computer samples the
heart rate over several cycles and determines the average R to R
interval and imaging time per frame.   Data acquisition is begun as
the tracer is injected as a bolus.   Acquisition is terminated when
the activity is seen within the pulmonary capillary bed and before
the tracer has reached the left heart.   The result is a composite
right heart cardiac cycle which is the average of 6-10 heart beats.
This composite cycle can then be analyzed as described below.

     In some patients, it is possible to acquire a levophase
multigated first-pass study immediately following the right heart
study using similar technique.

2.   Clinical Applications

A.   Measurement of Global Right Ventricular Function.   A composite right heart image is created by adding all of the individual right heart frames.   Regions-of-interest are created over the right ventricle and a periventricular background area. High-frequency time-activity curves are generated for both ventricular and background regions and the background curve subtracted from the ventricular curve.   The peaks of the background-subtracted ventricular time-activity curve represent ventricular activity at end-diastole and the nadirs activity at end-systole (Figure 3).   If there has been complete mixing of tracer and blood, ventricular activity should be proportional to ventricular volume (38) and ejection fraction may be calculated as follows:

$$EF = \frac{\text{End-diastolic counts} - \text{End-systolic counts}}{\text{End-diastolic counts}}$$

Right ventricular ejection fraction is usually measured from the average end-diastolic and end-systolic counts over several heart beats.   Alternatively, corresponding frames from several consecutive cycles may be added to create an average or composite cardiac cycle.   RVEF may then be measured from the time-activity curve generated from this composite cycle.   Right ventricular wall motion may be evaluated by observing an endless-loop cinematic display of the composite cycle images and by superimposing the ventricular boundaries at end-diastole and end-systole.   Right ventricular volume cannot be accurately measured from the first-pass study.

Failure to deliver an adequate bolus, arrhythmias during the study, and an inability to separate right atrial activity from right ventricular activity in the anterior projection are potential sources of error in the first-pass measurement of RVEF.

B.   Measurement of Left Ventricular Performance.   Left ventricular ejection performance can be evaluated from the first-pass study in a manner identical to that described for the right ventricle (77,115).   In summary, ventricular and background regions-of-interest are identified using a composite left heart image.   High-frequency time-activity curves are generated for both regions and the left ventricular curve corrected for background (18,51,67,103).   Left ventricular ejection fraction is measured from the average maximum and average minimum counts from several consecutive cardiac cycles.   Alternatively, corresponding frames from several cycles are added to create a composite, average cardiac cycle (13,14).   Left ventricular ejection fraction and other ejection and relaxation parameters may be measured from the time-activity curve generated from this data set (Figure 3 and 4).

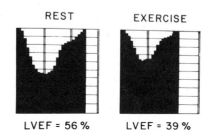

Figure 4. High frequency representative cardiac cycles obtained at
    30 frames/sec in a patient with coronary artery disease. Note
    the fine detail of the relative ventricular volume curves.
    Left ventricular ejection fraction fell with exercise.
    Reproduced from Reference 14 by permission of author and
    publisher.

        Left ventricular wall motion may be evaluated from a cinematic
display of the composite cycle frames or by superimposition of end-
diastolic and end-systolic boundaries (67). Left ventricular
volumes may be calculated using the area-length
technique (59,61,93,100).

        Failure to deliver an adequate bolus, arrhythmias during the
study, selection of an inappropriate detector, and delayed right
ventricular emptying are causes of potential error in first-pass
measurements of LVEF.

        Numerous studies utilizing both single crystal and
multicrystal scintillation cameras have demonstrated good agreement
between ejection fraction measured by first-pass radionuclide
angiocardiography and contrast ventriculography (13,14,67,77), as
well as those by first-pass and multiple gated cardiac blood pool
imaging (Figure 5).

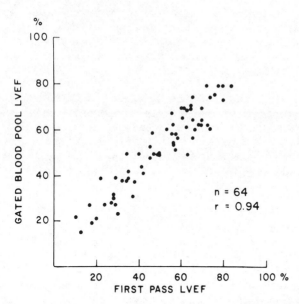

Figure 5. Left ventricular ejection fraction (LVEF) obtained in 64
    patients initially by first-pass technique and then by
    multiple gated cardiac blood pool imaging. Note the excellent
    correlation between the 2 methods over a wide range of
    ejection fractions. Reproduced from Reference 116 by
    permission of author and publisher.

Equilibrium Radionuclide Ventriculography

1. Radioactive Tracers. Equilibrium blood pool imaging is
performed with a tracer which remains within the intravascular
space throughout the acquisition period. The tracer of choice for
equilibrium imaging is Tc-99m labeled red blood cells. Several
methods of red blood cell labeling are in common use. The in-vivo
method is the simplest (85). Approximately 1 mg of stannous ion
(usually in the form of stannous pyrophosphate prepared from a
standard kit) is injected intravenously and followed some 20-30
minutes later by the injection of 15-30 mCi of Tc-99m-
pertechnetate. The in-vitro method employs a tin containing kit to
which the patient's blood is added (40). The reaction vial is then
incubated for 15 minutes and the blood re-injected. A combination
method has also been described. Twenty minutes following the
intravenous injection of 1 mg of stannous ion, 5-10 ml blood is
withdrawn through a large bore catheter into a shielded syringe
containing 15-30 mCi Tc-99m-pertechnetate. The catheter line
should contain saline with a total of 10-20 units of heparin. The
blood is allowed to incubate for 5-10 minutes with gentle inversion
of the syringe at 30 second intervals. The labeled blood is then

re-injected. Acceptable images are obtained with each of these methods. The in-vitro and combination methods, however, usually produce images with better ratios of blood pool to background activity. Serial images can usually be obtained for up to 6 hours following red blood cell labeling.

2. Technique. Images of the labeled cardiovascular blood pool are usually obtained with a single detector. Acquisition of the images is most commonly synchronized with some physiologic trigger. Synchronization of image acquisition with the R-wave of the electrocardiogram allows the acquisition of images corresponding to end-diastole and end-systole or to multiple segments of the cardiac cycle.

     A. Two Frame End-diastolic and End-systolic Imaging. The original technique described by Strauss allowed images to be acquired at only two points in the cardiac cycle (112). An end-diastolic image is recorded by triggering acquisition during the 50 msec interval immediately preceding the R-wave. An end-systolic image is recorded during the 50 msec interval following the T-wave. Since the number of events detected during a single 50 msec interval is small, acquisition is continued over many cardiac cycles to build the composite end-diastolic and end-systolic images.

     B. Multigated Acquisition (MUGA). Multigated acquisition allows the recording of multiple images of the cardiac blood pool throughout the cardiac cycle (49). A dedicated computer system is used to sample the patient's electrocardiogram. The R to R interval is divided into 14-64 discrete time intervals (50). During acquisition, the image data coming from the detector is stored as sequential images in separate areas of computer memory according to time elapsed since the R wave. Again, since the number of events detected in any one time interval of a single cardiac cycle is small, acquisition is continued over many cardiac cycles to build composite images of multiple discrete time intervals during the cardiac cycle (Figures 6 and 7).

     There are several requirements for successful multigated blood pool imaging (111): (1) cardiac function should be constant during recording; (2) patient and diaphragmatic motion must be minimized; (3) the relationship between the triggering signal and cardiac function should be fixed during recording; (4) the tracer should remain confined to the vascular space; (5) the number of frames per cardiac cycle must be adequate to characterize the parameter of cardiac function being evaluated; (6) the time per individual frame must be sufficiently short to effectively stop cardiac motion; (7) information density must be adequate for both visual interpretation and quantitative analysis; (8) spatial resolution

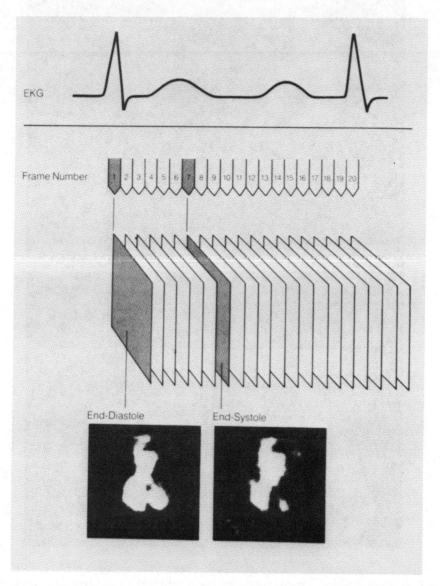

Figure 6. Multigated acquisition (MUGA) dynamic imaging approach
    to evaluation of ventricular function. Note that counts are
    accumulated throughout the cardiac cycle for several hundred
    beats.   It is possible to play back the dynamic myocardial
    scintigram in a cine-style format.

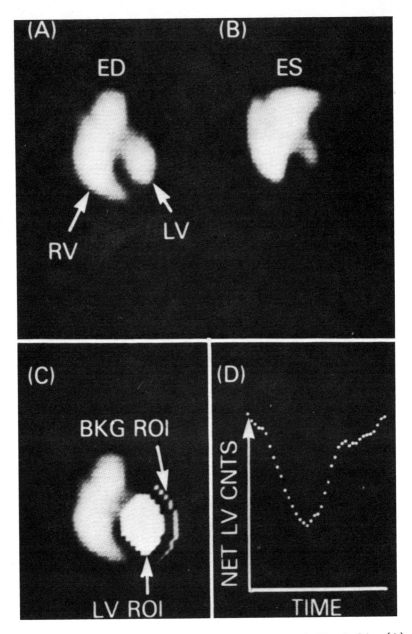

Figure 7. Modified left anterior oblique end-diastolic (A) and
           end-systolic images (B) from a multiple gated equilibrium
           blood pool scan in a patient with normal function at rest. In
           (C) a left ventricular (LV) and background (BKG) region of
           interest (ROI) have been identified. In (D) these regions are
           used to plot LV counts (CNTS) against time. Reproduced from
           Reference 14 by permission of author and publisher.

should be sufficient to depict the smallest significant wall motion abnormality; and (9) a sufficient number of views must be recorded to ensure that each chamber is adequately visualized.

Subjective analysis of multigated equilibrium blood pool images is best performed using an endless-loop cinematic display. Many computer systems allow the simultaneous display of 2 or 4 different projections. Quantitative analysis includes the measurement of right and left ventricular ejection fraction, characterization of the ventricular and atrial time-activity curves, and determination of ventricular volumes (37,107).

Quantitative analysis of the left atrium and left ventricle is best performed from data acquired in a modified left anterior oblique projection. The degree of obliquity is selected for each patient as that view which optimizes visualization of the interventricular septum. The detector is then positioned with 5-15° of caudal angulation in order to separate left atrial from left ventricular activity. Left ventricular time-activity curves are generated from manually or automatically selected regions-of-interest (ROI) and are corrected for background in the manner described for analysis of first-pass studies. Global left ventricular ejection fraction is calculated from the ventricular counts at end-diastole and end-systole using the following formula:

$$\frac{EDC - ESC}{EDC}$$

where EDC and ESC are background corrected end-diastolic and end-systolic counts, respectively. Measurement of LVEF using these methods correlate well with results obtained by contrast venticulography (6,37).

Left ventricular volumes may be measured by the conventional area-length method (61,100) or by a nongeometric technique developed recently (36,107). After background subtraction, a ROI is constructed over the left ventricle at end-diastole and end-systole and the number of counts determined. Left ventricular volumes are calculated from the radionuclide activity over the left ventricle normalized for the radionuclide activity per milliliter of peripheral venous blood and corrected for acquisition time per frame, and decay of the radioisotope. We use the following equation for scintigraphic volume calculations:

$$\frac{\dfrac{\text{Background Corrected LV Counts}}{\dfrac{\%\ \text{cycle acquired}}{\#\ \text{of frames gated}}}\ X\ T_{total}}{\text{Peripheral Blood Activity } X\ e^{-\lambda t}}$$

where $e^{-\lambda t}$ is the general equation for isotope decay, $\lambda = 693/T\frac{1}{2}$, t = time in minutes from counting the peripheral blood sample to the midpoint of the gated study, and $T\frac{1}{2}$ for technetium-99m is 360 minutes. Scintigraphic determination of left ventricular volumes has correlated well with contrast ventriculography (Figures 8 and 9) (35,107). Right ventricular volumes also may be measured accurately with this methodology using slant hole collimation and a more shallow left anterior oblique projection (34).

3. <u>Clinical Applications</u>. Radionuclide ventriculography may be used to estimate global and segmental function at rest and during stress, including upright or supine exercise and pharmacologic interventions. Ventricular volumes and ejection fraction may be estimated accurately and the severity of regurgitant lesions and the detection of sizable left to right shunts are accomplished using this methodology. Particular clinical applications are described elsewhere and in more detail below (2-4,7,9,13,15, 20-28,30-37,41,42,47,54,57,63,68,74,84,87,89-92,95-98,101,102,105-109,113,114,117,119).

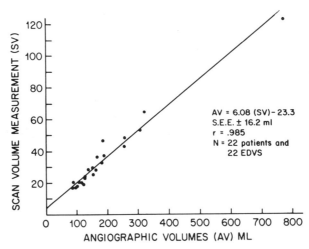

Figure 8.   Relation   between   scintigraphic   (SV)   and angiographic (AV)   end-diastolic   volumes   (EDVS)   in milliliters (ML). Reproduced from Reference 37 by permission of author and publisher.

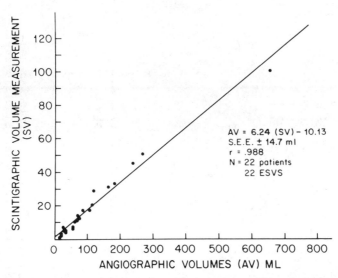

Figure 9. Relation between scintigraphic (SV) and angiographic (AV) end-systolic volumes (ESVS) in milliliters (ML). Reproduced from Reference 37 by permission of author and publisher.

A. Assessment of A Patient with Chest Pain and Detection of Significant Coronary Arterial Disease. The detection of physiologically significant coronary arterial stenosis represents one of the most important uses of rest and exercise radionuclide ventriculography (22,24,36,58,82). In normal subjects without evidence of cardiac disease, the normal exercise response is an increase in left ventricular ejection fraction of 5 ejection fraction units, a reduction in left ventricular end-systolic volume, and homogenously improved segmental wall motion (10,15,93) (Figure 10).

Patients with 2 or 3 vessel coronary arterial stenosis usually demonstrate either no change or a fall in left ventricular ejection fraction and an increase in left ventricular end-systolic volume at peak exercise (22,36) (Figure 11). Patients with single vessel disease may not demonstrate an abnormal response to peak exercise, unless they have proximal left anterior descending artery disease (36) (Figure 12 and 13). Abnormal LVEF responses to stress also may be caused by cardiomyopathy (117), valvular heart disease (21,33,54), aging (89), and any other process that causes extensive ventricular damage.

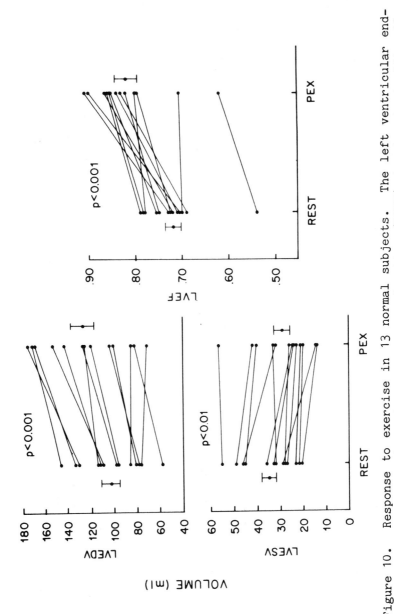

Figure 10. Response to exercise in 13 normal subjects. The left ventricular end-diastolic volume (LVEDV) and ejection fraction (LVEF) increased significantly from rest to peak exercise (PEX), while left ventricular end-systolic volume (LVESV) decreased significantly. The bars show mean $\pm$ SEM. Reproduced from Reference 36 by permission of author and publisher.

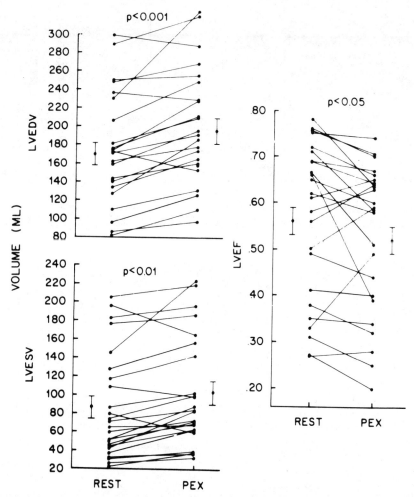

Figure 11.   In 24 patients with 2 or 3 vessel disease, left
    ventricular end-diastolic volume (LVEDV) and end-systolic
    volume (LVESV) increased at peak exercise (PEX), while
    ejection fraction (LVEF) decreased.   Reproduced from
    Reference 36 by permission of author and publisher.

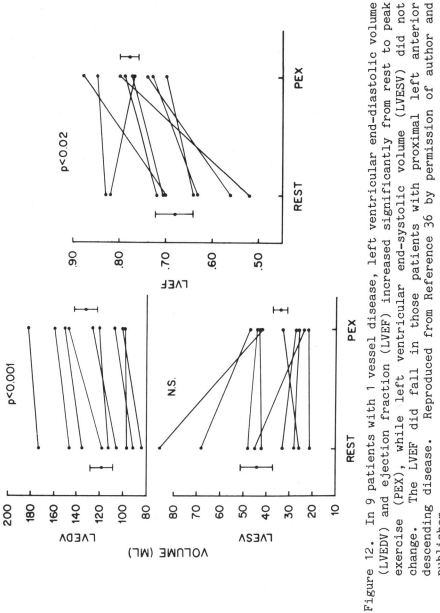

Figure 12. In 9 patients with 1 vessel disease, left ventricular end-diastolic volume (LVEDV) and ejection fraction (LVEF) increased significantly from rest to peak exercise (PEX), while left ventricular end-systolic volume (LVESV) did not change. The LVEF did fall in those patients with proximal left anterior descending disease. Reproduced from Reference 36 by permission of author and publisher.

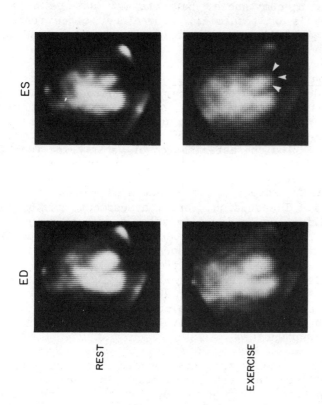

Figure 13. Modified left anterior oblique projection of end-diastolic and end-systolic images at rest and exercise in a patient with significant coronary artery disease. Note deterioration in wall motion excursion at peak exercise in the apical septal, apical and apical lateral segments (arrows).

The sensitivity of exercise radionuclide venticulography for the detection of anatomically important coronary arterial stenosis is approximately 90% with a specificity of approximately 50% compared to a sensitivity of 64% and a specificity of 90% for exercise electrocardiography (15,22,24,58,82,93). Regional wall motion abnormalities are relatively specific for coronary arterial disease and the greater the fall in ejection fraction at peak exercise the greater the extent of significant coronary arterial stenoses (36,58) (Figure 13).

Under certain circumstances, patients may not be able to exercise on a bicycle or treadmill. Therefore, other forms of stress have been employed including isometric handgrip and cold pressor stimulation (19,58,59,86,117).

B. <u>Evaluation of Patients with Acute Myocardial Infarction</u>. Resting radionuclide ventriculograms may be used to determine the functional impairment caused by acute (and/or previous) myocardial infarction and the resultant effect on right and left ventricular ejection fraction, ventricular volumes and regional wall motion (96,97,101,102,105). The characterization of ventricular function by radionuclide ventriculography provides a better assessment of the functional impact of myocardial infarction than Killip classification, chest radiograms, and the presence of rales or gallop sounds (101). In addition, serial assessments may be made throughout hospitalization to identify infarct extension (91) and the efficacy of pharmacological interventions. Radionuclide ventriculography in patients with shock may direct appropriate medical therapy, especially by differentiating acute right ventricular and left ventricular myocardial infarction; such differentiation is of critical importance therapeutically (91). Radionuclide scintigraphy also may allow the identification of mechanical problems including acute valvular regurgitation or acute ventricular septal rupture (14).

Radionuclide ventriculography has demonstrated that anterior transmural myocardial infarction results in greater left ventricular dysfunction as evidenced by lower left ventricular ejection fraction than inferior wall myocardial infarction. Right ventricular dysfunction occurs primarily in patients with transmural inferior wall myocardial infarction (Figure 14) (91,96,97,101,105,113). Recent studies have emphasized the prognostic importance of the resting left ventricular ejection fraction as a predictor of post myocardial infarction complications such as sudden death, early mortality or congestive heart failure (104,105). Acute left ventricular rupture after myocardial infarction also may be detected by radionuclide scintigraphy (81).

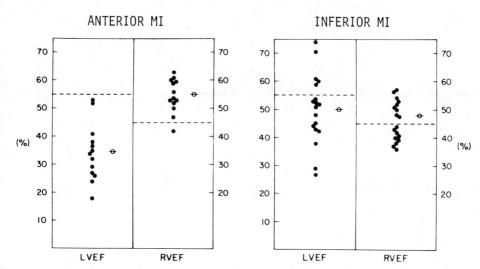

Figure 14.   Left ventricular (LV) and right ventricular (RV)
    ejection fraction (EF) in 31 patients with acute transmural
    myocardial infarctions (MI).   The RVEF was normal in 12 of 13
    patients with anterior infarction, but was abnormal in 9 of 18
    with inferior infarction.   Lower limits of normal are shown by
    dashed horizontal lines.   Reproduced from Reference 91 by
    permission of author and publisher.

     Submaximal exercise performed 2 to 3 weeks after myocardial
infarction   coupled   to   radionuclide   ventriculography   may
(1) demonstrate alterations in ejection fraction response and wall
motion   abnormalities   prior   to   or   without   electrocardiographic
changes and (2) provide valuable prognostic information by allowing
identification of patients at high risk for ischemic events in the
ensuing   6   months   (31,90).   Patients   demonstrating   an   abnormal
response   to   submaximal   exercise   testing,   after   myocardial
infarction, as evidenced by a failure to increase left ventricular
ejection fraction by 5 ejection fraction units, increases in left
ventricular   end-systolic   volume   index,   new   wall   motion
abnormalities, or an abnormal peak systolic blood pressure-left
ventricular end-systolic volume index ratio (Figure 15) (36,99) are
at high risk for sudden death, recurrent myocardial infarction,
unstable angina, and persistent congestive heart failure in the
ensuing 6 months.   However, 80 to 90% of patients demonstrating
normal LVEF and end-systolic volume response to submaximal exercise
at the time of hospital discharge do not develop cardiac events in
the following 6 months (31).

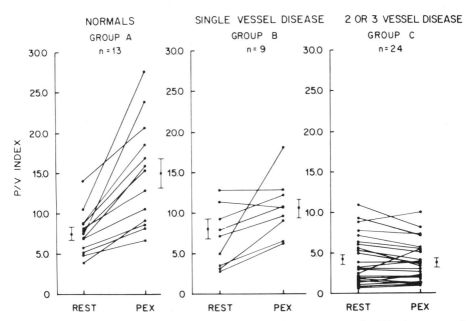

Figure 15.   Changes in the pressure-volume index (P/V) in normal
    subjects and patients with coronary artery disease.   The
    resting P/V index was lower in Group C (2 or 3 vessel disease)
    patients and the response to exercise was markedly blunted.
    PEX = peak exercise.   Reproduced from Reference 36 by
    permission of author and publisher.

    C.   Detection of Congestive Heart Failure.   Patients with
congestive heart failure can have the severity of ventricular
dysfunction   detected   and   quantitated   by   radionuclide
ventriculography.   In this manner, assessment of right and left
ventricular function may allow one to differentiate cardiac
dysfunction from pulmonary abnormalities.   In addition, it allows
one to distinguish between regional left ventricular dysfunction
(aneurysm),   and   diffuse   left   ventricular   dysfunction   (80)
(Figure 16).   It also may help assess and differentiate patients
with cardiomyopathies (congestive, hypertrophic, and ischemic)
(28).   Patients with ischemic heart disease usually have more
prominent segmental than global wall motion abnormalities (28).

    D.   Valvular Heart Disease.   Rest and exercise radionuclide
ventriculography has been used to evaluate patients with chronic
mitral or aortic valvular regurgitation.   In asymptomatic patients
with chronic aortic regurgitation, radionuclide scintigraphy has
demonstrated normal left ventricular function at rest but a
heterogeneous response to exercise (Figures 17 and 18) (21,33).

ED ES

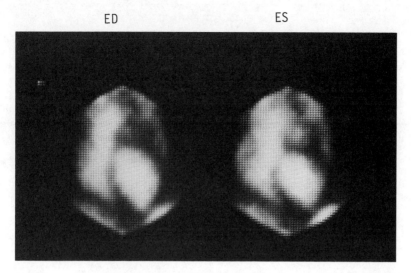

Figure 16. Modified left anterior oblique projection of end-diastolic and end-systolic images at rest in a patient with an idiopathic cardiomyopathy. Note global left ventricular hypokinesis.

ED ES

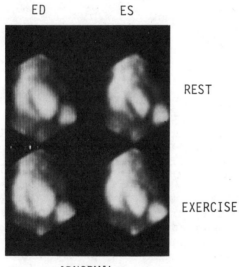

REST

EXERCISE

ABNORMAL
RESPONSE

Figure 17. Modified left anterior oblique projection of end-diastolic and end-systolic images at rest and peak exercise in a patient with chronic aortic regurgitation. Note increase in end-systolic volume at peak exercise.

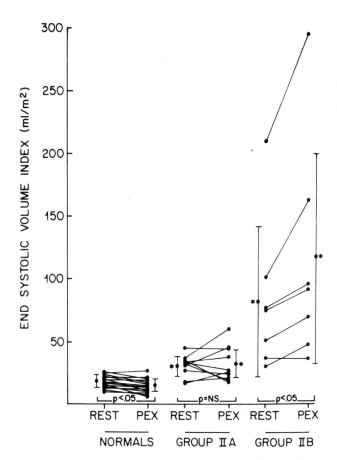

Figure 18.   Left ventricular end-systolic volume index decreases
     during   exercise   in   normal   subjects   but   increased   in
     symptomatic   patients   with   chronic   aortic   regurgitation
     (Group IIB), and shows a heterogeneous response in those
     patients   with   minimal   symptoms   and   chronic   aortic
     regurgitation.   Reproduced from Reference 33 by permission of
     author and publisher.

Some patients demonstrate normal left ventricular reserve with an increase in left ventricular ejection fraction and a fall in left ventricular end-systolic volume, whereas others have abnormal left ventricular reserve with no change or a fall in left ventricular ejection fraction and an increase in left ventricular end-systolic volume index. In addition, it appears that the response to exercise as evaluated with scintigraphy identifies detection of left ventricular dysfunction earlier than echocardiography and resting measurements of left ventricular volumes (54). After aortic valve replacement, abnormal exercise responses may revert to normal (25,27).

E.   Assessment of Right Ventricular Function.   Left ventricular function is usually normal in patients with chronic obstructive pulmonary disease, whereas pulmonary artery hypertension generally causes abnormalities in right ventricular function (17). The degree of resting right venticular dysfunction is related to the severity of arterial hypoxemia and ventilatory impairment. Abnormal right ventricular function has been shown to be the forerunner of subsequent cardiopulmonary decompensation in patients with chronic obstructive pulmonary disease and in ambulatory young adults with cystic fibrosis (11,12,72).

The abnormal right ventricular exercise response found in patients with chronic obstructive pulmonary disease probably represents altered afterload due to pulmonary vasoconstriction or changes in intrathoracic pressures (71).

F.   Assessment of Intracardiac Shunts.   The first pass method provides the best means to detect intracardiac shunts since the tracer can be followed through the cardiac chambers by virtue of temporal and anatomic separation of cardiac chambers. Computer-derived time activity curves provide both qualitative and quantitative information (114). However, accurate assessment of shunt location and size can be made only when ventricular function is relatively normal and when the bolus injection is compact. If ventricular dysfunction is present, pulmonary transit may be prolonged resulting in a false impression of a left-to-right shunt.

G.   Assessment of Drug Therapy.   The radionuclide scintigraphic assessment of global ejection fraction as well as left ventricular volumes can evaluate the influence of pharmacologic intervention (and other training or surgical procedures) on ventricular function. Some of the agents evaluated have included vasodilator therapy with nitroglycerin (23,98), and prazosin (47), the myocardial inotropic agents digitalis (42,76), and amrinone (119), the beta blocker propranolol (32,70,71), the slow channel calcium antagonist, verapamil (20,57), the bronchodilator aminophyllin (73), and the pulmonary vasodilator oxygen (84). Serial analysis of left ventricular function has allowed the detection of ventricular dysfunction caused by potentially cardiotoxic chemotherapeutic agent, such as doxorubicin (3,30,48), thus making it possible to identify patients at risk for the development of congestive heart failure and those who may receive higher cumulative doses of the agent.

SUMMARY

Developments over the past decade have allowed one to visualize the right and left ventricles using radionuclide techniques and to study the influence of a wide range of physiologic, pharmacologic and surgical interventions on global and regional ventricular function thereby providing important diagnostic insight and improved therapeutic capabilities. These tests are relatively non-invasive, they can be performed serially, they may be performed in patients that are seriously ill, and they have no recognized risk other than low level radiation exposure. With continued improvement in noninvasive imaging and processing and in the sophistication of associated computer systems, one may expect significant and wide ranging additional contributions in the assessment of myocardial function using radionuclide ventriculographic techniques.

REFERENCES

1. ADAM, W.E., TARKOWSKA, A., BITTER, F., STAUCH, M. & GEFFER H. Equilibrium (gated) radionuclide ventriculography. Cardiovascular Radiology 2, 161-173 (1979).

2. ALAZRAKI, N.P., ASHBURN, W.L., HAGAN, A., & FRIEDMAN, W.F. Detection of left-to-right cardiac shunts with the scintillation camera pulmonary dilution curve. Journal of Nuclear Medicine 13, 142 (1972).

3. ALEXANDER, R.S., DAINIAK, N., BERGER, H.J., GOLDMAN, L., JOHNSTONE, D., REDUTO, L., DUFFY, T., SCHWARTZ, P., GOTTSCHALK, A. & ZARET, B.L. Serial assessment of doxorubicin cardiotoxicity with quantitative radionuclide angiocardiography. New England Journal of Medicine 300, 278-283 (1979).

4. ANDERSON, P.A., JONES, R.H. & SABISTON, D.C. Quantification of left-to-right cardiac shunts with radionuclide angiography. Circulation 49, 512-516, (1974).

5. ANDREAS, R., ZIERLER, K.L., ANDERSON, H.M., STAINSBY, W.N., CADER, G., GHRAYYIB, A.S. & LILIENTHAL, J.L. Measurement of blood flow and volume in the forearm of man with notes on the

therapy of indicator-dilution and on the production of turbulence, hemolysis, and vasodilation by invascular injection. Journal of Clinical Investigation **33**, 482-504 (1954).

6. ASHBURN, W.L., SCHELBERT, H.R. & VERBA, J. Left ventricular ejection fraction--a review of several radionuclide angiographic approaches using the scintillation camera. Progress in Cardiovascular Diseases **20**, 267-284 (1978).

7. ASKENAZI, J., AHNBERG, D.S., KORNGOLD, E., LaFARGE, C.G., MALTZ, D.L., & TREVES, S. Quantitative radionuclide angiography: detection and quantification of left to right shunts. American Journal of Cardiology **37**, 382-387 (1976).

8. BACHARACH, S.L., GREEN, M.V., BORER, J.S., DOUGLAS, M.A., OSTROW, H.G. & JOHNSTON, G.S. A real-time system for multi-image gated cardiac studies. Journal of Nuclear Medicine **18**, 79-84 (1977).

9. BERGER, H.J., GOTTSCHALK, A. & ZARET, B.L. Radionuclide assessment of left and right ventricular performance. Radiologic Clinics of North America **18**, 441-466 (1980).

10. BERGER, H.J., JOHNSTONE, D.E., SANDS, J.M., GOTTSCHALK, A. & ZARET, B.L. Response of right ventricular ejection fraction to upright bicycle exercise in coronary artery disease. Circulation **60**, 1292-1300 (1979).

11. BERGER, H.J. & MATTHAY, R.A. Noninvasive radiographic assessment of cardiovascular function in acute and chronic respiratory failure. American Journal of Cardiology **47**, 950-962 (1981).

12. BERGER, H.J., MATTHAY, R.A., LOKE, J., MARSHALL, R.G., GOTTSCHALK, A. & ZARET, B.L. Assessment of cardiac performance with quantitative radionuclide angiocardiography: right ventricular ejection fraction with reference to findings in chronic obstructive pulmonary disease. American Journal of Cardiology **41**, 897-905 (1978).

13. BERGER, H.J., MATTHAY, R.A. & PYTLIK, L.M. Ventricular performance in patients with cardiac and pulmonary disease. In Cardiovascular Medicine, Freeman, L.M. and Blaufox, M.D., Eds., Grune & Stratton, New York (1980).

14. BERGER, H.J., MATTHAY, R.A., PYTLIK, GOTTSCHALK, A. & ZARET, B.L. First-pass radionuclide assessment of right and left ventricular performance in patients with cardiac and pulmonary disease. Seminars in Nuclear Medicine **9**, 275-295 (1979).

15. BERGER, H.J., REDUTO, L.A., JOHNSTONE, D.E., BORKOWSKI, H., SANDS, M.J., COHEN, L.S., LANGOU, E.A., GOTTSCHALK, A. & ZARET, B.L. Global and regional left ventricular response to bicycle exercise in coronary artery disease. Assessment by quantitative radionuclide angiocardiography. American Journal of Medicine **66**, 13-21 (1979).

16. BERGER, H.J., SANDS, M.J., DAVIES, R.A., WACKER, F.J., ALEXANDER, J., LACHMAN, A.S., WILLIAMS, B.W. & ZARET, B.L. Exercise left ventricular performance in patients with chest pain, ischemic-appearing exercise electrocardiograms, and angiographically normal coronary arteries. Annals of Internal Medicine **94**, 186-191 (1981).

17. BERGER, H.J. & ZARET, B.L. Noninvasive radionuclide assessment of right ventricular performance in man. In Nuclear Cardiology, Willerson, J.T., Ed., p. 91, F.A. Davis Company, Philadelphia (1980).

18. BODENHEIMER, M.M., BANKA, V.S., FOOSHEE, C.M., HERMANN, G.A. & HELFANT, R.H. Quantitative radionuclide angiography in the right anterior oblique view: Comparison with contrast ventriculography. American Journal of Cardiology **41**, 718-732 (1978).

19. BODENHEIMER, M.M., BANKA, V.S., FOOSHEE, C.M., GILLESPIE, J.A. & HELFANT, R.H. Detection of coronary heart disease using radionuclide determined regional ejection fraction at rest and during handgrip exercise: correlation with coronary arteriography. Circulation **58**, 640-648 (1978).

20. BONOW, R.O., LEON, M.B., ROSING, D.R., KENT, K.M., LIPSON, L.C., BACHARACH, S.L., GREEN, M.V. & EPSTEIN, S.E. Effect of propranolol and verapamil on left ventricular diastolic filling in patients with coronary artery disease. Circulation (Abstract) **62**, 85 (1980).

21. BORER, J.S., BACHARACH, S.L., GREEN, M.V., KENT, K.M., HENRY, W.L., ROSING, D.R., SEIDES, S.F., JOHNSTON, G.S. & EPSTEIN, S.E. Exercise-induced left ventricular dysfunction in symptomatic and asymptomatic patients with aortic regurgitation: assessment with radionuclide cineangiography. American Journal of Cardiology **42**, 351-357 (1978).

22. BORER, J.S., BACHARACH, S.L. GREEN, M.V., KENT, K.M., EPSTEIN, S.E. & JOHNSTON, G.S. Real-time radionuclide cineangiography in the noninvasive evaluation of global and regional left ventricular function at rest and during exercise in patients with coronary artery disease. New England Journal of Medicine **296**, 839-844 (1977).

23. BORER, J.S., BACHARACH, S.L., GREEN, M.V., KENT, K.M.,
     JOHNSTON, G.S. & EPSTEIN, S.E. Effects of nitroglycerin on
     exercise-induced abnormalities of left ventricular regional
     function and ejection fraction in coronary artery disease:
     assessment by radionuclide cineangiography in symptomatic and
     asymptomatic patients. Circulation **57,** 314-320 (1978).

24. BORER, J.S., KENT, K.M., BACHARACH, S.L., GREEN, M.V., ROSING,
     D.R., SEIDES, S.F., EPSTEIN, S.E. & JOHNSTON, G.S.
     Sensitivity, specificity and predictive accuracy of
     radionuclide cineangiography during exercise in patients with
     coronary artery disease: comparison with exercise electro-
     cardiography. Circulation **60,** 572-580 (1979).

25. BORER, J.S., ROSING, D.R., KENT, K.M., BACHARACH, S.L., GREEN,
     M.V., McINTOSH, C.J., MORROW, A.G. & EPSTEIN, S.E. Left
     ventricular function at rest and during exercise after aortic
     valve replacement in patients with aortic regurgitation.
     American Journal of Cardiology **44,** 1297-1305 (1979).

26. BORER, J.S., ROSING, D.R., MILLER, R.H., STARK, R.M., KENT,
     K.M., BACHARACH, S.L., GREEN, M.V., LAKE, C.R., COHEN, H.,
     HOLMES, D., DONOHUE, D., BAKER, W. & EPSTEIN, S.E. Natural
     history of left ventricular function during 1 year after acute
     myocardial infarction: comparison with clinical electrocar-
     diographic and biochemical determinations. American Journal
     of Cardiology **46,** 1-12 (1980).

27. BOUCHER, C.A., BINGHAM, J.B., OSBAKKEN, M.D., OKADA, R.D.,
     STRAUSS, H.W., BLOCK, P.C., LEVINE, F.H., PHILLIPS, H.R. &
     POHOST, G.M. Early changes in left ventricular size and
     function after correction of left ventricular volume overload.
     American Journal of Cardiology **47,** 991-1004 (1981).

28. BUCKLEY, B.H., HUTCHINS, G.M., BAILEY, I., STRAUSS, H.W. &
     PITT, B. Thallium-201 imaging and gated cardiac blood pool
     scans in patients with ischemic and congestive cardiomyopathy:
     a clinical and pathologic study. Circulation **55,**
     753-760 (1977).

29. BURROW, R.D., STRAUSS, H.W., SINGLETON, R., POND, P., REHN,
     T., BAILEY, I.K., GRIFFITH, L.C., NICKOLOFF, E. & PITT B.
     Analysis of left ventricular function from multiple gated
     acquisition cardiac blood pool imaging: comparison to
     contract angiography. Circulation **56,** 1024-1028 (1977).

30. CHOI, W., BERGER, H., ALEXANDER, J., SCHWARTZ, P., WACKERS, F.
     & ZARET, G. Serial radionuclide assessment of doxorubicin
     cardiotoxicity in cancer patients with abnormal baseline

resting left ventricular performance. American Journal of Cardiology (Abstract) **47,** 474 (1981).

31. CORBETT, J.R., DEHMER, G.J., LEWIS, S.E., WOODWARD, W., HENDERSON, E., PARKEY, R.W., BLOMQVIST, C.G. & WILLERSON, J.T. The prognostic value of submaximal exercise testing with radionuclide ventriculography before hospital discharge in patients with recent myocardial infarction. Circulation **64,** 535-544 (1981).

32. DEHMER, G.J., FALKOFF, M., LEWIS, S.E., HILLIS, L.D., PARKEY, R. & WILLERSON, J.T. Effect of oral propranolol on rest and exercise left ventricular ejection fraction, volumes and segmental wall motion in patients with angina petoris: assessment with equilibrium gated blood pool imaging. British Heart Journal **45(6),** 656-666 (1981).

33. DEHMER, G.J., FIRTH, B.G., HILLIS, L.D., CORBETT, J.R., LEWIS, S.E., PARKEY, R.W., & WILLERSON, J.T. Alterations in left ventricular volumes and ejection fraction at rest and during exercise in patients with aortic regurgitation. American Journal of Cardiology **48,** 17-27 (1981).

34. DEHMER, G.J., FIRTH, B.G., HILLIS, L.D., NICOD, P., WILLERSON, J.T. & LEWIS, S.E. Nongeometric determination of right ventricular volumes from equilibrium blood pool scans. American Journal of Cardiology **49,** 78-84 (1982).

35. DEHMER, G.J., FIRTH, B.G., LEWIS, S.E., WILLERSON, J.T. & HILLIS, L.D. Direct measurement of cardiac output by gated equilibrium blood pool scintigraphy: validation of scintigraphic volume measurements by a non-geometric technique. American Journal of Cardiology **47,** 1061-1067 (1981).

36. DEHMER, G.J., LEWIS, S.E., HILLIS, L.D., CORBETT, J.R., PARKEY, R.W. & WILLERSON, J.T. Exercise-induced alterations in left ventricular volumes and the pressure-volume relationship: a sensitive indicator of left ventricular dysfunction in patients with coronary artery disease. Circulation **63,** 1008-1018 (1981).

37. DEHMER, G.J., LEWIS, S.E., HILLIS, L.D., TWIEG, D., FALKOFF, M., PARKEY R.W. & WILLERSON, J.T. Nongeometric determination of left ventricular volumes from equilibrium blood pool scans. American Journal of Cardiology **45,** 293-300 (1980).

38. DONATO, L. Basic concepts of radiocardiography. Seminars in Nuclear Medicine **3,** 111-130 (1973).

39. DONATO, L., ROCHESTER, D.F., LEWIS, M.L., DURAND, J., PARKER,
     J.O. & HARVEY, R.M.   Quantitative radiocardiography.   II.
     Technic and analysis of curves.   Circulation **26**,
     183-188 (1962).

40. ECKELMAN, W., RICHARDS, P. & HAUSER, W.   Technetium-labeled
     red blood cells.   Journal of Nuclear Medicine **12**,
     22-24 (1971).

41. FLAHERTY, J.T., CANENT, R.V., BOINEAU, J.P., ANDERSON, P.A.W.,
     LEVIN, A.R.   & SPACH, M.S.   Use of externally recorded
     radioisotope-dilution curves for quantitation of left-to-
     right shunts.   American Journal of Cardiology **20**,
     341-345 (1967).

42. FIRTH, B.G., DEHMER, G.J., CORBETT, J.R., LEWIS, S.E., PARKEY,
     R.W. & WILLERSON, J.T.   Effect of chronic oral digoxin therapy
     on ventricular function at rest and peak exercise in patients
     with ischemic heart disease.   American Journal of Cardiology
     46, 481-490 (1980).

43. FOLLAND, E.D., HAMILTON, G.W., LARSON, S.M., KENNEDY, W.J.,
     WILLIAMS, D.L.   & RITCHIE, J.L.   The radionuclide ejection
     fraction: A comparison of three radionuclide techniques with
     contrast angiography.   Journal of Nuclear Medicine **18**,
     1159-1166 (1977).

44. FREEMAN, M.R., BERMAN, D.S., STANILOFF, H.M., WAXMAN, A.D.,
     MADDAHI, J., BUCHBINDER, N.A., FORRESTER, J.S. & SWAN, H.J.C.
     Improved assessment of inferior segmental wall motion by the
     addition of a 70-degree left anterior oblique view in multiple
     gated equilibrium scintigraphy.   American Heart Journal **101**,
     169-173 (1981).

46. GIBBONS, R.H., LEE, J.L., COBB, F.R. & JONES, R.H.   Ejection
     fraction response to exercise in patients with chest pain and
     normal coronary arteriograms.   Circulation **64**, 952-957 (1981).

47. GOLDMAN, S.A., JOHNSON, L.L., ESCALA, E., CANNON, P.J. &
     WEISS, M.B.   Improved exercise ejection fraction with long
     term prazosin therapy in patients with heart failure.
     American Journal of Medicine **68**, 36-42 (1980).

48. GOTTDIENER, J.B., MATHISEN, D.J., BORER, J.S., BONOW, R.O.,
     MYERS, C.E., BARR, L.H., SCHWARTZ, D.E., BACHARACH, S.L.,
     GREEN, M.V. & ROSENBERG, S.A.   Doxorubicin cardiotoxicity:
     assessment of late left ventricular dysfunction by
     radionuclide cineangiography.   Annals of Internal Medicine **94**,
     430-435 (1981).

49. GREEN, M.V., OSTROW, H.G., DOUGLAS, M.A., MYERS, R.W., SCOTT, R.N., BAILEY J.J. & JOHNSTON, G.S. High temporal resolution ECG-gated scintigraphic angiocardiography. Journal of Nuclear Medicine **16**, 95-98 (1975).

50. HAMILTON, G.W., WILLIAMS, G.L. & GOULD, L. Selection of appropriate frame rates for radionuclide angiography. Journal of Nuclear Medicine (Abstract) **17**, 556 (1976).

51. HENNING, H., SCHELBERT, H., CRAWFORD, M.H., KARLINER, J.S., ASHBURN, W.L., O'ROURKE, R.A. Left ventricular performance assessed by radionuclide angiocardiography and echocardiography in patiens with previous myocardial infarction. Circulation **52**, 1069-1075 (1975).

52. HOLMAN, B.L., WYNNE, J., ZIELONKA, J.S. & IDOINE, J.D. A simplified technique for measuring right ventricular ejection fraction using the equilibrium radionuclide angiocardiogram and the slant-hole collimator. Radiology **138**, 429-435 (1981).

53. HUNG, J., HARRIS, P.J., UREN, R.F., TILLER, D.J. & KELLY, D.T. Uremic cardiomyopathy--effect of hemodialysis on left ventricular function in end stage renal failure. New England Journal of Medicine **302**, 547-551 (1980).

54. HUXLEY, R.L., GAFFNEY, F.A., CORBETT, J.R., PESHOCK, R., FIRTH, B.G., NICOD, P., LEWIS, S.E. & WILLERSON, J.T. Early detection of left ventricular dysfunction in patients with chronic aortic regurgitation: contrast angiographic, echocardiograhic and rest and exercise scintigraphic assessments (Submitted).

55. JENGO, J.A., MENA, I., BLAUFUSS, A. & CRILEY, J.M. Evaluation of left ventricular function (ejection fraction and segmental wall motion) by single pass radioisotope angiography. Circulation **57**, 326-332 (1978).

56. JENGO, J.A., OREN, V., CONANT, R., BRIZENDINE, M., NELSON, T., USZLER, J.M. & MENA, I. Effects of maximal exercise stress on left ventricular function in patients with coronary artery disease using first pass radionuclide angiocardiography: a rapid, noninvasive technique for determining ejection fraction and segmental wall motion. Circulation **59**, 60-65 (1979).

57. JOHNSON, S.M., MAURITSON, D.R., CORBETT, J.R., WOODWARD, W., WILLERSON, J.T. & HILLIS, L.D. Double blind, randomized, placebo-controlled comparison of propranolol and verapamil in the treatment of patients with stable angina pectoris. American Journal of Medicine **71**, 443-451 (1981).

58. JONES, R.H., McEWAN, P., NEWMAN, G., PORT, S., RERYCH, S.K., SCHOLZ, P.M., UPTON, MT., PETER, C.A., AUSTIN, E.H., LEONG, K., GIBBONS, R.J., COBB, F.R., COLEMAN, R.E. & SABISTON, D.C. The accuracy of diagnosis of coronary artery disease by radionuclide measurements of left ventricular function during rest and exercise. Circulation **64**, 586-601 (1981).

59. JONES, R.H., RERYCH, S.K., NEWMAN, G.E., SCHOLZ, P.M., HOWE, R., OLDHAM, N., GOODRICH, J.K. & SABISTON, D.C. Noninvasive radionuclide procedures for diagnosis and management of myocardial ischemia. World Journal of Surgery **2**, 811-824 (1978).

60. KELLY, M.J., GILES, R.W., SIMON, T.S., BERGER, H.J., LANGOU, R.A., ZARET, B.L. & WACKER, F.J. Multigated equilibrium radionuclide angiocardiography: Improved detection of left ventricular wall motion abnormalities and aneurysms by the addition of the left lateral view. Radiology **139**, 167-173 (1981).

61. KENNEDY, J.W., TRENHOLME, S.E. & KASSER, I.S. Left ventricular volume and mass from single plane cineangiocardiogram. A comparison of anteroposterior and right anterior oblique methods. American Heart Journal **80**, 343-352 (1970).

62. KENT, K.M., BORER, J.S., GREEN, M.V., BACHARACH, S.L., McINTOSH, C.L., CONKLE, D.M. & EPSTEIN, S.E. Effects of coronary-artery bypass on global and regional left ventricular function during exercise. New England Journal of Medicine **298**, 1434-1439 (1978).

63. KRISS, J.P. ENRIGHT, L.P., HAYDEN, W.G., WEXLER, L. & SHUMWAY, N.E. Radioisotopic angiocardiography: wide scope of applicability in diagnosis and evaluation of therapy in diseases of the heart and great vessels. Circulation **43**, 792-808 (1971).

64. LAM, W., PAVEL, D., BYROM, E., SHEIKH, A., BEST, D. & ROSEN, K. Radionuclide regurgitant index: value and limitations. American Journal of Cardiology **47**, 292-298 (1981).

65. LIBERTHSON, R.R., BOUCHER, C.A., STRAUSS, H.W., DINSMORE, R.E., McKUSICK, K.A. & POHOST, G.M. Right ventricular function in adult atrial septal defect: preoperative and postoperative assessment and clinical implications. American Journal of Cardiology **47**, 56-60 (1981).

66. LEWIS, S.E., DEHMER, G.J., FALKOFF, M., HILLIS, L.D. & WILLERSON, J.T. A nongeometric method for the scintigraphic

determination of left ventricular volume: contrast correlation. Journal of Nuclear Medicine (Abstract) **20**, 661 (1979).

67. MARSHALL, R.C., BERGER, H.J., COSTIN, J.C., FREEDMAN, G.S., WOLBERG, J., COHEN, L.S., GOTTSCHALK, A. & ZARET, B.L. Assessment of cardiac performance with quantitative radionuclide angiocardiography: Sequential left ventricular ejection fraction, normalized left ventricular ejection rate, and regional wall motion. Circulation **56**, 820-829 (1977).

68. MARSHALL, R.C., BERGER, H.J., REDUTO, L.A., COHEN, L.S., GOTTSCHALK, A. & ZARET, B.L. Assessment of cardiac performance with quantitative radionuclide angiography: effects of oral propranolol on global and regional left ventricular function in coronary artery disease. Circulation **58**, 808-814 (1978).

69. MARSHALL, R.C., BERGER, H.J., REDUTO, L.A., GOTTSCHALK, A. & ZARET, B.L. Variability in sequential measures of left ventricular performance assessed with radionuclide angiocardiography. American Journal of Cardiology **41**, 531-536 (1978).

70. MARSHALL, R.C., WISENBERG, G., SCHELBERT, H.R. & HENZE, E. Effect of oral propranolol on rest, exercise and post exercise left ventricular performance in normal subjects and patients with coronary artery disease. Circulation **63**, 572-583 (1981).

71. MATTHAY, R.A., BERGER, H.J., DAVIS, R.A., LOCKE, J., MAHLER, D.A., GOTTSCHALK, A. & ZARET, B.L. Right and left ventricular exercise performance in chronic obstructive pulmonary disease: radionuclide assessment. Annals of Internal Medicine **93**, 234-239 (1980).

72. MATTHAY, R.A., BERGER, H.J., LOKE, J., DOLAN, T.F., FAGENHOLZ, S.A., GOTTSCHALK, A. & ZARET, B.L. Right and left ventricular performance in ambulatory young adults with cystic fibrosis. British Heart Journal **43**, 474-480 (1980).

73. MATTHAY, R.A., BERGER, H.J., LOKE, J., GOTTSCHALK, A. & ZARET, B.L. Effects of aminophyllin upon right and left ventricular performance in chronic obstructive pulmonary disease: noninvasive assessment by radionuclide angiocardiography. American Journal of Medicine **65**, 903-910 (1978).

74. McKUSICK, K.A., BINGHAM, J.B., POHOST, G.M. & STRAUSS, H.W. The gated first-pass radionuclide angiogram: A method for

measurement of right ventricular ejection fraction. Circulation (Abstract) **57/58,** II-130 (1978).

75. MEIER, P. & ZIERLER, K.L. On the theory of the indicator-dilution method for measurement of blood flow and volume. Journal of Applied Physiology **6,** 731-744 (1954).

76. MORRISON, J., COROMILAS, J., ROBBINS, M., ONG, L., EISENBERG, S., STECHEL, R., ZEMA, M., REISER, P. & SHERR, L. Digitalis and myocardial infarction in man. Circulation **62,** 8-16 (1980).

77. MULLINS, C.B., MASON, D.T., ASHBURN, W.L. & ROSS, J. Determination of ventricular volume by radioisotope angiography. American Journal of Cardiology **24,** 72-78 (1969).

78. NEWMAN, G.E., GIBBONS, R.J. & RONES, R.H. Cardiac function during rest and exercise in patients with mitral valve prolapse: role of radionuclear angiocardiography. American Journal of Cardiology **47,** 14-19 (1981).

79. NEWMAN, G.F., RERYCH, S.K., UPTON, M.T., SABISTON, D.C., JR. & RONES, R.H. Comparison of electrocardiographic and left ventricular functional changes during exercise. Circulation **62,** 1204-1211 (1980).

80. NICHOLS, A.B., McKUSICK, K.A., STRAUSS, H.W., DINSMORE, R.E., BLOCK, P.C. & POHOST, G.M. Clinical utility of gated cardiac blood pool imaging in congestive left heart failure. American Journal of Medicine **65,** 785-793 (1978).

81. NICOD, P., CORBETT, J., LEACHMAN, R., CROYLE, P., REICH, S., PESHOCK, R., FARKAS R., RUDE, R., BUJA, L.M., MILLS, L., LEWIS, S. & WILLERSON, J.T. Myocardial rupture after myocardial infarction: Detection by multigated image acquisition scintigraphy. American Journal of Medicine (In press, 1982).

82. OKADA, R.D., BOUCHER, C.A., STRAUSS, H.W. & POHOST, G.M. Exercise radionuclide imaging approaches to coronary artery disease. American Journal of Cardiology **46,** 1188-1204 (1980).

83. OKADA, R.D., POHOST, G.M., KIRSHENBAUM, H.D., KUSHNER, F.G., BOUCHER, C.A., BLOCK, P.C. & STRAUSS, H.W. Radionuclide determined changes in pulmonary blood volume with exercise: improved sensitive of multigated blood-pool scanning in detecting coronary artery disease. New England Journal of Medicine **301,** 569-576 (1979).

84. OLVEY, S.K., REDUTO, L.A., STEVENS, P.M., DEATON, W.J. &
    MILLER, R.R. First pass radionuclide assessment of right and
    left ventricular ejection fraction in chronic pulmonary
    disease: effect of oxygen upon exercise response. Chest **78**,
    4-9 (1980).

85. PAVEL, D.G., ZIMMER, A.M. & PATTERSON, U.N. In vivo labeling
    of red blood cells with 99mTc: a new approach to blood pool
    visualization.   Journal   of   Nuclear   Medicine   **18**,
    305-308 (1977).

86. PETER, C.A. & JONES, R.H. Effects of isometric hand grip and
    dynamic exercise on left ventricular function. Journal of
    Nuclear Medicine **21**, 1131-1138 (1980).

87. POHOST, G.M., VIGNOLA, P.A., McKUSICK, K.E., BLOCK, P.C.,
    MYERS, G.S., WALKER, H.J., COPEN, D.L. & DINSMORE, R.E.
    Hypertrophic cardiomyopathy: evaluation by cardiac blood pool
    scanning. Circulation **55**, 92-99 (1977).

88. POLINER, L.R., DEHMER, G.J., LEWIS, S.E., PARKEY, R.W.,
    BLOMQVIST, C.G. & WILLERSON, J.T. Left ventricular
    performance in normal subjects: a comparison of the responses
    to exercise in the upright and supine positions. Circulation
    62, 528-534 (1980).

89. PORT, S., COBB, F.R., COLEMAN, R.E. & JONES, R.H. Effect of
    age on the response of the left ventricular fraction to
    exercise.   New   England   Journal   of   Medicine   **303**,
    1133-1137 (1980).

90. PULIDO, J.I., DOSS, J., TWIEG, D., BLOMQVIST, C.G., FAULKNER,
    D., HORN V., DeBATES, D., TOBEY, M., PARKEY, R.W., WILLERSON,
    J.T. Submaximal exercise testing after acute myocardial
    infarction: myocardial scintigraphic and electrocardiogr-
    aphic observations. American Journal of Cardiology **42**,
    19-28 (1978).

91. REDUTO, L.A., BERGER, H.J., COHEN, L.S., GOTTSCHALK, A. &
    ZARET, B.L. Sequential radionuclide assessment of left and
    right ventricular performance after acute transmural
    myocardial infarction. Annals of Internal Medicine **89**,
    441-447 (1978).

92. REDUTO, L.A., BERGER, H.J., JOHNSTONE, D.E., HELLENBRAND, W.,
    WACKERS, F., WHITTEMORE, R., COHEN, L.S., GOTTSCHALK, A. &
    ZARET, B.L. Radionuclide assessment of right and left
    ventricular exercise reserve after total correction of
    tetralogy of Fallot. American Journal of Cardiology
    45,1013-1018 (1980).

93. RERYCH, S.K., SCHOLZ, P.M., NEWMAN, G.E., SABISTON JR, D.C. &
     JONES, R.H. Cardiac function at rest and during exercise in
     normals and in patients with coronary heart disease:
     evaluation by radionuclide angiography. Annals of Surgery
     187, 449-464 (1978).

94. RERYCH, S.K., SCHOLZ, P.M., SABISTON, D.C., JR. & JONES, R.H.
     Effects of exercise training on left ventricular function in
     normal subjects: a longitudinal study by radionuclide
     angiography.   American   Journal   of   Cardiology
     45,244-252 (1980).

95. RIGO, P., ALDERSON, P.O., ROBERTSON, R.M., BECKER, L.C. &
     WAGNER, H.N., JR.   Measurement of aortic and mitral
     regurgitation by gated cardiac blood pool scans. Circulation
     60, 306-12 (1979).

96. RIGO, P., MURRAY, M., STRAUSS, H.W., TAYLOR, D., KELLY, D.,
     WEISFELDT, M. & PITT, B. Left ventricular ejection fraction
     in acute myocardial infarction evaluated by gated
     scintigraphy. Circulation **50**, 678-684 (1974).

97. RIGO, P., MURRAY, M., TAYLOR, D.R., WEISFELDT, M.L., KELLY,
     D.T., STRAUSS, H.W. & PITT, B. Right ventricular dysfunction
     detected by gated scintigraphy in patients with acute inferior
     myocardial infarction. Circulation **52**, 268-274 (1975).

98. RITCHIE, J.L., SORENSEN, S.G., KENNEDY, J.W. & HAMILTON, G.W.
     Radionuclide angiography: noninvasive assessment of
     hemodynamic changes after administration of nitroglycerin.
     American Journal of Cardiology **43**, 278-284 (1979).

99. SAGAWA, K., SUGA, H., SHOUKAS, A.A., BAKALAR, K.M.   End-
     systolic pressure/volume ratio: A new index of ventricular
     contractility. American Journal of Cardiology **40**, 748 (1977).

100. SANDLER, H. & DODGE, H.T.   Use of single plane
     angiocardiograms for the calculation of left ventricular
     volumes in man. American Heart Journal **75**, 325-334 (1968).

101. SANFORD, C.F., CORBETT, J.R., NICOD, P., CURRY, G.L., LEWIS,
     S.E., DEHMER, G.J., ANDERSON, A., MOSES, B. & WILLERSON, J.T.
     Value of radionuclide ventriculography in the immediate
     characterization of patients with acute myocardial infarction.
     American Journal of Cardiology **49**, 637-644 (1982).

102. SCHELBERT, H.R., HENNING, H., ASHBURN, W.L., VERBA, J.W.,
     KARLINER J.S. & O'ROURKE, R.A. Serial measurements of left
     ventricular ejection fraction by radionuclide angiography

early and late after myocardial infarction. American Journal of Cardiology **38**, 407-415 (1976).

103. SCHELBERT, H.R., VERBA, J.W., JOHNSON, A.D., BROCK, G.W., ALAZRACKI, N.P., ROSE, F.J. & ASHBURN, W.L. Nontraumatic determination of left ventricular ejection fraction by radionuclide angiocardiography. Circulation **51**, 902-909 (1975).

104. SCHULZE JR, R.A., STRAUSS, H.W. & PITT, B. Sudden death in the year following myocardial infarction: relation to ventricular premature contractions in the late hospital phase and left ventricular ejection fraction. American Journal of Medicine **62**, 192-199 (1977).

105. SHAH, P.K., PICHLER, M., BERMAN, D.S., SINGH, B.N. & SWAY, H.J.C. Left ventricular ejection fraction and first third ejection fraction determined by radionuclide ventriculography in early stages of first transmural myocardial infarction: relation to short-term prognosis. American Journal of Cardiology **45**, 542-546 (1980).

107. SLUTSKY, R., KARLINER, J., RICCI, D., KAISER, R., PFISTERER, M., GORDON, D., PETERSON K. & ASHBURN, W. Left ventricular volumes by gated equilibrium radionuclide angiography: a new method. Circulation **60**, 556-564 (1979).

108. SORENSON, S.G., O'ROURKE, R.A. & CHADHURI, T.K. Noninvasive quantitation of valvular regurgitation by gated equilibrium radionuclide angiography. Circulation **62**, 1089-1098 (1980).

109. STEELE, P., LeFREE, M. & KIRCH, D. Measurement of left ventricular mean circumferential fiber shortening velocity and systolic ejection rate by computerized radionuclide angiocardiography. American Journal of Cardiology **37**, 388-393 (1976).

110. STOKELY, E.M., PARKEY, R.W., BONTE, F.J., GRAHAM, K.D., STONE, M.J. & WILLERSON, J.T. Gated blood pool imaging following technetium-99m pyrophosphate imaging. Radiology **120**, 433-434 (1976).

111. STRAUSS, H.W. & PITT, B. Cardiovascular Nuclear Medicine (2nd Edition), pp. 126-139. St. Louis: C.V. Mosby (1979).

112. STRAUSS, H.W., ZARET, B.L., HURLEY, P.J., NATARAJAN, T.K. & PITT, B. A scintiphotographic method for measuring left ventricular ejection fraction in man without cardiac catheterization. American Journal of Cardiology **28**, 575-580 (1971).

113. TOBINICK, E., SCHELBERT, H.R., HENNING, H., LeWINTER, M., TAYLOR, A., ASHBURN, W.L. & KARLINER, J.S. Right ventricular ejection fraction in patients with acute inferior and anterior myocardial infarction assessed by radionuclide angiocardiography. Circulation **57**, 1078-1084 (1978).

114. TREVES, S. & PARKER, J.A. Detection and quantification of intracardiac shunts. In Cardiovascular Nuclear Medicine, Strauss, H.W. and Pitt, B., Eds., pp. 148-161. St. Louis, C.V. Mosby (1979).

115. VANDYKE, D., ANGER, H.O., SULLIVAN, R.W., VETTER, W.R., YANO, Y. & PARKER, H.G. Cardiac evaluation from radioisotope dynamics. Journal of Nuclear Medicine **13**, 585-592 (1972).

116. WACKERS, F.J., BERGER,H.J., JOHNSTONE, D.E., GOLDMAN, L., REDUTO, L.A., LANGOU, R.A., GOTTSCHALK, A. & ZARET, B.L. Multiple gated cardiac blood pool imaging for left ventricular ejection fraction: Validation of the technique and assessment of variability. American Journal of Cardiology **43**, 1159-1166 (1979).

117. WAINWRIGHT, R.J., BRENNAND-ROPER, D.A., CUENI, T., SOWTON, E., HILSON, A.J.W. & MAISEY, M.N. Cold pressor test in detection of coronary heart disease and cardiomyopathy using technetium-99m gated blood pool imaging. Lancet **2**, 320-323 (1979).

118. WATSON, D.D., NELSON, J.P. & GOTTLIEB, S. Rapid bolus injection of radioisotopes. Radiology **106**, 347-352 (1973).

119. WYNNE, J., MALACOFF, R.F., BENOTTI, J.R., CURFMAN, G.D., GROSSMAN, W., HOLMAN, B.L., SMITH, T.W. & BRAUNWALD, E. Oral amrinone in refractory congestive heart failure. American Journal of Cardiology **45**, 1245-1249 (1980).

120. ZARET, B.L., STRAUSS, H.W., HURLEY, P.J., NATARAJAN, T.K. & PITT, B. A noninvasive scintiphotographic method for detecting regional ventricular dysfunction in man. New England Journal of Medicine **284**, 1165-1170 (1971).

ENERGY PRODUCTION AND UTILIZATION IN CONTRACTILE FAILURE DUE TO INTRACELLULAR CALCIUM OVERLOAD*

N.S. Dhalla, J.N. Singh, D.B. McNamara, A. Bernatsky, A. Singh and J.A.C. Harrow

Experimental Cardiology Laboratory, Department of Physiology, Faculty of Medicine, University of Manitoba Winnipeg, Canada R3E 0W3

INTRODUCTION

Intracellular calcium overload has been suggested to cause myocardial cell damage and contractile failure (6,7,10); however, the mechanisms of the calcium-induced pathophysiologic changes are poorly understood. Recently, intracellular calcium overload has been demonstrated to occur upon reperfusing rat hearts following a few minutes of perfusion with Ca^{2+}-free medium (1). Reperfusion of the Ca^{2+}-deprived hearts with a normal medium failed to restore their ability to generate contractile force and caused a further deterioration of cardiac ultrastructure (12,22,26,27). Furthermore, dramatic alterations in the abilities of mitochondrial and sarcoplasmic reticular (microsomal) fractions to transport calcium have been observed upon reperfusing the Ca^{2+}-deprived hearts (2, 13). Although high energy phosphate stores, creatine phosphate (CrP) and ATP, have been found to be depressed in reperfused hearts (3,4,5,14,20,21), the exact reason for these metabolic changes is not clear at present. It is generally believed that an overstimulation of the myofibrillar ATPase due to intracellular calcium overload results in depletion of myocardial high energy phosphate stores but an adequate information on the status of other systems involved in energy utilization is not available in the literature. In addition, virtually nothing is known about changes in the process of energy production upon reperfusing the Ca^{2+}-deprived hearts. This study was therefore undertaken to

---

*This work was supported by a grant from the Manitoba Heart Foundation.

investigate alterations in myocardial energy metabolism due to an intracellular calcium overload.

METHODS

Male rats each weighing about 300 g were sacrificed by decapitation, the heart rapidly removed, placed in ice cold oxygenated Krebs - Henseleit bicarbonate buffer and freed from adipose and connective tissue. The aorta was tied to a cannula of the perfusion apparatus for coronary perfusion by the Langendorff technique as described elsewhere (8). After equilibrating the hearts for 15 min with normal medium, the hearts were perfused with a Ca^{2+}-free medium for different intervals and then these Ca^{2+}- deprived hearts were perfused with normal medium containing 1.25 mM Ca^{2+} for a period of 10 min. In some experiments perfusion with Mg^{2+}-free medium was carried out for the purpose of comparison. Control hearts were perfused with normal medium for comparable lengths of times. It should be mentioned that the temperature of the perfusion medium was maintained at 37°C and the coronary flow was kept at a rate of 10 ml/min with a peristaltic pump. When Ca^{2+} or Mg^{2+} was omitted from the medium, the osmolarity was maintained by adding an appropriate amount of sucrose. The perfusion medium was equilibrated with 95% O_2 and 5% CO_2 gas mixture and the pH of the medium was 7.4. The contractile force of myocardium was recorded on a Grass Polygraph by using a force displacement transducer (FT. 03). In one set of experiments, the hearts were frozen with a Wollenberger clamp, precooled in liquid N , for biochemical determinations. Adenine nucleotides and creatine phosphate were analyzed enzymatically using the fluorometric methods of Estabrook and Maitra (9). In all other experiments performed in this study unfrozen hearts were used for isolating cellular components.

Myofibrils were isolated from the control, calcium-deprived and reperfused hearts and their ATPase activities were measured according to the methods of Muir et. al. (19). The total ATPase activity of the myofibrillar fraction (0.5 - 1 mg protein/ml) was determined in a medium containing 10 mM histidine, pH 6.8, 5 mM sodium azide, 60 mM KC1, 3 mM MgCl and either 0.1 mM CaCl or 4 mM EGTA at 37°C. The myofibrillar ATPase in the presence of EGTA was taken to be due to the basal ATPase (Mg^{2+} ATPase) whereas the difference between the total and basal activities was taken to be due to the Ca^{2+} stimulated ATPase activity. The method employed for isolating mitochondria was the same as that described by Sordahl and Schwartz (23) whereas the microsomal fraction was isolated according to the method of Harigaya and Schwartz (11). The oxidative phosphorylation activities of mitochondria were determined by employing Clark oxygen electrode and Gilson oxygraph (23). The incubation medium employed for this purpose contained 0.25 M sucrose, 10 mM Tris-HC1, pH 7.4, 1.5 mM pyruvate and 0.5 mM malate. The total ATPase activity of the mitochondrial or micro-

Table 1. High energy phosphate stores in rat hearts perfused with
          Ca^{2+}-free medium for 5 or 10 min as well as reperfused
          with medium containing 1.25 mM Ca^{2+} for 10 min

Conditions	High energy phosphate contents (μmoles/g dry heart wt)	
	CrP	ATP
A. Control	31.4 ± 1.67	19.2 ± 0.23
B. 5 min Ca^{2+}-free perfusion:		
$\quad$ Ca^{2+}-free	30.6 ± 1.93	19.6 ± 0.34
$\quad$ Reperfused	11.2 ± 2.10*	13.7 ± 1.33*
C. 10 min Ca^{2+}-free perfusion:		
$\quad$ Ca^{2+}-free	32.8 ± 1.76	20.4 ± 0.51
$\quad$ Reperfused	5.7 ± 0.81*	7.5 ± 1.08*

Each value is a mean ± S.E. of 4 to 6 experiments. Control hearts
were perfused for 5 to 20 min with normal medium. * - Significantly different ($P < 0.05$) from the control values.

somal fraction was determined at 37°C in a medium containing 100
mM KCl, 4 mM $MgCl_2$, 0.1 mM $CaCl_2$, 20 mM Tris-HCl, pH 7.0, except
that 4 mM potassium oxalate was also present for estimating the
total ATPase activity of the microsomal fraction. The basal ATP-
ase activities (Mg^{2+} ATPase) of the mitochondrial and microsomal
fractions were measured in the same medium as for the total ATPase
activities except that 0.1 mM $CaCl_2$ was omitted and 1 mM EGTA was
added in the medium. The difference between the total and basal
ATPase activities was taken to represent Ca^{2+}-stimulated ATPase
activity. The methods for determining the mitochondrial and
microsomal ATPase activities are similar to those described earlier
(24). The mitochondrial and microsomal Ca^{2+} ATPase activities
were determined in the medium for Mg^{2+} ATPase except that 4 mM
$CaCl_2$ was used instead of 4 mM $MgCl_2$.

    The sarcolemmal fraction was isolated from the myocardium by
the hypotonic shock-LiBr treatment method (17,18). The adenylate
cyclase activity of the sarcolemmal preparation was determined by
incubating 50-60 μg of membrane protein in a total volume of 0.15
ml containing Tris-HCl, pH 8.5, 8 mM caffeine, 2 mM cyclic AMP,
5 mM KCl, 20 mM phosphoenolpyruvate, 15 mM MgCl , 130 μg/ml pyruvate kinase and 0.4 mM ATP - ^{14}C at 37°C. On the other hand, the
sarcolemmal Mg^{2+} ATPase and Ca^{2+} ATPase activities were determined
by incubating this fraction (60-100 μg membrane protein/ml) in a
medium containing 50 mM Tris-HCl, pH 7.4, and 4 mM ATP in the

Table 2. Myofibrillar ATPase activities in rat hearts perfused
          with Ca^{2+}-free medium for 5 to 10 min as well as reper-
          fused with medium containing 1.25 mM Ca^{2+} for 10 min

Conditions	Myofibrillar ATPase activity (μmoles Pi/mg protein/min)	
	Mg^{2+}-ATPase	Ca^{2+}-stimulated ATPase
A. Control	0.19 ± 0.02	0.16 ± 0.01
B. 5 min Ca^{2+}-free perfusion:		
Ca^{2+}-free perfused	0.20 ± 0.02	0.15 ± 0.02
Reperfused	0.19 ± 0.01	0.14 ± 0.02
C. 10 min Ca^{2+}-free perfusion:		
Ca^{2+}-free perfused	0.18 ± 0.03	0.14 ± 0.02
Reperfused	0.17 ± 0.02	0.16 ± 0.03

Each value is a mean ± S.E. of 4 to 6 experiments. Control hearts
were perfused for 5 to 20 min with normal medium.

absence and presence of 4 mM $MgCl_2$ or 4 mM $CaCl_2$ at 37°C. The
sarcolemmal $Na^+ - K^+$ ATPase activity was estimated by finding the
difference between ATP hydrolysis in absence or presence of 100
mM NaCl and 10 mM KCl in a medium containing 50 mM Tris-HCl, pH
7.4, 4 mM $MgCl_2$, 4 mM ATP and 60-100 μg membrane protein/ml at
37°C. These methods for determining sarcolemmal bound enzyme
activities have been described in detail previously (17,18). The
estimations of Pi and protein concentration were carried out by
the methods of Taussky and Shorr (25) and Lowry et. al. (16)
respectively. It should be noted that the control and experimental preparations were made simultaneously under identical conditions.
In some experiments, the ventricular tissue was dried to a constant
weight by keeping it in an oven at 100°C. Student's t - test was
used to analyze the statistical significance of differences in
control and experimental data.

RESULTS

     The high energy phosphate stores, CrP and ATP were determined
in hearts upon perfusion with Ca^{2+}-free medium as well as upon
reperfusion with normal medium. No changes (P > 0.05) in the CrP
and ATP contents were seen upon perfusion with Ca^{2+}-free medium
for 5 or 10 min; however, reperfusing the Ca^{2+}-deprived hearts
with normal medium for 10 min was found to decrease (P < 0.05)
their contents (Table 1). By employing 2 hearts for each time
interval, an appreciable (15 to 30%) fall in both CrP and ATP

Table 3. Mitochondrial respiratory and oxidative phosphorylation activities in rat hearts perfused with Ca^{2+}-free medium for 5 to 10 min as well as reperfused with medium containing 1.25 mM Ca^{2+} for 10 min

Conditions	ADP:0 ratio	Phosphorylation rate (μmoles ADP phosphorylated /min/g protein)	Respiratory rates (μatoms O/min/g protein)		RCl
			State 3	State 4	
A. Control	2.8 ± 0.02	456 ± 13.0	160 ± 5.0	19.8 ± 0.8	8.1 ± 0.36
B. 5 min Ca^{2+}-free perfusion:					
Ca2+-free	2.8 ± 0.01	460 ± 10.0	160 ± 3.4	19.8 ± 0.2	8.1 ± 0.26
Reperfused	2.5 ± 0.04*	216 ± 17.8*	88 ± 6.6*	15.4 ± 0.6*	5.8 ± 0.58*
C. 10 min Ca^{2+}-free perfusion:					
Ca2+-free	2.7 ± 0.05	450 ± 22.8	168 ± 7.0	20.2 ± 0.4	8.3 ± 0.35
Reperfused	2.3 ± 0.1*	146 ± 56.0*	58 ± 21.4*	11.8 ± 2.8*	4.1 ± 0.78*

Each value is a mean ± S.E. of 4-6 experiments. Control hearts were perfused for 5 to 20 min with normal medium. * - Significantly different (P < 0.05) from the control values. The state 3 respiration was initiated by the addition of 250 nmoles ADP whereas state 4 refers to a condition when all the ADP in the medium was phosphorylated. The respiratory control index (RCl) was calculated as the ratio of oxygen consumption during state 3 and 4 whereas the phosphorylation rate was calculated by multiplying the values for ADP:0 ratio and state 3 respiration rate.

Table 4. Mitochondrial and microsomal ATPase activities in rat
          hearts perfused with Ca^{2+}-free medium for 10 min as well
          as reperfused with medium containing 1.25 mM Ca^{2+} for
          10 min

Conditions	ATPase activities (μmoles Pi/mg protein/hr)		
	Ca^{2+} ATPase	Mg^{2+} ATPase	Ca^{2+}-stimulated ATPase
A. Mitochondria:			
Control	72.3 ± 4.1	80.5 ± 5.1	N.D.
Ca^{2+}-free	73.7 ± 3.2	76.9 ± 4.4	N.D.
Reperfused	74.2 ± 2.6	78.6 ± 4.5	N.D.
B. Microsomes:			
Control	105.4 ± 5.4	117.6 ± 6.3	12.0 ± 1.13
Ca^{2+}-free	103.6 ± 4.6	112.3 ± 4.2	9.4 ± 0.86
Reperfused	100.5 ± 5.8	108.2 ± 4.9	6.3 ± 0.75*

Each value is a mean ± S.E. of 3 experiments. N.D. - not detectable. * - Significantly different (P < 0.05) from the control
value. Control hearts were perfused for 10 to 20 min with normal
medium.

levels was seen at 1 and 2 min of starting reperfusion (data not
shown). The concentrations of both ADP and AMP were 1.5 to 4
times higher at 1 and 2 min but were not significantly different
at 5 and 10 min of reperfusion with normal medium following Ca^{2+}-
free perfusion for 5 min. Myofibrillar Mg^{2+} ATPase and Ca^{2+}-stim-
ulated ATPase activities in the Ca^{2+} - deprived or reperfused
hearts were not different (P > 0.05) from the control preparations
(Table 2). The mitochondrial oxidative phosphorylation activities
were also examined in hearts perfused for 5 and 10 min with Ca^{2+}-
free medium as well as upon reperfusing these Ca^{2+}- deprived
hearts with normal medium containing 1.25 mM Ca^{2+} for 10 min. The
results in Table 3 indicate no significant (P > 0.05) effect of
Ca^{2+}free perfusion upon different parameters of the mitochondrial
respiratory and oxidative phosphorylation activities; however,
reperfusion was found to depress ADP:0 ratio, phosphorylation rate,
respiratory rates in states 3 and 4, and RCl significantly (P <
0.05). Mitochondrial and microsomal Ca^{2+} ATPase and Mg^{2+} ATPase
activities from Ca^{2+}- deprived hearts or reperfused hearts were
not different (P > 0.05) from the control preparations except
that microsomal Ca^{2+}-stimulated ATPase activity was decreased in
reperfused hearts (Table 4). Similar results were obtained when
both mitochondrial (1,000 - 10,000 x g) and microsomal (10,000 -

Table 5. Sarcolemmal Mg^{2+} ATPase and Na^+-K^+ ATPase activities in
rat hearts perfused with Ca^{2+}-free medium for 5 or 10
min as well as reperfused with medium containing 1.25
mM Ca^{2+} for 10 min

Conditions	ATPase activities (μmoles Pi/mg protein/hr)	
	Mg^{2+} ATPase	Na^+-K^+ ATPase
A. Control	25.2 ± 1.3	11.1 ± 0.55
B. 5 min Ca^{2+}-free perfusion:		
Ca^{2+}-free	23.8 ± 1.4	9.7 ± 0.66
Reperfused	17.5 ± 0.7*	5.4 ± 0.31*
C. 10 min Ca^{2+}-free perfusion:		
Ca^{2+}-free	20.3 ± 1.2*	8.0 ± 0.52*
Reperfused	14.0 ± 0.5*	4.3 ± 0.21*

Each value is a mean + S.E. of 4 to 6 experiments. Control hearts
were perfused for 5 to 20 min with normal medium. * - Significantly different (P < 0.05) from the control values.

40,000 x g) fractions were isolated from the same heart homogenates
according to the method described elsewhere (24).

As shown previously (26), the rat hearts perfused with Ca^{2+}-
free medium for 5 min or more were unable to recover their ability
to generate contractile force upon reperfusion with normal medium
containing 1.25 Ca^{2+}. In order to demonstrate the effects of
reperfusion on the sarcolemmal enzyme activities, the hearts were
perfused for 5 or 10 min with Ca^{2+}-free medium and then reperfused
for a period of 10 min with normal medium. The data from these
experiments are shown in Tables 5 and 6. Significant (P < 0.05)
decreases in the sarcolemmal Mg^{2+} ATPase and Na^+ - K^+ ATPase activities were observed upon perfusing the Ca^{2+} - deprived hearts
with medium containing calcium (Table 5). Likewise,sarcolemmal
Ca^{2+} ATPase and adenylate cyclase activities were also decreased
upon reperfusing the Ca^{2+}-deprived hearts with a normal medium
(Table 6). On the other hand, reperfusing the hearts with normal
medium for 10 min after a 10 min perfusion with Mg^{2+} -free medium
had no effect upon the sarcolemmal bound enzyme activities.

DISCUSSION

It was interesting to observe that the hearts were unable to

Table 6.   Sarcolemmal adenylate cyclase and Ca^{2+}-ATPase activities
           in hearts perfused with Ca^{2+}-free medium for 5 or 10 min
           as well as with medium containing 1.25 mM Ca^{2+} for 10 min

Conditions	Adenylate cyclase activity (pmoles cyclic AMP/mg protein/min)	Ca^{2+}-ATPase activity (μmoles Pi/mg protein/hr)
A. Control	375 ± 15	29.2 ± 1.9
B. 5 min Ca^{2+}-free perfusion:		
$\quad$ Ca^{2+}-free	$305 \pm 12^*$	28.7 ± 1.2
$\quad$ Reperfused	$203 \pm 19^*$	$22.6 \pm 0.9^*$
C. 10 min Ca^{2+}-free perfusion:		
$\quad$ Ca^{2+}-free	$268 \pm 15^*$	26.8 ± 1.6
$\quad$ Reperfused	$158 \pm 14^*$	$21.0 \pm 0.5^*$

Each value is a mean $\pm$ S.E. of 4 to 6 experiments. * - Significantly different (P < 0.05) from the control values. Control
hearts were perfused for 5 to 20 min with normal medium.

recover its ability to generate contractile force upon reperfusion
with normal medium following a brief period of Ca^{2+}-free perfusion
and the sarcolemmal Ca^{2+} ATPase activity was depressed whereas the
sarcolemmal adenylate cyclase, Mg^{2+} ATPase and Na^+ - K^+ ATPase
activities were decreased further. Since reperfusion of the Ca^{2+}-
deprived hearts with normal medium has been shown to produce an
intracellular calcium overload and dramatic changes in the myocardial ultrastructure (1,15,26), it is likely that the observed
changes are due to this or some other associated event. It is
noteworthy that the intracellular calcium overload produced under
the experimental conditions described in this study was found to
depress mitochondrial respiratory and oxidative phosphorylation
activities without any changes in the mitochondrial and microsomal
ATPase activities. In this regard it should be pointed out that
the ATP-supported calcium accumulation by mitochondria was augmented and that by microsomes was decreased (2,13). While the depression in the mitochondrial respiratory and oxidative phosphorylation activities can be considered to be due to an increased accumulation of calcium within these organelles (15), the exact mechanisms for the observed changes in the sarcolemmal enzyme activities
and the microsomal calcium accumulation are a matter of speculation.
At any rate, these results demonstrate that the intracellular calcium overload is capable of producing dramatic changes in certain
functions of the sarcolemmal, mitochondrial and microsomal membranes and thus can be seen to produce alterations in the process

of energy production and utilization in the myocardium.

Although $\underline{in\ vitro}$ myofibrillar, mitochrondrial and microsomal ATPase activities of the control, and reperfused hearts were
not different from each other, it is conceivable that intracellular calcium overload is associated with an increased ATP hydrolysis by these systems under $\underline{in\ vivo}$ conditions. However, in this
regard it is pointed out that the myofibrillar ATPase activity
curve is of bell shape and it is rather likely that an excessive amount of calcium in the cytoplasm may in fact depress the
myofibrillar ATPase activity under $\underline{in\ vivo}$ situation employed
in this study. Thus the contribution of myofibrils in hydrolyz-
ing ATP under the condition of intracellular calcium overload
remains to be a matter of speculation. On the other hand, less
ATP will be utilized by sarcolemmal Ca^{2+} ATPase, Mg^{2+} ATPase, Na^+
- K^+ ATPase and adenylate cyclase during intracellular calcium
overload because the activities of these enzyme systems were depressed under these conditions. Likewise, less ATP will be utilized by calcium pump mechanism at the sarcoplasmic reticulum as
Ca^{2+}-stimulated ATPase activity of the microsomal fraction was
decreased in the reperfused hearts. ATP production by mitochondria in the reperfused hearts would be expected to decrease because the mitochondrial oxidative phosphorylation activity was
markedly depressed under the conditions of intracellular calcium
overload. Decreased adenylate cyclase activity in Ca^{2+} -deprived
and reperfused hearts would be associated with decreased production of cyclic AMP which will result in decreased mobilization of
both glycogen and triglyceride stores. On the other hand, elevated levels of intracellular calcium in reperfused hearts would
enhance the mobilization of glycogen and triglycerides through
some cyclic AMP - independent mechanisms. At any rate, the high
energy phosphate stores, CrP and ATP were unchanged upon Ca^{2+}-
free perfusion but were decreased during intracellular calcium
overload. The major problem facing the myocardium during calcium
free perfusion (intracellular calcium deficiency) seems to be an
insufficient utilization of ATP due to a lack of the coupling
factor between ATP and systems responsible for its hydrolysis.
On the other hand, during intracellular calcium overload there
is a depletion of ATP stores due to decreased energy production
mainly while increased energy utilization by myofibrils, if any,
may contribute to a smaller extent. This view is further supported by the fact that the heart is unable to recover its ability
to generate contractile force upon reperfusion and thus the contribution of energy utilized for the purpose of cardiac contraction is negligible.

SUMMARY

      Intracellular calcium overload was produced by perfusing the
Ca^{2+}- deprived rat hearts for 5 or 10 min with normal medium con-

taining 1.25 mM Ca^{2+} for 10 min and changes in the myofibrillar and membrane ATPase, sarcolemmal adenylate cyclase, mitochondrial oxidative phosphorylation and high energy phosphate stores in failing hearts were examined. Myocardial creatine phosphate and ATP were decreased by the intracellular calcium overload whereas the myofibrillar, mitochondrial and microsomal ATPase activities were not altered. The intracellular calcium overload markedly depressed the mitochondrial oxidative phosphorylation as well as sarcolemmal Ca^{2+} ATPase, Mg^{2+} ATPase, $Na^+ - K^+$ ATPase and adenylate cyclase. These results suggest that abnormalities in the process of energy production rather than energy utilization may primarily account for the depressed energy state of hearts failing due to an intracellular calcium overload.

REFERENCES

1. ALTO, L.E. & DHALLA, N.S. Myocardial cation contents during induction of calcium paradox. Am. J. Physiol. 237, H713-H719 (1979).
2. ALTO, L.E. & DHALLA, N.S. Role of changes in microsomal calcium uptake in the effects of reperfusion of Ca^{2+}-deprived rat hearts. Circ. Res. 48, 17-24 (1981).
3. ASHRAF, M., ONDA, M., BENEDICT, J.B. & MILLARD, R.W. Prevention of calcium paradox-related myocardial cell injury with dilitiazem, a calcium channel blocking agent. Am. J. Cardiol. 49, 1675-1681 (1982).
4. BOINK, A.B.T.J., RUIGROK, T.J.C., MAAS, A.H.J. & ZIMMERMAN, A.N.E. Changes in high-energy phosphate compounds of isolated rat hearts during Ca^{2+}-free perfusion and reperfusion with Ca^{2+}. J. Mol. Cell. Cardiol. 8, 973-979 (1976).
5. BUCKLEY, B.H., NUNNALLY, R.L. & HOLLIS, D.P. Calcium paradox and the effect of varied temperature on its development. Lab. Invest. 39, 133-140 (1978).
6. DHALLA, N.S., DAS, P.K. & SHARMA, G.P. Subcellular basis of cardiac contractile failure. J. Mol. Cell. Cardiol. 10, 363-385 (1978).
7. DHALLA, N.S., PIERCE, G.N., PANAGIA, V., SINGAL, P.K. & BEAMISH, R.E. Calcium movements in relation to heart function. Basic. Res. Cardiol. 77, 117-139 (1982).
8. DHALLA, N.S., YATES, J.C., WALZ, D.A., MCDONALD, V.A. & OLSON, R.E. Correlation between changes in the endogenous energy stores and myocardial function due to hypoxia in the isolated perfused rat heart. Can. J. Physiol. Pharmacol. 50, 333-345 (1972).
9. ESTABROOK, R.W. & MAITRA, P.K. A fluorometric method for the quantitative microanalysis of adenine and pyridine nucleotides. Anal. Biochem. 3, 369-382 (1962).
10. FLECKENSTEIN, A., JANKE, J., DORING, H.J. & LEADER, O. Myocardial fiber necrosis due to intracellular Ca^{2+} overload - a new principle in cardiac pathophysiology. In Recent

Advances in Studies on Cardiac Structure and Metabolism, Volume 4, N.S. Dhalla, Ed. pp. 563-580, Baltimore: University Park Press (1975).

11. HARIGAYA, S. & SCHWARTZ, A. Rate of calcium binding and uptake in normal animal and failing human cardiac muscle. Membrane vesicles (relaxing system) and mitochondria. Circ. Res. 25, 781-794 (1969).

12. HOLLAND, C.E., JR. & OLSON, R.E. Prevention by hypothermia of paradoxical calcium necrosis in cardiac muscle. J. Mol. Cell. Cardiol. 7, 917-928 (1975).

13. LEE, S.L. & DHALLA, N.S. Subcellular calcium transport in failing hearts due to calcium deficiency and overload. Am. J. Physiol. 231, 1159-1165 (1976).

14. LEE, Y.C.P. & VISSCHER, M.B. Perfusate cations and contracture and Ca, Cr. PCr and ATP in rabbit myocardium. Am. J. Physiol. 219, 1637-1641 (1970).

15. LEHNINGER, A.L. Mitochondria and calcium ion transport. Biochem. J. 119, 129-138 (1970).

16. LOWRY, O.H., ROSEBROUGH, N.J., FARR, A.L. & RANDALL, R.J. Protein measurement with Folin phenol reagent. J. Biol. Chem. 193, 265-275 (1951).

17. MCNAMARA, D.B., SINGH, J.N. & DHALLA, N.S. Properties of some heart sarcolemmal-bound enzymes. J. Biochem. 76, 603-609 (1974).

18. MCNAMARA, D.B., SULAKHE, P.V., SINGH, J.N. & DHALLA, N.S. Properties of heart sarcolemmal $Na^+ - K^+$ ATPase. J. Biochem. 75, 795-803 (1974).

19. MUIR, J.R., WEBER, A. & OLSON, R.E. Cardiac myofibrillar ATPase: A comparison with that of fast skeletal actomyosin in its native and in an altered conformation. Biochim. Biophys. Acta 234, 199-209 (1971).

20. OHHARA, H., KANAIDE, H. & NAKAMURA, M. A protective effect of verapamil on the calcium paradox in the isolated perfused rat heart. J. Mol. Cell. Cardiol. 14, 13-20 (1982).

21. RUIGROK, T.J.C., BOINK, A.B.T.J., SPIES, F., BLOK, F.J., MAAS, A.H.J. & ZIMMERMAN, A.N.E. Energy dependence of the calcium paradox. J. Mol. Cell. Cardiol. 10, 991-1002 (1978).

22. SINGAL, P.K., MATSUKUBO, M.P. & DHALLA, N.S. Calcium-related changes in the ultrastructure of mammalian myocardium. Br. J. Exp. Pathol. 60, 96-106 (1979).

23. SORDAHL, L.A. & SCHWARTZ, A. Effects of dipyridamole on heart muscle mitochondria. Mol. Pharmacol. 3, 509-515 (1967).

24. SULAKHE, P.V. & DHALLA, N.S. Excitation-contraction coupling in heart VII. Calcium accumulation in subcellular particles in congestive heart failure. J. Clin. Invest. 50, 1019-1027 (1970).

25. TAUSSKY, H.H. & SHORR, E.A. A microclorimetric method for the determination of inorganiz phosphorus. J. Biol. Chem. 202, 675-685 (1953).

26. YATES, J.C. & DHALLA, N.S. Structural and functional changes

associated with failure and recovery of hearts after perfusion with Ca^{2+} - free medium. J. Mol. Cell. Cardiol. 7, 91-103 (1975).

27. ZIMMERMAN, A.N.E., DAEMS, W., HULSMANN, W.C., SNIJDER, J., WISSE, E. & DURRER, D. Morphological changes of heart muscle caused by successive perfusion with calcium-free and calcium-containing solutions (calcium paradox). Cardiovasc. Res. 1, 201-209 (1967).

AORTIC PERFUSION PRESSURE AND PROTEIN SYNTHESIS*

Yuji Kira, Pamela Kochel and Howard E. Morgan

Department of Physiology
The Milton S. Hershey Medical Center
The Pennsylvania State University
Hershey, PA   17033

INTRODUCTION

Cardiac hypertrophy is a compensatory mechanism utilized when the heart must do additional work. Immediately after imposition of an increased pressure load, an acceleration in the rate of protein synthesis must depend upon increased efficiency because sufficient time has not elapsed to allow for synthesis of increased numbers of ribosomes and other components of the pathway. Efficiency of synthesis refers to the rate at which amino acids are incorporated into protein when expressed as a function of tissue RNA, whereas capacity refers to the quantity of RNA present within the heart (Waterlow et al., 1978). When the effects of increased pressure load were studied in vitro, incorporation of amino acids into heart protein was accelerated by higher work loads in working heart preparations or by increased perfusion pressure in Langendorff preparations (Schreiber et al., 1966; Hjalmarson and Isaksson, 1972a; Morgan et al., 1980). In these circumstances, increased synthesis was thought to be related to development of higher levels of ventricular pressure. In working hearts supplied glucose as substrate, increased protein synthesis appeared to involve prevention of the development of a block in peptide-chain initiation that developed in Langendorff preparations that were supplied glucose and developed low levels of ventricular pressure (Hjalmarson and Isaksson, 1972b; Morgan et al., 1980). A higher pressure load, but not a higher volume load,

*Supported by a grant from the National Heart, Lung and Blood Institute (HL-20388).

resulted in accelerated rates of protein synthesis (Hjalmarson and
Isaksson, 1972a; Schreiber et al., 1975).

The parameter that most closely relates increased pressure
load to acceleration of protein synthesis remains unresolved. The
observation that tetrodotoxin could stop all mechanical activity
of aerobic Langendorff preparations without reducing the rate of
protein synthesis suggested that protein synthesis was not
dependent upon contraction, per se (Jefferson et al., 1971). When
contractile activity was inhibited by induction of anoxia,
however, protein synthesis was reduced. These findings were
confirmed by Schreiber et al. (1977) in K^+-arrested hearts and
extended to show that the inhibitory effects of anoxia were
minimized by K^+-arrest. In recent studies, Takala (1981) found
that an increase in perfusion pressure from 60 to 150 mmHg in
Langendorff preparations supplied glucose accelerated
phenylalanine incorporation not only in beating hearts, but also
K^+-arrested hearts in which intraventricular pressure was adjusted
to zero. These findings indicate that not only the "basic" rate
of protein synthesis (Schreiber et al., 1977), but also the
increased rate induced by a pressure load was independent of
cardiac contraction (Takala, 1981). When higher perfusion
pressures were imposed on beating Langendorff preparations, more
intraventricular pressure was developed and myocardial oxygen
consumption increased (Opie, 1965; Neely et al., 1967; Arnold et
al., 1968). Arnold et al. (1968) presented additional data
showing that an elevation of perfusion pressure from 60 to 160
mmHg in empty beating hearts increased oxygen consumption from 6.1
to 12.2 ml/min · 100 g; in K^+-arrested hearts, the same increase
in perfusion pressure raised oxygen consumption from 2.8 to 4.5
ml/min · 100 g. These findings were postulated to indicate that
the increased perfusion pressure in the coronary arteries had
stretched the vessels, the so-called "garden-hose effect", and
secondarily had stretched the heart muscle fibers. These findings
were consistent with the observation of Peterson and Lesch (1972)
that stretch of the right ventricular papillary muscle would
increase phenylalanine incorporation. Taken together, these
findings appear to rule out cardiac work, intraventricular
pressure development, and contraction, per se as parameters
associated with increased protein synthesis in hearts subjected to
a pressure load and to focus attention on the relationship between
wall tension and the synthetic rate.

The purpose of the present experiments has been to explore
further the relationship between coronary perfusion pressure and
protein synthesis in 1) Langendorff preparations and working
hearts that are developing varying levels of intraventricular
pressure, 2) Langendorff preparations that are beating but
developing no intraventricular pressure, and 3) Langendorff
preparations in which all mechanical activity has been inhibited

with tetrodotoxin and intraventricular pressure maintained at zero.

MATERIALS AND METHODS

Animals

Sprague-Dawley strain, male rats, weighing about 300 g were provided with food and water, ad libitum, until killed. The rats were injected intraperitoneally with heparin (300 units/100 g body weight) and sodium pentobarbital (8 mg/100 g body weight) prior to removal of the heart.

Perfusion

Hearts were removed and dropped into ice-cold saline, and perfusion was initiated as either Langendorff preparations or working hearts as described previously (Neely et al., 1967; Morgan et al., 1980). During the first 10 minutes of perfusion, Krebs-Henseleit bicarbonate buffer containing normal plasma levels of 19 amino acids (Williams et al., 1980), 0.4 mM phenylalanine, and 15 mM glucose was allowed to pass through the heart a single time at a pressure of 40 mmHg. The perfusate was maintained at $37°$ and was gassed with $O_2:CO_2$ (95:5%). Following this period of preliminary perfusion, 30 ml of the same buffer containing [U-^{14}C]phenylalanine (0.2 µCi/ml) and 0.2% bovine serum albumin (American Research Product Co., Fraction V, Diagnostic grade) were recirculated through the heart for periods up to 2 hours. The perfusion pressure of Langendorff preparations was either 60, 90 or 120 mmHg. In some experiments, the left ventricular apex was cannulated with a Teflon tube (18 gauge, 5 mm long) to eliminate intraventricular pressure development. In some experiments, tetrodotoxin (final concentration, 9 µg/ml; Sankyo Co., Japan) was employed to arrest all mechanical activity (Jefferson et al., 1971). In working hearts, a 20 gauge needle was placed in the aortic outflow tract.

Intraventricular Pressure Measurement

Intraventricular pressure in the left ventricle was measured through an 18 gauge needle inserted in the apex. The needle was attached to a pressure transducer (Statham P23A) connected to a recorder (Beckman Type RB Dynograph).

Oxygen Consumption

When oxygen consumption was measured, the pulmonary artery was cannulated with a 14 gauge needle to measure pulmonary artery flow and to allow for collection of a sample for measurement of O_2

tension. Since about 20% of coronary flow is drained from the
right atrium in Langendorff preparations perfused with a high
aortic pressure, coronary flow was estimated by collecting the
perfusate from the pulmonary artery and from the surface of the
heart (Neely et al., 1967). Arterial samples of perfusate were
collected from the tube supplying perfusate to the heart with a
syringe. Oxygen tension was measured using a pH/blood gas
analyzer (Corning, Model 165/2), and oxygen consumption was
calculated as described previously (Neely et al., 1967).

Estimation of the Rate of Protein Synthesis

Rates of protein synthesis were estimated by measuring the
rate of incorporation of [^{14}C]phenylalanine into cardiac protein.
The radioactivity was added to the recirculation buffer either
after 10 or 70 minutes of perfusion. Incorporation of
[^{14}C]phenylalanine was measured over the next 60 or 120 minutes.
At the phenylalanine concentration that was employed (0.4 mM), the
specific activity of phenylalanine in the perfusate, intracellular
water, and bound to tRNA were equal (McKee et al., 1978). Tissue
protein was purified, as described earlier (Morgan et al., 1971a)
from a perchloric acid pellet and solubilized in 1 ml of NCS
tissue solubilizer (New England Nuclear). Radioactivity was
estimated by liquid scintillation spectroscopy and protein content
was determined by weighing. Rates of synthesis are expressed as
nmol phenylalanine incorporated/g dry heart; protein content of
dry heart averaged 750 mg/g (Morgan et al., 1980).

Heart Extraction

Frozen hearts (approximately 1.3 g) were weighed and powdered
in porcelain mortars cooled to the temperature of liquid nitrogen.
A sample (approximately 150 mg) of the heart powder was removed,
weighed immediately in a cup of aluminum foil, and dried at 105°C
to determine dry weight/wet weight ratio. Three ml of 1.66 M
perchloric acid were pipetted into a beaker half-filled with
liquid nitrogen. The resulting perchloric acid ice ball was
powdered along with the heart in the liquid nitrogen cooled mortar
and mixed thoroughly. The mixture of powder was poured into a
porcelain mortar at room temperature and allowed to thaw while
being ground with a pestle. The homogenate was centrifuged at
12,000 g for 10 min at 4°C. The pellets were used to determine
radioactivity of heart protein. An aliquot of the supernatant was
weighed and 0.2 ml of 1M morpholinopropanesulfonic acid, pH 6.7,
was added. The supernatant was neutralized with KOH, weighed, and
recentrifuged as above to remove the precipitated KClO$_4$. The
neutralized extract was assayed using standard enzymatic methods
to determine the content of ATP and creatine phosphate.

Table 1. Protein Synthesis in Langendorff Preparations and Working Hearts

Preparation	Perfusion Pressure	Protein Synthesis, %	
		10-70 min	70-130 min
Langendorff	60 mmHg	100 ± 0.9(6)	81 ± 1.5(12)*†
Langendorff	120 mmHg	95 ± 2.6(6)	113 ± 4.6(11)*†
Working	145/77 mmHg	110 ± 3.8(7)*	99 ± 4.8(6)

Hearts were perfused for the period indicated as described in Materials and Methods. Values are expressed as % of the rate in Langendorff preparations between 10 and 70 min of perfusion (701 ± 6 nmol phenylalanine/g · h) and are given as mean ± S.E. The number of observations is shown in parentheses. *p < 0.05 versus Langendorff, 60 mmHg, 10-70 min. †p < 0.05 versus 10-70 min, same condition.

Statistical Analysis

For comparison of differences between means, Student's t test was employed.

RESULTS AND DISCUSSION

Aortic Perfusion Pressure and Protein Synthesis in Hearts Developing Intraventricular Pressure

During the first hour of perfusion, an increase in aortic pressure from 60 to 120 mmHg in the Langendorff preparation did not significantly affect the rate of protein synthesis (Table 1). In working hearts, protein synthesis increased as compared to Langendorff preparations perfused at 60 mmHg during this period. Intraventricular pressures (systolic/diastolic) in Langendorff preparations perfused with aortic pressures of 60 and 120 mmHg were 67 ± 3/0 and 121 ± 7/0 mmHg, respectively. In working hearts, the aortic pressure was 145/77 mmHg (Morgan et al., 1980).

The rate of protein synthesis fell significantly (p < 0.001) in the second hour in Langendorff preparations perfused at 60 mmHg. When aortic pressure was raised to 120 mmHg, protein synthesis was significantly higher than in the first hour at this pressure and also was higher than in Langendorff preparations perfused with an aortic pressure of 60 mmHg (70-130 min). In working hearts, the rate of synthesis was not changed significantly from that observed in the first hour.

When glucose alone was provided as oxidative substrate, the decrease in the rate of protein synthesis in Langendorff preparations perfused with an aortic pressure of 60 mmHg was due to development of a block in peptide chain initiation, as indicated by loss of polysomes and accumulation of ribosomal subunits (Morgan et al., 1971b, 1980). Induction of cardiac work increased the synthetic rate and the content of polysomes, indicating that development of the initiation block had been prevented (Hjalmarson and Isaksson, 1972b; Morgan et al., 1980). The increased rate of synthesis in Langendorff preparations perfused with an aortic pressure of 120 mmHg also probably involved prevention of the initiation block, but this point has not been explored by measuring ribosomal subunits and polysomes.

These studies confirmed earlier experiments (Schreiber et al., 1966, 1975; Hjalmarson and Isaksson, 1972a, 1972b; Morgan et al., 1980; Takala, 1981) in showing that an increased aortic pressure in Langendorff preparations or development of higher levels of aortic pressure in working hearts would increase protein synthesis in hearts supplied glucose as oxidizable substrate.

Aortic Perfusion Pressure and Protein Synthesis in Hearts with a
Ventricular Drain or Arrested with Tetrodotoxin

The next series of experiments were undertaken to differentiate between the various parameters of contractile activity that might correlate with an increase in protein synthesis. Intraventricular pressure development was prevented in either beating or tetrodotoxin-arrested hearts by insertion of a ventricular drain. Measurement of intraventricular pressure through a separate needle inserted into the ventricle revealed that no pressure developed in either preparation (data not shown). Rates of protein synthesis were measured during the second hour of perfusion to enhance the effects of aortic pressure on protein synthesis (Table 2).

In Langendorff preparations perfused with an aortic pressure of 60 mmHg, prevention of intraventricular pressure development by insertion of a drain or cessation of beating and intraventricular pressure development by addition of tetrodotoxin and insertion of a drain had no effect on the rate of protein synthesis. These results are in agreement with earlier studies from this (Jefferson et al., 1971) and other laboratories (Schreiber et al., 1977; Takala, 1981). Myocardial oxygen consumption was not reduced by insertion of a drain, but fell almost 60% when contractile activity was terminated.

When aortic pressure was increased to 120 mmHg, protein synthesis increased 46% in Langendorff preparations that were developing intraventricular pressure. Prevention of pressure

Table 2. Relationship Between Rates of Protein Synthesis, Ventricular Pressure Development and Oxygen Consumption

Preparation	Perfusion Pressure, mmHg	Protein Synthesis, %	Oxygen Consumption, %
Langendorff	60	100 ± 3.1(18)	100 ± 7.6 (8)
	120	146 ± 2.5 (10)†	185 ± 13 (8)†
+ Ventricular	60	99.4 ± 3.1(6)	99.2 ± 5.0(9)
Drain	120	156 ± 9.0(6)†	162 ± 13(9)†
+ Tetrodotoxin	60	107 ± 5.9(6)	42.9 ± 3.4(4)*†
and Drain	120	156 ± 5.0(6)†	42.9 ± 5.0(3)*†

Hearts were perfused as described in Materials and Methods and protein synthesis was measured during the second hour of perfusion. Values are expressed as % of the rate of protein synthesis (524 ± 16 nmol/g · h) or oxygen consumption (1.19 ± .09 mmol/g · h) found in Langendorff preparations with an aortic pressure of 60 mmHg. Values represent mean ± S.E. *p < 0.05 versus Langendorff preparation, same pressure. †p < 0.05 versus Langendorff preparation, 60 mmHg.

development or cessation of contractile activity had no effect on the stimulatory effect of aortic pressure on protein synthesis (Table 2). An increase in aortic pressure also raised myocardial oxygen consumption by 85%. Insertion of a ventricular drain did not reduce oxygen consumption significantly at 120 mmHg aortic pressure but cessation of beating in tetrodotoxin-treated hearts reduced oxygen consumption to the value observed in arrested hearts perfused with an aortic pressure of 60 mmHg. ATP and creatine phosphate contents were not significantly different among the groups of hearts perfused at 60 and 120 mmHg (data not shown). These results confirm the finding of Takala (1981) in showing no relationship between intraventricular pressure development, myocardial oxygen consumption, or contractile activity and a faster rate of protein synthesis induced by elevation of aortic pressure. Maintenance of the same rate of oxygen consumption in hearts containing a ventricular drain is consistent with the observations of Arnold et al. (1968). These workers postulated that the higher rates of oxygen consumption observed with increased aortic pressures were due to increased wall tension that resulted from the "garden-hose effect".

Although coronary flow rates in beating hearts perfused with an aortic pressure of 60 mmHg were less than those in beating hearts perfused at 120 mmHg, the coronary flows in arrested hearts perfused at 120 mmHg were not significantly different from those in beating hearts perfused at 60 mmHg (data not shown). These results are consistent with the findings of Hjalmarson and Isaksson (1972a) and Schreiber et al. (1975) in suggesting that coronary flow itself had no effect on protein synthesis in pressure-loaded hearts. Similarly, coronary perfusion pressure and not coronary flow was correlated with myocardial oxygen consumption and increased ventricular pressure development (Opie, 1965; Arnold et al., 1968).

From the studies reported in this paper and those of Takala (1981), it appears that coronary perfusion pressure per se has a stimulatory effect on protein synthesis. This effect may be mediated by stretching of the ventricular wall. This suggestion is consistent with the observation of Peterson and Lesch (1972) that stretch of a ventricular papillary muscle would accelerate protein synthesis.

SUMMARY

The effect of increased pressure load on cardiac protein synthesis has been studied in Langendorff preparations and working hearts supplied glucose as substrate. During the second hour of perfusion, elevation of perfusion pressure from 60 to 120 mmHg in Langendorff preparations accelerated protein synthesis by approximately 40% while induction of cardiac work and development of a systolic pressure of 145 mmHg increased synthesis by 22%, as compared to a Langendorff preparation perfused at 60 mmHg. In Langendorff preparations, increased perfusion pressure still accelerated protein synthesis when a drain was placed in the ventricle and intraventricular pressure development was prevented or when the heart was arrested with tetrodotoxin and the ventricle drained. These results suggest that the enhancement of protein synthesis with a pressure load may be induced by passive stretch of the cardiac muscle cell secondary to increased perfusion pressure.

REFERENCES

Arnold, G., Kosche, F., Messner, E., Neitzert, A., and Lochner, W., 1968, The importance of the perfusion pressure in the coronary arteries for the contractility and oxygen consumption of the heart, Pflugers Archiv., 299:339.
Hjalmarson, A., and Isaksson, O., 1972a, In vitro work load and rat heart metabolism. I. Effect on protein synthesis, Acta Physiol. Scand., 86:126.

Hjalmarson, A., and Isaksson, O., 1972b, In vitro work load and rat heart metabolism. III. Effect on ribosomal aggregation, Acta Physiol. Scand., 86:342.

Jefferson, L. S., Wolpert, E. B., Giger, K. E., and Morgan, H. E., 1971, Regulation of protein synthesis in heart muscle. III. Effect of anoxia on protein synthesis, J. Biol. Chem., 246:2171.

McKee, E. E., Cheung, J. Y., Rannels, D. E., and Morgan, H. E., 1978, Measurement of the rate of protein synthesis and compartmentation of heart phenylalanine, J. Biol. Chem., 253:1030.

Morgan, H. E., Chua, B. H. L., Fuller, E. O., and Siehl, D., 1980, Regulation of protein synthesis and degradation during in vitro cardiac work, Am. J. Physiol., 238:E431.

Morgan, H. E., Earl, D. C. N., Broadus, A., Wolpert, E. B., Giger, K. E., and Jefferson, L. S., 1971a, Regulation of protein synthesis in heart muscle. I. Effect of amino acid levels on protein synthesis, J. Biol. Chem., 246:2152.

Morgan, H. E., Jefferson, L. S., Wolpert, E. B., and Rannels, D. E., 1971b, Regulation of protein synthesis in heart muscle. II. Effect of amino acids and insulin on ribosomal aggregation, J. Biol. Chem., 246:2163.

Neely, J. R., Liebermeister, H., Battersby, E. J., and Morgan, H. E., 1967, Effect of pressure development on oxygen consumption by isolated rat heart, Am. J. Physiol., 212:804.

Opie, L. H., 1965, Coronary flow rate and perfusion pressure as determinants of mechanical function and oxidative metabolism of isolated perfused rat heart, J. Physiol., 180:529.

Peterson, M. B., and Lesch, M., 1972, Protein synthesis and amino acid transport in the isolated rabbit right ventricular papillary muscle, Circ. Res., 31:317.

Schreiber, S. S., Hearse, D., J., Oratz, M., and Rothschild, M. A., 1977, Protein synthesis in prolonged cardiac arrest, J. Mol. Cell. Cardiol., 9:87.

Schreiber, S. S., Oratz, M., and Rothschild, M. A., 1966, Protein synthesis in the overloaded mammalian heart, Am. J. Physiol., 211:314.

Schreiber, S. S., Rothschild, M. A., Evans, C., Reff, F., and Oratz, M., 1975, The effect of pressure or flow stress on right ventricular protein synthesis in the face of constant and restricted coronary perfusion, J. Clin. Invest., 55:1.

Takala, T., 1981, Protein synthesis in the isolated perfused rat heart, Basic Res. Cardiol., 76:44.

Waterlow, J. C., Garlick, P. J., and Millward, D. J., 1978, "Protein Turnover in Mammalian Tissues and in the Whole Body," North Holland, New York.

Williams, I. H., Chua, B. H. L., Sahms, R. H., Siehl, D., and Morgan, H. E., 1980, Effects of diabetes on protein turnover in cardiac muscle, Am. J. Physiol., 239:E178.

THE EFFECT OF 5-HYDROXYTRYPTAMINE AND ARTERIAL BLOOD WITHDRAWAL ON CEREBRAL MICROCIRCULATION IN THE CAT, ARTERIAL PERMEABILITY IN THE RABBIT

R. J. Bing, Bing-Lo Chang, G. Santillan and M. Sato

Department of Experimental Cardiology, Huntington Medical Research Institutes, The Huntington Memorial Hospital, and the California Institute of Technology Pasadena, California 91105, U.S.A.

Abstract: Studies dealing with the effect of 5-HT on cerebral cortical microcirculation of cats and on permeability of femoral arteries to RISA of rabbits are presented. The effect of 5-HT on cerebral cortical microcirculation was compared to that of arterial blood withdrawal and blood reinfusion. The effect of topical administration of 5-HT was also studied. Cortical microcirculation was observed by transillumination using a microtransilluminator. Motion pictures were taken at a speed of 400 frames/sec. and a magnification of 3000X. Permeability was investigated using arterial RISA uptake in vessels perfused in vitro, with continuous recording of perfusion pressure.

Microcirculatory studies revealed that arterial blood withdrawal and injection of 5-HT diminished red cell velocity, although to a different degree. With blood withdrawal and reinjection, good correlation existed between blood pressure and red cell velocity. In contrast, no correlation between blood pressure and red cell velocity was found after intracarotid injection of 5-HT. Reactive hyperemia was noted during reinfusion of blood. Both arterial blood withdrawal and 5-HT injection resulted in disappearance of red cells in individual vessels (unperfused channels). Good correlation of blood pressure with capillary red cell velocity during arterial blood withdrawal suggests absence of autoregulation in this portion of the microcirculation. Topical administration of 5-HT caused general vasoconstriction. Permeability to 5-HT to RISA followed a parabolic curve. With slight arterial vasoconstriction, permeability declined, while it rose with severe vasoconstriction.

INTRODUCTION

Recent clinical observations on vascular spasm have aroused considerable interest in substances which may be responsible for vasoconstriction occurring in various circulatory areas, particularly the coronary and cerebral circulation (22,26). It has been proposed for example that vasospasm in coronary arteries may lead to more permanent vascular damage and to atherosclerosis. Thus Marzilli and co-workers (25) discovered clinical evidence that spontaneously concurring coronary arterial spasm can progress to fixed arteriosclerotic narrowing. Although vascular spasm appears to be an ubiquitous phenomenon, there exists considerable inhomogeneity in the response of individual vascular beds to vasoactive drugs. Bohr in 1965, (3) discovered that one of the most outstanding characteristics of smooth muscle is the individuality of the contractile response. Vascular spasm also plays an important role in the production of cerebral ischemia (28). Direct observations of the cerebral cortical microcirculation have recently been made possible by a new approach, employing transillumination of the cerebral cortex (8,29). This report is concerned with two different experimental approaches: the first deals with the effect of 5-HT on the cerebral cortical microcirculation of the cat. The second is concerned with the effect of 5-HT on the permeability of femoral arteries of rabbits to radioiodinated serum albumin (RISA).

In the study on the cerebral microcirculation three aspects were considered: 1) Response of red cell velocity (RCV) to arterial withdrawal of blood as compared to 5-HT; 2) Evidence for autoregulation in the capillaries of cerebral cortex under these conditions; 3) Changes in circulation resulting in conversion of functional vessels into non-functional unperfused channels. The aim of studies on the permeability of femoral arteries was to relate the changes observed during perfusion with 5-HT to the degree of vascular spasm, as reflected in an increase in perfusion pressure.

MATERIAL AND METHODS

I. Studies on the Cerebral Microcirculation

Thirty cats of either sex weighing from 2.3 to 4.5 kg were sedated with ketamine hydrochloride (18 mg/kg body weight). Sodium pentothal, not exceeding a total dose of 25 mg/kg body weight, was injected intravenously at intervals required to maintain a good level of anesthesia. A flexible catheter (4.0 FR, Malinckrodt) was inserted into a femoral artery. The second catheter was placed in the right carotic artery, with the tip facing cephalad. A third flexible catheter was placed into a femoral vein for injection of 5-HT. A tracheotomy was performed and the animals were ventilated with room air through an infant ventilator (LS104-150, Bourns, Inc.). Body

temperature was determined by an intrarectal thermocouple and maintained at about 37.5°C by means of heating pad. Arterial blood
pressure was continuously monitored and recorded with a polygraph
(Electronics for Medicine, Honeywell, Inc.). Arterial blood gasses
and pH were measured occasionally with a microanalyzer (Radiometer).
Values were within the range of awake cats (pH=7.3±0.07; pO_2=94mm Hg
pCo_2 = 30 ± 3.1). After anesthesia the head was fixed in a surgical
head holder (David Kopf Instruments). Craniotomy was performed by
means of a turbine drill. Following this the dura was radially incised and folded back, the cerebral surface was kept moist with frequent application of Ringer-Tyrode solution gassed with 5% CO_2 and
95% O_2 and warmed to 37°C.

Visualization of the cortex was carried out by means of transillumination with a microtransilluminator described in previous publications (8, 29). Essentially the transilluminator consists of a
hollow seamless steel tubing with an outer diameter of 0.7mm and a
length of 45 mm (8, 29). An inner coated optical fiber of a diameter
of 381 μm was then inserted into the lumen of the steel tubing. The
steel tubing is cut at a right angle at one end and the other end is
ground to a 20° bevel. One end of the optical fiber was cut at a
right angle and the other end at 45°; it was aluminized to reflect
light upwards into the tissue through a window that was drilled in
the steel tubing. The light source consisted of a pulsed short gap
300-W Xenon illuminator (Varian/Eimac), which contained a series of
heat filters to eliminate ultraviolet and heat radiation. It also
provided strobe impulses at rates between 50 and 400 flashes per second for TV monitoring. The strobe was triggered by the operation of
the Milliken camera. Each film strip was taken for approximately 3
seconds.

Previous results have shown that the injury to the tissues resulting from the introduction of the microtransilluminator is minimal
(28). The microtransilluminator was inserted parallel to the cortical
surface (suprasylvian and ectosylvian region) at a depth of at least
800 μm by means of a multiple joint manipulator. The depth of the
cortical area under observation was approximately 200-500 μm.

The transmitted light was then conducted through the objective
of a microscope (X32) to the optical system of an intravital microscope to a Milliken camera. Films were taken at a speed of 400
frames/sec. The red cell velocity was determined by frame to frame
analysis (20). Magnification of the screen was 3000X for the medium
objective (32X).

Effect of hydroxytryptamine (5-HT): After three control observations 5μg/kg of hydroxytryptamine were injected through carotid catheter. Additional films were taken whenever noticeable changes in
blood pressure occurred. The total number of film strips was usually
8.

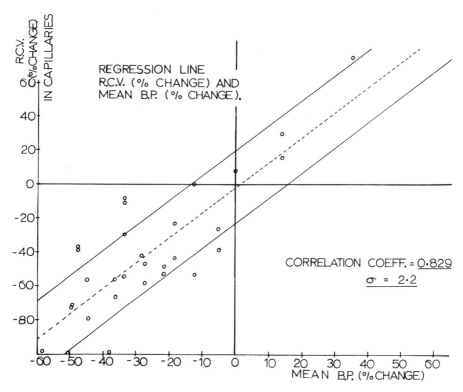

Figure 1.   Relationship between mean arterial blood pressure
            (abscissa) and percentage change in red cell velocity
            (RCV) in cortical capillaries during arterial blood
            withdrawl and reinfusion of blood. A direct relation-
            ship exists (correlation coefficient 0.82).

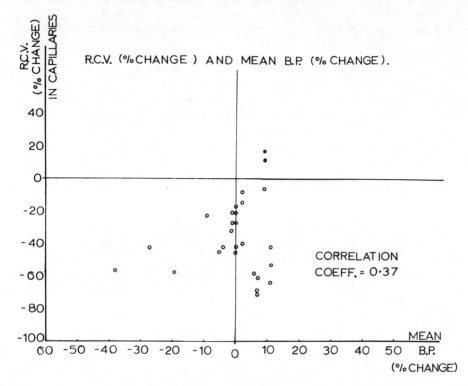

Figure 2.   Relationsip between mean arterial blood pressure
(abscissa) and percent change in RCV during and following intracarotid injection of 5-HT.   Despite minor
changes in blood pressure, RCV markedly decreased. There
is no relationship between percent change in RCV and
blood pressure (correlation coefficient of 0.37).

Arterial blood withdrawal: To study the effect of changes in blood pressure on the cerebral microcirculation, with particular ref erence to autoregulation, blood was withdrawn through the catheter inserted into the left femoral artery with a Harvard pump, at a spee of 3.82 ml/min. Changes in blood pressure were continuously recorde After 3 short strips of film had been taken during the control perio several additional films were recorded during removal of the blood, usually during the periods when major changes in blood pressure oc- curred. Following withdrawal, the blood was reinjected at the same speed and blood pressure and film strips were again recorded.

In a number of vessels removal of blood or injection of 5-HT re sulted in disappearance of red cells. We have termed these vessels unperfused channels. In order to quantitate these findings, a contr volume for each of these vessels was chosen and its volume was cal- culated. (Volume = L x $\frac{\pi d^2}{4}$). Since each control volume varied in length and diameter, the absolute volume differed in individual ves- sels. The effect of topically applied 5-HT (10^{-4}M) was observed by dropping 0.5 ml of this solution on the exposed cortical surface.

II. Studies on Perfused Arteries

Vascular permeability to RISA induced by 5-HT (10^{-5}M) was inves igated in arteries undergoing vascular spasm. 14 white New Zealand rabbits were used. The rabbits ranged in weight from 1.9 to 3.2 kgs The arteries were dissected clear of the surrounding tissue and all side branches were tied. They were then washed with Krebs-Henseleit solution. Two arterial segments about 7-18 mm long were cannulated on both ends with polyethylene tubing (1 mm internal diameter). The two segments were connected to a perfusion pump, maintaining the in vivo direction of flow. Perfusion pressure was determined by strain gauges (Gould-Statham pressure transducers Model P23 ID). Since, in the perfusion system used here, flow is maintained constant, the de- gree of rate of constriction is reflected by changes in perfusion pressure, as measured proximal to the perfused vessel. The degree of vasoconstriction induced by 5-HT is calculated as follows: degre of vasoconstriction = highest value of pressure - control pressure (ΔP). Perfusion was carried out by means of a Cole-Palmer variable pump set at a perfusion pressure of 50 mm Hg and a flow rate of 13.0 ml/min. The arteries were maintained in a bath of continuously oxy- genated Krebs-Henseleit solution at 37°C. Evans Blue (.001% final concentration) was prepared as follows: 10 μCi. of RISA were added to 100 mls of Krebs-Henseleit solution. After thorough mixing, the solution was divided into 2 equal parts: to one volume, 5-HT was added, to make a final concentration of 10^{-5}M. To the other, (con- trol) an identical amount of Krebs-Henseleit solution was added. Pe fusion was carried out for 1 hour prior to addition of 5-HT and RISA This period was chosen since Caro et al had demonstrated that the average permeability coefficient in the rabbit artery in situ become steady about 30 minutes after the injection of RISA (6).

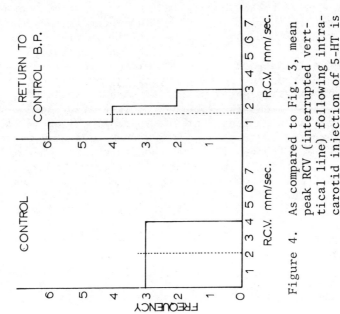

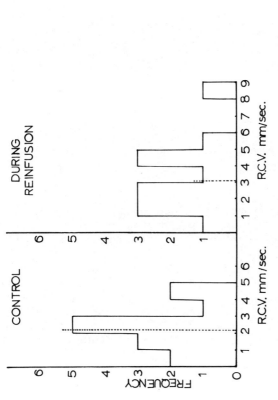

Figure 4. As compared to Fig. 3, mean peak RCV (interrupted vertical line) following intracarotid injection of 5-HT is slightly shifted to the left.

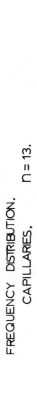

Figure 3. Frequency distribution of red cell velocity after reinfusion of arterial blood. As compared to the control, mean peak of RCB (interrupted vertical line) is shifted to the right, illustrating reactive hyperemia.

Aliquots of the bathing solution were collected every 5 minutes throughout the experiment to determine whether leakage of RISA into the bathing solution had occurred. After 15 minutes perfusion with 5-HT, the perfusate was replaced with Krebs-Henseleit solution and perfusion was continued for an additional minute. The arteries were then severed from the cannulae, avoiding any damage to the endothelial layer. All arteries were opened and washed extensively with 150 ml saline and the lumen was exposed. Surface area was determined from the diameter and the length of the segment. Excess liquid was removed from the arteries by gently pressing them against 2 pieces of filter paper; they were then quickly weighed to obtain wet weight. After the above measurements, the arterial activity was counted using a Packard Tandem gamma counter. Specific activity was determined by weight (CPM/gram) and by surface area (CPM/mm^2). Permeability was corrected for weight (CPM/g) or for surface area (CPM/mm^2).

$$\text{Permeability Coefficient} = \frac{\text{specific activity of artery (CPM/g or CPM/mm}^2)}{\text{specific activity of perfusate (CPM/ml x 15 minute)}}$$

For statistical analysis, paired t test and χ^2 were calculated (36).

RESULTS

I. Studies on the Cerebral Microcirculation

Table I describes the average results obtained during the withdrawal of arterial blood and during reinfusion. It can be seen that in all experiments, totalling 153 individual observations, mean blood pressure and red cell velocity declined significantly during blood withdrawal, while changes in vascular diameter were not significant. These alterations were noticed in capillaries, arterioles and venules alike. During reinfusion of blood, mean blood pressure rose significantly above its control value. In many vessels, red cell velocity also demonstrated an overshoot, indicating reactive hyperemia (Table I).

Table I illustrates the changes induced by 5-HT in 79 observations. The changes in mean blood pressure were not significant, and the range of change was less; in many experiments a biphasic response to 5-HT was noticed with an initial slight decline in mean blood pressure. Red cell velocity fell significantly in all vessels, often remaining below control values at the termination of the experiment. Changes in vascular diameter were statistically not significant, except in the case of arterioles in which the increase was significant.

Topical application of 5-HT (10^{-4}M) causes an average fall in RCV of: capillaries 1338 µm/sec; arterioles 3405 µm/sec; vessels 1170 µm/sec. Average changes in vascular diameter were: capillaries

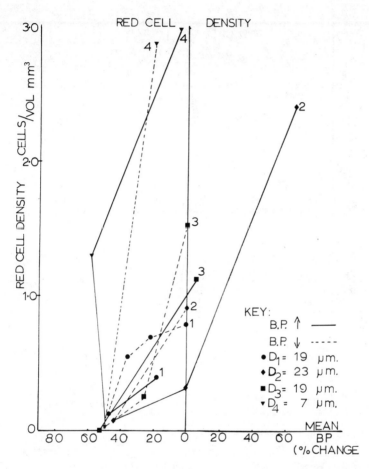

Figure 5.   Percent change in blood pressure is plotted against red
cell density in microcirculatory vessels during with-
drawls of arterial blood. As blood pressure falls, red
cell density in these vessels becomes zero (4 out of
19 observations).

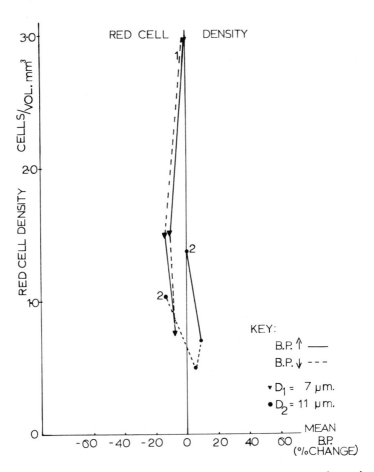

Figure 6.   Percent change in blood pressure is plotted against red
cell density during intracarotid injection of 5-HT.
Red cell density becomes zero (2 out of 22 observations
only).

TABLE I

Statistical Analysis (232 Observations) Control and Macimal Change
Arterial Blood Withdrawl, Reinfusion of 5-HT

EXP.	MEAN BLOOD PRESSURE mm Hg	CAPILLARIES		VENULES		ARTERIOLES	
		R.C.V. µm/sec.	DIAM. µm	R.C.V. µm/sec.	DIAM. µm	R.C.V. µm/sec.	DIAM. µm
ART. BLOOD WITHDRAWAL	p<0.001 *	p<0.01 *	n.s. p>0.05 *	p<0.01 *	n.s. p>0.05 *	p<0.01 *	n.s. p>0.05 *
MEAN MAXIMUM CHANGE FROM CONTROL	(-54.9)	(-1902.9)	(+1.125)	(-1692.4)	(+3.0)	(-3281.6)	(+1.8)
ART. BLOOD REINFUSION	p<0.01 *	p<0.01 *	n.s. p>0.4 *	p<0.01 *	n.s. p>0.05 *	p<0.05 *	n.s. p>0.5 *
MEAN MAXIMUM CHANGE FROM CONTROL	(+28.5)	(+613)	(-0.375)	(+3665)	(-2.2)	(+765)	(-0.4)
EFFECT OF 5-HT	n.s. p>0.05 *	p<0.001 *	n.s. p>0.2 *	p<0.001 *	n.s. p>0.05 *	p<0.02 *	p<0.05 *
MEAN MAXIMUM CHANGE FROM CONTROL	(-8.5)	(-998.0)	(+0.5)	(-684.5)	(0.3)	(-1116.0)	(+4.0)

* AS COMPARED TO CONTROL

1.7 µm; arterioles 4 µm; and vessels 2.8µm.

Clumping of red cells in all vessels was a common occurrence, especially following the injection of 5-HT. Another finding was the disappearance of red cells. This occurred more frequently during removal of arterial blood than following 5-HT injection.

II. Studies on Vascular Permeability

Fig. 7 shows per cent change in the permeability coefficient of RISA in 12 perfused isolated rabbit arteries. With slight rise in the difference (ΔP) between control and maximal rise in perfusion of pressure (from 0 to 20 mm Hg) permeability coefficient markedly decreased. However, with large ΔP (from 40 to 100 mm Hg) the permeability increased. Values calculated for wet weight did not differ essentially from those obtained for surface area.

DISCUSSION

I. Studies on the Cortical Microcirculation

One of the main goals of this investigation is the analysis of the response of the cortical microcirculation of the cat in vivo to a vasoactive drug, 5-Hydroxytryptamine (5-HT) and a comparison with the changes resulting from alterations in systemic blood pressure induced by withdrawal of arterial blood. Such a comparison is helpful in studying the behavior of the microcirculation with respect to autoregulation, local vasomotion and to development of unperfused or underperfused vascular channels.

Several marked differences are noted between 5-HT and arterial blood withdrawal (Table I). For example, the change in systemic blood pressure after 5-HT injection is not significant and the mean difference between control value and the maximal change in red cell velocity (RCV) is considerably less for 5-HT as compared to blood withdrawal (Table I). Despite relative constancy of arterial pressure, however, changes induced by 5-HT in red cell velocity and maximal changes from the mean are highly significant (Table I). In contrast following arterial blood withdrawal, both blood pressure and RCV decline significantly.

Topical application of 5-HT causes general marked constriction and a reduction in RCV in all cortical microcirculatory vessels visualized. It is known that agents which when topically applied to the cerebral surface cause marked vasoconstriction, but have only slight effects on cerebral vessels when injected into the systemic circulation (13,32). The difference may well be due to the blood brain barrier. A distinction therefore, has to be made between reports in the literature describing the effects of topically applied 5-HT from our data in which the drug was injected directly into the carotid

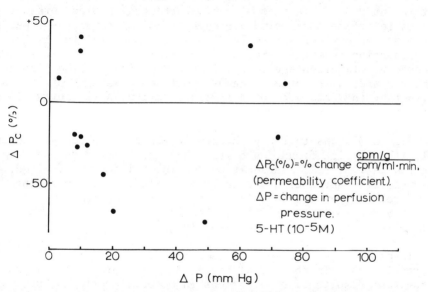

Figure 7.   Describes the relationship between percentile change in
perfusion pressure versus percentile changes in permeability. The curve, constructed according to the best
fit, is either quadratic or cubic.

artery. Edvinsson and Burrows (5, 11) have shown that the response
of topically applied 5-HT is variable as vessel size increases. Ves
sels of over 200 μm always respond to constriction while vessels le
than 70 μm consistently dilate. Topically applied, therefore, the
effect of 5-HT depends on the initial vascular tone (11). The tone
may be affected by such diverse factors as blood pressure, blood ga
or vasomotor tone (5). It is also to be recalled that Edvinsson st
ied pial vessels while we observed cortical vessels (11).

Figures 1 and 2 further show the difference between intraarter
injection of 5-HT and arterial blood withdrawal. Figure 1 shows go
linear correlation between percentile changes in mean blood pressur
and red cell velocity (correlation coefficient 0.829). With 5-HT o
the other hand (Fig. 2) a lack of correlation is evident (correlati
coefficient 0.37). Thus despite minor changes in blood pressure,
changes in red cell velocity are marked. A Chi-square test was per
formed on the data presented in Figure 2. Essential to this test i
the assumption that the percentage change in red cell velocity is
independent of percentage change in blood pressure. The informatio
indicates that with better than 99% confidence we may reject the hy
thesis that the data are not normally distributed (χ^2 for 99.5% con
fidence is 11.84; experimental is 8.14).

Figure 3 shows that the changes in red cell velocity induced b
5-HT although significant, are less than those noted during blood
withdrawal (Table I). In addition, during reinfusion of blood, red
cell velocity increases above control levels in all experiments, de
noting reactive hyperemia. As a result, the mean red cell velocity
after blood withdrawal shifts to the right while with 5-HT mean red
cell velocity is skewed to the left (Fig. 4).

Several of these observations are difficult to reconcile with
autoregulation. In the normal brain, cerebral blood flow is mainta
ed constant despite wide variations in cerebral perfusion pressure.
This mechanism is the result of an active vascular response; arter
iolar constriction results from increase in perfusion pressure and
arteriolar dilation from a pressure decrease (23). Table I indicat
that a fall in blood pressure resulting from withdrawal of blood,
causes no significant change in arteriolar diameter of cerebral cor
cal vessels. The finding that percentage changes in blood pressure
correlate well over a wide range with those in red cell velocity
(Fig. 1), further argue against autoregulation.

Autoregulation has been previously demonstrated only when tota
cerebral blood flow was correlated with changes in systemic blood
pressure (21, 23). Autoregulation in normotensive man is present
between pressures of from a mean of 60 to a mean of 130 mm Hg (23),
It is due to an inherent intrinsic feature of many organs (12), and
results from independent response of the vascular bed probably reg
ulated by myogenic responses (12,2).

Using 85 Kr clearance techniques, Harper (19) found no significant difference in flow among the frontal and the parieteal cortex.
It is known, however, that the flow rate in the white matter of the
dog is higher than the gray (18, 33). Failure to detect autoregulation in our preparation may be due to several causes. In the first
place, the region under observation may differ substantially from
other cerebral areas, where maintenance of flow is a more important
safeguard. It is also conceivable that all the seemingly irregular
and different quantums of capillary red cell velocities may, when
total cerebral blood flow is measured, appear as a homogenous system
possessing amongst others the property of autoregulation. Other
factors which must be considered are injury to the tissue by the
technique employed and the effect of anesthesia. The former has been
ruled out in extensive studies by Pawlik et al (29). It is also unlikely that anesthesia is responsible. Although cerebral blood flow
may be reduced in proportion to the depth of barbiturate anesthesia
(27,30,33,39), Ketamine used conjointly increases cerebral blood flow
while Atropin has little effect (17)

The fact remains that for whatever reason with the techniques
employed here, autoregulation of the microcirculation in the cerebral
cortex cannot be demonstrated. Related to this finding is the fact
that red cell velocity differs in different vessels of the microcirculation in a single frame, even at the same mean blood pressure.
This is the case during and after arterial blood withdrawal as well
as after the injection of 5-HT (Table I).

In several instances disappearance of red cells in capillaries,
arterioles and venules can be observed, resulting in unperfused channels (Figures 5 and 6). Figures 5 and 6 relate the percentile changes
in systemic blood pressure to density of red cells (number of cells/
unit volume) in these vessels. In 4 out of 19 observations, a fall in
blood pressure is accompanied by a lack of red cells. This occurs
less frequently during the injection of 5-HT (2 out of 22 observations). Pawlik et al (29) mentioned irregular flow pattern occurring
without changes in blood pressure. However, these oscillations lasted
only for a few milliseconds. Cobb in 1938 was impressed by the variety of stimuli that could increase the number of open pial capillaries (9). In our experiments, non-perfused vessels were visualized
for several minutes. Our observation must also be distinguished from
the intermittent, stochastic or spurt flow (29, 32) which has been
ascribed to topographical factors, thus altering fluid mechanics (16).
The appearance of non-perfused channels is probably the result of
alterations in metabolic demands of cortical tissue, induced by
changes in systemic blood pressure. The dependency of regional cerebral flow on regional metabolic activity has been demonstrated in man
by Reivich (31). It appears also that local cerebral glucose utilization is related to physiological function and therefore to regional
cerebral blood flow (37).

II. Studies on Perfused Arteries

The results illustrated in Figure 7 show parabolic response of permeability in the femoral artery to 5-HT. The results calculated for wet weight did not differ essentially from those obtained for surface area. With a slight increase in ΔP (the difference in pressure between control pressure and its maximal rise) vascular permeability index diminishes, but with large changes in ΔP the permeability index increases again, (Fig. 7). Caro and co-workers (6) have established that transport of labelled albumin across the arterial wall is a steady state process, with the arterial media providing a relatively high diffusional resistance. Previously Duncan et al have shown that elevation in blood pressure markedly increases vascular permeability (10). Bratzler (4) found that albumin mass transfer resistance in the intimal endothelium of the rabbit aorta was one order of magnitude greater than that associated with the media. It is therefore evident that damage to the endothelium alters the result obtained. Using the method of Schwartz (34) to study endothelial structure by histological means, intact endothelium was found by the EM and light microscopy. It also has been discovered that static pressure elevates protein flux via associated wall stretch (1,7,15) Majno and co-workers (24) found that 5-HT as well as histamine always causes vascular leakage on the venous side of the circulation between endothelial cells which become disconnected while the basement membrane remains intact and filters the plasma which escapes through the openings.

The work of Bratzler and of Majno and co-workers and of Sifling (4,24,35), indicates that the blood wall interface, specifically the endothelium is responsible for uptake of macromolecules by the arterial wall. It is possible that this occurs through endothelial inter cell clefts or through pinocytosis (14, 38). Bratzler concluded that the resistance residing in the intimal endothelium is presumably caused by a low diffusive permeability to macromolecules (4). Although the exact mechanism of the uptake of this material by the endothelium is not yet clear, it is possible that our findings reported in Fig. 7 are due to combined action of 5-HT and intravascular pressure. The downward portion of the parabola in Fig. 7 is due to the action of 5-HT, while the upward portion of the curve results from increases in perfusion pressure. Whether 5-HT diminishes the diameter of inter-cell clefts, or inhibits pinocytosis, or in some other way hinders uptake of macromolecules is not yet clear. These factors are important in the light of data published by Marzilli et al (25) who believe that vascular spasm can be an antecedent leading to the later development of atherosclerotic changes. The hypothesis is based on clinical observation on human coronary arteries in situ, while our studies are restricted to rabbit femoral arteries perfused in vitro.

REFERENCES

1. BATTEN, R. J. & NEWMAN, D.L. Influence of static and oscillatory
    pressure/strain on I^{131} albumin uptake by the wall of the isolated
    pig moracic aorta. Cardiovascular Research 14, 590-600 (1980).
2. BAYLISS, W. M. On the local actions of the arterial wall to
    changes of internal pressure. Journal of Physiology 28, 220-231
    (1902).
3. BOHR, D. F. Vascular smooth muscle: Dual effect of calcium.
    Science 139, 597-599 (1963).
4. BRATZLER, R. L., CHISOLM, G. M., COTTON, C. K., SMITH, K. A.,
    ZILVERSMITH, D. B. & LEES, R. S. The distribution of labeled
    albumin across the rabbit thoracic aorta in vivo. Circulation
    Research 40, 182-190 (1877).
5. BURROWS , M. E. & VANHOUTTE, P. Pharmacology of arterioles:
    Some aspects of variability in response to norepinephrine, hist-
    amine and 5-hydroxytryptamine. Journal of Cardiovascular Pharm-
    acology 3, 1370-1380 (1980).
6. CARO, C. G., LEVER, M. J., LAVER-RUDICH, Z., MEYER, F., LIRON, M.,
    EBEL, W., PARKER, K. H. & WINLOVE, C. P. Net albumin transport
    across the wall of the rabbit common carotid artery perfused in
    situ. Atherosclerosis 37, 497-511 (1980).
7. CARO, C. G., FITZGERALD, J. M. & SCHROTER, R. C. Arterial wall
    shear and distribution of early atheroma in man. Nature 223, 1159-
    1161 (1969).
8. CHANG, B. L., YAMAKAWA, T., NUCCIO, J., PACE, R. & BING, R. J.
    Microcirculation of left atrial muscle cerebral cortex and mes-
    entery of the cat: A comparative analysis. Circulation Research
    50, 240-249 (1982).
9. COBB, S. Cerebral circulation: A critical discussion of the sym-
    posium. Proceedings of the Association of Research in Nervous
    and Mental Diseases 18, 719-720 (1938).
10. DUNCAN, L. E. JR., CORNFIELD, J. & BUCK, K. The effect of blood
    pressure on the passage of labeled plasma albumin into canine
    aorta wall. Journal of Clinical Investigation 41, 1537-1545
    (1962).
11. EDVINSSON, L., HARDEBO, J. E., MACKENZIE, E. T. & STEWART, M.
    Dual action of serotonin on pial arterioles in situ and the
    effect of propranolol on the response. Blood Vessels 14, 366-
    371 (1977).
12. EDVINSSON, L. & MACKENZIE, E. T. Amine mechanisms in the cerebral
    circulation. Pharmacological Reviews 28, 275-348 (1977).
13. FLOREY, J. Microscopical observations on the circulation of the
    blood in the cerebral cortex. Brain 48, 43-64 (1925).
14. FLOREY, LORD & SHEPPARD, B. L. The permeability of arterial
    endothelium to horseradish peroxidase. Proceedings of the Royal
    Society of London, Series B, 174 435-443 (1970).

15. FRY, D. L. Responses of the arterial wall to certain physical factors. Atherosclerosis: Initiating Factors. Ciba Foundation Symposium 12, 93-125. Amsterdam, Associated Scientific Publishers (1973).

16. FUNG, Y. C. Stochastic flow in capillary blood vessels, Microvascular Research 5, 34-48 (1973).

17. GILMAN, A. G., GOODMAN, L. S., GILMAN, A. (Eds.) The Pharmacological Basis of Therapeutics, ed. 6. New York, Macmillan Publishing Co. (1980).

18. HAGGERDAL, E., MILSSON, N. J. & MORBACK, B. Effect of blood corpuscle concentration on cerebral blood flow. Acta Chirurgica Scandinavica - supplements 364, 13-21 (1966).

19. HARPER, A. M., GLASS, H. I. & GLOVER, M. M. Measurement of blood flow in the cerebral cortex of dogs by the clearance of 85 Kr. Scottish Medical Journal 6, 12-17 (1961).

20. HELLBERG, K., WAYLAND, H., RICKART, A. & BING, R. J. Studies on the coronary microcirculation by direct visualization. American Journal of Cardiology 19, 593-597 (1972).

21. HERNANDEZ, M. J. BRENNAN, R. W. & BOWMAN, G. S. Cerebral blood flow autoregulation in the rat. Stroke 9, 150-155 (1978).

22. KAPP, J. P., MAHALEY, M. S. JR. & ODOM G. I. Cerebral arterial spasm, Part 2. Experimental evaluation of mechanical and humoral factors in pathogenesis. Journal of Neurosurgery 29, 339-341 (1968).

23. LASSEN, M. A. & CHRISTENSEN, M. S. Physiology of cerebral blood flow. British Journal of Anesthesia 48, 719-734 (1976).

24. MAJNO, G., PALADE, G. E. & SCHOEFL, G. I. The site of action of histamine and serotonin along the vascular tree: A topographic study. The Journal of Biophysical and Biochemical Cytology 11, 607-626 (1961).

25. MARZILLI, M., GOLDSTEIN, S., TRIVELLA, M. A., PALUMBO, C. & MASERI, A. Some clinical considerations regarding the relation of coronary vasospasm to coronary atherosclerosis: A hypothetical pathogenesis. American Journal of Cardiology 45, 882-886 (1980).

26. MASERI, A. Pathogenic mechanism of angina pectons: expanding view. British Heart Journal 40, 648-660 (1980).

27. MCDOWALL, D. G. The effects of general anaesthetics on cerebral blood flow and cerebral metabolism. British Journal of Anaesthesiology 37, 236-245 (1965).

28. NOEL, M., SOKOL, M. D., DAVIES, L. R. & HENRIQUEZ, E. Vascular spasm in cat cerebral cortex following ischemia. Stroke 9, 52-57 (1978).

29. PAWLIK, G., RACKL, A. & BING, R. J. Quantitative capillary topography and blood flow in the cerebral cortex of cats: An in vivo microscopic study. Brain Research 208, 35-58 (1981).

30. PIERCE, E. C., LANEITSEN, C. J., DEUTSCH, S., CHASE, P. E., LIN, H. W., DRIPPS, R. D. & PIERCE, H. L. Cerebral circulation and metabolism during thiopental anaesthetic and hyperventilation i man. Journal of Clinical Investigation 41, 1664-1671 (1962).

31. REIVICH, M.   Blood flow metabolism couple vs. brain, Plum, F.
    (Ed.) Brain disfunction in metabolic disorders. Research Put-
    lication, Association of Nervous and Mental Diseases 53, 125-140
    (1974).
32. ROSENBLUM, W. I. & ZWEIFACH, B. W.   Cerebral microcirculation in
    the mouse brain. Archives of Neurology (Chicago) 9, 102-111
    (1963).
33. ROTH, J. A., GREENFIELD, A. J., KAIHARA, S. & WAGNER, H. N. JR.,
    Total and regional cerebral blood flow in unanesthetized dogs.
    American Journal of Physiology 219, 96-101 (1970).
34. SCHWARTZ, S. M. & BENDITT, E. P.   Structure and permeability of
    rat thoracic aortic intima. American Journal of Pathology 66,
    241-264 (1972).
35. SIFLINGER, A. PARKER, K. & CARO, C. G.   Uptake of ^{125}I albumin by
    the endothelial surface of the isolated dog common coratid artery:
    effect of certain physical factors and metabolic inhibitors.
    Cardiovascular Research 9, 478-489 (1975).
36. SNEDECOR, G.   Statistical Methods, 4th edition. Ames, Iowa,
    Iowa State College Press (1946).
37. SOKOLOFF, L.   Relation between physiological function and energy
    metabolism in the central nervous system. Journal of Neurochem-
    istry 29, 13-26 (1977).
38. STEIN, Y. & STEIN, O.   An electron microscopic study of the trans-
    port of peroxidases in the endothelium of mouse aorta. Zeitsch-
    rift fur Zellforschung und Mickroskopische Anatomie 133, 211-222
    (1972).
39. WOLLMAN, H., ALEXANDER, C., COHEN, P. J., SMITH, T. C., CHASE,
    P. E. & VAN DER MOTEN, R.   Cerebral circulation during general
    anesthesia and hyperventilation in man. Anesthesiology 26, 329-
    334 (1965).

LIPID PEROXIDATION AND ACUTE MYOCARDIAL ISCHEMIA

Parinam S. Rao and Hiltrud S. Mueller

Department of Medicine, Montefiore Hospital and Albert
Einstein College of Medicine, Bronx, New York   10467 USA

Lipid peroxides (LP) and free radicals (FR) have recently been identified by us as metabolic intermediates during acute myocardial ischemia. The mechanism of lipid peroxidation is not clearly understood. We hypothesize: 1) FR production increases during ischemia
due to alteration in the redox state of the mitochondria and due to
interaction between metabolites and O_2; 2) FR foster increased formation of LP with a concomitant decrease in protective antioxidants
such as glutathione peroxidase (GP) and ascorbic acid (ASC). To
test this hypothesis, we first studied animal models, rat and dog.
In the rat, 48 hrs post coronary occlusion (CO), the lipid peroxide
content in the infarcted left ventricular tissue (LV) measured as
its product malondialdehyde (MDA) increased from 0.31 to 0.58 nm/
mg P (p<.001), an increase of 87% while GP decreased from 62 to 21
nm/min/mg P (p<.001). Superoxide dismutase contents decreased from
81 to 63 µg/g (p<.001). The polyunsaturated fatty acid (PUFA) contents diminished significantly (arachidonic acid from 19 to 16%,
p<.001). In the dog, sequential transcardiac changes in blood showed very early increase of both FR as studied by electron spin resonance spectrometry in lyophilized samples and catecholamines (norepinephrine, NE, and epinephrine, E). The FR contents increased
from 3.3 to 5.6 nm/ml in coronary sinus blood (CS) at its peak
level (10 min) and remained elevated thereafter. Forty-five min
p̄ CO, the FR contents in the ischemic LV tissue increased from 9.3
to 12.8 nm/g, NE and E increased from 4.2 to 3.0 to 5.6 and 5.5 ng/g.
ASC fell from 1.03 to 0.85 nm/g (p<.01). On the other hand, MDA
increased from 0.94 to 1.27 nm/mg P (p<.001) and GP decreased from
19.7 to 14.7 nm/min/mg P (p<.01). We have tentatively identified
the FR produced as semidehydroascorbate and protein radical. They
are obtained by interaction of ascorbic acid with free radicals
like ubisemiquinone, superoxide and catecholamines and with Cu-

347

proteins like ceruloplasmin. In order to relate the above changes in FR and LP and their release into CS blood in humans, we studied 10 patients with acute myocardial infarction (MI) within 5 hrs after onset of pain and 10 patients with normal coronary arteries. In patients with MI, the arterial FR content averaged 18 nm/ml and CS 22 nm/ml (p<.01). In all patients, the CS FR content is higher than the arterial content suggesting increased production of FR by the myocardium. Lipid peroxide contents (MDA) averaged 2.8 nm/ml in both arterial and CS blood in normal patients. On the other hand, in patients with MI, the A averaged 4.5 and CS 8.07 nm/ml (p<.001) indicating enhanced lipid peroxidation across the myocardium. In conclusion: 1) FR are produced during MI and appear in CS blood; 2) LP is enhanced during MI as indicated by increase in MDA, and 3) increases in production of FR and catecholamines occurs first, followed by decrease in ascorbic acid. These changes possibly trigger secondary events such as lipid peroxidation and depletion of protective enzymes.

Key Words: Free radicals; Superoxide; Lipid peroxide; Myocardial ischemia; Myocardial infarction; Glutathione peroxidase.

INTRODUCTION

Free radicals have recently gained increasing interest as metabolic intermediates in acute myocardial ischemia. Yamamoto[1] observed during exercise an increase in plasma free radical contents in patients with coronary insufficiency in contrast to a decrease in normal volunteers. Akiyama[2] demonstrated an increase of free radical contents in coronary venous blood during experimental myocardial ischemia in dogs. Suzuki[3] showed an increase in mitochondrial free radical contents two hours after coronary ligation in an experimental dog model. The mechanisms by which evolving myocardial ischemia initiates free radical production are unclear. Based on studies in vitro, it is feasible to consider the following pathways contributing to free radical production in infarction of left ventricular tissue: (a) disturbance and dissociation of intramitochondrial electron transport system with release of ubisemiquinone, flavoprotein and superoxide free radicals; (b) accumulation and increased release of intracellular metabolites like NADH, lactates, flavoproteins, and catecholamines, which react between themselves and with oxygen; (c) acute inflammatory response with increased chemotactic activity of neutrophils; and, (d) interaction of the metabolic product hypoxanthine with O_2 in the presence of xanthine oxidase. An important question arises whether there is sufficient oxygen in ischemic tissue to support ongoing free radical reactions. Based on detailed radiobiological studies[4] the free radical reactions are shown to be enhanced even at very low O_2 tension. As shown in Figure 1, free radical production was increased by 83% at an O_2 tension of 6 mmHg and by 50% at an O_2 tension of 1 mmHg. Smith[5] demonstrate

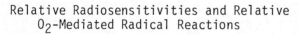

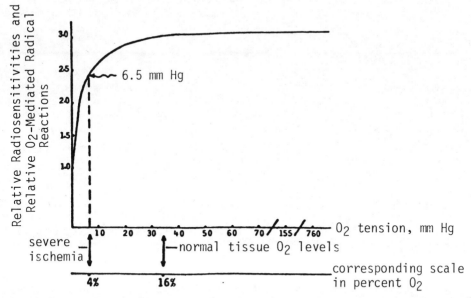

FIGURE 1.   Free radical production at low tissue O_2 contents (PO_2)[24]

that free radical peroxidation takes place quite rapidly in rat
brain homogenates incubated in gas mixtures that contained only 5%
O_2.

The free radicals thus produced initiate and enhance lipid peroxidation by attacking polyunsaturated membrane lipids (PUFA). PUFA
are thus selectively lost from membrane phospholipids during ischemia.
Lipid peroxides (LP) formed are toxic and the potential consequences
of FR membrane damage may result in adverse effects on key membrane
enzymes, loss of membrane fluidity and possible development of occlu-
sions in the microcirculation. Tappel[6] has shown extensive LP damage
to cell components in rat tissue. Myers[7] has demonstrated a significant role for LP in cardiac toxicity and tumor response. Wills[8] observed that LP inhibit the activity of certain enzymes predominantly
by oxidation of thiol groups. Lipid peroxides also impair circulation of blood and promote atherosclerosis and blood clot formation[9].

The present study was designed in the attempt to answer the
following questions: (1) Does production of free radicals increase
during myocardial ischemia and enhance formation of lipid peroxides?
(2) Does lipid peroxidation reach sufficient levels to reduce contents of antioxidant enzymes? and (3) Is there a time interval be-

tween production of free radicals and of lipid peroxides? Studies
were performed in experimental myocardial ischemia in the rat and
in dog. Subsequently, preliminary data were obtained during evolving myocardial infarction in man and compared to results obtained
in patients with normal coronary arteries and normal cardiac function.

METHODS AND MATERIALS

Animal Models

Rat: Twelve rats underwent ligation of the left coronary artery
2 mm from its origin; they were sacrificed 48 hrs after coronary
ligation. 500 mg of normal and infarcted left ventricular tissue
were removed immediately, frozen in liquid N_2 for analysis as described.

Dog: Ten mongrel dogs of both sexes, weighing between 15 and 20 kg,
were anesthetized with intravenous bolus injection of 10 mg/kg sodium
pentobarbital, intubated and connected to an animal respirator. Following left lateral thoracotomy, a 2.0 silk suture was placed around
the left descending coronary artery approximately 1 cm below the
first marginal branch for later ligation. Catheters were placed into the coronary sinus close to the great cardiac vein and into the
aorta. Arterial pressure and electrocardiogram were continuously
monitored. Blood samples from the aorta and the coronary sinus were
obtained according to protocol. Forty-five minutes after coronary
ligation the animals were sacrificed and tissue samples taken according to protocol.

Schedule of Blood Sampling. Before, immediately, and 30 minutes after opening of the chest; 1,3,5,10,15,30 and 45 minutes
p̄ coronary occlusion. 2 ml of blood were frozen immediately
in liquid N_2 for free radical determination; 5 ml of blood
were taken into a heparanized tube for measurements of MDA,
GP, ASC and H_2O_2.

Preparation of Tissue for Analysis. The animals were sacrificed with 5 ml of an euthanasia drug (T-61, Hoechst Health Division, NJ); tissue samples (2g) from the normal and ischemic
areas of the left ventricle were obtained immediately and frozen in liquid N_2: (i) 1 g of frozen tissue in liquid N_2 was
used for lyophilization (24 hours); 200 mg of lyophilized powder was homogenized in 5 ml $HClO_4$ (1 M) for tissue lactate
measurements; 50 mg for polyunsaturated fatty acids and the
rest for free radical measurements. (ii) 300 mg were homogenized in 5 ml $HClO_4$ (0.1 M) for tissue catecholamine measurements. (iii) 300 mg were homogenized in tris buffer (0.10 M)
containing EGTA (0.001 M), pH 7.4 for MDA, GP, H_2O_2 and protein determinations.

Human

Two groups of patients were studied: (1) ten patients with acute
myocardial infarction within 5 hrs of clinical onset. Age (47-69
yrs), sex (8M, 2F) and site of infarct (5 anterior, 5 inferior).
Patients received lidocaine (2 mg/min), nitroglycerin and morphine
as needed. (2) ten patients with normal coronary arteries and
normal cardiac function who underwent coronary arteriography because of atypical chest pains. Age (42-67 yrs), sex (5M, 5F).

Biochemical Assays

Free Radicals: 2 ml of blood frozen in liquid N_2 was smashed to a
pulp and lyophilized for 24 hrs. The lyophilized powder was packed
into 4 mm quartz tubes up to a height of 40 mm and stored at -20°C
until analysis. Electron spin resonance (ESR) signals were measured
with E109E varian ESR Spectrometer at rt°C, g = 2.005 (H = 3240 ±
400 gauss). The modulation amplitude was 2 gauss and the microwave
power 5 mw. Standard pitch and potassium superoxide were used to
identify the free radical and O_2 spectra. Hydroxyl radicals were
identified using the spin trap, 5,5-dimethyl-1 pyrroline-N-oxide
(DMPO). The O_2^- formed was distinguished from free radical (falvin
semiquinone, FADH) spectra by its shape and by warming the tube to
-40° where O_2^- disappears and then reappears on cooling to -168° .
Free radical intensities were calibrated using the spin label 4-hy-
droxy 2,2,6,6-tetramethylpiperidinoxy radical (H-TMPO). The relative spin concentrations were obtained by double integration of the
spectra by means of planimeter. The coefficient of variation
for duplicate assays was 3.5% (n = 13).

Malondialydehyde and Hydrogen Peroxide: Malondialdehyde was
assayed by the method of Satoh[10]. The coefficient of variation for
duplicate determinations averaged 1.4% (n = 10). H_2O_2 was assayed
by the method of Hildebrandt et al[11]. The reproducibility of assay
for duplicates was 1.3% (n = 13).

Glutathione peroxidase: Glutathione peroxidase (GP) was determined
according to the method of Rotruck[12]. The mean coefficient of variation for duplicates using this method was 3.34% (n = 13).

Superoxide dismutase: Superoxide dismutase was determined in tissue
homogenates by the method of Elstner et al[13].

Ascorbic acid: The plasma and tissue homogenates were analyzed by
the method of day et al[14], based on the reduction of ferric chloride
by ascorbic acid with the resulting ferrous ion quantitated by 2,4,
6-tripyridyl-S-triazine to form a purple color (595 nm).

Oxidation-reduction (Red-ox) capacity of blood: Total red-ox capacity of blood was measured using nitroblue tetrazolium (NBT) as indicator and capacity for superoxide radical (O_2^-) formation using
superoxide dismutase (SOD) as scavenger along with NBT. Total
sulfhydryl (T-SH) contents of plasma were determined by the method
of Sedlock-Lindsay[15].

Polyunsaturated fatty acids: Linoleic, arachidonic, eicosapentaenoic
and decosahexaenoic acids in phospholipids were measured by the extraction procedure of Crossman et al[16] and analyzed by Jordi's[17] high
pressure liquid chromatography method. The coefficient of variation
for duplicate assays was 5.8% (n = 10).

Catecholamines: Norepinephrine (NE) and epinephrine (E) concentrations in tissue and plasma were measured by high pressure liquid
chromatography using LC-4 electrochemical detection. Three ml of
blood were drawn into tubes kept in ice containing 50 μl Na meta-
bisulfite (2 M) and 750 μl EDTA (1%). The tubes were centrifuged
immediately; to 1 ml of plasma, 400 μl $HClO_4$ (4 M) was added to
precipitate protein and centrifuged. The catecholamines were eluted
from the plasma into alumina at pH 8.6. The alumina was washed three
times with water, dried by suction and the catecholamines were eluted
into 100 μl $HClO_4$ (0.5 M) using micro filters. Twenty μl were then
injected into a Waters 6000 A high pressure liquid chromatograph,
the individual catecholamines separated with a μ-Bondapak C_{18} column
and detected by LC-4 Electrochemical detector (Bioanalytical Systems,
West Lafayette, Indiana). Standards containing 200 pg/ml of NE and
E were run along each batch of samples. In our laboratory, plasma
catecholamines of 13 normal volunteers (after 20 min rest in supine
position) averaged NE 168 ± 41 (SD) pg/ml; and E 47 ± 17. The coefficient of variation for duplicates was (n = 13) 2.1% NE and 4.5% E

RESULTS

Rat: a) Lipid Peroxide Production: Forty-eight hrs p̄ coronary
occlusion, left ventricular (LV) tissue lipid peroxide contents, as
measured by its product malondialydehyde, had increased in the infarcted LV from 0.31 nm/mg P to 0.58 (p<.001) (Figure 2), an increase of 87%. The non-specific end product H_2O_2 had increased from
54 to 63 μm/g wet weight (p<.01). On the other hand, the antioxidant enzymes, superoxide dismutase (SOD, O_2^- scavenger) and glutathione peroxidase (GP, lipid peroxide scavenger) were reduced. SOD
decreased from 81 to 63 μg/g (p<.001), while GP contents diminished
from 62 to 21 nm/min/mg p (p<.001) (Figure 2). The reducing capacity of the infarcted LV tissue, as measured by its total sulfhydryl
contents had also decreased from 15 to 7.8 μm/g (p<.001).

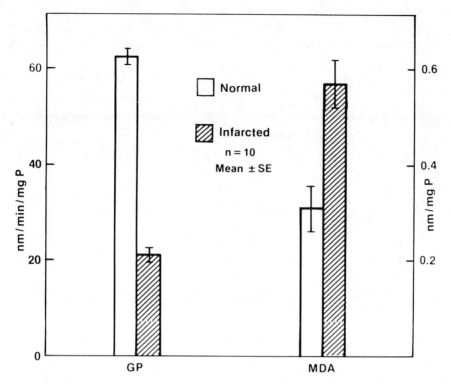

FIGURE 2.   Glutathione peroxidase and malondialdehyde contents in
rat myocardium.

b)   PUFA Reduction: The PUFA contents in normal and infarcted LV
were measured to evaluate if lipid peroxidation was associated with
lipid loss.   Results are shown in Figure 3.   In the normal myocardium, linoleic acid averaged 20% of total PUFA; arachidonic acid
(AA) 19%, eicosapentaenoic acid (EPA) 1% and decosahexaenoic acid
(DCH) 13%.   In the infarcted LV tissue, the mean % of linoleic acid
increased from 20 to 25% (p<.001), probably due to blockage of the
desaturation step to AA.   The remaining PUFA's decreased, AA from
19 to 16% (p<.001), EPA from 1.0 to 0.69% (p<.02) and DCH from 13
to 8% (p<.001).

Dog: FR Production: Results are shown in Table I.   Forty-five min
p̄ coronary occlusion, FR contents in LV ischemic tissue increased
from 9.3 to 12.8 μm/g (p<.01), NE and E increased from 4.2 and 3.0
ng/g to 5.6 and 5.5 ng/g (p<.001) respectively.   Ascorbic acid fell
from 1.03 to 0.85 μm/g (p<.01) MDA increased from 0.94 to 1.27 nm/
mg (p<.001).   GP decreased from 19.7 to 14.7 nm/min/mg P (p<.01).

FR were released into coronary sinus blood within minutes after
coronary ligation and reached peak levels within 10 min.   FR contents

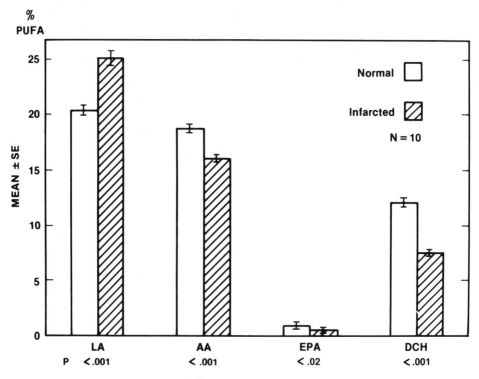

FIGURE 3.   Polyunsaturated fatty acid contents in rat myocardium.

TABLE I.   Free radical, catecholamine, lipid peroxide and anti-oxidant contents in left ventricular tissue.

Mean (n = 10)	FR nm/g	NE ng/g	E ng/g	ASA nm/g	MDA nm/mgP	GP nm/min/mgP
Normal	9.3	3.0	4.2	1.03	0.94	19.7
45 min p̄ occlusion	12.8	5.5	5.6	0.83	1.27	14.7
p	<.01	<.001	<.001	<.01	<.001	<.01

of CS blood increased from 3.3 to 5.6 nm/ml, 10 min after ligation and remained elevated thereafter. At 45 min p̄ CO, before sacrifice of the dog, the level was 5.3 ± 1.3 nm/ml. Preliminary data also showed increase of E (3x) and NE (2x) contents in CS blood which peaked within 5 min.

Human: a) FR and LP Production: In patients with normal coronary arteries, both arterial and coronary sinus contents of FR were simi-lar, averaging 4.98 and 5.05 nm/ml respectively (Figure 4). On the other hand, in patients with myocardial infarction, the FR contents in the coronary sinus were higher than in arterial blood averaging 22 and 18 nm/ml (p<.01). This increase in CS FR contents is sugges-tive for production of FR by the myocardium. The plasma lipid per-oxide (MDA) contents averaged the same in patients with normal

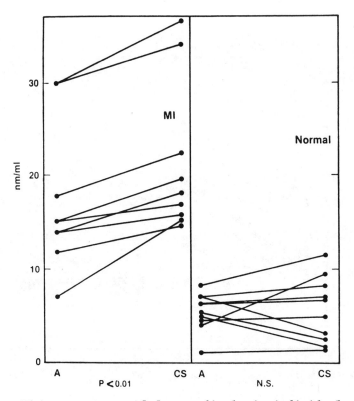

FIGURE 4. Plasma contents of free radicals in individual patients.

coronary arteries, 2.8 nm/ml (Figure 5) while in patients with MI,
the A averaged 4.49 and CS 8.07 nm/ml (p<.001). This increased MDA
production across the myocardium is indicative of enhanced lipid
peroxidation. H_2O_2 also increased from 21 to 26 nm/ml (p<.05) in
MI patients.

b) <u>Systemic and Myocardial Oxidation-Reduction (Red-ox) Processes</u>:
Results are shown in Table II. (1) the total reducing capacity of
arterial blood in patients with normal coronary arteries averaged
284 nm/ml and in CS blood 434 nm/ml (p<.001). In patients with MI,
the increase was less, mean values in A and CS blood were 277 and
347 nm/ml (p<.001) respectively. (2) the total sulfhydryl contents
in normal volunteers averaged the same, 480 (Arterial) and 460 (CS)
nm/ml while in MI patients their mean values fell in both A and CS
blood to 340 and 330 nm/ml respectively. (3) the capacity for superoxide formation in MI patients increased in both A (130 to 165 nm/ml

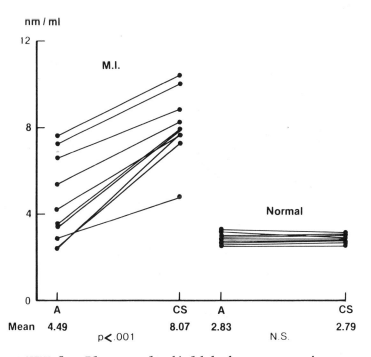

FIGURE 5. Plasma malondialdehyde contents in man.

TABLE II: Total reducing capacity, (TRC by NBT reduction), total sulfhydryl contents (T-SH) in plasma and capacity of superoxide formation (C-O$_2^-$) of blood across the myocardium during myocardial infarction.

nm/ml	TRC			T-SH		C-O$_2^-$		
	A	CS	(A-CS)	A	CS	A	CS	(A-CS)
(n = 10)								
Normal	284*	434	-141	480	460	130*	33	83
MI	277*	347	- 70	340	330	165*	65	100

p<.001*, P<.02°
A, Arterial; CS, Coronary Sinus

and CS (33 to 65 nm/ml, p<.001) blood compared to normal volunteers. Thus, during myocardial infarction, the Red-ox capacity of blood is diminished in general (total sulfhydryl) and across the heart (total reducing capacity). Conversely, capacity of O$_2^-$ formation is increased in general and in coronary sinus blood. These results suggest shifts in Red-ox systems leading to increased formation of toxic metabolites.

DISCUSSION

The data suggests that free radicals are produced and released early from the ischemic myocardium and initiate lipid-free radical reactions over a period of time. The early and concurrent increase of 1-norepinephrine and free radicals suggests that the two might be related.

1) Identity of Free Radicals

In order to elucidate the mechanism of lipid-free radical reactions further, it is very important to identify the free radicals produced after lyophilization. We observed that the two electron spin resonance (ESR) peaks (Figure 6) located at and near g = 2.005 do not belong to the same species since the peak at g = 2.005 saturates faster and is strongly influenced by O$_2$. We have tentatively identified them as semidehydroascorbate (SDA) radical (1) and a protein

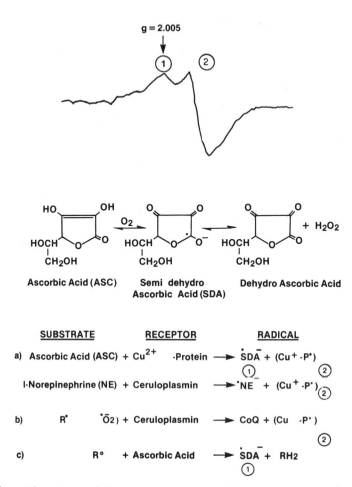

FIGURE 6. Identity of free radicals by ESR spectrometry (top) and the mechanism of production of free radicals (bottom).

radical (2) from our experiments where several oxidizing-reducing agents were added to plasma. Only ascorbic acid showed an increase in ESR peak at g = 2.005. The other ESR peak observed at a slightly higher field is identified as the well established protein radical[18]. During the interaction between ascorbic acid and Cu-proteins the protein moity may be reduced to a paramagnetic species while ascorbic acid is oxidized to a SDA radical. This reaction is catalyzed by Cu^{2+} in the protein. The production and stability of the two radical species depends on O_2 and is favored under anaerobic conditions. Normally, SDA radical appears as a doublet instead of the observed singlet. This is probably due to change in relaxation time caused by the interaction between ascorbic acid and its receptors (Cu containing proteins namely ceruloplasmin, cytochrome-C oxidase and others). Lohman et al[18] have established the identity of SDA and protein radicals in leukemic blood and have shown them to be distinct and separate from lipid, lipid peroxy, superoxide, Fe^{2+} chelated cytochromes, myoglobins, nonheme iron, amino acid and nucleic acid free radicals. Ascorbic acid is very unstable with a moderately high redox potential ($E°^1 = +.05$) and SDA radical can be readily formed both enzymatically and nonenzymatically and by interaction with all other free radicals such as semiquinones, superoxide, and lipid peroxy produced in tissue/blood due to their lower redox potentials. Another source of SDA radical may be catecholamines which serve as substrates for ceruloplasmin[19] producing catecholamine radical which, in the presence of ascorbate, produces SDA radical. Thus, SDA radical can serve as a marker for all free radical reactions.

2) Limitation of Methods for Free Radical Determination

One should be careful in interpreting the free radical data obtained especially after lyophilization. Our initial experiments using known FR scavengers such as tetranitromethane, nitroblue tetrazolium and superoxide dismutase for direct assay of free radicals in tissue blood yielded small and unreliable data. Recently developed techniques like FR spin traps using 5,5-dimethyl-1 pyrroline-N-oxide (DMPO)[20] and 4-hyodroxy-N-acetylamino flourene[21] are unsuccessful in our hands when applied to blood and tissue. Freshly frozen tissue/blood sample in liquid N_2, on the other hand, yielded a weak but distinct ESR signal at g = 2.005 and at the limit of sensitivity of the instrument (gain 10 x 10^4). However, after lyophilization for 24 hrs, the same ESR signal increased twenty fold. This suggests: 1) increased reactivity among metabolic intermediates resulting in increased FR formation; and/or 2) possible enrichment of FR concentration during lyophilization enhancing the otherwise too small a signal to detect in frozen media. One should not, however, rule out the increased formation of FR by homolytic cleavage of covalent bonds especially organic C-H linkages of proteins during lyophilization. If this is the case, bovine albumin itself should produce a big signal and the degree/mode of lyophilization should effect the ESR signal. We have observed, however, only a very small ESR signal with bovine serum albumin (0.2%); on the other hand, our lyophilization technique is very reproducible (CV 3.5% for duplicates, n = 35). We were unable to identify any direct formation of superoxide radical probably because: a) O_2^- reacts rapidly with ascorbic acid; or 2) the alternate pathways proposed play an important role in the free radical-induced lipid peroxidation processes.

Work is in progress to make direct measurements of free radicals using: a) special ESR technique (CAT) with a stop flow cell; b) spin labels, and c) photosensitive radical scavengers and dyes.

3) Lipid Peroxides

The mechanism by which lipid peroxidation is initiated is not clear. There are several indications that free radicals and SDA radical initiate the oxidation process. Harmon and Piette[22] have speculated that peroxidation of serum lipoprotein occurs, possibly sensitized in part by free radicals formed in the oxidation of compounds such as epinephrine, ascorbic acid as well as by metals such as Cu and Fe in the proteins. The expected lipid peroxy radical signal (g = 2.015) was not detected apparently because they react so rapidly with ascorbate to yield a radical at g = 2.005. The indirect evidence for free radical production in myocardial ischemia includes: (1) loss of polyunsaturated fatty acids from membrane phospholipids, at periods that are far beyond the temporary activation of phospholipase A_2; (2) the increase in lipid peroxide production as studied by malondialdehyde; (3) the depletion of glutathione peroxidase, and (4) consumption of ascorbic acid. Spector[23] has demonstrated this loss of ascorbate in central nervous systems as due to free radical formation. Lipid peroxidation may be an important process for cell damage during myocardial infarction. The depletion of polyunsaturated fatty acids, especially arachidonic acid (the substrate for prostaglandins) from the membrane results in loss of membrane stability and possible vascular damage.

One other potential consequence of membrane lipid free radical reaction involves the endothelial cells. Arachidonic acid is present in large quantities in platelets, and cyclo-oxygenase oxidizes it to prostaglandin endoperoxide PGG_2 through a free radical mechanism[24]. PGG_2 is in turn converted to PGH_2 (producing a superoxide radical) which yields: (a) prostaglandins E, F; (b) thromboxane A_2, and (c) prostacyclin PGI_2, as products. TxA_2 is an extremely potent platelet aggregator, whereas PGI_2 prevents the aggregation and promotes the disaggregation of platelets. The balance between TxA_2 and PGI_2 is critical for homeostasis. Harland[25] has observed LP to selectively inhibit PGI_2 and result in platelet induced micro-occlusion. Demopoulos[24] has confirmed this result by examining the microcirculation in brain ischemic tissue using scanning electron microscopy.

4) Protective Antioxidants

Cardiac muscle tissue can be protected from FR and LP damage by protective enzymes, superoxide dismutase, glutathione peroxidase (GP) and antioxidants ascorbic acid (ASC) and glutathione (GSH). However, the heart lacks a full complement of these antioxidant enzymes as demonstrated by Doroshow[26]. Demopoulos[24] observed depletion of antioxidant ascorbic acid and GP much before lipid loss and it appears to be an important factor in establishing the free radical nature of some of the pathological changes. Acute myocardial ischemia which leads to increased FR and LP production also results in depletion of cardiac antioxidant enzymes[27,28,29].

Free radical scavengers such as α-tocopherol can protect the ischemic myocardium and have proven effective in lessening the acute pathologic changes observed in mouse and rat hearts[30]. Glutathione peroxidase (containing selenium) provides a major enzymatic pathway for the removal of FR, LP and O_2 metabolites from the heart. McCoy[31] has shown that GP may exert its effect by directly preventing FR attack on PUFA membrane lipids. Doroshow[25] demonstrated that selenium deficiency with a concomitant decrease in cardiac GP markedly augmented lipid peroxidation by doxorubicin in mouse hearts. Jaakkola[32] has observed that α-tocopherol administration along with selenium has a beneficial effect in patients with ischemic heart disease. Demopoulos[24] treated cats with regional cerebral ischemia using large doses of methohexital, a short acting lipid soluble barbiturate. Methohexital prevented: (a) lipid-free radical changes; (b) pathological consumption of ascorbic acid; (c) microcirculatory pathology; (d) gross and histological evidence of cerebral infarction, and (e) ubisemiquinone radical formation.

Results obtained in man suggest that free radical and lipid peroxide production plays an important role in causing irreversible damage during acute myocardial ischemia. However, many well-designed experiments are needed to elucidate the role of free radicals and lipid peroxides in the pathogenesis of cell death in myocardial tissues. Systematic work is in progress now in our laboratories to: (1) make direct measurement of free radicals without lyophilization; (2) to study the time sequence of FR release relative to indices of cell death, and (3) use of specific FR scavengers in salvaging ischemic myocardium.

REFERENCES

1. YAMAMOTO, H. Studies on clinical applications of electron spin resonance (ESR) spectrometry: Application to diagnosis of ischemic heart disease. Japan. Circ. J. 35, 1257-1258 (1971).
2. AKIYAMA, K. Studies on myocardial metabolism in the ischemic heart. Part II. Studies by the method of electron spin resonance. Japan. Circ. J. 33, 146-147 (1969).

3. SUZUKI, Y. Studies on the free radicals in myocardial mitochondria by electron spin resonance (ESR) spectrometry (Studies on experimental infarction dogs). Japan. Circ. J. 39, 683-691 (1975).

4. HALL, E.T. The oxygen effect, in: Radiobiology for the radiologist. p. 48, New York, Harper and Row 1973).

5. SMITH, D.S., REHNCRONA, S. & SIESJO, BO K. Barbiturates as protective agents in brain ischemia and as free radical scavengers in vitro. Acta Physiol. Scand. Suppl. 492, 129-134 (1980).

6. TAPPEL, A. Free radical lipid peroxidation and its inhibition by vitamin E and selenium. Federation Proc. 24, 73-78 (1965).

7. MYERS, C.E., MCGUIRE, W.P., LISS, R.H., IFRIM, I., GROTZINGER, V., & YOUNG, R.C. Adriamycin: The role of lipid peroxidation in cardiac toxicity and tumor response. Science 197, 165-167 (1977).

8. WILLS, E.D. Effect of unsaturated fatty acids and their peroxides on enzymes. Biochem. Pharmacol. 7, 7-16 (1961).

9. OKUMA, M., TAKAYAMA, H., & UCHINO, H. Generation of prostacyclin-like substance and lipid peroxidation in vitamin E deficient rats. Prostaglandins, 19, 527 (1980).

10. SATOH, K. Serum lipid peroxide in cerebrovascular disorders determined by a new colorometric method. Clin. Chim. Acta 90, 37-43 (1978).

11. HILDEBRANT, A.G., & ROOTS, I. Reduced nicotinamide adenine dinucleotide phosphate (NADPH) dependent formation and breakdown of hydrogen peroxide during mixed function oxidation reactions in liver microsomes. Arch. Biochem. Biophys. 171, 385-397 (1975).

12. ROTRUCK, J.T., POPE, A.L., GANTHER, H.E., SWANSON, A.B., HAFEMAN, D.G., & HOEKSTRA, W.G. Selenium: Biochemical role as a component of glutathione peroxidase. Science, 179, 588-590 (1973).

13. ELSTNER, E.R., & HEUPEL, A. Inhibition of nitrite formation from hydroxylammonium cholride. A simple assay for superoxide dismutase. Anal. Biochem. 70, 616-620 (1976).

14. DAY, B.R., WILLIAMS, D.R., & MARSH, C.A. A rapid manual method for routine assay of ascorbic acid in serum and plasma. Clin. Biochem. 12, 22 (1979).

15. SEDLOCK, J., & LINDSAY, R.H. Estimation of total, protein bound and nonprotein sulfhydryl groups in tissue with Ellman's reagent. Anal. Biochem. 25, 192 (1968).

16. CROSSMAN, M.W., & HIRSCHBERG, C.B. Biosynthesis of phytospingosine by the rat. J. Biol. Chem. 252, 5815-5819 (1977).

17. JORDI, H.C. Separation of long and short chain fatty acid as naphthacyl and substituted phenacyl esters by high performance liquid chromatography. J. Liq. Chromat. 1(2), 215-230 (1978).

18. LOHMANN, W., SCHREIBER, J., & GREULICH, W. On the possible involvement of ascorbic acid and copper proteins in leukemia. IV. ESR investigations on the interaction between ascorbic acid and some copper proteins. Z. Naturforsch. 34, 550-554 (1979).

19. WALAAS, E., LOVSTAD, R., & WALAAS, O. Free radical formation of catecholamines by the action of ceruloplasmin. Proc. Biochem. Soc. J92, 18P-19P (1964).

20. JANZEN, E.G. Spin traps and ESR spectrometry. Acc. Chem. Res. 4, 31-42 (1971).

21. FLOYD, R.A., SOONG, L.M., WALKER, R.N., & STUART, M. Lipid hydroperoxide activation in N-hydroxyl N-acetylaminoflourene via a free radical route. Cancer Res. 36, 2761-2767 (1976).

22. HARMON, D., & PIETTE, L. Free radical theory of aging. Free radical reactions in serum. J. Gerontol. 21(4), 560-565 (1966).

23. SPECTOR, R. Vitamin homeostasis in the central nervous system. New Eng. J. Med. 296, 1393 (1977).

24. DEMOPOULOS, H.B., FLAMM, E.S., PIETRONIGRO, D.D., & SELIGMAN, M.L. The free radical pathology and the microcirculation in the major central nervous system disorders. Acta Physiol. Scand. Suppl. 492, 91-119 (1980).

25. HARLAND, W.A., GILBERT, J.D., & BROOKS, C.J.W. Lipids of human atheroma. VII. Oxidized derivatives of cholesteryl linoleate. Biochem. Biophys. Acta 316, 378-385 (1973).

26. DOROSHOW, J.H., LOCKER, G.Y., & MYERS, C.E. Enzymatic defenses of the mouse heart against reactive oxygen metabolites. Alterations produced by doxorubicin. J. Clin. Invest. 65, 128-135 (1980).

27. RAO, P.S., & MUELLER, H.S. Lipid peroxide production and glutathione peroxidase depletion in rat myocardium after acute infarction. Clin. Chem. 27, 1027 (1981).

28. RAO, P.S., RAO, P.B., BROCK, R.E., & MUELLER, H.S. Patterns of free radicals across the heart during acute myocardial infarct. Clin. Res. 28, 758A (1980).

29. RAO, P.S., EVANS, R.G., & MUELLER, H.S. Sequential transcardiac changes in free radicals, catecholamines and lipid peroxides in early experimental myocardial infarction. Clin. Res. 30, 214A (1982).

30. SONNEVELD, P. Effect of α-tocopherol on the cardiotoxicity of adriamycin in the rat. Cancer Treat. Rep. 62, 1033-1036 (1978).

31. MCCOY, P.B., GIBSON, D.D., FONG, K., & HORNBROOK, K.R. Effect of glutathione peroxidase on lipid peroxidation in biological membranes. Biochem. Biophys. Acta 431, 459-468 (1976).

32. JAAKKOLA, K. Administration of vitamin E along with selenium to patients with ischemic heart disease. Prevention, 33(9), 97 (1981).

OXYGEN RADICALS AND VASCULAR DAMAGE

H. A. Kontos and M. L. Hess

Department of Medicine
Medical College of Virginia
Richmond, Virginia

ABSTRACT

The effects of topical application of agents which produce oxygen radicals on cerebral arterioles were studied in anesthetized cats. Xanthine oxidase plus xanthine, which produced superoxide anion radical, hydrogen peroxide, and hydrogen peroxide plus ferrous sulfate, which produced the free hydroxyl radical, induced sustained dilation, reduced responsiveness to the vasoconstrictor effect of hypocapnia, and destructive lesions of the endothelium and of the vascular smooth muscle. Similar effects were produced by arachidonate, 15-HPETE, and PGG_2. The effect of arachidonate was inhibited by mannitol, a free hydroxyl radical scavenger, the effect of PGG_2 was inhibited by SOD, the effect of 15-HPETE was inhibited by either catalase or SOD. These results suggest that these cerebral vascular abnormalities were produced by a single destructive free radical, probably the hydroxyl free radical, generated via interaction of superoxide and hydrogen peroxide. Cerebral vascular abnormalities similar to those produced by oxygen radicals were also seen after experimental concussive brain injury or after acute hypertension. After brain injury, activation of phospholipase C and increased brain prostaglandin concentration were demonstrated. The vascular effects of brain injury and acute hypertension were inhibited by free radical scavengers. The results suggest that, in these conditions, vascular damage is induced by oxygen radicals generated from arachidonate in association with increased prostaglandin synthesis.

INTRODUCTION

Vascular abnormalities are a prominent feature of a number of pathological processes including prolonged ischemia, arterial hypertension, inflammation and trauma. The mechanisms by which vascular damage is mediated in these conditions are poorly understood. It is usually postulated that the vessels are injured by toxic substances released within the involved tissues. Oxygen radicals are suitable candidates for mediating vascular damage for a number of reasons. These radicals are very reactive (7) and have been shown to kill cells (2, 13, 19, 26), to destroy cell membranes (22) and to inactivate enzymes and other important cellular components (1, 12, 26). Oxygen radicals are produced in tissues but their concentration is, under normal conditions, kept very low by effective scavenging mechanisms (7). It is conceivable that, under certain pathological conditions, these protective mechanisms may fail either because oxygen radical production increases or because the protective mechanisms themselves are altered.

We consider below four aspects of oxygen radical induced damage to blood vessels: 1) The effects of oxygen radicals on the caliber, functional behavior, and morphology of cerebral vessels in vivo; 2) The effects of oxygen radicals on the metabolism of cerebral vessels in vitro; 3) The effects of oxygen radicals on calcium uptake by vascular sarcoplasmic reticulum; and 4) The involvement of oxygen radicals in the pathogenesis of the vascular damage seen in experimental brain injury and acute hypertension.

Effects of Oxygen Radicals on Cerebral Arterioles in Vivo

We studied the effects of oxygen radicals on cerebral vessels in anesthetized cats and, to a lesser extent, to unanesthetized rabbits equipped with cranial windows for the observation of the pial microcirculation (21). The experimental approach involved introduction of agents which generate oxygen radicals under a cranial window for 15 minutes followed by washout of these agents with fresh artificial cerebrospinal fluid (CSF). Observations were made before, during the application of the agents, and 1 hour after washout. After termination of the functional studies, the vessels were fixed by perfusion, harvested, and examined by scanning and transmission electron microscopy. Table 1 lists the oxygen radicals studied as well as the agents used to generate them. The xanthine oxidase reaction is known to generate superoxide anion radical (23). The combination of hydrogen peroxide and ferrous sulfate (Fenton reagent) generates the free hydroxyl radical (7). Arachidonate is metabolized via the cyclooxygenase pathway to the endoperoxide G_2 (PGG_2) or via the lipoxygenase pathway to hydroperoxy-eicosatetraenoic acid. These products are then peroxidized via the hydroperoxidase activity of cyclooxygenase to PGH_2 or hydroxy-eicosatetraenoic acid. In the process of this peroxidation, an oxygen radical is generated whose identity is not known with certainty (17). This radical is a powerful oxidant and is very similar, if not identical, to the free hydroxyl radical.

Table 1. Agents Used to Generate Oxygen Radicals

Oxygen Radical	Source of Radical
Superoxide Anion Radical	Xanthine plus Xanthine Oxidase
Hydrogen Peroxide	Hydrogen Peroxide
Free Hydroxyl	Hydrogen Peroxide plus Ferrous Sulfate
Unknown; probably free hydroxyl radical	Arachidonic Acid
Unknown; probably free hydroxyl radical	15-Hydroperoxy-eicosatetraenoic Acid
Unknown; probably free hydroxyl radical	Prostaglandin G_2

All the agents used produced arteriolar dilation and reduced responsiveness to vasoconstrictor agents, such as arterial hypocapnia, during their application. The vasodilation and reduced responsiveness were sustained after washing the free radical generating agents off the brain surface. Electron microscopy demonstrated localized destructive lesions of the endothelium. These lesions were mostly localized in the junctions between cells and consisted mostly of crater-like lesions of variable density. Examination of a large number of these lesions showed that they began as a localized destruction of the cell which formed a vacuole. When the vacuole burst through the cell membrane into the lumen of the vessel, the lesion took the appearance of a crater. The vascular smooth muscle of the affected vessels also showed abnormalities which consisted of necrosis of individual smooth muscle cells, increased density of cells, presence of inclusion bodies and myelin figures. Occasionally, there was more extensive necrosis. All vessels which displayed sustained dilation had vascular smooth muscle abnormalities, but the number of smooth muscle cells affected in any one vessel was relatively small.

Topical application of arachidonate also produced vasodilation in unanesthetized rabbits. These animals were equipped with chronically implanted windows (21) and were also examined 24 hours after the application of arachidonate. At that time, there was pronounced vasodilation and marked accumulation of leukocytes at the site of application of arachidonate, presumably because of production of chemotactic products from arachidonate.

It should be noted that dilation is not the only response to the application of oxygen radical generating agents. For example, Rosenblum (25) found that a number of unsaturated fatty acids, including arachidonate, induced transient vasoconstriction of cerebral arterioles in mice. DelMaestro et al. (3) found that oxygen radicals generated from the xanthine oxidase reaction induced increased endothelial permeability to macromolecules in vessels of the cheek pouch of the hamster associated with arteriolar constriction.

Inhibition of Cerebral Vascular Effects of Oxygen Radicals

Table 2 shows the agents which have been found to effectively inhibit the cerebral vascular effects of oxygen radicals. Inhibition of the effects of oxygen radicals was judged by reduction in the residual vasodilation observed 1 hour after washout of the free radical generating agent, preservation of normal responsiveness to vasoconstrictor agents and absence or reduction in the density of endothelial lesions. Indomethacin inhibited the effects of arachidonate presumably because it inhibits cyclooxygenase, suggesting that the origin of the free radical from arachidonate metabolism comes from the cyclooxygenase pathway. As expected, superoxide dismutase (SOD), which eliminates the superoxide anion radical, is effective in inhibiting the effects of xanthine oxidase. The effects of 15-HPETE were inhibited by either SOD or catalase. This suggests that the agent immediately responsible for vascular damage is the hydroxyl free

Table 2. Agents Which Inhibit the Cerebral Vascular Effects of Oxygen Radicals

Source of Radical	Inhibitor
Xanthine plus Xanthine Oxidase	Superoxide Dismutase
Arachidonic Acid	Indomethacin; Mannitol
15-Hydroperoxy- eicosatetraenoic	Superoxide Dismutase; Catalase
Prostaglandin G_2	Superoxide Dismutase

radical which is generated by the interaction of superoxide anion
radical and hydrogen peroxide via the Haber-Weiss reaction (9).
Consistent with this view is the finding that mannitol, a free hydroxyl radical scavenger, also inhibited the vascular damage from
arachidonate (15). The damage from PGG_2 was partially inhibited by
SOD (15). These results suggest that arachidonate and its metabolites are capable of releasing superoxide anion radical and that this
leads to the generation of the free hydroxyl radical.

Effects of Oxygen Radicals on Metabolism of Cerebral Vessel Metabolism in Vitro

We studied the effects of oxygen radical generating agents on
cerebral vessel oxygen metabolism in vitro. Cerebral arterioles were
removed from the brain of cats, divided in several segments, and
incubated for 15 minutes with various oxygen radical generating
agents (20). The vessels were then washed and placed in the
Cartesian diver microrespirometer where their oxygen consumption rates
were determined for several hours. Xanthine oxidase, acting on
acetaldehyde as substrate, 15-HPETE and arachidonate, were all found
to depress severely oxygen consumption of cerebral arterioles. This
effect was inhbited by the combination of SOD and catalase but not by
each one of these enzymes separately, nor by mannitol. These findings suggest that the oxygen radicals, either superoxide anion
radical, hydrogen peroxide, and the hydroxyl free radical, are each
one by itself damaging to vascular tissue or that the initially generated oxygen radicals interact and generate a final destructive
radical, such as the hydroxyl radical. The reduced oxygen consumption caused by oxygen radicals is probably due to damage to mitochondrial membranes and alterations of mitochondrial enzymes.

Effects of Oxygen Radicals on Vascular Sarcoplasmic Reticulum

One of the potential mechanisms by which oxygen radicals can
interfere with the capacity of vascular smooth muscle to generate
tension is via effects on sarcoplasmic reticulum. For this reason,
we studied the effects of superoxide anion radical generated via the
xanthine oxidase reaction on aortic sarcoplasmic reticulum. The
vesicular fraction of vascular smooth muscle was prepared from
ascending aorta of cows by a variation of the procedure originally
described by Hess and Ford (11). Figure 1 shows calcium accumulation monitored by following the loss of ^{45}Ca from the incubation
medium using Millipore filtration to stop the reaction. It is seen
that calcium uptake was inhibited by xanthine oxidase plus xanthine
at both pH 7.0 and pH 6.4. This effect of xanthine oxidase was inhibited by SOD only at pH 6.4 but not at pH 7.0. The absence of an
effect of SOD at the higher pH may be the result of pH-dependent
modification of the amounts of superoxide generated by xanthine
oxidase.

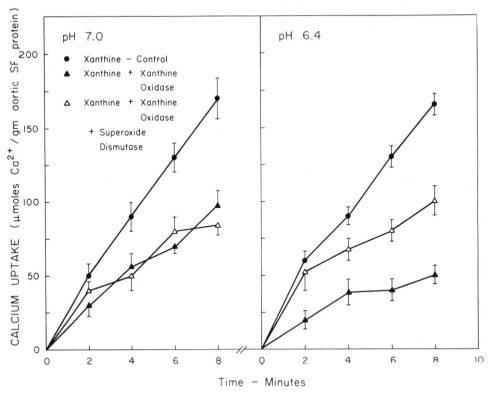

Figure 1. Effect of oxygen radicals generated by the xanthine oxidase reaction on calcium uptake by aortic SR at pH 7.0 (A) and at pH 6.4 (B). Note that xanthine oxidase + xanthine reduced calcium uptake at both pH levels. Superoxide dismutase partially reversed the effect of oxygen radicals only at pH 6.4.

Involvement of Arachidonate-Derived Oxygen Radicals in Cerebral Vascular Abnormalities

In view of the effects of oxygen radicals on cerebral blood vessels described above, it would appear profitable to examine the participation of these agents in conditions associated with abnormal vasodilation and reduced responsiveness of the cerebral circulation. A number of conditions have been described in which these circumstances occur. These include ischemia (18), acute severe intracranial hypertension (31), repeated seizures (16), acute severe arterial hypertension (14) and experimental traumatic brain injury (29).

Gaudet et al. (8) found that brain ischemia in gerbils was associated with an increase in tissue concentration of free arachidonate. When perfusion was reestablished, arachidonate concentration decreased, and there was a corresponding increase in the concentration of cyclooxygenase products. These results show that under these conditions there is activation of phospholipases resulting in increased arachidonate availability. The consequent increase in prostaglandin synthesis and the associated production of oxygen radicals might be responsible for some of the vascular changes which occur during ischemia (4).

Experimental brain injury brought about by fluid percussion in cats (29) or acute hypertension induced in cats by intravenous administration of vasoconstrictor agents (14) produce cerebral vascular abnormalities that are very similar to those induced by free radical generation on the brain surface. After percussion injury or after acute hypertension, the cerebral arterioles displayed sustained dilation for several hours, reduced or absent responsiveness to the vasoconstrictor effects of arterial hypocapnia and reduced ability to respond to changes in arterial blood pressure. Electron microscopic examination of the vessels which showed these abnormalities disclosed discrete endothelial destructive lesions morphologically similar to those found from the action of free radicals as well as abnormalities of the vascular smooth muscle. Such vessels had reduced oxygen consumption in vitro when compared to vessels of comparable size from normal animals (14, 29). Although spontaneous platelet aggregation was rare, platelet aggregation in response to other interventions was enhanced (24).

The pathogenesis of the abnormalities in both brain injury and hypertension is similar. Immediately following percussion type brain injury, there is a marked increase in arterial blood pressure which is short-lasting. This acute hypertensive episode was found to be essential for the production of the vascular abnormalities outlined above. When the blood pressure increase was prevented, the vessels remained unchanged in caliber, they were normally responsive functionally and morphologically intact (29).

The functional and morphological abnormalities after brain injury and after acute hypertension were inhibited by agents which inhibit cyclooxygenase, such as indomethacin or sodium amfenac, showing that the abnormalities were dependent on activation of arachidonate metabolism via cyclooxygenase (14,29). These abnormalities were also inhibited partially or completely by SOD, mannitol or by nitroblue tetrazolium, a dye which is a free radical scavenger (14, 28). These results show that the immediate cause of the injury is the generation of oxygen radicals.

The sequence of events which account for the vascular changes in experimental brain injury and acute hypertension is as follows: The initial essential step seems to be a marked increase in arterial blood pressure. The rise in arterial blood pressure causes phospholipase activation and release of free arachidonate. A increase in

phospholipase C activity in the brain following brain injury was
demonstrated (27). No comparable studies have yet been carried out
in acute hypertension from vasoconstrictor agents. The precise
mechanism by which the rise in blood pressure activates phospholipas
is not known. It may involve an increase in vascular permeability
and entry of blood constituents into the vessel wall and into the
brain parenchyma, or release of normal constituents of the brain
tissue which activate phospholipase. A number of polypeptides are
capable of doing this and some of these are present in the brain (3C
The increase in concentration of free arachidonate stimulates prost
glandin synthesis. A rise in prostaglandin concentration in the bra
tissue was demonstrated shortly after injury in cats (6).

If the increase in prostaglandin synthesis occurs in a burst of
very high intensity. it is conceivable that the associated production of free radicals might overcome the normal defenses of the
tissues and that these may then escape into the extracellular fluid.
Once this occurs, a chain reaction might begin with sequential production of new radicals which eventually destroy cell membranes and
cause the vascular abnormalities we observed. The endothelial
destructive lesions can be explained as a result of the action of
free radicals generated in this manner upon the membrane of endothelial cells. The localized nature of the lesions is of interest,
but the reasons for this localization are not clear. The loci of
damage may represent particularly vulnerable portions of the cell
or they may represent the location of enzymes involved in the production of radicals. The enhancement of platelet aggregation may
be explained by the fact that oxygen radicals have been shown to
selectively destroy prostacyclin synthetase (10).

The vascular smooth muscle abnormalities including relaxation
and unresponsiveness can probably be explained by the damage done
by oxygen radicals to the vascular smooth muscle. Whether the
morphological lesions are sufficiently extensive to explain the
marked vasodilation and unresponsiveness is not known with certainty
If, however, one assumes that those smooth muscle cells that have
been damaged are less able to develop tension, then the proper conditions would exist for heterogeneous internal contraction of
contractile element within the vessel wall. Since the vascular
smooth muscle cells are in series, shortening of one smooth muscle
cell may produce lengthening of another (14). It is known that
vascular smooth muscle activated at long length in vitro may display
reduced ability to generate tension (5). At times, agents which
cause contraction of vascular smooth muscle, such as norepinephrine,
may actually cause dilation of the vessels under these circumstances
(57). This phenomenon has been explained as due to an unequal short
ening of contractile elements in series and is known under the name
of attenuation. It seems to be a plausible explanation for the
abnormalities we observed.

ACKNOWLEDGEMENT

This work was supported by Grants HL 21851 and NS 12587.

REFERENCES

1. Armstrong, D. A. & Buchanan, J. D. Reactions of $\cdot O_2^-$, H_2O_2 and other oxidants with sulfhydryl enzymes. Photochem. Photobiol. 28, 743-755 (1978).
2. Babior, B. M. Oxygen-dependent microbial killing by phagocytes. New Engl. J. Med. 298, 659-688 (1978).
3. Del Maestro, R. F., Thaw, H. H., Björk, J., Planker, M. & Arfors, K. E. Free radicals as mediators of tissue injury. Acta Physiol. Scand., Suppl. 492, 43-57 (1980).
4. Demopoulos, H. B., Flamm, E. S., Pietronigro, D. D. & Seligman, M. L. The free radical pathology and the microcirculation in the major central nervous system disorders. Acta Physiol. Scand. Suppl. 492, 91-118 (1980).
5. Dobrin, P. B. Influence of initial length of length-tension relationship of vascular smooth muscle. Am. J. Physiol. 225, 664-670 (1973).
6. Ellis, E. F., Wright, K. F., Wei, E. P. & Kontos, H. A. Cyclo-oxygenase products of arachidonic acid metabolism in cat cerebral cortex after experimental concussive brain injury. J. Neurochem. 37, 892-896 (1981).
7. Fridovich, I. The biology of oxygen radicals. Science 201, 875-880 (1978).
8. Gaudet, R. J., Alam, I. & Levine, L. Accumulation of cyclooxy-genase products of arachidonic acid metabolism in gerbil brain during reperfusion after bilateral common carotid artery occlu-sion. J. Neurochem. 35, 653-658 (1980).
9. Haber, F. & Weiss, J. The catalytic decomposition of hydrogen peroxide by iron salts. Proc. Roy. Soc. London A147, 332-351 (1934).
10. Ham, E. A., Egan, R. W., Soderman, D. D., Gale, P. H. & Kuehl, F. A., Jr. Peroxidase-dependent deactivation of prostacyclin synthetase. J. Biol. Chem. 254, 2191-2194 (1979).
11. Hess, M. L. & Ford, G. D. Calcium accumulation by subcellular fractions from vascular smooth muscle. J. Mol. Cell. Cardiol. 6, 275-282 (1974).
12. Kellogg, E. W., III & Fridovich, I. Superoxide, hydrogen per-oxide and singlet oxygen in lipid peroxide by a xanthine oxidase system. J. Biol. Chem. 250, 8812-8817 (1975).
13. Kellogg, E. W., III & Fridovich, I. Liposome oxidation and erythrocyte lysis by enzymically generated superoxide and hydro-gen peroxide. J. Biol. Chem. 252, 6721-6728 (1977).
14. Kontos, H. A., Wei, E. P., Dietrich, W. D., Navari, R. M., Povlishock, J. T., Ghatak, N. R., Ellis, E. F. & Patterson, J. L., Jr. Mechanism of cerebral arteriolar abnormalities after acute hypertension. Am. J. Physiol. 240, H511-H527 (1981).

15. Kontos, H. A., Wei, E. P., Povlishock, J. T., Dietrich, W. D., Magiera, C. J. & Ellis, E. F. Cerebral arteriolar damage by arachidonic acid and prostaglandin G_2. Science 209, 1242-1245 (1980).

16. Kontos, H. A., Wei, E. P., Raper, A. J., Rosenblum, W. I., Navari, R. M. & Patterson, J. L., Jr. Role of tissue hypoxia i local regulation of cerebral microcirculation. Am. J. Physiol. 234, H582-H591 (1978).

17. Kuehl, F. A., Jr., Humes, J. L., Ham, E. A., Egan, R. W. & Dougherty, H. W. Inflammation: The role of peroxidase-derived products. Advances in Prostaglandin and Thromboxane Research (B. Sammuelsson, P. W. Ramwell and R. Paoletti eds.), vol. 6, pp. 77-86. Raven Press, New York.

18. Lassen, N. A. Luxury-perfusion syndrome and its possible relation to acute metabolic acidosis localized within the brain. Lancet 2, 1113-1115 (1966).

19. Lavelle, F., Michelson, A. M. & Dimitrijevic, L. Biological protection by superoxide dismutase. Biochem. Biophys. Res. Commun. 55, 350-357 (1973).

20. Levasseur, J. E., Kontos, H. A. & Ellis, E. F. Effect of free oxygen radicals on cerebral arteriolar oxygen consumption. Microvasc. Res. 21, 249 (abstract) (1981).

21. Levasseur, J. E., Wei, E. P., Raper, A. J., Kontos, H. A., & Patterson, J. L., Jr. Detailed description of a cranial window technique for acute and chronic experiments. Stroke 8, 308-317 (1975).

22. Lynch, R. E. & Fridovich, I. Effects of superoxide anion on th erythrocyte membrane. J. Biol. Chem. 253, 1838-1845 (1978).

23. McCord, J. M. & Fridovich, I. The reduction of cytochrome c by mild xanthine oxidase. J. Biol. Chem. 243, 5753-5760 (1968).

24. Rosenblum, W. F., Wei, E. P., & Kontos, H. A. Platelet aggrega tion in cerebral arterioles is more likely provoked after percussive brain trauma. Cardiovasc. Dis., (In Press).

25. Rosenblum,W. I. Unsaturated fatty acids and cyclooxygenase inhibitors: effects of pial arterioles. Am. J. Physiol. 242, H629-H632 (1982).

26. Van Hemmen, J. J. & Meuling, W. J. A. Inactivation of biologically active DNA by x-ray induced superoxide radicals and their dismutation products: singlet molecular oxygen and hydrogen peroxide. Biochim. Biophys. Acta 402, 133-141 (1975).

27. Wei, E. P., Lamb, P. G. & Kontos, H. A. Increased phospholipas C activity after experimental brain injury. J. Neurosurg. (In Press).

28. Wei, E. P., Kontos, H. A., Dietrich, W. D., Povlishock, J. T. & Ellis, E. F. Inhibition by free radical scavengers and by cycl oxygenase inhibitors of pial arteriolar abnormalities from concussive brain injury in cats. Circ. Res. 48, 95-103 (1981).

29. Wei, E. P., Dietrich, W. D., Povlishock, J. T., Navari, R. M. & Kontos, H. A. Functional, morphological, and metabolic abnorma ties of the cerebral microcirculation after concussive brain

injury in cats. <u>Circ</u>. <u>Res</u>. 46, 37-47 (1980).

30. Wei, E. P., Kontos, H. A. & Said, S. I. Mechanism of action of vasoactive intestinal polypeptide on cerebral arterioles. <u>Am</u>. <u>J</u>. <u>Physiol</u>. 239, H765-H768 (1980).

31. Zwetnow, N. N. Effects of increased cerebrospinal fluid pressure on the blood flow and on the energy metabolism of the brain. <u>Acta</u> <u>Physiol</u>. <u>Scand</u>. Suppl. 339, 1-31 (1970).

MEDIATION OF SARCOPLASMIC RETICULUM DISRUPTION IN THE ISCHEMIC MYOCARDIUM: PROPOSED MECHANISM BY THE INTERACTION OF HYDROGEN IONS AND OXYGEN FREE RADICALS

M. L. Hess, Steven Krause and H. A. Kontos

Departments of Medicine (Cardiology) and Physiology
Medical College of Virginia
Richmond, Virginia

ABSTRACT

Acute myocardial ischemia results in a decrease in developed tension and an increase in resting tension. A breakdown of the excitation-contraction coupling system can explain the behavior of the ischemic muscle at a subcellular level. We have identified a specific defect in the sarcoplasmic reticulum (SR) from the ischemic myocardium; i.e., the uncoupling of calcium transport from ATP hydrolysis. The mediators of this excitation-contraction uncoupling process have not been identified. It is now established that the intracellular pH of the ischemic myocardium is in the range of 6.4 but the role of protons and potential role of free radicals have not been identified. We have hypothesized that protons and free radicals may interact to produce the excitation-contraction uncoupling of the ischemic myocardium. Cardiac SR was isolated from the wall of canine left ventricle and calcium uptake velocity and Ca^{2+} stimulated-Mg^{2+} dependent ATPase activity determined. Increasing proton concentration between pH 7.0 and 6.4 significantly reduced calcium uptake rates (pH 7.0 = 0.95 $\pm$ 0.02; 6.4 = 0.50 $\pm$ 0.02 µmoles Ca^{2+}/mg-min; p<0.01) with no effect on ATPase activity. Calculated coupling ratios (µmoles Ca^{2+}/µmoles P_i) decreased from 0.87 $\pm$ 0.06 at pH 7.0 to 0.51 $\pm$ 0.05 at pH 6.4. At pH 7.0, the generation of exogenous free radicals from the xanthine-xanthine oxidase system significantly depressed both calcium uptake rates (Control = 0.95 $\pm$ 0.02; X+XO = 0.15 $\pm$ 0.02) and ATPase activity (Control = 1.05 $\pm$ 0.02; X+XO + 0.30 $\pm$ 0.01 µmoles P_i/mg-min; p<0.01). The decreases in calcium uptake and in ATPase activity were completely reversible with superoxide dismutase (SOD). At pH 6.4 in the presence of xanthine and xanthine oxidase, there is a further depression of calcium uptake rates (Control = 0.50 $\pm$ 0.02; X+XO = 0.11 $\pm$ 0.01; p<0.05) but there

377

is no SOD reversible component. The addition of SOD + 20mM mannitol
normalized calcium transport at pH 6.4. The calculated coupling
ratio at pH 6.4 in the presence of free radicals was 0.13. In contrast sarcoplasmic reticulum isolated from ischemic myocardium
demonstrated a significant depression of calcium uptake rates at pH
7.1 which was further accentuated at pH 6.4. Ca^{2+}-ATPase was significantly depressed at pH 7.1 but there was no accentuation at pH
6.4. It is concluded that no single species of free radical can
explain the intarcellular excitation-contraction uncoupling of the
ischemic myocardium. The system can be explained by the interaction
of hydrogen ions and superoxide anions producing both injury to the
sarcoplasmic reticulum and the formation of lipid free radicals with
hydroxyl-like activity.

INTRODUCTION

     Acute myocardial ischemia produces a rapid decline in develop-
ed tension and subsequent increase in resting tension (14, 25). If
the ischemic episode is prolonged, or if reperfusion occurs after
prolonged ischemia, there is a loss of viable myocardial tissue,
developed tension remains depressed and resting tension increases.
The increase in resting tension is probably due to the breakdown
of cell membrane barriers to calcium and resultant intracellular
calcium overload (29).

     This laboratory and others (25) are investigating the hypothesis
that this progression of ischemia from a reversible to irreversible
phase involves a breakdown of the excitation-contraction coupling
system. This defect has been characterized as an uncoupling of calcium transport from ATP hydrolysis. The mediators of this uncoupling
process in the ischemic myocardium have not been conclusively identified.

     A significant process that would fuel this cascade and lead to
reduced myocardial contractility during ischemia is the generation
of protons. There is abundant evidence that during ischemia, there
is a switch from aerobic to anaerobic metabolism with increased rates
of glycolysis and, therefore, the generation of protons at an increased rate (11). The accumulation of these hydrogen ions leads to
a decrease in intramyocardial pH, a finding now documented by
direct intracellular pH measurements (4) and nuclear magnetic resonance studies (10).

     A second potential mediator contributing to the ischemic pro-
cess is the generated free radical. Under ischemic conditions,
because of the decreased concentration of oxygen, there is a large
increase in reducing equivalents (8). Under these conditions, the
univalent reduction of oxygen is more likely and therefore, the production of superoxide anion and other free radicals is favored. In
this environment, reoxygenation may result in a burst of free radical

in a high enough concentration to exceed the capacity of the tissue to eliminate them. Any free radical generated during myocardial ischemia would readily interact with the unsaturated fatty acids of phospholipid membranes (3). This interaction may then generate new radicals in a chain reaction which might lead to the extensive cellular damage at the sarcolemma, sarcoplasmic reticulum and mito-chondria that has been documented during the course of myocardial ischemia (19, 23, 26).

There are only scattered reports of the possible role of the generation of free radicals during the course of myocardial ischemia. In the isolated rat heart following prolonged hypoxia and reoxygena-tion, Guarnieri et al. (12) found a decrease in SOD and glutathione peroxidase activity incriminating a role for free oxygen radicals. In skeletal muscle, Arkhipenko et al., (1, 2) found an increase in lipid peroxidation products and disturbed calcium transport during limb tourniquet ischemia.

What has not been done to date is the integration of the con-cepts of free radical generation and increase in proton concentration that one would expect in the ischemic myocardium. Within the past year, this laboratory has seriously addressed the question based on the assumption that it is possible that acidosis and free oxygen radicals or the processes that lead to their production may interact in a way such that the damage induced by free radicals may be en-hanced by the presence of acidosis.

METHODS

Healthy, adult filaria-free dogs were anesthetized with sodium pentobarbital (25 mg/kg iv), and the heart was rapidly excised and placed in $4^{o}C$ saline. All subsequent procedures were carried out in a $4^{o}C$ cold room. The free wall of the left ventricle was cleaned of connective tissue and epicardial vessels, diced with scissors, and homogenized in a Sorvall Omnimixer for 1 minute at top speed with 3 volumes of 10 mM imidazole, pH 7.0.

A) Sarcoplasmic Reticulum (SR)

An aliquot from this procedure was saved and designated as whole heart homogenate. Calcium transport was studied under conditions that optimized sarcoplasmic reticulum calcium uptake as previously described by Solaro and Briggs (27). The homogenate was then centri-fuged at 4,080 g max x 20 minutes, filtered through cheesecloth and centrifuged at 51,000 g max x 60 minutes. The resultant pellet was then resuspended in 1 M KCL + 10 mM imidazole, pH 7.0 and centri-fuged at 198,000 g max for 60 minutes. The final pellet, designated SR, was then resuspended in 5 volumes of 30% sucrose + 20 mM imida-zole, pH 7.0. Protein concentration was determined by the method of

Lowry (22). The velocity of calcium uptake by the SR was determined in the presence of oxalate using the Millipore filtration
technique. All incubations were carried out at 37°C. The composition of the standard incubation solution was 100 mM KCL, 18 mM
imidazole, pH 7.0, 10 mM K-oxalate, 5 mM MgCl$_2$, 5 mM ATP, 0.18 mM
CaCl$_2$ with 0.05 µCi/ml ^{45}CaCl$_2$. The reaction was started by the
addition of 0.15 mg/ml SR protein and aliquots taken at various
intervals over two minutes, filtered through Millipore filters of
0.45 µ pore diameter and the filtrate counted in a liquid scintillation spectrometer. The velocity of calcium uptake is presented
as the mean ± one SEM of the specific activity (µmoles Ca^{2+}/mg
protein). The reaction is linear over a 2-minute period. Calcium-
stimulated, magnesium-dependent adenosine triphosphatase (ATPase)
activity of the vesicular fraction was determined utilizing the
same medium as SR calcium uptake activity except ^{45}CaCl$_2$ was omitted. ATPase activity was determined as the rate at which inorganic
phosphate was liberated during the incubation. Samples were analyzed for inorganic phosphate by the method of King (20). The ATP
hydrolysis, associated with the uptake of calcium, was calculated
as the difference between the ATPase activity in the presence and
in the absence of 0.02 M EGTA (ethyleneglycol bis (oxyethylene
nitrilo) tetraacetic acid) and is presented as µmoles P$_i$/mg protein.

B) Generation of Free Radicals and Use of Free Radical Scavengers

Free oxygen radicals were generated by xanthine oxidase (0.2 mg/
ml; Vega Biochemicals, Tucson, AZ) acting on xanthine as a substrate.
It has been shown that xanthine oxidase generates superoxide anion
radical ($\cdot O_2^-$) according to the following reaction (9):

$$\text{xanthine} \xrightarrow{\text{xanthine oxidase}} \text{urate} + \cdot O_2^- \qquad \text{(Equation 1)}$$

$\cdot O_2^-$ produces hydrogen peroxide (H_2O_2) according to the dismutation reaction:

$$\cdot O_2^- + \cdot O_2^- + 2H^+ \xrightarrow{\text{SOD}} H_2O_2 + O_2 \qquad \text{(Equation 2)}$$

This reaction can proceed spontaneously or it can be catalyzed
by superoxide dismutase (SOD). Superoxide anion radical and H_2O_2
interact to generate free hydroxyl radical ($\cdot OH$) according to the
following reaction (13, 24):

$$\cdot O_2^- + H_2O_2 \longrightarrow O_2 + OH^- + \cdot OH \qquad \text{(Equation 3)}$$

We used SOD, 10 µg/ml (Biotics Research, Houston, TX) to
scavenge $\cdot O^-$ and mannitol (20 mM) to scavenge $\cdot OH$ (Dorfman and
Adams, 1973).

C. Myocardial Ischemia

Normothermic, global, canine myocardial ischemia of thirty
minutes duration was produced following the method of Hess et al.
(17). The free wall of the left ventricle was removed, diced and
homogenized in 4 vols. of 10 mM imidazole pH 7.0. The sarcoplasmic
reticulum was isolated and SR calcium uptake, calcium stimulated,
Mg dependent ATPase activity and calcium permeability determined
as described in sections B, C, and D.

RESULTS

Figure 1 presents cardiac sarcoplasmic reticulum calcium uptake
rates and calcium stimulated, magnesium dependent ATPase activity
from the control (n=4) and ischemic (n=4) groups. Control calcium
uptake rates demonstrated a significant depression at pH 6.4. Thirty
minutes of normothermic ischemia resulted in a significant depression
of calcium uptake rate when performed at pH 7.1 that was further
accentuated at pH 6.4. Control Ca-ATPase activity was also significantly depressed at pH 6.4. Ca-ATPase from the ischemic group
demonstrated a similar significant depression at pH 7.1 but was not
further significantly depressed at pH 6.4. Calculation of the coupling ratios (μmoles Ca^{2+} transported μmole ATP hydrolyzed) yielded
a control value at pH 7.1 of 0.53 and at pH 6.4 of 0.50. In the
ischemic SR, the coupling ratio at pH 7.1 was found to be 0.50 and at
pH 6.4, 0.22. Therefore, at pH 6.4, cardiac sarcoplasmic reticulum
isolated from the ischemic myocardium demonstrated a significant
degree of uncoupling of calcium transport from ATP hydrolysis that
was not observed in control SR or in ischemic SR at pH 7.1.

Table 1 presents the effect of increasing hydrogen ion concentration between pH 6.4 and 7.0 on normal canine cardiac sarcoplasmic reticulum (SR) calcium uptake velocity. There was no
difference in SR calcium uptake rates between pH 6.8 and 7.0 but
at pH 6.6, there was a significant decrease in SR calcium uptake
which was even further depressed at pH 6.4.

This depression of SR calcium transport by decreasing pH is
also demonstrable in the whole heart homogenate. Table 2 demonstrates that the SR calcium transport in the whole heart homogenate
is even more sensitive to pH than the isolated SR. In the whole
heart homogenate, pH 6.8 produced a significant decrease in calcium
transport that was not observed in the isolated SR. At pH 6.6, there
was a 40 percent depression of SR calcium uptake in the whole heart
homogenate compared to 24 percent depression in the isolated SR and
pH 6.4 produced a 66 percent depression compared to a 44 percent
depression in the isolated SR.

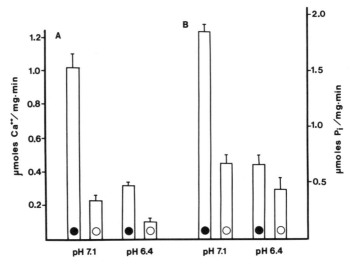

Figure 1. Calcium uptake velocity and calcium stimulated, magnesium dependent ATPase activity of cardiac sarcoplasmic reticulum at pH 7.1 and pH 6.4 from controls (N=4, 0) and from ischemic myocardium (N=4, 0). The bar represents the mean of 12-16 determinations and the error bar ± one SEM.

TABLE 1.   Sarcoplasmic Reticulum Activity at Varying pH

pH	6.4	6.6	6.8	7.0
Ca^{2+} uptake activity (μmoles Ca^{2+}/mg-min)	0.55±0.02	0.78±0.02	0.92±0.03	0.99±0.02

TABLE 2.   Whole Heart Homogenate Calcium Uptake at Varying pH

pH	6.4	6.6	6.8	7.0
Ca^{2+} uptake velocity (μmoles Ca^{2+}/g-min)	4.1±0.2	6.5±0.2	8.0±0.3	10.9±0.4

Having established that decreasing pH can produce a defect in SR calcium transport, we next turned to the effects of exogenously generated free radicals on calcium transport function of isolated cardiac SR. Table 3 presents the effects of superoxide anion generation from a xanthine-xanthine oxidase system at pH 7.0 on SR calcium transport function. At pH 7.0, the coupling ratio (μmoles Ca^{2+} transported/μmole ATP hydrolyzed was 0.855 - a coupling ratio in good agreement with previously reported work from our own laboratory (7). Xanthine alone has no effect on our system. With the generation of the superoxide anion, there is a significant depression of both SR calcium uptake rates and ATPase activity with a degree of uncoupling resulting in a coupling ratio of 0.479. Superoxide dismutase significantly inhibited the effects of the xanthine-xanthine oxidase system. SR ATPase activity and calcium uptake were significantly protected with the resulting coupling ratio of 0.755.

Table 4 presents the effects of the xanthine-xanthine oxidase system on SR calcium transport function at pH 6.4. Control studies at pH 6.4 resulted in a significant depression of SR calcium uptake with no significant effect on ATPase activity. Xanthine had no effect on this system. In the presence of the xanthine-xanthine oxidase system, there was a further significant depression of calcium uptake rates, no effect on ATPase activity resulting in a marked uncoupling of calcium transport from ATP hydrolysis with a resultant coupling ratio of 0.134. In contrast to the studies at pH 7.0, SOD had no effect on this system and mannitol alone had no effect on this system. But, in the presence of both SOD and mannitol, calcium uptake rates were normalized to pH 6.4 control values and the coupling ratio returned to 0.50. Having established that free radicals can disrupt isolated SR calcium transport, we ask the question, can the xanthine-xanthine oxidase system disrupt SR calcium transport in the whole heart homogenate?

TABLE 3. The Effect of Superoxide Anion on Sarcoplasmic Reticulum Calcium Transport at pH 7.0

	Control	Xanthine	Xanthine+ Xanthine Oxidase	Xanthine + Xanthine Oxidase + SOD
Ca^{2+} Uptake (μmoles Ca^{2+}/mg-min)	0.94+0.02	0.88+0.03	0.23+0.05	0.83+0.04
ATPase Activity (μmoles P_i/mg-min)	1.10+0.05	1.16+0.06	0.48+0.05	1.10+0.08
Coupling Ratio (μmoles Ca^{2+}/μmoles P_i)	.855	.759	.479	.755

TABLE 4.   The Effect of Hydroxyl Radicals on Sarcoplasmic
           Reticulum Calcium Transport at pH 6.4

	Control	Xanthine	Xanthine + Xanthine Oxidase	Xanthine + Xanthine Oxidase + SOD + Mannitol
Ca^{2+} Uptake (μmoles Ca^{2+}/mg-min)	0.53±0.02	0.54±0.03	0.15±0.02	0.60±0.03
ATPase Activity (μmoles P_i/mg-min)	1.06±0.05	1.04±0.08	1.12±0.05	1.20±0.05
Coupling Ratio ($\frac{\mu moles\ Ca^{2+}}{\mu moles\ P_i}$)	0.500	0.519	0.134	0.500

Table 5 presents the results of this study. At pH 7.0, the
xanthine-xanthine oxidase system produced a significant depression of
SR calcium transport in the whole heart homogenate that was SOD
reversible. At pH 6.4, there was a direct effect of pH. In the
presence of xanthine-xanthine oxidase system, there was a further
depression of calcium transport that was unaffected by either SOD or
mannitol alone. In the presence of both SOD and mannitol, there was
a significant reversal of the inhibitory effects of free radicals.

TABLE 5.   The Effect of Free Radicals on Homogenate Calcium Uptake
           Velocity[1]

	Control	Xanthine	Xanthine + Xanthine Oxidase	Xanthine + Xanthine Oxidase + SOD	Xanthine + Xanthine Oxidase + SOD + Mannitol
pH 7.0	11±0.2	10.8±1.4	6.8±0.9	10.6±0.9	10.9±0.4
pH 6.4	4.5±0.2	5.2±0.5	3.0±0.4	3.2±0.6	5.0±0.7

[1]Ca^{2+} Uptake expressed as μmoles Ca^{2+}/g-min.

DISCUSSION

It has now been demonstrated that the onset of myocardial ischemia is associated with a significant decrease in intracellular
pH (4, 10). The mechanisms coupling the increase in intracellular
proton concentrations to the decrease in developed tension during
ischemia have not been elucidated. The sarcoplasmic reticulum (SR)
of cardiac muscle has been demonstrated to serve as an intracellular
source and sink for activator calcium in the excitation-contraction
coupling system of cardiac muscle (6). This laboratory has identified a specific defect in the sarcoplasmic reticulum from the ischemic
myocardium which could directly lead to a decrease in tension development during ischemia. An uncoupling of SR calcium transport from
ATP hydrolysis has been identified in prolonged normothermic global
ischemia (7), hypothermic global ischemia (15, 17) and ischemic/
reperfusion injury (16). This defect in sarcoplasmic reticulum
function has also been observed by Arkhipenko et al., (1) during the
course of skeletal muscle ischemia. By simulating the intracellular
pH of the ischemic myocardium, this study has demonstrated a significant uncoupling of SR calcium transport from ATP hydrolysis at pH
6.4, but this increase in proton concentration produces a coupling
ratio that is larger than that following prolonged myocardial ischemia
in the canine heart. Therefore, increasing acidosis does not appear
to be solely responsible for the intracellular damage to the SR arising during global ischemia.

The generation of oxygen free radicals would appear to be another
likely candidate for an intracellular mediator of the ischemic process.
Tappel et al., (28) postulated that ischemia reperfusion injury can be
partially attributed to free radical production which enhances lipid
peroxidation at the cell membrane. Lipid peroxidation, in turn, leads
to membrane alterations from phospholipid depletion and also leads to
the inhibition of membrane associated enzymes (18). Further, the
generation of free radicals from the metabolic pathways of arachidonic acid could also result in the formation of lipid peroxides
which act as vasoconstrictors of the coronary vasculature and contribute to the ischemic process. Other indirect evidence for the
role of free radicals comes from the protective effect of free radical scavengers during the course of myocardial ischemia. Lefer et
al. (21) using the antioxidant MK-447, demonstrated preservation of
contractile force and dF/dt in the ischemia isolated perfused cat
heart. Guarnieri et al., (12) found that the antioxidant α-tocopherol not only reduced the ischemic induced increase in resting
tension, but also resulted in a decreased release of lactate.

With the implication of both free radical production and a
decrease in pH as intracellular mediators of the ischemic process,
we designed our study to examine the combined efforts of both
free radicals and protons on the sarcoplasmic reticulum of cardiac
muscle. We found the following significant points: Isolated

cardiac sarcoplasmic reticulum from the ischemic myocardium is characterized by a depression of calcium uptake rates and Ca-ATPase activity
at pH 7.0 and at pH 6.4, the isolated SR demonstrated a significant
degree of uncoupling of calcium transport from ATP hydrolysis. We
interpret this finding as a defect in the phospholipid permeability
barrier of the SR to calcium. In an attempt to simulate this system in vitro, we found that a decrease in pH from 7.0 to 6.4 uncouples
calcium transport from ATP hydrolysis. However, the decrease in pH
does not significantly decrease the coupling ratio; therefore, it is
unlikely that protons alone are mediating the damage.

Using the xanthine-xanthine oxidase system at pH 7.0 which
results in the generation of the superoxide anion (9), we found both
a depression and uncoupling of the SR calcium transport system. With
the generation of the superoxide anion, the coupling ratio decreased
from 0.85 to 0.479 and this 44 percent reduction in the coupling
ratio connotates a significant degree of uncoupling.

However, the pH of the ischemic myocardium is not 7.0 but is in
the range of 6.0-6.4 (4, 10). At this pH we have previously shown
that the dominant free radical species generated by the xanthine-
xanthine oxidase system is either a perhydroxyl or an hydroxyl radical. In our isolated SR studies at pH 6.4, the xanthine-xanthine
oxidase system produced a significant depression of calcium uptake,
no effect on ATPase activity and a 73 percent decrease in the
coupling ratio.

Given this data, it is difficult to incriminate a single free
radical species as the mediator of the intracellular excitation-
contraction uncoupling of the ischemic myocardium. Of the free
principle species of free radicals, H_2O_2, $\cdot O_2^-$, and $\cdot OH$ we can probably effectively eliminate H_2O_2 as a mediator. Although H_2O_2 is the
principle free radical species generated by leukocytes, Del Maestro
has claimed that it is highly unlikely that intracellular fluxes to
H_2O_2 ever become large enough to exert a cytotoxic effect. Further,
in our laboratory, the direct addition of H_2O_2 produces results
very similar to the calcium ionophore A23187 with absolutely no
effect on the Ca-ATPase activity. This then leaves us with the
superoxide anion and the hydroxyl radical. In a recent study from
this laboratory, we have demonstrated in the whole heart homogenate
that reduction in pH from 7.0 to 6.4 results first in the production of the superoxide anion and then with continued acidosis, the
production of a species of hydroxyl radical. The hydroxyl radical
per se is probably not the single, cytotoxic species. Sing has
stated that hydroxyl radicals in biological systems must be generated and have a site of action within 10 Å. Cardiac SR does not
appear to have the capability to do this. Cytochrome P 450 is not
present in cardiac SR (Hess, unpublished) and myeloperoxidase systems
are not present. A very plausible scheme that can explain our findings in both the ischemic myocardium and the exogenous free radical

system at pH 6.4 would have the superoxide anion serving as a pivi-
tol role. With the onset of ischemia and the increase in reducing
equivalents there would be a backup of electron transport. This
would result in the transport of reducing equivalents outside of the
mitochondria with the cytosolic generation of the superoxide anion.
The dismutation reaction would produce hydrogen peroxide and then by
Fenton reactions result in the local production of hydroxyl radicals.
The combination of either the hydroxyl radicals or more likely the
superoxide anions could result in the formation of lipid free radicals with hydroxyl-like activity and further are quite capable of
initiating a chain reaction resulting in lipid peroxidation, conju-
gated dienes and membrane dysfunction. This hypothesis could explain
both the depression and uncoupling of SR calcium transport in the
acidotic environment of the ischemic myocardium.

ACKNOWLEDGEMENT

This work was supported by HL24917 from the National Institutes
of Health.

REFERENCES

1. Arkhipenko, V., Bilenko, M. V., Dobrina, S. K., Kagan, V. E.,
    Kozlou, Y. P. & Shelenkoua, L. N. Ischemic damage to sarco-
    plasmic reticulum of skeletal muscle: role of lipid peroxidation.
    Bull. Exp. Biol. Med. 83, 683-686 (1977).
2. Arkhipenko, V., Gazdarou, A. K., Kagan, V. E., Kozlou, Y. P. &
    Spirichev, V. B. Lipid peroxidation and disturbances in Ca^{2+}
    transport through membranes of sarcoplasmic reticulum in
    E-vitaminosis. Bull. Exp. Biol. Med. 82, 1540-1543 (1976).
3. Boime, J., Smith, E. E. & Hunter, F. E. The role of fatty acids
    in mitochondrial changes during liver ischemia. Arch. Biochem.
    139, 425-443 (1970).
4. Cobbe, S. M. & Poole-Wilson, P. A. The time of onset and sever-
    ity of acidosis in myocardial ischemia. J. Mol. Cell. Cardiol.
    12, 745-760 (1980).
5. Dorfman, L. M. & Adams, G. E. Reactivity of hydroxyl free radi-
    cals in aqueous solutions. NSRDS N135, No. 46, United States
    Department of Commerce, National Bureau of Standards (1973).
6. Fabiato, A. & Fabiato, F. Calcium and cardiac excitation-
    contraction coupling. Ann. Rev. Physiol. 41, 473-484 (1979).
7. Feher, J., Briggs, F. N. & Hess, M. L. Characterization of
    cardiac sarcoplasmic reticulum from ischemic myocardium: compari-
    son of isolated sarcoplasmic reticulum with unfractionated
    homogenates. J. Mol. Cell. Cardiol. 12, 427-432 (1980).
8. Fridovich, I. Hypoxia and oxygen toxicity. Adv. Neurol. 26,
    255-275 (1979).

9. Fridovich, I. Quantitative aspects of the production of super-
    oxide anion radical by milk xanthine oxidase. J. Biol.
    Chemistry 245, 4053-4057 (1970).
10. Garlick, P. A., Radda, G. K. & Seeley, J. P. Studies of acid-
    osis in the ischemic heart by phosphorus nuclear magnetic
    resonance. Biochem. J. 184, 547-554 (1979).
11. Gevers, J. A. Generation of protons by metabolic processes in
    heart cells. J. Mol. Cell. Cardiol. 11, 867-877 (1977).
12. Guarnieri, C., Flamigni, F. & Caldarera, C. M. Role of oxygen
    in the cellular damage induced by re-oxygenation of hypoxic
    heart. J. Mol. Cell. Cardiol. 12, 797-808 (1980).
13. Haber, F. & Weiss, J. The catalytic decomposition of hydrogen
    peroxide by ion salts. J. Proc. Royal Soc. 147, 332-351 (1934).
14. Hearse, D. J. Reperfusion of the ischemic myocardium. J. Mol.
    Cell. Cardiol. 9, 605-616 (1977).
15. Hess, M. L., Krause, S. M., Robbins, A. D. & Greenfield, L. J.
    Excitation-contraction coupling in hypothermic ischemic myo-
    cardium. Am. J. Physiol. 240, H336-H341 (1981a).
16. Hess, M. L., Warner, M. F., Robbins, A. D., Crute, S. &
    Greenfield, L. J. Characterization of the excitation-contrac-
    tion coupling system of the hypothermic myocardium following
    ischemia and reperfusion. Cardiovasc. Res. 15, 390-397 (1981b).
17. Hess, M. L., Krause, S. M. & Greenfield, L. J. Assessment of
    hypothermic cardioplegic protection of the global ischemic
    myocardium. J. Thorac. Cardiovasc. Surg. 80, 293-301 (1980).
18. Hochstein, P. & Jain, S. K. Association of lipid peroxida-
    tion and polymerization of membrane proteins with erythrocyte
    aging. Fed. Proc. 40, 183-188 (1981).
19. Jennings, R. B. & Ganote, C. E. Structural changes in myo-
    cardium during acute ischemia. Circ. Res. (Suppl III) 35,
    156-172 (1974).
20. King, E. J. Colorimetric determinations of phosphorous.
    Biochem. J. 26, 292-297 (1932).
21. Lefer, A. M., Araki, H. & Okamatsu, S. Beneficial actions of a
    free radical scavenger in traumatic shock and myocardial
    ischemia. Circ. Shock 8, 273-282 (1981).
22. Lowry, O. H., Rosenbrough, N. J., Farr, A. L. & Randall, R. J.
    Protein measurement with the Folin phenol reagent. J. Biol.
    Chem. 193, 265 (1951).
23. McCallister, L. P., Daiello, D. C. & Tyers, G. F. O. Morpho-
    metric observations of the effects of normothermic ischemic
    arrest on dog myocardial ultrastructure. J. Mol. Cell. Cardiol.
    10, 67-80 (1978).
24. McCord, J. M. & Fridovich, I. The reduction of cytochrome C
    by milk xanthine oxidase. J. Biol. Chem. 243, 5753-5760 (1968).
25. Nayler, W. G., Poole-Wilson, P. A. & Williams, A. Hypoxia and
    calcium. J. Mol. Cell. Cardiol. 11, 683-706 (1979).
26. Schwartz, A., Wood, J. M., Allen, J. C. & Bornet, E. P., et al.
    Biochemical and morphological correlates of cardiac ischemia.
    Am. J. Cardiol. 32, 46-61 (1973).

27. Solaro, R. J. & Briggs, F. N. Estimating the functional capabilities of sarcoplasmic reticulum in cardiac muscle. Circ. Res. 34, 531-539 (1974).

28. Tappel, A. L. Lipid peroxidation damage to cell components. Fed. Proc. 32, 1870 (1973).

29. Zimmerman, A. R. E., Dames, W., Hulsmann, W. D., Snijder, J., Wisse, E. & Durrer, D. Morphological changes of heart muscle caused by successive perfusion with calcium free and calcium containing solutions (Calcium paradox). Cardiovasc. Res. 1, 201-209 (1967).

POTENTIAL OXIDATIVE PATHWAYS OF CATECHOLAMINES IN THE FORMATION OF

LIPID PEROXIDES AND GENESIS OF HEART DISEASE

Pawan K. Singal*, Robert E. Beamish and Naranjan S.
Dhalla

Experimental Cardiology Section, Department of
Physiology, Faculty of Medicine, University of Manitoba
Winnipeg, Canada   R3E 0W3

INTRODUCTION

Results of clinical and experimental animal studies have shown
that unusually high levels of catecholamines in the blood cause a
variety of morphological and functional changes in the heart (1,
18,22,25,28). The endogenous stores of adenine triphosphate and
creatine phosphate are depleted (8,25,26) and mitochondrial structure-function is impaired (7,15). Intracellular increase in calcium has been considered to be a determinant factor in this as well
as in variety of other models of heart cell damage (8,21). In
this regard catecholamine-induced cardiomyopathy, has been shown
to be accompanied by a significant increase in the myocardial calcium content (8,15) indicating changes in the membrane permeability. Strong evidence for the alterations in the permeability of
sarcolemma due to isoproterenol treatment was provided by the
intracellular diffusion of horseradish peroxidase, an extracellular
protein tracer, following the drug injection (19).

Since biological membranes are rich in polyunsaturated fatty
acids, these structure can be expected to be more susceptible to
oxidative changes thereby compromising the semipermeable characteristics of the membrane. This may be particularly true during a
relative increase in the oxidative capacity in the cell membranes

---
*Research Scholar of the Canadian Heart Foundation. This work was
 supported by Grants from the Manitoba Heart Foundation and the
 Great West Life Assurance Company.

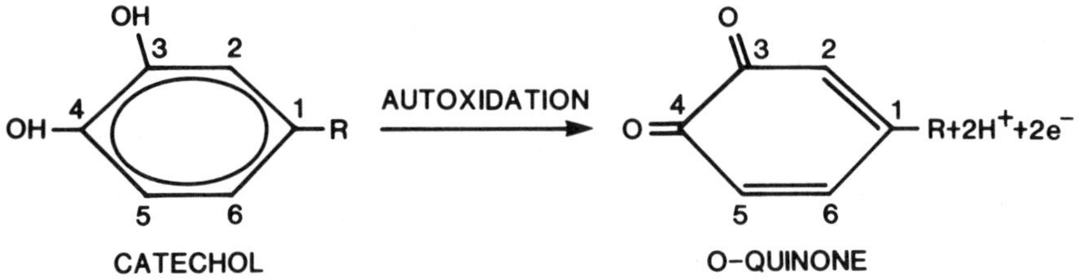

Where R = CH(OH) CH$_2$ NH CH$_3$ (EPINEPHRINE)

CH(OH) CH$_2$ NH$_2$ (NOREPINEPHRINE)

CH(OH) CH$_2$ NHC$_3$H$_7$ (ISOPROTERENOL)

Fig. 1. Autoxidation of catecholamines.

such as may be produced due to increased free radical activity subsequent to the production of electrons by autoxidation of catecholamines according to the scheme shown in Fig. 1.

The electrons thus produced can be captured by molecular oxygen to produce a superoxide radical which is capable of initiating and propagating free radical chain reactions through the formation of hydrogen peroxide as well as hydroxy radicals. The hydroxy radicals may initiate peroxidation of polyunsaturated fatty acyl groups of phospholipids in the hydrophobic region of the membrane, compromising its structural and functional integrity.

If catecholamine-induced myocardial cell damage is mediated by the peroxidation processes it follows that isoproterenol administration should increase lipid peroxide activity in the heart. Furthermore, fat-soluble antioxidants, such as a α-tocopherol (vitamin E), administered in vivo should protect the membrane from the effects of free-radical mediated catecholamine induced changes. This hypothesis has been tested by studying the isoproterenol effects on the malondialdehyde content in the myocardium of rats pretreated with vitamin E and in animals maintained on vitamin E deficient diet.

METHODS

Male Sprague-Dawley rats weighing 350-400 gm. were used. All rats were maintained in our animal holding facilities and were given access to standard rat chow and water ad libitum until the day of the experiment. For vitamin E treatment, the animals were given intraperitoneal injections of α-tocopherol acetate for two weeks (10 mg/kg per day). In vitamin E deficiency studies, animals were kept on a special diet lacking in vitamin E for 8 weeks. On recovery studies, vitamin E deficient animals were put on a normal diet and were also given intraperitoneal injections of 10 mg/kg per day of α-tocopherol acetate for two weeks. These differently treated experimental as well as control animals were then challenged with isoproterenol. For isoproterenol treatment, animals received subcutaneous injections of 40 mg/kg of the drug daily for two days for a cumulative dose of 80 mg/kg. Appropriate vehicle control experiments were also carried out for each study. Animals were employed in further studies 24 hours after the last injection.

Lipid peroxide formation was followed by modification of the thiobarbituric acid method for estimating malondialdehyde (10). Heart homogenate (10% W/V) was prepared in 0.2 M tris - 0.16 M KCl buffer of pH 7.4 (17) and incubated for 1 hr at 37°C in a water bath. A 1- ml aliquot was withdrawn from the incubation mixture and pipetted into an 8- ml Pyrex tube. This was followed by the addition of 0.5 ml of 40% trichloroacetic acid and 0.25 ml of 5 N HCl. After mixing, 0.25 ml of 2% sodium α-thiobarbiturate was added promptly. The tubes were boiled for 15 minutes and cooled in a bucket of ice. One ml of 70% trichloroacetic acid was then added and tubes were allowed to stand for 20 minutes, centrifuged at 2500 r.p.m. for 10-15 minutes, and the color read at 532 mμ. The standard tubes contained 1 μM of malondialdehyde.

RESULTS

Although myocardial changes in the ultrastructure as well as high energy phosphate contents due to isoproterenol treatment (80 mg/kg given over two days in equal doses) have been described recently (22,25), for the sake of clarity and completeness these changes as well as the effects of vitamin E are briefly described in the following section.

Ultrastructure and High Energy Phosphates

Isoproterenol treatment caused arrhythmias and 25 per cent mortality within 24 hrs of the last injection. Both adenosine triphosphate and creatine phosphate levels were markedly decreased in hearts from animals treated with isoproterenol. The ultrastructural changes typical of catecholamine-induced cardiomyopathy

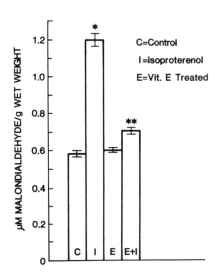

Fig. 2. Effects of vitamin E treatment on isoproterenol-induced
changes in the MDA content in the rat heart. *significantly different from C (P < 0.05). **significantly
different from C, I and E (P < 0.05). Each value is a
mean ± S.E. of 4-6 experiments.

were seen in the subendocardium and in focal areas of the subepicardium. These changes included disruption of mitochondria as
well as accumulation of calcium granules in these organelles.
Loss of myofibrils, fibrosis, cell necrosis and infiltration of
the damaged tissue by scavenger cells was also seen. Pretreatment
of the animals with vitamin E as described in the Methods' section
was found to protect these hearts from isoproterenol-induced
changes. Vitamin E deficient diet reduced the dose of isoproterenol required to produce the type and level of changes described
above. This increase in sensitivity to isoproterenol-induced

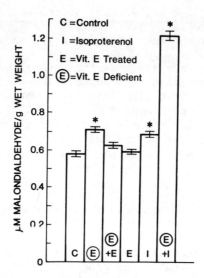

Fig. 3.   Effects of vitamin E deficient diet on isoproterenol-in-
          duced changes in the MDA content in the rat heart. *Sig-
          nificantly different from C (P < 0.05). Each value is a
          mean ± S.E. of 4-6 experiments.

damage due to vitamin E deficiency was reversible upon refeeding
the animals with a normal diet coupled with vitamin E treatment
(22,25).

Malondialdehyde Content

     Effects of isoproterenol and vitamin E treatment on the malon-
dialdehyde (MDA) content in the heart were determined and the results are shown in Fig. 2. There was a significant increase in
the MDA content of the hearts following the isoproterenol treatment. This increase in the MDA levels due to isoproterenol was

significantly less in animals pretreated with vitamin E for two
weeks. Vitamin E alone had no effect on the MDA content.

Since our previous studies of the rat electrocardiogram, mortality and myocardial high energy phosphates as well as ultrastructure have revealed that vitamin E deficient animals were more sen-
itive to isoproterenol (25), studies on the MDA content in vitamin
E deficient animals were done by employing a lower concentration of
isoproterenol (20 mg/kg) and the results are shown in Fig. 3.

Vitamin E deficiency alone caused a small but significant increase in the MDA content of the heart. These changes were reversed in two weeks when these vitamin E deficient animals were fed a
normal diet and were supplemented with vitamin E. Treatment of
the control animals with isoproterenol (20 mg/kg) resulted in
about 15 percent increase in the MDA content. However, vitamin E
deficient animals when given 20 mg/kg isoproterenol showed more
than 100 percent increase in their MDA content of the heart.

DISCUSSION

Although the molecular mechanisms responsible for lipid peroxidation are not fully understood and the breakdown pathways for
these peroxidized lipids are even less clear, it suffices here to
state that one of the stable end products is MDA (2). Furthermore,
it has been shown that there is stoichiometric relationship between
the amount of MDA formed and the fatty acid oxidized (13). The
data presented here clearly show that lipid peroxide activity in
the myocardium increases in response to isoproterenol treatment
and this effect is prevented by pretreatment of the animals with
vitamin E - a membrane soluble antioxidant. It is possible that
increased superoxide radical activity due to autoxidation of
catecholamines promotes inorganic as well as organic free radical
chains in the hydrophobic region of the biological membranes as
shown schematically in Figure 4. These chain reactions can then
lead to the formation of lipid peroxides.

The scheme of events proposed in Fig. 4 is supported by the
present study as well as by reports published elsewhere. In this
regard free radicals are known to be produced during autoxidation
of catecholamines (5,9,20). Peroxidation of lipids in the myocardium due to excess release of catecholamines in severe emotional
and painful stress has also been reported (14). Since introduction
of peroxidation products in the membranes has been considered to
affect semipermeable characteristics of the membrane (4,16), increased lipid peroxide activity observed in this study may also
explain the occurrence of intracellular calcium overload (8,15) as
well as intracellular diffusion of extracellular protein tracers
(19) after isoproterenol treatment. The protective effect of
vitamin E against catecholamine-induced rhythm changes, myocardial

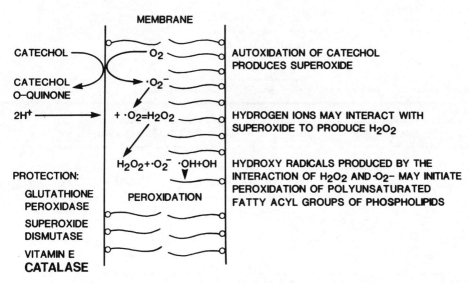

Fig. 4.   Scheme of steps involved in catecholamine (CATECHOL) in-
          duced lipid peroxidation in the membrane. Some of the
          naturally occurring protecting agents capable of inhibit-
          ing or slowing down the process of peroxidation have been
          listed in the lower half of the left column.

cell damage, decline in high energy phosphates and mortality reported earlier (25) may also have been due to a reduction in the
lipid peroxide content in the vitamin E protected heart. This
argument is further supported by the observation of increased sensitivity of vitamin E deficient animals to isoproterenol induced
myocardial changes. Obviously the antioxidant capacity in these
animals was markedly reduced due to a lack of vitamin E leading
to increased lipid peroxide formation at a lower dose of isoproterenol.

    In order to asses the full potential of oxidative pathways of
catecholamines one must also consider the fate and role of catechol
0-quinone - another major product of the autoxidation process
(Fig. 1). Since 0-quinone is an electron deficient metabolite,
it is highly reactive with sulphydryl groups. Original 0-quinone
can also be rereduced to the parent catecholamine by endogenous
reductants. Intracyclization of this species can also take place
near neutral pH yielding aminochromes e.g. adrenochrome. In a
study on the isolated rat hearts perfused with adrenochrome in the
presence of variety of reducing agents we have demonstrated the
occurrence of myocardial cell damage and contractile failure,

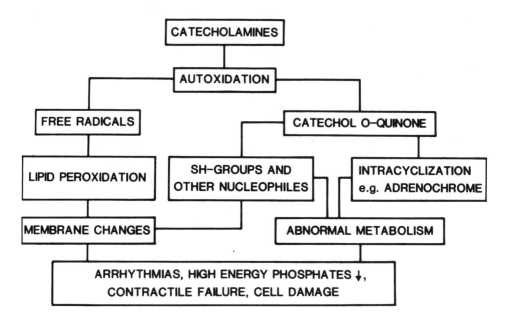

Fig. 5.   Scheme of events mediating catecholamine-induced heart
          disease.

probably by an interaction of this agent with sulphydryl group
(23).   Further oxidation products of adrenochrome were found to
be ineffective in producing these changes. In vivo administration
of adrenochrome has been shown to cause both arrhythmias and myocardial cell damage in a dose dependent manner (3,24).   Subcellular
membrane systems in the isolated rat heart have also been shown
to be effected by perfusion with adrenochrome (27) and oxidized
isoproterenol (6) indicating abnormalities of the cell metabolism
during exposure to oxidation products of catecholamines.   An overview of the potential role of the oxidative pathways in the genesis
of heart disease has been indicated in Fig. 5.

It should be recognized that the possibility of oxidative
pathways of catecholamines proposed here become great when the
usual monoamine oxidase or catechol 0 methyl transferase degradation processes are exceeded during situations leading to a chronic
increase in plasma catecholamines as has been reported in patients
after myocardial infarction (11,28) and other stressful situations
(12).

SUMMARY

Effects of vitamin E, a fat soluble antioxidant, on the isoproterenol-induced changes in the lipid peroxide activity as determined by a quantitation of malondialdehyde (MDA) content in the myocardium were examined. Isoproterenol treatment (80 mg/kg given over two days in two equal doses) caused more than 100 percent increase in the MDA content which was prevented by pretreatment of the animals with vitamin E (α-tocopherol acetate, 10 mg/kg) for two weeks. Animals maintained on vitamin E deficient diet for 8 weeks were found to be more sensitive to isoproterenol-induced increase in the MDA content. A small increase in MDA content was also seen due to vitamin E deficiency alone. These changes were found to be reversible upon a 2 week feeding of the animals on the normal diet coupled with vitamin E treatment. Based on these data it is proposed that free radical mediated increase in lipid peroxide activity may have a role in catecholamine-induced heart disease.

REFERENCES

1. AVIADO, D.M., WNUCK, A.L. & DE BEER, E.J. Cardiovascular effects of sympathomimetic bronchodilators: epinephrine, ephedrine, pseudoephedrine, isoproterenol, methoxyphenamine and isoprophenamine. J. Pharmacol. Exp. Therap. 122, 406-417 (1958).

2. BARBER, A.A. & BERNHEIM, F. Lipid peroxidation: its measurement, occurrence and significance in animal tissue. Adv. Gerontal. Res. 2, 355-403 (1967).

3. BEAMISH, R.E., DHILLON, K.S., SINGAL, P.K. & DHALLA, N.S. Protective effect of sulfinpyrazone against catecholamine metabolite adrenochrome-induced arrhythmias. Am. Heart. J. 102, 149-152 (1981).

4. CHANCE, B., SEISS, H. & BOVERIS, A. Hydroperoxide metabolism in mammalian organs. Physiol. Rev. 59, 527-605 (1979).

5. COHEN, G. & HEIKKILA, R.E. The generation of hydrogen peroxide, superoxide radical and hydroxyl radical by 6-hydroxydopamine, dialuric acid and related cytotoxic agents. J. Biol. Chem. 249, 2447-2452 (1974).

6. DHALLA, N.S., YATES, J.C., LEE, S.L. & SINGH, A. Functional and subcellular changes in the isolated rat heart perfused with oxidized isoproterenol. J. Mol. Cell. Cardiol. 10, 31-41 (1978).

7. DHALLA, N.S., SINGAL, P.K. & DHILLON, K. Mitochondrial functions and drug-induced heart disease. In: Drug-Induced Heart Disease, Vol. 5 (Bristow, M.R., ed.) North-Holland Biomedical Press, New York, 39-61 (1980).

8. FLECKENSTEIN, A., JANKE, T., DOERING, H.J. & PACHINGOER, O. Ca overload as the determinant factor in the production of catecholamine-induced myocardial lesions. Recent Advances in Studies on Cardiac Structure and Metabolism. 2, 455-466 (1973).

9. GRAHAM, D.G., TIFFANY, S.M., BELL, W.R. & GUTKNECTH, W.F. Autoxidation versus covalent binding of quinones as the mecha-

nism of toxicity of dopamine, 6-hydroxydopamine and related
compounds toward C 1300 neuroblastoma cells in vitro. Mol.
Pharmacol. 14, 644-653 (1978).

10. HUNTER, F.E., GEBICKI, J.M., HOFFSTEN, P.E., WEINSTEIN, J. &
     SCOTT, A. Swelling and lysis of rat liver mitochondria in-
     duced by ferrous ions. J. Biol. Chem. 238, 828-835 (1963).

11. JEQUIER, E. & PERRET, C. Urinary excretions of catecholamines
     and their main metabolites after myocardial infarction relat-
     ionship to the clinical syndrome. Eur. J. Clin. Invest. 1,
     77-82 (1970).

12. LEVI, L. Neuroendocrinology of anxiety. In: Studies of Anx-
     iety (Lader, M.H., ed.) Headley, London, P. 40 (1970).

13. MAY, H.E. & McCAY, P.B. Reduced triphosphopyridine nucleotide
     oxidase-catalyzed alterations of membrane phospholipids. J.
     Biol. Chem. 243, 2296-2305 (1968).

14. MEERSON, F.Z. Disturbances of metabolism and cardiac function
     under the action of emotional painful stress and their prophy-
     laxis. Basic. Res. Cardiol. 75, 479-500 (1980).

15. NIRDLINGER, E.L. & BRAMANTE, P.O. Subcellular myocardial
     ionic shifts and mitochondrial alterations in the course of
     isoproterenol-induced cardiomyopathy of the rat. J. Mol. Cell.
     Cardiol. 6, 49-60 (1974).

16. PLAA, G.L. & WITSCHE, H. Chemicals, drugs and lipid peroxida-
     tion. Ann. Rev. Pharmacol. 16, 125-141 (1976).

17. PLACER, Z.A., CUSHMAN, L.L. & JOHNSON, B.C. Estimation of
     product of lipid peroxidation (Malonyl dialdehyde) in bio-
     chemical systems. Anal. Biochem. 16, 359-365 (1966).

18. RONA, G., CHAPPEL, C.I., BALAZS, T. & GAUDRY, R. An infarct-
     like myocardial lesion and other toxic manifestations produc-
     ed by isoproterenol in the rat. A.M.A. Archiv. Pathol. 67,
     443-455 (1959).

19. RONA, G., HUTTNER, I., BOUTET, M. & BADONNEL, M.-C. Coronary
     microcirculatory factors in cardiac muscle cell injury. Re-
     cent Advances in Studies on Cardiac Structure and Metabolism.
     12, 559-571 (1978).

20. SACHS, C. & JONSSON, G. Mechanisms of action of 6-hydroxy-
     dopamine. Biochem. Pharmacol. 24, 1-8 (1975).

21. SINGAL, P.K., MATSUKUBO, M.P. & DHALLA, N.S. Calcium-related
     changes in the ultrastructure of mammalian myocardium. Br.
     J. Exp. Pathol. 60, 96-106 (1979).

22. SINGAL, P.K., DHILLON, K.S., BEAMISH, R.E. & DHALLA, N.S.
     Protective effect of zinc against catecholamine-induced myo-
     cardiac changes: Electrocardiographic and ultrastructural
     studies. Lab. Invest. 44, 426-433 (1981).

23. SINGAL, P.K., YATES, J.C., BEAMISH, R.E. & DHALLA, N.S.
     Influence of reducing agents on adrenochrome-induced changes
     in the heart. Arch. Pathol. Lab. Med. 105, 664-669 (1981).

24. SINGAL, P.K., DHILLON, K.S., BEAMISH, R.E., KAPUR, N. &
     DHALLA, N.S. Myocardial cell damage and cardiovascular
     changes due to I.V. infusion of adrenochrome in rats. Brit.

J. Exp. Pathol. 63, 167-176 (1982).

25. SINGAL, P.K., KAPUR, N., DHILLON, K.S., BEAMISH, R.E. & DHALLA, N.S. Role of free radicals in catecholamine-induced cardio-myopathy. Can. J. Physiol. Pharmacol.(1982, in press).

26. TAKENAKA, F. & HUGUCHI, M. High-energy phosphate contents of subendocardium and supepicardium in the rat treated with iso-proterenol and some other drugs. J. Mol. Cell. Cardiol. 6, 123-135 (1974).

27. TAKEO, S., TAAM, G.M.L., BEAMISH, R.E. & DHALLA, N.S. Effect of adrenochrome on calcium accumulation by heart mitochondria. Biochem. Pharmacol. 30, 157-163 (1981).

28. VALORI, C., THOMAS, M., SHILLINGFORD, J. Free noradrenaline and adrenaline excretion in relation to clinical syndromes following myocardial infarction. Am. J. Cardiol. 20, 605-609 (1967).

HIGH ENERGY PHOSPHATES, ANAEROBIC GLYCOLYSIS AND IRREVERSIBILITY IN ISCHEMIA

Robert B. Jennings, Keith A. Reimer, Robert N. Jones and Robert B. Peyton

Departments of Pathology and Surgery*
Duke University Medical Center
Durham, N.C.

Results of recent studies of energy production in severe or total ischemia in the dog heart have shown a striking relationship between deficient supplies of high energy phosphate and the loss of much of the adenine nucleotide pool.[1,2] The depletion of the adenine nucleotide pool in ischemia occurs because the ischemic tissue utilizes high energy phosphate at a greater rate than it can produce it by anaerobic glycolysis.[2-6] Some of the interrelationships among anaerobic glycolysis, energy metabolism, and cell death will be reviewed in this paper.

ADENINE NUCLEOTIDE POOL IN SEVERE REGIONAL ISCHEMIA:

The effect of severe ischemia on ATP and the adenine nucleotide pool (ΣAd) of left ventricular myocardium is shown in Fig. 1. Groups of 4-6 open-chest dogs anesthetized with pentobarbital were subjected to 0, 15, 30, 40, 60, 120, and 240 minutes of ischemia. Pure samples of ischemic myocardium were taken with the aid of thioflavine S to identify accurately that the tissue being assayed was severely ischemic. The results showed that both ATP and the ΣAd pool decreased rapidly until, at 40 minutes, virtually all the ATP and much of the ΣAd had disappeared. At this time, the injury to most of the myocytes in this region is irreversible.

Evidence for irreversibility in ischemic injury includes failure to salvage ischemic cells by reperfusion with arterial blood[1] as well as the presence of characteristic ultrastructural

*This work was supported in part by grants HL 23138 and HL 27416 from the National Heart, Lung and Blood Institute of the National Institutes of Health.

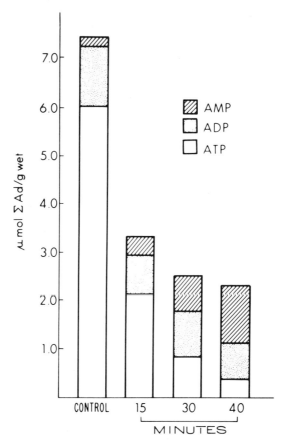

Figure 1. The ΣAd of normal and severely ischemic myocardium (mean of 3-5 dogs ±S.E. of mean) of dogs subjected to proximal occlusion of the circumflex branch of the left coronary artery are shown. Control data was pooled. Normal or mildly ischemic cells were excluded from the ischemic samples with intravenous thioflavine S (see text). After 40 minutes of ischemia, when most myocytes in the sample are irreversibly injured, only 6% of the initial ATP and 31% of the ΣAd remained in the tissue. (The data is plotted from Table 2 of reference 1.)

and functional evidence of severe cellular damage[1,2]. The unexpectedly close association between marked ATP depletion and the early phase of irreversibility may be a cause and effect relationship. However, proof of causality requires identification of the reaction or reactions requiring ATP, the absence of which leads to the development of irreversibility. To date, such a reaction or reactions have not been identified.[2]

In addition to being associated with low ATP, irreversibility is associated with a high tissue lactate. In the experiments described above, lactate was increased 25-30 times above control (Fig. 2) early in the irreversibile phase. Moreover, once tissue lactate reached 50-60 µmol/g wet, anaerobic glycolysis (lactate production) ceased.[2,3]

ENERGY PRODUCTION AND UTILIZATION OF ATP IN ISCHEMIA

Fig. 3 shows the reactions which produce and utilize ATP in ischemia.[2] In the absence of oxygen, oxidative phosphorylation produces no high energy phosphate (HEP) and in the absence of a continuous supply of substrate, substrate level phosphorylation also produces no significant ATP. This leaves only 20-22 µmoles of reserve HEP present in dog myocardium (5.6 µmol ATP x 2 + 1.2 µmol of ADP + 8 µmoles of CP or 20.8 total µmol HEP plus new ATP produced by anaerobic glycolysis). About 44 µmoles/g of glucose equivalents of glycogen also are present. If all the glycogen were converted to lactate by anaerobic glycolysis, then 3 net µmoles of HEP would be produced per µmole of glucose converted to lactate which yields a net of 44 x 3 = 132 µmoles of ATP.[3,7] Thus, the maximum amount of HEP which can be produced and utilized in zones of low-flow or total ischemia is 132 + 20.8 = 152.8 µmole HEP.

The reactions which utilize HEP in ischemia are shown in the lower half of Fig 3. The size of the arrows indicates the theoretical magnitude of the contribution of each reaction. Contraction is the major function utilizing HEP in healthy myocardium; continued contraction for the first few seconds of ischemia utilizes much of the reserve HEP of the myocyte, but, for unknown reasons, after 15-30 seconds of ischemia, effective contractions cease. In contrast to skeletal muscle, little reserve HEP is present in heart, and in fact Morgan and Neely (8) have shown that the reserve supply can support less than a minute of contractile activity. On theoretical grounds, the major reactions using ATP in the ischemic myocytes are the Na^+, K^+ ATPase of the sarcolemma and the Ca^{2+} activated ATPase of the sarcoplasmic reticulum. These ATPases, plus adenyl cyclase, fatty CoA synthetase, and probably other ATPases are considered to be the principal reactions using ATP in acutely ischemic myocardium.

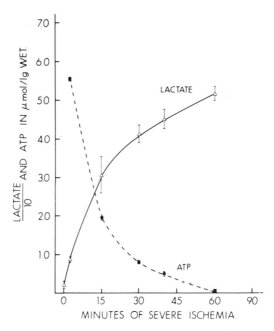

Figure 2. The inverse relationship between tissue ATP and lactate
in the zone of severe ischemia is plotted in this figure (Fig. 9
illustrates this relationship in total ischemia). Both ATP and
lactate results are considered to be asymptotic at 60 minutes because results of total ischemia experiments, in which all tissue is
equally injured, show that no further lactate is produced when the
ATP has fallen to only 0.18 μmole/g of wet tissue as noted at 60
minutes of ischemia in this figure. Thus, although not shown,
anaerobic glycolysis and lactate production have virtually ceased
at 60 minutes. After 4 and 24 hours of severe regional ischemia,
ATP is unchanged and lactate has fallen to 45 and 7 μmoles/g
respectively. The decrease in tissue lactate is due to diffusion of
this anion from the ischemic tissue to the systemic circulation.
(This graph was plotted from data reported in reference 1 as well as
from unpublished data from this experiment.)

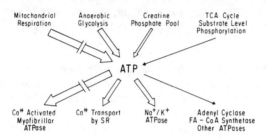

Figure 3. The principal reactions producing and utilizing HEP in ischemic tissue are illustrated. In severe ischemia, aerobic respiration is abolished. The preexisting stores of HEP, in the form of creatine phosphate (CP), ATP, or ADP are relatively small. Thus, anaerobic glycolysis becomes the principal source of energy, producing 80-90% of the high-energy phosphate bonds that can be utilized by ischemic tissue. Energy utilization also is markedly reduced during ischemia. Cardiac contraction, which is mediated by the Ca^{2+} activated myofibrillar ATPase, consumes much of the ATP produced in aerobic myocardium. However, contraction is abolished or severely depressed in areas of severe ischemia. Nevertheless, ATP continues to be required to remove Na^+ from the cell, to keep Ca^{2+} sequestered in the sarcoplasmic reticulum, and for a variety of other cellular processes that may continue to compete for the remaining ATP. The width of the arrows indicates the estimated quantitative importance of the various reactions. Substrate level phosphorylation of α-ketoglutarate in the mitochondria does not require O_2, but the tissue content of substrates which can be shuttled to α-ketoglutarate is small. Thus, these mechanisms do not produce a significant quantity of new ATP. (This figure is reproduced from reference 2 with permission of the publishers.)

RELATION BETWEEN ADENINE NUCLEOTIDE POOL DEGRADATION AND ENERGY
PRODUCTION IN TOTAL ISCHEMIA:

The relationship between energy production from anaerobic glycolysis and the adenine nucleotide pool is difficult to study in
regional ischemia both because only small quantities of tissue are
available for analysis and because of variation in the severity of
ischemia from dog to dog as a function of variable collateral flow.
For this reason, we have analyzed these processes in total
ischemia, i.e., in tissue receiving no arterial flow[9] and have
found that virtually the same changes are produced in total ischemia as are observed in severe ischemia in vivo, but on a slower
time scale.[3,4]

Total ischemia is produced by incubating excised hearts of
normal dogs in a moist environment at 37°C. The data in Fig. 4
shows that the totally ischemic myocardium exhibits progressive
depletion of ATP and parallel degradation of adenine nucleotides.
Note that the ATP and ΣAd pool depletion are parallel processes for
the first 60-90 minutes but that later, the degradation of the ΣAd
pool slows and AMP begins to accumulate. The lost nucleotides can
be recovered stoichiometrically as the nucleosides and bases, i.e.,
adenosine, inosine, hypoxanthine and xanthine (Fig. 5).

If one assumes that anaerobic glycolysis remains coupled with
phosphorylation of ADP and that alternate sources of high energy
phosphate production are insignificant in total ischemia, then one
can estimate high energy phosphate production during severe or
total ischemia from the lactate produced by anaerobic glycolysis.
This technique of assessment of production and utilization is shown
in Fig. 6. During the first 1-3 minutes of ischemia there was rapid
consumption of high energy phosphate and a burst of anaerobic glycolysis. Thereafter, both lactate production and high energy phosphate bond production and utilization slowed but continued at a
constant rate until 50-60 μmoles of lactate had accumulated within
the tissue. At about this time, virtually all of the reserve high
energy phosphate had been split and anaerobic glycolysis ceased.

Note that the rate of high energy phosphate production and
utilization is faster during ischemia in vivo. Presumably this is
due to the continued electrical and perhaps, slight mechanical activity of the low-flow ischemic myocardium in vivo.

The initial acceleration of the rate of glycolysis presumably
is due to and to the conversion of phosphorylase b to a, thereby
promoting rapid glycogenolysis,[10,11] and to removal of allosteric
inhibition of phosporylase b and rate limiting steps of glycolysis.
The phosphorylase conversion is stimulated by ischemia induced catecholamine release and the consequent formation of cyclic AMP. The
normal inhibition of phosphorylase b is reduced because of the

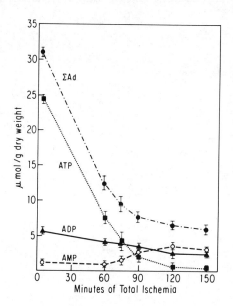

Figure 4. The progressive degradation of total adenine nucleotides
(ΣAd) in parallel with the depletion of ATP during total ischemia is
illustrated. Adenosine diphosphate (ADP) content decreased slowly
throughout 150 minutes of total ischemia. Adenosine monophosphate
(AMP) content was unchanged at 60 minutes but increased between 60
and 120 minutes, suggesting either that 5'-nucleotidase was becoming inhibited or that AMP was being sequestered in a compartment in-
accessible to this enzyme. (This figure is reproduced from reference 4 with permission of the publishers.)

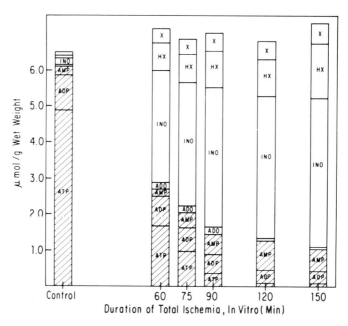

Figure 5.   The decrease in ATP, ADP, and ΣAd (ATP, ADP, plus AMP)
that occurs as a function of the period of total ischemia is illustrated.   The decrease in the ΣAd is accounted for by a marked
increase in the content of inosine (INO), hypoxanthine (HX), and
xanthine (X).   (This figure is reproduced from reference 3 with
permission of the publishers.)

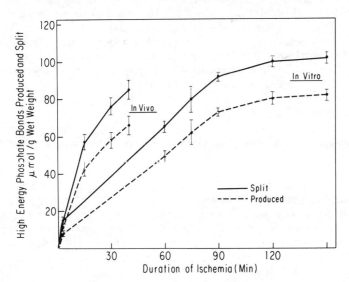

Figure 6.   The rates of high-energy phosphate bond utilization
(split) and production via anaerobic glycolysis (estimated from
lactate accumulation on the basis Δ lactate x 1.5 = μmoles ATP
produced from anaerobic glycolysis) in severe ischemia in vivo or
total ischemia in vitro are plotted as a function of the duration of
ischemia. Both the rate of production and the rate of utilization
were much higher in vivo than in vitro.   The temperature of the
heart was 37° C in both experiments.   (This figure is reproduced
from reference 3 with permission of the publishers.

reduced sarcoplasmic ATP and increased AMP and inorganic phosphate. Phosphofructokinase (PFK) is activated by the increased quantities of the allosteric effectors ADP, AMP and inorganic phosphate, and by reduction in the inhibition of this enzyme by ATP during ischemia.[11,12] Increased hexokinase and pyruvate kinase activity also contribute to the acceleration of anaerobic glycolysis characteristic of the early phase of ischemia.[13]

The slowing of the glycolytic rate observed shortly after the onset of total ischemia has been observed previously in rat hearts subjected to low-flow ischemia.[5,6,14] In these hearts, a rapid initial burst of anaerobic glycolysis was followed by contractile failure, slow lactate production, and depletion of high energy phosphates and adenine nucleotides. The mechanism (s) causing the slowing of the glycolytic rate after the initial burst of anaerobic glycolysis probably are related to inhibition of glyceraldehyde-3-phosphate dehydrogenase because of excessive levels of NADH and lactate and insufficent pyruvate. In addition, PFK is inhibited by acidosis and by the accumulation of lactate.[14]

The explanation for the cessation of glycolysis is not known. In our studies, it occurred at a time when 25-30% of the glycogen still was present in the heart[15] and when glucose-6-phosphate content had increased to 3-4.5 μmoles/g wet weight. Thus, it seems likely that glycolysis ceased because of low sarcoplasmic ATP. Kubler and Spieckerman[13] have noted a similar phenomenon in the isolated perfused anoxic rat heart. The low sarcoplasmic ATP limits the conversion of fructose-6-phosphate to fructose 1,6 diphosphate; glucose-6-phosphate accumulates as a consequence of inhibition of PFK. On the other hand, inactivation of glycolytic enzymes, loss of cofactors critical for glycolysis through the damaged sarcolemma of the irreversibly injured cells or other events also could explain why glycolysis ceased. The virtual cessation of glycolysis as well as the low ATP and high lactate all occurred at or about the same time as signs of irreversible injury became detectable.

The faster rate of depletion of high energy phosphate in severe ischemia in contrast to total ischemia was associated with a greater rate of lactate production, an observation which suggests that the rate of anaerobic glycolysis in ischemia continues to be modulated in part by the demand for high energy phosphate, and presumably is mediated by the relative concentrations of ATP, ADP, AMP, and inorganic phosphate.

In neither form of ischemia can the rate of HEP production keep up with the rate of utilization of ATP; consequently the ADP concentration in the tissue increases and myokinase becomes active (Fig. 7). The activity of myokinase in the ischemic myocytes is

CRITICAL SEQUENCE IN ISCHEMIA

ATP Utilization > ATP Production

Result --   ADP ↑ MYOKINASE
                    ACTIVE

ATP and AMP PRODUCED

AMP DESTROYED BY 5' NUCLEOTIDASE
    with production of ADENOSINE

ADENOSINE diffuses to extracellular
    space and is lost from myocyte

Figure 7. This figure summarizes the critical sequence in ischemia
in terms of the destruction of adenine nucleotide pool.

critical in that it permits recovery of the second high energy phosphate bond of ADP. However, the AMP which results is further
catabolized by 5' nucleotidase. Since the cell membrane is im-
perme able to nucleotides and permeable to nucleosides and bases,
the adenosine produced is lost from the myocyte and the result is
depletion of the total adenine nucleotide pool. Further degradation of adenosine follows the reaction sequence shown in Fig. 8. It
should be noted that AMP also is produced from ATP by other reactions, such as adenyl cyclase.

INTERVENTIONS DESIGNED TO ALTER THE RATE OF ATP UTILIZATION:

        Analysis of the reactions producing and utilizing ATP in
ischemia (Fig. 2) suggests that one could maintain higher net ATP
levels by interventions which either improved ATP production or
inhibited ATP utilization. The effect of hypothermia and of inhibition of anaerobic glycolysis on these processes will be presented
in this section.
        We have investigated the effect of temperature on the rate of
production, utilization and destruction of high energy phosphate in
the totally ischemic, potassium-arrested dog heart using a recently
described in vitro model in which the onset and full development of
contracture-rigor were detected through pressure changes in a bal-
loon in the cavity of the left ventricle.[15,16] Three degree centi-
grade decrements in temperature progressively slowed ATP utilization and also the production of ATP by anaerobic glycolysis. The

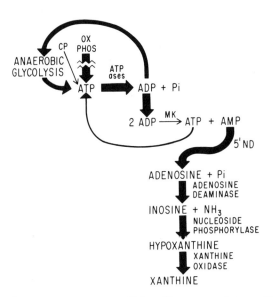

Figure 8.   The large arrows on this diagram shows the theoretical
route through which the adenine nucleotide pool is destroyed in
ischemia.   The inadequate supply of ATP in the ischemic tissue leads
to elevated ADP and activation of myokinase (MK).   The ATP formed
from ADP by myokinase is reutilized and the AMP is converted to
adenosine by 5' nucleotidase (5'ND).   Some AMP also is generated by
reactions such as adenyl cyclase or fatty acid CoA synthetase.   As
noted in Fig. 5, inosine and hypoxanthine are the principal end
products.   When ATP has fallen to 1-2% of control, more than 80% of
the adenine nucleotide pool can be recovered as inosine and hypoxanthine.

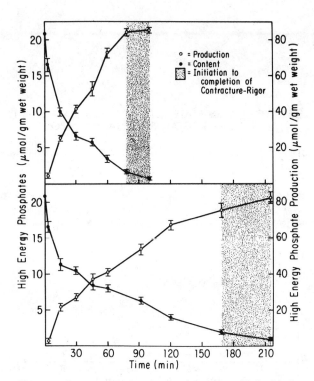

Figure 9.   Effect of temperature on myocardial high-energy phosphate production and depletion during total ischemia.   The total
myocardial content of high-energy phosphates and cumulative high-
energy phosphate production from anaerobic glycolysis at 37° and
28°C are compared in 9 hearts in each group by the technique described in Fig. 6.   Brackets indicate the standard errors of the
mean.   Although hypothermia delayed high-energy phosphate depletion, it also slowed high-energy phosphate production via anaerobic
glycolysis.   In all groups, lactate accumulation plateaued (and
high-energy phosphate production ceased) concurrent with the development of contracture-rigor and depletion of 95% of the ATP and
total high-energy phosphate reserves of the tissue. This figure is reproduced from reference 16 with permission of the publishers.

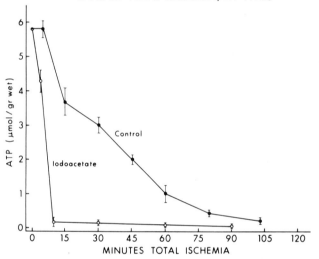

EFFECT OF IODOACETATE ON MYOCARDIAL ATP CONTENT
DURING TOTAL ISCHEMIA, IN VITRO

Figure 10.   The accelerated utilization of reserves of high energy
phosphate in hearts poisoned with sodium iodoacetate is shown.
Virtually all the ATP is gone in less than 8 minutes at $37^{\circ}C$ in
totally ischemic potassium arrested dog hearts in which anaerobic
glycolysis is completely inhibited.   The data on this graph is from
reference 17.

onset of contracture-rigor (Fig. 9) was delayed but was not pre-vented. Reserve supplies of high energy phosphates were utilized and much of the adenine nucleotide pool was destroyed at all temperatures studied. Anaerobic glycolysis provided more than 80% of the high energy phosphate utilized by the ischemic cell at all temperatures studied (between 28 and 40°C, but always ceased when ATP levels decreased to 1-2% of control (Fig. 9). Thus, it is clear that one can influence the speed of production and utilization of ATP by temperature and that the rates of the multi-enzyme processes involved both in the production of ATP and in the destruction of the adenine nucleotide pool seem to be affected to the same extent. Moreover, the rate of production of ATP by anaerobic glycolysis remains inversely related to the rate of destruction of ATP.

Since 80% of the HEP produced and utilized by the ischemic cell arises via anaerobic glycolysis, one would expect inhibition of anaerobic glycolysis to have a devastating effect on the ATP con-tent of ischemic myocardium. Fig. 10 shows that inhibition of anaerobic glycolysis by iodoacetate in totally ischemic myocardium causes the myocardial ATP supply to fall to less than 10% of control in only 8 minutes. Much of the adenine nucleotide pool is destroyed as well, and the hearts simultaneously develop full contracture-rigor.[17]

The results shown in Fig. 10 dramatically demonstrate the im-portance of anaerobic glycolysis in providing ATP to the ischemic heart as well as how small the reserves of HEP are in myocardium and how quickly they can be exhausted by the continued demand of the ischemic tissue for HEP.

SUMMARY

The effects of severe regional myocardial ischemia in vivo and total ischemia in vitro on energy production by anaerobic gly-colysis in dogs are described. The critical feature of ischemic injury in terms of the adenine nucleotide pool is the fact that the demand of severely or totally ischemic tissue for HEP exceeds the capacity of the damaged myocytes to produce it. The consequent depletion of ATP to very low levels and the destruction of the adenine nucleotide pool are associated with, or may be causally related to, the loss of cellular viability.

REFERENCES

1. Jennings, R.B., Hawkins, H.K., Lowe, J.E., Hill, M.L., Klotman, S., and Reimer, K.A: Relation between high energy phosphate and lethal injury in myocardial ischemia in the dog. Am. J. Path. 92:187–214 (1978).

2. Jennings, R.B. and Reimer, K.A.: Lethal myocardial ischemic injury. Am. J. Path. 102:241–255 (1981).

3. Jennings, R.B., Reimer, K.A., Hill, M.L, and Mayer, S.E.: Total myocardial ischemia, in vitro. I. Comparison of high energy phosphate production, utilization and depletion and of adenine nucleotide catabolism in total ischemia in vitro vs. severe ischemia in vivo. Circ. Res. 49:892–900 (1981).

4. Reimer, K.A., Jennings, R.B., and Hill, M.L.: Total myocardial ischemia, in vitro. II. High energy phosphate depletion and associated defects in energy metabolism, cell volume regulation, and sarcolemmal integrity. Circ. Res. 49:901–911 (1981).

5. Rovetto, M.J., Whitmer, J.T., and Neely, J.R.: Comparison of the effects of anoxia and whole–heart ischemia on carbohydrate utilization in isolated working rat heart. Circ. Res. 32:699–711 (1973).

6. Rovetto, M.J., Lamberton, W.F., and Neely, J.R.: Mechanisms of glycolytic inhibition in ischemic rat hearts. Circ. Res. 37:742–751 (1975).

7. Scheuer, J. and Stezoski, S.W.: Protective role of increased myocardial glycogen stores in cardiac anoxia in the rat. Circ. Res. 27:835–849 (1970).

8. Morgan, H.E. and Neely, J.R.: Metabolic regulation and myocardial function. In The Heart, J.W. Hurst, Ed., pp. 128–142. Baltimore:McGraw Hill Co. (1981).

9. Jennings, R.B.: Myocardial ischemia—observations, definitions and speculations (Editorial). J. Mol. Cell. Cardiol. 1:345–349 (1970).

10. Mayer, S.E., Williams, B.J., and Smith, J.M.: Adrenergic mechanisms in glycogen metabolism. Ann. N.Y. Acad. Sci. 139:682–702 (1967).

11. Wollenberger, A. and Krause, E.: Metabolic control characteristics of the acutely ischemic myocardium. Am. J. Cardiol. 22:349–359 (1968).

12.   Williamson, J.R.:   Glycolytic Control Mechanisms.   II. Kinetics of intermediate changes during the aerobic-anoxic transition in perfused rat heart. J. Biol. Chem. 241:5026–5036 (1966).

13.   Kübler, W. and Spieckermann, P.G.:   Regulation of glycolysis in the ischemic and anoxic myocardium.   J. Mol. Cell. Cardiol. 1:351–377 (1970).

14.   Neely, J.R. and Morgan, H.E.:   Relationship between carbohydrate and lipid metabolism and the energy balance of heart muscle. Ann. Rev. Physiol. 36:413–459 (1974).

15.   Jones, R.N., Reimer, K.A., Hill, M.L., and Jennings, R.B.: Effect of hypothermia on changes in high energy phsopahte production and utilization in total ischemia.   In press, J. Mol. Cell. Cardiol.

16.   Jones, R.N., Hill, M.L., Reimer, K.A., Wechsler, A.S., and Jennings, R.B.:   Effect of hypothermia on the relationship between adenosine triphosphate depletion and membrane damage. Surg. Forum XXXII 250–253 (1981).

17.   Peyton, R.B., Jones, R.M., Reimer, K.A., Wechsler, A., and Jennings, R.B.:   Inhibition of anaerobic glycolysis in total ischemia. Fed. Proc. 40:751 (1981).

MEMBRANE DAMAGE IN ISCHEMIA

L. Maximilian Buja, Kenneth R. Chien, Karen P. Burton*,
Herbert K. Hagler, Amal Mukherjee and James T. Willerson

Departments of Pathology and Internal Medicine (Cardiac
Division), The University of Texas Health Science Center
at Dallas, Dallas, Texas and *Department of Pharmacology
The University of South Alabama College of Medicine
Mobile, Alabama

INTRODUCTION

Our studies have evaluated the hypothesis that progressive
membrane damage, particularly to the plasma membrane, is a major
factor in the evolution of myocardial ischemic and hypoxic injury
and in particular the conversion from reversible to irreversible
injury. A proposed schema of progressive membrane injury involves
sequential changes characterized by: a) altered flux and distribution of monovalent ions and water leading to loss of cellular
potassium, increase in cell sodium, chloride and water, and cell
swelling and edema; b) altered flux and distribution of polyvalent
ions, including calcium, associated with further impairment in
cellular integrity, and c) physical defects in membrane integrity
in severely damaged cells [4,28]. The first two alterations (a
and b) could involve alterations in specific membrane transport
systems or, conversely, non-specific changes in membrane permeability.
The former catagory includes potential alterations in sodium-potassium ATPase, the slow calcium channel, the sodium-calcium exchange
system, and other such specific membrane systems. Alternatively,
the pathophysiologic changes could result from progressive increases
in membrane fluidity and permeability induced by changes in the
phospholipid bilayer of the membrane.

LANTHANUM PROBE STUDIES

We developed an ionic lanthanum probe technique for the study

421

of altered membrane integrity in isolated cardiac muscle preparations [6-8]. Lanthanum is an electron-dense, trivalent ion with
properties similar to those of calcium. Since lanthanum retains
an extracellular location in normal muscle, intracellular lanthanum
accumulation can serve as a marker of altered membrane permeability.
The general procedure is to subject isolated cardiac muscle to
control or experimental conditions and then to introduce 2-5mM
lanthanum choloride in buffer for a short time interval prior to
fixation for ultrastructural examination. The technique has been
used to evaluate membrane permeability changes during the course
of hypoxia with and without reoxygenation in isolated cat papillary
muscle [6,8] and ischemia with reflow in the perfused rabbit interventricular septal preparation [7].

In the isolated cat papillary muscle preparations, after 75
minutes of hypoxia, many muscle cells showed only mild alteration
of ultrastructure but exhibited abnormal intracellular deposition
of lanthanum along the I-bands of the myofibrils and within the
mitochondria [6]. If reoxygenation was provided after 75 minutes
of hypoxia, significant structural and functional recovery occurred
and abnormal lanthanum accumulation was not observed. However, if
hypoxia was continued for 2-3 hours, or if 75 minutes of hypoxia was
combined with glucose deprivation, reoxygenation was associated
with continued functional depression and severe ultrastructural
injury with prominant intracellular lanthanum in many muscle cells
[6,8].

Further studies were performed in the isolated perfused rabbit
interventricular septal preparation, in which ischemia was induced
for periods of 1, 1½ and 2 hours followed by reflow for 1 hour [7].
After 1 hour of ischemia, the septa contained a mixed population of
muscle cells with mild structural injury, characterized by mild
cytoplasmic and organellar edema and glycogen loss, and those with
severe ultrastructural injury, characterized by clumping of the
chromatin and severe alterations of the mitochondria. At this
time interval, intracellular lanthanum accumulation was limited to
the muscle cells with severe structural damage. After 1½ hours of
ischemia and 1 hour of reflow, the percentages of mildly damaged
and severely damaged cells were increased. At this time interval,
abnormal lanthanum accumulation indicative of altered movement of
polyvalent ions was found, not only in severely damaged muscle cells,
but also in a significant proportion of the muscle cells with only
mild structural damage. After 2 hours of ischemia and reflow, the
septa had a large percentage of severely damaged myocytes, most
of which contain intracellular lanthanum [7].

The lanthanum probe findings also correlated with evidence of
functional recovery. Rate of tension development (+ dT/dt) showed
good recovery after 1 hour of ischemia and reflow, an intermediate
return of function after 1½ hours and very poor functional recovery

after 2 hours of ischemia and reflow. Resting tension showed a
return to a near normal level after 1 hour of ischemia and reflow,
a moderate persistent elevation after 1½ hours, and a greater persistent elevation after 2 hours of ischemia and reflow. From these
studies we concluded that abnormal intracellular lanthanum accumulation serves as a sensitive marker of an important membrane defect
to polyvalent ions which develops at a transitional stage in the
progression from reversible to irreversible injury [6-8].

ELECTRON PROBE X-RAY MICROANALYSIS

We have modified the perfused rabbit interventicular septal
preparation to leave the small right ventricular papillary muscles
attached to the septum for subsequent quick freezing, cryosectioning
and elemental analysis by the technique of energy dispersive x-ray
microanalysis [5,17]. When one subjects freeze-dried cryosections
to electron probe x-ray microanalysis, one obtains a spectrum containing specific elemental peaks of all of the various elements of
biological interest within small microregions of the cells. These
peaks from the test spectra are converted to elemental concentrations
using suitable elemental standards which we have prepared.

We have performed microanalyses on control papillary muscles
from non-perfused and perfused, oxygenated septa and also on papillary muscles from septa subjected to hypoxic perfusion for 60-90
minutes [5,17]. Little difference was measured in elemental concentration between non-perfused and perfused controls. Analysis of the
hypoxic muscles revealed two populations of muscle cells. The majority of the muscle cells exhibited significant loss of cytoplasmic
and mitochondrial potassium and increase in sodium without a measurable change in calcium. These myocytes also exhibited a decrease in
phosphorus probably reflecting a breakdown in high energy phosphates. A minority of the cells exhibited even further reductions
in mitochondrial and cytosolic potassium and increases in sodium.
These muscle cells, however, exhibited evidence of overloading with
calcium and inorganic phosphate which was characterized by the formation of electron dense inclusions and very prominant calcium and
phosphorus peaks in the mitochondria [5, 17]. The levels of calcium
and phosphorus which accumulated in the mitochondria exceeded the
levels which have been previously shown to produce severe damage
to isolated mitochondrial preparations [21].

MYOCARDIAL TISSUE SLICE STUDIES

We have also explored the pathophysiology of membrane injury
in the setting of regional myocardial ischemia in vivo [4]. The
left circumflex coronary artery was ligated in anesthetized mongrel
dogs for 30 or 60 minutes. Transmural blocks of tissue from the

control anterior myocardium and the ischemic (cyanotic) posterior
myocardium were obtained and divided into subepicardial, subendocardial and papillary muscle regions. Thin tissue slices were prepared and incubated in Krebs-Ringer - phosphate-succinate medium
containing trace amounts of ^{14}C-inulin. They were incubated either
at 0°C for 60 minutes, 37°C for 120 minutes, or were first subjected
to cold shock (0°C for 60 minutes) followed by rewarming (37°C for
60 minutes). Slices were processed to obtain wet weight, dry weight
and inulin space measurements. Inulin is a 5,000 molecular weight,
non-metabolizable polysaccharide, which is generally excluded from
normal cells. From these measurements, total tissue water, inulin
impermeable space and inulin diffusible space were calculated.

The response of control tissue to cold shock was characterized
by increase in the total tissue water and inulin impermeable space
without a change in inulin diffusible space. These measurements
were indicative of intracellular swelling following cold-induced
inhibition of energy-dependent membrane pumps. Upon rewarming, the
increases in total tissue water and inulin impermeable space were
reversed. In contrast, the ischemic tissue slices exhibited increases
in total tissue water, inulin impermeable space and inulin diffusible
space upon rewarming. Mild but significant increases in total tissue
water, inulin impermeable space, and inulin diffusible space were
present in all slices (subepicardial, subendocardial, papillary
muscle) after 30 minutes of coronary occlusion. After 60 minutes
of coronary occlusion, there were further increases in the alterations, and these increases were greatest in the ischemic papillary
muscle. The interpretation of these results is as follows: a) the
persistent elevation of total tissue water content after cold shock
and rewarming is consistent with defective cell volume regulation,
and b) the defective cell volume regulation is accompanied by increased membrane permeability reflected by expansion of the inulin
diffusible space [4].

To further define the nature of the membrane injury, control
and ischemic myocardial slices were incubated in isosmolar medium
as well as incubated in hyperosmolar media containing 40 milliosmolar mannitol, 100 milliosmolar mannitol or 50 milliosmolar polyethelene glycol [4]. All of the hyperosmolar agents produced significant reductions in the total tissue water, and this was accomplished
primarily by a shrinkage of the inulin impermeable space, with
minimal change in the inulin diffusible space. The 50 milliosmolar
polyethelyene glycol, a relatively large molecular weight compound
(6,000), was more effective than either 40 or 100 milliosmolar
mannitol, which has a molecular weight of 182.

On electron microscopic examination, control slices showed
minimal ultrastructural change whereas ischemic slices inucbated
in isomolar medium had many swollen myocytes. After incubation
in hyperosmolar media, particularly polyethelene glycol, two popula-

tions of myocytes were identified. Some myocytes had structurally
intact plasma membranes and showed little or no swelling after exposure to the polyethelyene glycol, whereas other myocytes had breaks
in the plasma membranes and remained swollen.

From the tissue slice studies we reached the following conclusions [4]. First, myocardial tissue slices from areas of in vivo
ischemia exhibit defective cell volume regulation and increased
membrane permeability after 30 minutes of coronary occlusion. The
alterations are most severe in slices obtained from ischemic papillary
muscle and subendocardium, but also occur in subepicardial slices.
Second, abnormal volume regulation in tissue slices from ischemic
myocardium can be partially modified since incubation in hyperosmolar solutions retards total fluid accumulation, but does not
produce a major reduction in increased inulin permeability. Polyethylene glycol, a larger molecule, exerts a greater reduction in
fluid accumulation than does mannitol. Third, the data suggest
that early ischemic injury results in a mixed population of myocytes,
including those with reversible alterations, as well as those with
severe irreversible alterations, in volume regulation and membrane
integrity.

ALTERATIONS IN ADRENERGIC RECEPTORS

Another potential consequence of altered membrane integrity in
ischemic myocardium is an alteration of one or more classes of membrane receptors involved in the regulation of various physiological
functions of the cell. We have recently been interested in evaluating
the effects of ischemic injury on adrenergic receptors [18,26]. We
measured the binding of the potent beta adrenergic antagonist, (-)
tritiated dihydroalprenolol, in membrane homogenates from control
and ischemic canine myocardium after ligation of the left anterior
descending coronary artery and in sham preparations [19,20]. Control
preparations gave typical binding curves for beta adrenergic receptors. No regional differences were detected in the left ventricles
of sham-operated dogs. However, after 1 hour of coronary occlusion,
ischemic myocardium exhibited an approximately 60% increase in the
number (B max) of beta adrenergic receptors without a change in
receptor affinity (K_D). We also showed that, when the increased
numbers of beta adrenergic receptors in ischemic myocardium were
stimulated by isoproterenol or epinephrine infusion, the ischemic
tissue developed increased levels of cyclic AMP and phosphorylase
activation (b to a conversion). Corr et al. have reported that the
number of alpha adrenergic receptors in feline heart increases after
30 minutes of coronary occlusion [13]. No change in muscarinic
cholinergic receptors was measured [19,20]. Further work is in
progress to characterize the potential significance of this change
in adrenergic receptors, which we feel may be a manifestation of
altered membrane function in ischemic myocytes. Furthermore, we feel

that this change may have physiologic significance, since as we
have previously shown, the degree of cell damage after early coronary
occlusion is variable such that some injured but viable myocytes
retain metabolic integrity after this period of coronary occlusion.

EFFECTS OF MEMBRANE INJURY

    It is important to consider the pathophysiologic consequences
of altered membrane function on the myocytes, since these consequences
will mediate the effects of altered membrane function in leading to
progressive cell injury. Altered monovalent ion and water accumulation leads to cell swelling, which in turn could alter oxygen transport distances, access to metabolites, transport distances for ions,
access to enzyme systems, and produce effects on organellar function
[4,21,28]. Altered flux of calcium ions has the potential for even-
tual net intracellular accumulation of calcium, direct toxic effects
on various membranes and enzymes, activation of degredative enzymes,
stimulation of ATP-dependent reactions leading to ATP depletion,
hypercontraction and eventually disruption of the cells [6-8,14,16,
22,23]. It is important to indicate that the magnitude of these
changes is dependent upon access to extracellular fluid. Thus, these
changes in ion and water content of cells will be most dramatic in
the setting of reperfusion injury [27], but also can be seen with
permanent coronary occlusion, particularly at the periphery of the
evolving infarct [3]. The changes in total content of water and ions,
however, are known to be minimal in the central ischemic zone [27].
Nevertheless, subtle shifts of ions and water from extracellular to
intracellular regions as well as intracellular redistribution may be
sufficient to produce these toxic effects.

MECHANISMS OF MEMBRANE DYSFUNCTION

    As mentioned above, the changes in monovalent ion, water, and
polyvalent ion flux could be mediated either by changes in specific
membrane pump systems or by progressive increases in non-specific
membrane permeability. We, as well as others, have obtained evidence
for depressed sodium-potassium ATPase activity during a relatively
early stage of cell injury [1,28]. We performed studies in an
isolated blood perfused canine heart preparation [28]. Following
60 minutes of permanent coronary occlusion, as well as temporary
occlusion and reflow, significant inhibition of sodium-potassium
ATPase activity in membrane homogenates was measured in both the
ischemic subendocardium and subepicardium. These results were confirmed by evidence of reduced tritiated ouabain binding in the
homogenates. The decreased sodium-potassium ATPase activity was
associated with multifocal swelling of myocytes but occurred prior
to the onset of extensive cell necrosis, as judged by morphologic
criteria and by the lack of reduction of ischemic tissue creatine

kinase activity. Other specific membrane transport systems may be
involved during the evolution of cell injury [25]. The mechanisms
of inhibition of sodium-potassium ATPase activity and possibly other
membrane transport systems is uncertain, but could involve progressive
depletion of a critical residual ATP pool as an energy source, or
enzymatic inhibition by various toxic metabolites which accumulate
in the ischemic cell.

Another hypothesis for progressive alterations in membrane function is a non-specific increase in membrane permeability related
to a change in membrane phospholipid composition [9,12,14]. Activation of membrane-associated phospholipases may be triggered by a
relatively small increase in cytosolic calcium secondary to derangements in specific calcium transport mechanisms at the level of the
sarcolemma, sarcoplasmic reticulum or mitochondria [16,22,23]. Phos-
pholipase-induced changes in membrane phospholipids may lead to
significant changes in membrane permeability with the potential for
marked calcium influx. Available evidence favors such a change in
membrane permeability rather than involvement of a specific membrane
transport system in the gross derangements of calcium homeostasis
which can accompany advanced stages of myocardial injury [2,15].

ALTERATIONS OF MEMBRANE PHOSPHOLIPIDS

The phospholipid hypothesis was stimulated by the work of
Farber, Chien and their associates [9,14], who studied phospholipid
metabolism in the setting of ischemic injury in the rat liver. They
found rapid and prominent depletion of the phospholipid content of
whole liver homogenates, which correlated with the onset of irreversible injury and massive calcium influx. Similar findings regarding
phospholipid depletion were recorded for isolated membrane homogenates.

Subsequently, Chien et al. [12] performed similar studies in
a model in which coronary occlusion was produced for various periods
of time in anesthetized dogs with or without reflow. Some animals
were injected with technetium-99m pyrophosphate, a scintigraphic
marker which has been shown previously to correlate with the development of irreversible myocardial injury [3]. After 1 hour of permanent coronary occlusion, there was an overall 3.3% reduction in total
phospholipids in the ischemic subendocardium which was associated
with a 5% decrease in phosphatidyl ethanolamine, a slight decrease
in phosphatidyl choline, and no change in cardiolipin. After 3 hours
of coronary occlusion, there was an overall 10.8% decrease in phospholipids which was associated with 11.6% decreases in both phosphatidyl ethanolamine and phosphatidyl choline and a slight decrease
in cardiolipin. Under our assay conditions and extraction procedures, we measured no or only slight increases in lysophospholipids.
In the animals subjected to temporary coronary occlusion and reper-

fusion, significant temporal and topographical correlations were
found between phospholipid degredation and accumulation of techne-
tium-99m pyrophosphate [12]. Similar correlations with metabolites
of fatty acids were not observed [10,11].

It must be stated that the alterations in phospholipid content
in ischemic canine myocardium were not as dramatic as those observed
in the setting of rat liver ischemia [9,12]. This may be due to
more active phospholipase activity in the liver model. However,
the temporal and topographical correlations with technetium-99m
pyrophosphate uptake suggest that either minimal changes in membrane
phospholipid composition or changes more subtle than changes in total
content could produce significant membrane dysfunction. To further
test this hypothesis, microsomal vesicles were prepared from canine
myocardium and loaded with ^{45}Ca by sodium-calcium exchange [12].
We then followed the effects on calcium efflux in these vesicles after
treatment with phospholipases. Treatment of the vesicles with
phospholipase C (0.01 mg per ml) produced a significant acceleration
of calcium efflux. Treatment with a similar concentration of phospholipase A produced a greater acceleration of calcium efflux. The
prominent changes in calcium flux were associated with a slight
decrease in the content of phosphatidyl choline, a slight increase in
lysophosphatidyl choline and minimal change in total phospholipid
composition of the microsomes. Thus, these studies suggest that
marked changes in membrane permeability properties can occur with
minimal alterations in total phospholipid content [12].

Additional evidence regarding the role of membrane phospholipids
has come from the studies of Farber and Chien and associates [9,14],
who tested the protective effects of chlorpromazine, a phenothiazine
with local anesthetic properties and the capability of blocking
degredation of membrane phospholipids. These workers showed that
chlorpromazine exerted a marked protective effect on phospholipid
degredation and markedly retarded ischemic injury in rat liver and
heart. We have recently evaluated the effect of choloropromazine
pretreatment on the course of ischemic injury and abnormal lanthanum
accumulation in the isolated rabbit interventricular septal preparation [7]. In this study three groups of rabbits were examined, i.e.,
rabbits pretreated in vivo with 15 or 25 mg. per kg of choloproma-
zine and non-treated rabbits. The perfused interventricular septal
preparations from the three groups were subjected to 1½ hours of
in vitro, no flow ischemia followed by 1 hour of reflow with subsequent exposure to lanthanum prior to fixation. Samples were processed from the same two anatomic sites from each muscle and a total
of 200 cell profiles from each muscle were examined for ultrastructural alterations and abnormal intracellular lanthanum accumulation.
Non-treated septa showed extensive injury with abnormal intracellular
lanthanum accumulation in muscle cells with mild as well as severe
structural damage. The chlorpromazine-pretreated muscles showed
less extensive ultrastructural alterations and marked reduction in

intracellular lanthanum accumulation. Chlorpromazine pretreatment
also had a beneficial effect on recovery of cardiac contractile
function.

These studies support the conclusion that a membrane defect
associated with altered phospholipid integrity and abnormal lanthanum
accumulation, and by implication abnormal calcium flux, has an important role in the progression of ischemic myocardial injury. Recently,
Peyton et al. [24] have tested the effects of cholorpromazine in a
global no flow ischemia model and failed to find a protective effect.
The discrepancies in these studies with cholorpromazine do not per se
negate the phospholipid hypothesis.

CONCLUSIONS

On the basis of the work reviewed above, we have reached the
following general conclusions. First, in myocardium subjected to
ischemia or related forms of injury, progressive dysfunction of the
sarcolemma produces major derrangements in cellular homeostasis,
including altered cell volume regulation, altered calcium flux and
multiple secondary effects resulting from altered electrolyte and
water balance. Second, the membrane injury is induced by ischemic
or related forms of injury per se, whereas the severity of cellular
edema, electrolyte shifts and calcium accumulation is determined by
the level of access to extracellular fluid provided by reperfusion
or collateral perfusion. Third, the irreversible phase of injury
may be produced by a severe alteration in membrane permeability,
which is characterized by the potential for increased net intracellular influx of calcium ions, and which appears to be linked to an
altered membrane phospholipid composition. Fourth, future work should
be directed at further elucidation of the nature and mechanisms
responsible for ischemic injury as well as optimal methods of pre-
serving membrane integrity.

REFERENCES

1. Beller, G.A., Conroy, J. & Smith, T.W. Ischemic-induced altera-
    tions in myocardial ($Na^+ + K^+$)- ATPase and cardiac glycoside
    binding. Journal of Clinical Investigation 57, 341-350, (1976).
2. Bourdillon, P.D. & Poole-Wilson, P.A. The effects of verapamil,
    quiescence, and cardioplegia on calcium exchange and mechanical
    function in ischemic rabbit myocardium. Circulation Research 50,
    360-368 (1982).
3. Buja, L.M., Tofe, A.J., Kulkarni, P.V., Mukherjee, A., Parkey,
    R.W., Francis, M.D., Bonte, F.J. & Willerson, J.T. Sites and
    mechanisms of localization of technetium-99m phosphorus radio-
    pharmaceuticals in acute myocardial infarcts and other tissues.
    Journal of Clinical Investigation 60, 724-740 (1977).

4.   Buja, L.M. & Willerson, J.T. Abnormalities of volume regulation
     and membrane integrity in myocardial tissue slices after early
     ischemic injury in the dog: effects of mannitol, polyethylene
     glycol, and propranolol. American Journal of Pathology 103, 79-95
     (1981).

5.   Burton, K.P., Hagler, H.K., Greico, C.A., Willerson, J.T. & Buja,
     L.M. Electron probe x-ray microanalysis of cryosectioned normal
     and hypoxic myocardium (Abstract). Federation Proceedings 39,
     276 (1980).

6.   Burton, K.P., Hagler, H.K., Templeton, G.H., Willerson, J.T. &
     Buja, L.M. Lanthanum probe studies of cellular pathophysiology
     induced by hypoxia in isolated cardiac muscle. Journal of Clini-
     cal Investigation 60, 1289-1302 (1977).

7.   Burton, K.P., Hagler, H.K., Willerson, J.T. & Buja, L.M. Rela-
     tionship of abnormal intracellular lanthanum accumulation to
     progression of ischemic injury in isolated perfused myocardium:
     effect of chlorpromazine. American Journal of Physiology: Heart
     and Circulatory Physiology 241, H714-H723 (1981).

8.   Burton, K.P., Templeton, G.H., Hagler, H.K., Willerson, J.T. &
     Buja, L.M. Effect of glucose availability on functional membrane
     integrity, ultrastructure and contractile performance following
     hypoxia and reoxygenation in isolated feline cardiac muscle.
     Journal of Molecular and Cellular Cardiology 12, 109-133 (1980).

9.   Chien, K.R., Abrams, J., Serroni, A., Martin, J.T. & Farber, J.L.
     Accelerated phospholipid degradation and associated membrane
     dysfunction in irreversible ischemic liver cell injury. Journal
     of Biological Chemistry 253, 4809-4817 (1978).

10. Chien, K.R., Buja, L.M., Mukherjee, A. & Willerson, J.T. Fatty
     acyl metabolites and membrane injury in ischemic canine myocar-
     dium: dissociation from a sarcolemmal Ca^{++} permeability defect
     and correlation with mitochondrial dysfunction (Abstract). Cir-
     culation 64 (Supplement LV), LV-153 (1981).

11. Chien, K.R., Buja, L.M. & Willerson, J.T. Induction of a revers-
     cardiac lipidosis and focal cardiomyopathy by a dietary long
     chain fatty acid: similarity to lipid accumulation in border
     zones of myocardial infarcts (Abstract). Clinical Research 30,
     480A (1982).

12. Chien, K.R., Reeves, J.P., Buja, L.M., Bonte, F., Parkey, R.W.
     & Willerson, J.T. Phospholipid alterations in canine ischemic
     myocardium. Temporal and topographical correlations with Tc-99m-
     PPi accumulation and an in vitro sarcolemmal Ca^{2+} permeability
     defect. Circulation Research 48, 711-719 (1981).

13. Corr, P.B., Shayman, J.A., Kramer, J.B. & Kipnis, R.J. Increased
     alpha adrenergic receptors in ischemic cat myocardium. Journal
     of Clinical Investigation 67, 1232-1236 (1981).

14. Farber, J.L., Chien, K.R. & Mittnacht, Jr., S. The pathogenesis
     of irreversible cell injury in ischemia. American Journal of
     Pathology. 102, 271-281 (1981).

15. Frank, J.S., Beydler, S., Kreman, M. & Rau, E.E. Structure of
     the freeze-fractured sarcolemma in the normal and anoxic rabbit

myocardium. Circulation Research 47, 131-143 (1980).

16. Jennings, R.B. & Reimer, K.A. Lethal myocardial ischemic injury.
    American Journal of Pathology 102, 241-255 (1981).

17. Hagler, H., Burton, K. & Buja, L. Electron probe x-ray micro-
    analysis of normal and injured myocardium: methods and results.
    In Microprobe Analysis of Biological Systems, T.E. Hutchinson &
    A.P. Somlyo, Eds, pp. 127-155. New York: Academic Press (1981).

18. Lefkowitz, R.J. Direct binding studies of adrenergic receptors:
    biochemical, physiologic, and clinical implications. Annals of
    Internal Medicine 91, 450-458 (1979).

19. Mukherjee, A., Bush, L.R., McCoy, K.E., Duke, R.J., Hagler, H.,
    Buja, L.M. & Willerson, J.T. Relationship between β-adrenergic
    recptor numbers and physiological responses during experimental
    canine myocardial ischemia. Circulation Research 50, 735-741
    (1982).

20. Mukherjee, A., Wong, T.M., Buja, L.M., Lefkowitz, R.J. & Willer-
    son, J.T. Beta adrenergic and muscarinic cholinergic receptors
    in canine myocardium: effects of ischemia. Journal of Clinical
    Investigation 64, 1423-1428 (1979).

21. Mukherjee, A., Wong, T.M., Templeton, G.H., Buja, L.M. & Willer-
    son, J.T. Influence of volume dilution, lactate, phosphate and
    calcium on mitochondrial functions. American Journal of Physiol-
    ogy: Heart and Circulatory Physiology 237, H224-H238 (1979).

22. Nayler, W.G. The role of calcium in the ischemic myocardium.
    American Journal of Pathology 102, 262-270 (1981).

23. Nayler, W.G., Poole-Wilson, P.A. & Williams, A. Hypoxia and
    calcium. Journal of Molecular and Cellular Cardiology 11, 683-
    706 (1979).

24. Peyton, R.B., Hill, M.L., Kinney, R.B., Reimer, K.A. & Jennings,
    R.B. The effect of chlorpromazine on myocardial injury in total
    ischemia (Abstract). Federation Proceedings 41:381 (1982).

25. Shine, K.I. Ionic events in ischemia and anoxia. American
    Journal of Pathology 102, 256-261 (1981).

26. Watanabe, A.M., Jones, L.R., Manalan, A.S. & Besch, Jr., H.R.
    Cardiac autonomic receptors: recent concepts from radiolabeled
    ligand-binding studies. Circulation Research 50, 161-174 (1982).

27. Whalen, D.A., Jr., Hamilton, D.G., Ganote, C.E. & Jennings, R.B.
    Effect of a transient period of ischemia on myocardial cells:
    I. Effects on cell volume regulation. American Journal of
    Pathology 74:381-398 (1974).

28. Willerson, J.T., Scales, F., Mukherjee, A., Platt, M., Temple-
    ton, G.H., Fink, G.S. & Buja, L.M. Abnormal myocardial fluid
    retention as an early manifestation of ischemic injury. Ameri-
    can Journal of Pathology 87, 159-188 (1977).

INTRACELLULAR CALCIUM HOMEOSTASIS WITH

EXTRAPOLATIONS TO CARDIAC ISCHEMIA

John R. Williamson, Suresh K. Joseph, Kathleen E. Coll,
James S. Marks, and Ronald H. Cooper

Department of Biochemistry and Biophysics
University of Pennsylvania
Philadelphia, Pennsylvania 19104

INTRODUCTION

The processes involved in the maintenance of intracellular
calcium homeostasis are complex and still poorly understood. Most
cells contain between 3 and 6 μmol total calcium per g dry wt, are
exposed to medium containing 1.25 mM free Ca^{2+} and yet maintain an
intracellular free Ca^{2+} concentration of 50 to 200 nM in the resting state[1-7]. Apart from calcium bound to the glycocalyx and head
groups of externally facing phospholipids of the plasma membrane,
which rapidly exchanges with the extracellular Ca^{2+}[8], most of the
intracellular calcium is present in bound form in mitochondria and
sarcoplasmic reticulum. $^{45}Ca^{2+}$ flux studies have shown that there
is a dynamic equilibrium between extracellular and intracellular
Ca^{2+} and between the different intracellular calcium pools[8,9].
However, $^{45}Ca^{2+}$ exchange studies and derived flux data are difficult to interpret, and provide misleading values for intracellular
pool sizes and no information concerning free Ca^{2+} concentrations
or ratios of bound to free Ca^{2+}.

Over the past few years our laboratory has been investigating
the topic of cellular calcium homeostasis from a different vantage
point, with emphasis being placed on the development of methods to
measure free Ca^{2+} concentrations in the cytosolic and mitochondrial
matrix spaces, the kinetics of Ca^{2+} cycling across the mitochondrial membrane and the distribution of total calcium between the
major intravesicular pools. To date these studies have focussed on
the use of isolated hepatocytes[3,10] and isolated liver and heart
mitochondria[11], but the methods in principle are applicable to any
isolated cell and studies are in progress with Ca^{2+}-resistant

myocytes.

In this paper we present some recent unpublished data on the regulation of Ca^{2+} cycling in liver mitochondria, the effect of mixing sarcoplasmic reticulum vesicles with mitochondria on steady state free Ca^{2+} concentrations and inter-organelle calcium flux, and a summary of our current knowledge of calcium homeostasis in the hepatocyte. Also included is a brief review of the mechanisms involved in regulating intracellular Ca^{2+} flux in the heart, and finally we present our working hypothesis concerning the physiological and pathological changes to intracellular calcium homeostasis that may be involved in the transition from reversible to irreversible ischemic injury.

EXPERIMENTAL PROCEDURES

Preparation of Hepatocytes, Mitochondria and Sarcoplasmic Reticulum

Hepatocytes were prepared from fed, male rats of the Sprague-Dawley strain (180-220 g) by modifications[12] of the method of Berry and Friend[13]. The cells were washed and resuspended in Ca^{2+} and Mg^{2+}-free Hank's medium containing 137 mM NaCl, 4.2 mM $NaHCO_3$, 5.4 mM KCl, 0.44 mM KH_2PO_4, 0.33 mM Na_2HPO_4 and 20 mM HEPES (4-(2-hydroxyethyl)-1-piperazine ethane sulfonic acid), pH 7.4, and were stored on ice prior to use. Different cellular calcium contents were obtained by incubating the cells in this medium at 0°C with $CaCl_2$ concentrations up to 10 mM for a period of 1 hr[14]. Similar incubations in the absence of added calcium were used to obtain cells depleted of calcium. Cell viability, as judged by Trypan Blue exclusion, was greater than 95% was not affected by the calcium loading or depletion procedures. ATP contents ranged from 8 to 10 nmol/mg dry wt.

Rat liver mitochondria were isolated by standard techniques used in this laboratory[11,15]. Mitochondria were depleted of their endogenous calcium (ranging from 5 to 15 nmol/mg protein) by incubation at a concentration of 2-5 mg protein/ml for 20 min at room temperature in medium containing 120 mM KCl, 20 mM HEPES, 0.1 mM $MgCl_2$ and 0.5 mM EGTA, pH 7.2. The mitochondria were washed twice with medium containing 225 mM mannitol, 75 mM sucrose, 20 mM HEPES and 20 µM EGTA, pH 7.2 and the final pellet was resuspended in the same medium at a protein concentration of 30-40 mg/ml. The mean calcium content of 9 batches of calcium-depleted liver mitochondria was 1.64 ± 0.19 nmol/mg protein. Sarcoplasmic reticulum was isolated from rabbit skeletal muscle according to the method described by Herbette et al[16].

Measurement of Free Ca^{2+} Concentration and Intracellular Calcium Distributions

The free Ca^{2+} concentration in suspensions of hepatocytes or mitochondria was measured spectrophotometrically in an Aminco DW2a Spectrophotometer by following the absorbance change of the Ca-arsenazo III complex using a wavelength pair of 675-685 nm[3,17]. For measurements of the extramitochondrial free Ca^{2+} concentration at equilibrium (the Ca^{2+} set point[18]), mitochondria (approximately 1 mg protein/ml) were incubated at 30°C in buffer containing 120 mM KCl, 20 mM HEPES and 40 µM arsenazo III, pH 7.2. This buffer was passed several times through Chelex 100 (Na^+ form) to reduce the contaminating Ca^{2+} to below 0.4 µM, and supplemented with 2 mM succinate and 1 µg/mg protein of rotenone. The free Ca^{2+} concentration in equilibrium with the Ca-arsenazo complex was calculated from a knowledge of the total concentrations of calcium and arsenazo III and the apparent dissociation constant of the Ca-arsenazo complex[3,19], which was 30 µM for the above medium. When Mg^{2+} ions were also present in the incubation medium, the free Ca^{2+} concentration was calculated using a computer program based on the reiterative algorithm described by Portzehl et al[20]. A value of 830 µM was used for the K'_d of the Mg-arsenazo complex[21]. Total mitochondrial or cellular calcium was measured by atomic absorption spectroscopy[3]. The hepatocyte cytosolic free Ca^{2+} concentration was measured by the digitonin null point titration technique as previously described[3]. Different vesicular intracellular calcium pools in intact hepatocytes were estimated by successive additions of 1 nmol/mg dry wt of FCCP (carbonyl cyanide p-trifluoromethoxyphenyl-hydrazone) and 2 nmol/mg dry wt of A23187. The uncoupling agent FCCP releases calcium from the mitochondrial pool[22] as a result of the collapse of the proton electrochemical gradient. The ionophore A23187 releases calcium from all vesicular pools[23], hence the term "A23187 minus FCCP releasable calcium" represents predominantly the calcium pool of the endoplasmic reticulum.

RESULTS AND DISCUSSION

Cellular Calcium Transport Mechanisms

Questions of fundamental importance for an understanding of cellular calcium homeostasis in the resting state as well as for its displacement from equilibrium during excitation-contraction coupling, stimulus-secretion coupling or hormone receptor-response coupling, relate to the identity of the subcellular organelle(s) responsible for maintaining a low resting cytosolic free Ca^{2+} concentration and the source of calcium responsible for the transient rise of the cytosolic free Ca^{2+} concentration when the cell is stimulated. Differences in intracellular calcium pool sizes and flux undoubtedly exist between different cell types because of their disparate functions, but there are clear similarities of the

Ca^{2+}-transporting systems present in the plasma membrane, mitochondria and reticular membranes between different tissues.

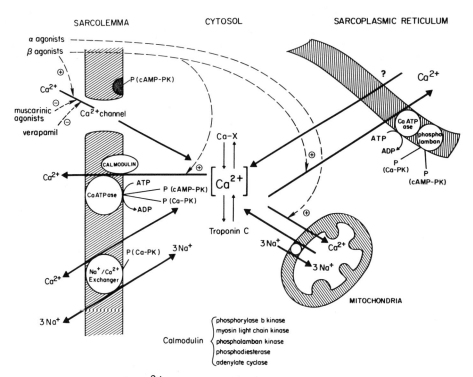

Fig. 1.   Scheme of Ca^{2+} fluxes and their regulation in cardiac muscle.

Figure 1 summarizes current knowledge concerning Ca^{2+} fluxes and their regulation in heart. During the normal heart beat, entry of Ca^{2+} into the cell probably occurs mainly by the voltage dependent Ca^{2+} channel during the plateau phase of the action potential[24]. Influx of Ca^{2+} through this channel is increased by β-adrenergic agents and is inhibited by activation of the muscarinic receptors and by Ca^{2+} blocking agents such as verapamil[24,25]. Its activity is apparently regulated by phosphorylation of a membrane protein by cAMP-dependent protein kinase[26]. The plasma membrane also contains an electrogenic Na^+-Ca^{2+} exchange system[27-30], which may be regulated by phosphorylation of a protein component by Ca^{2+}-dependent protein kinase[31]. Efflux of Ca^{2+} on this system is energetically favored at high membrane potentials. The third system in the plasma membrane for Ca^{2+} transport is a Ca^{2+}-ATPase, which is involved in Ca^{2+} efflux[32-35]. This enzyme is calmodulin-dependent and is also apparently regulated by phosphorylation involving both Ca^{2+}-dependent and cAMP-dependent protein kinases[34,35]. Calmodulin decreases the apparent K_m of the Ca-ATPase for Ca^{2+}, while phosphorylation increases the V_{max}. The Na^+-Ca^{2+} exchanger has a 30-fold greater V_{max} for Ca^{2+} transport than the Ca-ATPase and a 5-fold higher apparent K_m for Ca^{2+}[30,34]. Under normal physiological conditions, most of the Ca^{2+} efflux from the cell during the cardiac contraction cycle probably occurs via Na^+-Ca^{2+} exchange.

The amount of Ca^{2+} entering the cell by the voltage-dependent Ca^{2+} channel is not considered sufficient to elicit contraction via interaction with the troponin C-tropomyosin-actomyosin complex of the myofilaments, and is thought to trigger a greater release of "contractile calcium" from specialized portions of the sarcoplasmic reticulum by mechanisms which have not yet been thoroughly characterized[36,37]. Cytosolic free Ca^{2+} increases transiently to above 1 µM during contraction[2,4,5,6]. The amount of calcium which has to be mobilized to increase the cytosolic free Ca^{2+} by 10-fold may be an appreciable fraction of the sarcoplasmic reticulum pool because of Ca^{2+} binding to troponin C, calmodulin and other Ca^{2+}-binding sites designated as X in Figure 1, which buffer the cytosolic free Ca^{2+}. Calcium is removed from troponin C during the relaxation phase by sequestration into the sarcoplasmic reticulum via a high affinity Ca^{2+}-ATPase, which in cardiac muscle is regulated by phosphorylation of a separate protein (phospholamban) by both Ca^{2+} and cAMP-dependent protein kinases[38-42]. Thus, activation of adenylate cyclase by β-agonists with a consequent increase of cAMP levels increases phosphorylation of regulatory proteins which enhance the activities of the Ca^{2+}-ATPases of the plasma membrane and the sarcoplasmic reticulum as well as Ca^{2+} entry into the cell through the Ca^{2+} channel.

Mitochondria probably play a minor role in the overall process of Ca^{2+} uptake and release during the cardiac contraction-relaxation cycle[43]. Their role in the intact heart in relation to calcium homeostasis is presently unclear because of lack of knowledge of the *in situ* mitochondrial calcium content. Calcium uptake into mitochondria occurs by an electrophoretic process (Ca^{2+} uniport) involving a net transport of divalently charged calcium[44-46]. Uptake is energetically driven by the electrogenic proton pump of the respiratory chain, which establishes an electrical potential (negative inside) across the mitochondrial membrane. Under energized conditions associated with a high proton electrochemical gradient, Ca^{2+} uptake by the uniport mechanism is unidirectional since the gradient of free Ca^{2+} across the mitochondrial membrane never reaches equilibrium with the membrane potential[11,46]. However, collapse of the membrane potential is associated with a rapid Ca^{2+} efflux probably by reversal of the Ca^{2+} uniport. The V_{max} of Ca^{2+} uptake is very high and is normally limited by the rate of electron transport driven proton efflux[44]. The K_m of Ca^{2+} uptake varies somewhat with the species of mitochondria within the range of 2 to 10 μM, which is at least an order of magnitude higher than the basal cytosolic free Ca^{2+} concentration. The apparent K_m is increased even further by the presence of Mg^{2+} concentrations in the physiological range of 0.5 to 1 mM, which greatly enhances the sigmoidal nature of the Ca^{2+} uptake kinetics[47-49]. Efflux of calcium from energized mitochondria occurs by an electroneutral mechanism. In many mitochondrial species, including heart, Ca^{2+} is exchanged with Na^+ ions [50], while in liver mitochondria Ca^{2+} efflux is coupled primarily with proton influx[51]. The V_{max} for Ca^{2+} efflux is low (5 nmol/mg protein.min for liver and 10 nmol/mg protein.min for heart at 30°C), while the apparent K_m values for free Ca^{2+} are about 10 μM for liver mitochondria and 5 μM for heart mitochondria[11]. Recent studies from our laboratory have shown that most of the calcium present in the mitochondria is in the bound form such that 1 nmol of total calcium/mg protein corresponds to 1.05 μM free Ca^{2+} for liver mitochondria and 0.73 μM for heart mitochondria[11].

Mitochondrial Calcium Cycling
_____

In the steady state, Ca^{2+} cycles across the mitochondrial membrane and an equilibrium is achieved between extramitochondrial and intramitochondrial free Ca^{2+} concentrations. As a consequence of the different kinetic parameters of the separate Ca^{2+} uptake and efflux pathways of mitochondria, it has been proposed that they may play an important physiological role of buffering the cytosolic free Ca^{2+} against externally imposed changes associated with Ca^{2+} influx into the cell[18,45]. This phenomenon is illustrated by the experiment shown in Figure 2A. Liver mitochondria containing an initial calcium content of 12.5 nmol/mg protein were allowed to reach Ca^{2+} equilibration with Ca^{2+}-depleted buffer, and a value of about 0.2 μM was maintained for the extramitochondrial free Ca^{2+} concentration. Addition of a small pulse of calcium transiently increased the free Ca^{2+} to about 0.5 μM before it was transported into the mitochondria over 1 to 2 min. The final value for the extramitochondrial free Ca^{2+} was almost the same as that prior to the calcium pulse, and was also little affected by three further calcium pulses. Consequently, the conclusion is reached that the steady state value of the extramitochondrial free Ca^{2+}, or Ca^{2+} set point, is independent of the mitochondrial calcium content under conditions of calcium loading in the range from 10 to 60 nmol/mg protein[18]. However, this conclusion is not valid when the mitochondria contain very little calcium. In Figure 2B, liver mitochondria were depleted of calcium to a value of 1.5 nmol/mg protein and incubated as in Figure 2A. Their initial Ca^{2+} set point was lower, and the first three pulses of Ca^{2+} caused a marked increase of the

Ca^{2+} set point. Thus, whether or not mitochondria maintain a constant extramitochondrial free Ca^{2+} concentration depends on their calcium content.

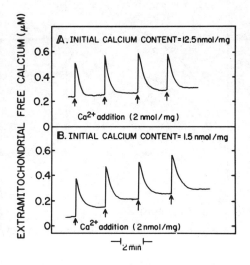

Fig. 2. Effects on the extramitochondrial free Ca^{2+} concentration of addition of 2 nmol/mg protein of calcium to liver mitochondria containing initially 12.5 nmol of calcium/mg protein (A) or 1.5 nmol of calcium/mg protein (B).

     The results of a large series of experiments similar to those of Figure 2, relating the steady state extramitochondrial free Ca^{2+} to the mitochondrial calcium content, are shown in Figure 3A. In the absence of added Mg^{2+} (control curve of Figure 3A), the Ca^{2+} set point of liver mitochondria was relatively independent of mitochondrial calcium above values of about 4 nmol/mg protein (4.2 μM intramitochondrial free Ca^{2+}), but varied with the calcium content below this value. Addition of 0.15 mM Mg^{2+} increased the Ca^{2+} set point 2 to 3-fold at all levels of mitochondrial calcium. Phosphate (1 mM) in the presence of Mg^{2+} had no effect on the Ca^{2+} set point (Figure 3A), (c.f. 52), but it was decreased to values slightly above those for control by the addition of 2 mM MgATP with 0.15 mM free Mg^{2+} (data not shown), in general agreement with the data of Becker[53]. These ion effects are presumably caused by alterations of the apparent K_m for Ca^{2+} influx. The Ca^{2+} uniporter is known to be inhibited by ruthenium red, and Figure 3B shows that the Ca^{2+} set point is shifted to higher values by suboptimal concentrations of ruthenium red. Thus, an increase of the apparent K_m for Ca^{2+} influx or a decrease of the V_{max} both increase the Ca^{2+} set point for a given mitochondrial calcium content. A stimulation of Ca^{2+} efflux will also increase the Ca^{2+} set point, as shown by addition of Na^+ (half maximum effect at about 4 mM) to heart or brain mitochondria[45].

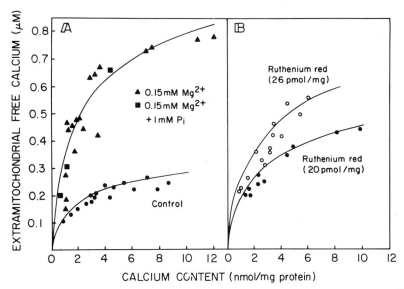

Fig. 3.   Relationships between the extramitochondrial free Ca^{2+} concentration and the calcium content of liver mitochondria.
In (A), mitochondria were incubated in the absence of Mg^{2+}
for control conditions or in the presence of 0.15 mM Mg^{2+}
or 0.15 mM Mg^{2+} plus 1 mM phosphate. In (B), mitochondria
were incubated in the absence of Mg^{2+} but with either 20
or 26 pmol of ruthenium red/mg protein to cause partial
inhibition of the Ca^{2+} uniporter.

From the above findings it appears that the relationship between the extramitochondrial and intramitochondrial free Ca^{2+} should
be defined by the kinetic parameters for Ca^{2+} influx and efflux on
the separate transport systems.   In the presence of Mg^{2+}, calcium
uptake follows sigmoidal kinetics with a Hill coefficient of approximately 2 [54].   The rate of Ca^{2+} uptake (v_1) can be described by
equation 1, where K_1 and V_1 are the apparent K_m and V_{max} of the uptake carrier and $[Ca^{2+}]_o$ is the extramitochondrial free Ca^{2+} concentration:

$$v_1 = \frac{V_1([Ca^{2+}]_o/K_1)^2}{1 + ([Ca^{2+}]_o/K_1)^2} \qquad (1)$$

Assuming that the Ca^{2+} efflux carrier obeys Michaelis–Menten
kinetics[11], the rate of Ca^{2+} efflux (v_2) is given by equation 2,
where K_2 and V_2 are the apparent K_m and V_{max} of the efflux carrier
and $[Ca^{2+}]_i$ is the intramitochondrial free Ca^{2+} concentration:

$$v_2 = \frac{V_2([Ca^{2+}]_i/K_2)}{1 + ([Ca^{2+}]_i/K_2)} \qquad (2)$$

Under steady state conditions of Ca^{2+} cycling, $v_1 = v_2$, and equations 1 and 2 can be rearranged and solved for $[Ca^{2+}]_o$ to give equation 3, which describes the steady state relationship between extra- and intramitochondrial free Ca^{2+} in terms of three independent kinetic parameters, namely K_1, K_2 and α, defined as the ratio V_2/V_1:

$$[Ca^{2+}]_o^2 = \frac{K_1^2\alpha([Ca^{2+}]_i/K_2)}{1 + ([Ca^{2+}]_i/K_2)(1-\alpha)} \qquad (3)$$

The lines drawn in Figure 3A are theoretical curves generated from the above equation. For the control Mg^{2+}-free condition, the follow-ing values for the kinetic parameters were used: 10 µM free Ca^{2+} for K_2 (the K'_m for Ca^{2+} efflux) together with a ratio of total/free Ca^{2+} of 7 x 10^{-4} for the matrix calcium[11], 1.6 µM for K_1 (the K'_m for Ca^{2+} influx) and 0.056 for α (the ratio V'_{max} efflux/V'_{max} influx). These values for K_1 and α were chosen on the basis of the results of a kinetic analysis of the data in Figure 3B[10]. The curve drawn through the points for the plus Mg^{2+} condition in Figure 3A was generated by increasing K_1 from 1.6 µM to 4.5 µM, leaving the other kinetic parameters the same. These values for the K'_m for Ca^{2+} influx in the absence and presence of Mg^{2+} are similar to those reported in the literature[49,55]. As seen from Figure 3 the fit of the theoreti-cal curves to the data points is rather close.

Figure 4 shows the calculated sensitivity of the steady state extramitochondrial free Ca^{2+} concentration to variations of the individual kinetic parameters in equation 3 and the Hill coefficient. For the data in Figure 4, a value of 10 µM was chosen for $[Ca^{2+}]_i$, but the results were qualitatively similar at lower values. It can be seen that $[Ca^{2+}]_o$ was much more sensitive to changes of the K'_m for Ca^{2+} influx than to changes of the K'_m for Ca^{2+} efflux, the Hill coefficient or changes in the ratio of the V_{max} values for Ca^{2+} efflux and influx. These data suggest that hormonal or other factors affecting the cytosolic free Ca^{2+} concentration may be mediated by regulation of the K_m for Ca^{2+} influx into mitochondria[46].

Intracellular Calcium Homeostasis

A question of fundamental importance in relation to intracel-lular calcium homeostasis is whether the cytosolic free Ca^{2+} con-centration of resting cells is determined by the kinetics of mito-chondrial Ca^{2+} cycling or whether the Ca^{2+} transport properties of other intracellular organelles and the plasma membrane exert a

primary influence on both the cytosolic free Ca^{2+} concentration and
the mitochondrial calcium content. Becker *et al*[56] using mixtures
of liver mitochondria and microsomes, and digitonized hepatocytes,
obtained evidence suggesting that the Ca^{2+}-ATPase activity of the
hepatic microsomes was responsible for lowering the Ca^{2+} set point
from the value of 0.45 µM observed with isolated mitochondria to
the cytosolic free Ca^{2+} concentration of about 0.2 µM observed with
intact hepatocytes[3]. Becker *et al*[56] also reported that in conjunction with the 2-fold lowering of the Ca^{2+} set point upon addition of
microsomes, the mitochondrial calcium content decreased from 18 to
10 nmol/mg protein. According to our own (Figure 3) as well as
other[18] studies, mitochondria should be able to buffer the extramitochondrial free Ca^{2+} concentration over this range of calcium
content, and the data of Becker *et al*[56] appears incompatible with
our results. Consequently, we reinvestigated the problem using
mixtures of liver mitochondria and either hepatic microsomes[10] or
rabbit skeletal muscle sarcoplasmic reticulum (Figure 5).

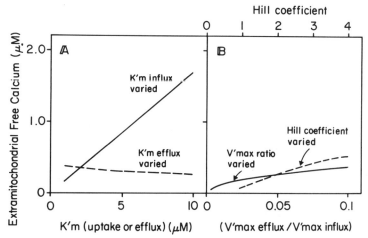

Figure 4.   Calculated sensitivity of the steady state extramito-
             chondrial free Ca^{2+} concentration to variation of indi-
             vidual kinetic parameters using equation 3 in the text.
             When fixed, the kinetic parameters used in the model
             were: K_1 = 1.6 µM, K_2 = 10 µM, $\alpha(V_2/V_1)$ = 0.056 and Hill
             coefficient = 2.

In Figure 5A, the response of the mitochondrial Ca^{2+} set point
to equivalent pulses of either Ca^{2+} or EGTA is illustrated. The
initial calcium content of the mitochondria was 8 nmol/mg protein
and the free Mg^{2+} concentration was about 200 µM, giving a Ca^{2+}
set point of 0.75 µM free Ca^{2+}. Under these conditions the half
time of Ca^{2+} uptake was twice that of Ca^{2+} efflux. Figure 5B shows

that addition of 90 µg of sarcoplasmic reticulum protein to 1.76 mg protein of liver mitochondria caused a rapid fall of the extramitochondrial free Ca^{2+} concentration from 0.75 µM to 0.5 µM followed by a slower rise back to the initial value. Measurements of the changes in the amounts of calcium present in the mitochondria and sarcoplasmic reticulum in separate experiments showed that the initial fall of extramitochondrial free Ca^{2+} was MgATP-dependent and was associated with uptake of Ca^{2+} from the medium into the sarcoplasmic reticulum.

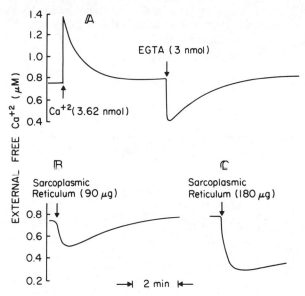

Fig. 5.   In A, B, and C, liver mitochondria (1.76 mg protein) containing initially 8 nmol of calcium/mg protein were incubated in Ca^{2+}-depleted medium containing 0.20 mM Mg^{2+} and 0.05 mM MgATP. A shows the effects of small additions of Ca^{2+} or EGTA on the steady state extramitochondrial free Ca^{2+} concentration. B and C show the effects of adding 90 and 180 µg protein, respectively, of rabbit skeletal muscle sarcoplasmic reticulum.

There was no further Ca^{2+} uptake when the capacity of the sarcoplasmic reticulum for Ca^{2+} sequestration was reached. This fall of the extramitochondrial free Ca^{2+} upset the Ca^{2+} cycling equilibrium of mitochondria, with the result that net Ca^{2+} efflux was stimulated, as after EGTA addition, until an equilibrium Ca^{2+} set point was restored. Thus, the mitochondria buffered the medium free Ca^{2+} concentration even in the presence of sarcoplasmic reticulum. In Figure 5C, twice the amount of sarcoplasmic reticulum protein was added to the mitochondria, and since the capacity for Ca^{2+}

uptake was greater, there was a larger fall of the extramitochondrial free Ca^{2+} concentration. The mitochondria released a greater amount of calcium than in Figure 5B until at equilibrium (not shown) the Ca^{2+} set point decreased below the original value of 0.8 µM. Addition of 360 µg of sarcoplasmic reticulum protein rapidly decreased the extramitochondrial free Ca^{2+} concentration essentially to zero, and decreased the mitochondrial calcium content to below 1 nmol/mg protein (data not shown). These data, and similar results with mixtures of mitochondria and liver microsomes[10] suggest that in the intact cell the Ca^{2+}-ATPase of the endo or sarcoplasmic reticulum will remove Ca^{2+} from the cytosol and the mitochondria until Ca^{2+} uptake by the reticular system becomes kinetically limiting or its maximum capacity to accumulate calcium is reached.

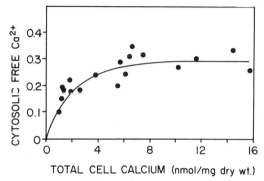

Fig. 6.   Cytosolic free Ca^{2+} concentration of isolated hepatocytes as a function of total cell calcium.

The relationship between the cytosolic free Ca^{2+} concentration and the distribution of intracellular calcium between the mitochondria and endoplasmic reticulum was investigated further as a function of total cell calcium using isolated hepatocytes. Figure 6 shows that the cytosolic free Ca^{2+} concentration increased from 0.1 µM at a cell calcium content of about 1 nmol/mg dry wt to a plateau value of 0.3 µM at cell calcium contents of 5 nmol/mg dry wt and above. It may be noted that this curve is remarkably similar to the relationship between the equilibrium value of the extramitochondrial free Ca^{2+} and the calcium content of isolated mitochondria (c.f. Figure 3), in agreement with the conclusion that Ca^{2+} cycling across the mitochondrial membrane determines the cytosolic free Ca^{2+}

concentration. The plateau value observed for the cytosolic free
Ca^{2+} in the hepatocytes presumably reflects the summation of ligand
binding effects (e.g. Mg^{2+}, MgATP, Pi) on the kinetic parameters of
Ca^{2+} recycling across the mitochondrial membrane.

The distribution of calcium between mitochondria and endoplasmic
reticulum in the liver cell as a function of total cell calcium was
determined by the sequential additions of the uncoupling agent FCCP
to release calcium from the mitochondrial pool, and the ionophore
A23187 to release calcium from the remaining intravesicular calcium
pools (Figure 7). We consider that this method is superior to the
rapid disruption method previously used[3], because there is less
possibility of redistribution of calcium between the organelles and
their environment prior to compartmental calcium measurements, as
discussed elsewhere[10]. High quality cells combined with addition of
ruthenium red to the cell suspension is essential, however, to
prevent artifacts introduced by an abnormal mitochondrial calcium
content of damaged cells. Figure 7 shows that at the lowest cell
calcium content of 1 nmol/mg cell dry wt, the endoplasmic reticulum
calcium pool (A23187 minus FCCP releasable calcium) was very small
and most of the cell calcium was in the mitochondria.

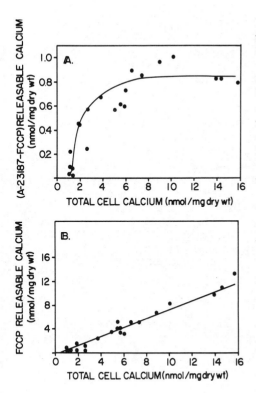

Fig. 7. Hepatocytes (2mg dry wt/
ml) containing different amounts
of total calcium were incubated
in Ca^{2+}-depleted medium containing
40 µM arsenazo III. The amount of
calcium released after addition
of the uncoupling agent FCCP was
measured to estimate the calcium
content of the mitochondrial pool.
The amount of calcium in the endoplasmic reticulum pool was estimated from the difference between
the separately measured A23187-
releasable and FCCP-releasable
calcium. The amounts of FCCP and
A23187 used were 1 and 2 nmol/mg
cell dry wt, respectively. The
total calcium content of the
hepatocytes was measured by atomic
absorption spectroscopy. Control
experiments showed that FCCP and
A23187 released the same amount
of calcium from isolated mitochondria and that A23187 but not
FCCP released all the calcium
from isolated hepatic microsomes.

The endoplasmic reticulum calcium pool became fully filled when the cell calcium was 6 nmol/mg dry wt, while the mitochondrial calcium pool increased linearly with cell calcium loading. For comparison with data using isolated mitochondria (Figure 3), it may be noted that at a total cell calcium content of 6 nmol/mg dry wt, the mitochondria contained 4 nmol/mg dry wt, which corresponds to a calcium content of 16 nmol/mg of mitochondrial protein since 1 g dry wt of cells contains approximately 250 mg of mitochondrial protein. At this level of calcium content, the mitochondria clearly buffer the cytosolic free Ca^{2+} concentration. In contrast, the maximum capacity of the endoplasmic reticulum calcium pool is 0.8 nmol/mg cell dry wt, which corresponds to about 10 nmol of calcium/mg of microsomal protein on the basis of about 10% of the total cellular protein being in the endoplasmic reticulum[10]. At an intermediate cell calcium content of 2 nmol/mg dry wt, the endoplasmic reticulum calcium pool is half-filled, the cytosolic free Ca^{2+} concentration is well below its final equilibrium value and the mitochondrial calcium content is about 2 nmol/mg mitochondrial protein, which according to Figure 3 is in the range where mitochondria are poor buffers of the extramitochondrial free Ca^{2+} concentration.

Normal liver contains 4 to 5 nmol of total calcium/mg dry wt, which from Figures 6 and 7 would indicate that the endoplasmic reticulum calcium pool is almost filled, and that mitochondria contain approximately 75% of the total cellular calcium and buffer the cytosolic free Ca^{2+} concentration at about 0.25 μM. The relative activities of the Ca^{2+} influx and efflux systems of the plasma membrane must determine the total tissue calcium content, while the intracellular calcium distribution is determined by the capacity and activity of the endoplasmic reticulum to accumulate calcium in relation to the kinetics of mitochondrial Ca^{2+} cycling. Upon hormonal stimulation of liver by α–adrenergic agents, vasopressin or angiotensin II, calcium is apparently released from both the mitochondrial and endoplasmic reticulum calcium pools [46] and the cytosolic free Ca^{2+} concentration rapidly increases leading to activation of phosphorylase a, while Ca^{2+} efflux from the cell is transiently stimulated[57]. As previously noted[46], a net fall of mitochondrial calcium content with an increase of the cytosolic free Ca^{2+} concentration implies a specific increase of the apparent K_m for Ca^{2+} influx into mitochondria (see also Figure 4). A hormonally induced net efflux of calcium from the endoplasmic reticulum suggests the existence of a physiologically active Ca^{2+} efflux pathway and the possibility of regulated Ca^{2+} cycling across the endoplasmic reticulum membrane. This was not observed with microsome vesicles prepared from either liver or rabbit skeletal muscle, suggesting that the calcium handling properties of these organelles *in vitro* are significantly different from those in the intact cell.

The heart also contains between 4 and 5 nmol of calcium/mg dry wt, but detailed studies of intracellular calcium distribution are presently not available. The principles of Ca^{2+} cycling across the mitochondrial membrane are similar in heart and liver, but the capacity of the sarcoplasmic reticulum for calcium uptake is much greater and the plasma membrane transport systems are probably different in detail as well as being more active. Consequently, at physiological levels of total calcium in the heart, the proportion of calcium in the mitochondria is probably less than in liver. At present it is not clear whether the calcium content of mitochondria in the intact heart is in the range to buffer the cytosolic free Ca^{2+} concentration or whether an increase of the intracellular steady state free Ca^{2+} concentration, e.g. during positive inotropic interventions, causes elevation of the mitochondrial calcium content and activation of intramitochondrial Ca^{2+}-sensitive enzymes such as pyruvate dehydrogenase phosphatase, NAD-linked isocitrate dehydrogenase and α-ketoglutarate dehydrogenase[58]. Our own studies to define the activity of α-ketoglutarate dehydrogenase in isolated heart mitochondria as a function of total and free Ca^{2+} have shown that mitochondria must contain less than 3 nmol of calcium/mg protein (2.2 μM free Ca^{2+}) for Ca^{2+}-dependent regulation of enzyme activity[11].

Breakdown of Cellular Calcium Homeostasis with Ischemic Injury: Hypothesis

In the following discussion, ischemia is considered to be associated with a cessation of coronary flow in certain regions of the heart even though in other regions flow is maintained. With absent or restricted coronary flow, delivery of substrates and oxygen, and removal of metabolically produced lactate, H^+ and CO_2 are curtailed. When the overall coronary flow is decreased below a critical limit, regional tissue anoxia develops even though other heterogeneous areas of the heart remain aerobic[59,60]. For convenience of discussion, the time sequence of events following the onset of ischemia is divided into three phases, although there is of necessity a continuity between them (c.f. 61). The first phase occurring within the first few minutes is associated with contractile failure, the second phase encompasses the following 15 to 30 minutes during which the metabolic and functional changes are essentially reversible following restoration of coronary flow and oxygen availability, while the third phase defines the chemical processes responsible for irreversible cellular injury.

One of the first consequences of decreased oxygen delivery to the myocardium in ischemia is an increase of the intracellular H^+ ion concentration[62-66]. Contractility falls rapidly because of decreased sensitivity of the myofibrillar ATPase for Ca^{2+} [67,68] presumably due to competition between H^+ and Ca^{2+} for the troponin-C Ca^{2+} binding sites of the actomyosin complex[69]. Increased H^+ ion concentration also causes an impairment of Ca^{2+} uptake and diminished Ca^{2+} release from the cardiac sarcoplasmic reticulum[68,70]. Although direct experimental proof is lacking, these effects are likely to increase the availability of cytosolic free Ca^{2+} concentration because of a decreased affinity of binding sites for Ca^{2+}. The mitochondria will attempt to buffer the cytosolic Ca^{2+} with the result that there is likely to be a redistribution of intracellular calcium from the sarcoplasmic reticulum to the mitochondria. Although electron transport flux ceases rapidly due to cellular anoxia, ATP synthesis still occurs because of accelerated glycogenolysis, although at a diminished rate, and ATP levels decline relatively slowly[71,72]. Consequently, it is likely that during the first phase of ischemia the cytosolic phosphorylation potential will be sufficient to keep the mitochondrial membrane potential high enough to retain calcium in the mitochondrial matrix.

During the second phase of ischemia, ATP levels fall gradually to about 20% of the aerobic values, and there is a commensurate loss of total nucleotides with accumulation of inosine and smaller quantities of hypoxanthine and xanthine due to the activities of AMP 5' nucleotidase, adenosine deaminase, nucleoside phosphorylase and xanthine oxidase[73,74]. Since the cytosolic phosphorylation potential is likely to remain in near equilibrium with the mitochondrial membrane potential[75], a fall of the former will decrease the latter and cause increased Ca^{2+} efflux from the mitochondria by reversal of the Ca^{2+} uniporter[44]. The intracellular mitochondrial Ca^{2+} set point is thus likely to increase, possibly to the region of 10 μM although it must be stressed that experimental proof is presently lacking. This estimate is based on the supposition that mitochondria release 10 nmol of calcium/mg protein, which on the basis of a mitochondrial content of 250 mg protein/g dry wt of heart and an intracellular volume of 2.5 ml/g dry wt will cause an increase of total calcium in the cytosol of 1 μmol/ml. Assuming an activity coefficient of 100 for cytosolic calcium, this will increase the cytosolic free Ca^{2+} by 10 μM. The postulated rise of the cytosolic free Ca^{2+} and fall of mitochondrial calcium content may be compounded by a deficiency of the plasma membrane Ca^{2+} efflux systems[61,76-79]. This may be caused by the decrease of the cytosolic ATP concentration, by H^+ ion competition for the Ca^{2+} binding sites on calmodulin and possibly also by dephosphorylation of regulatory proteins associated with the plasma membrane Ca^{2+}-ATPase and Na^+-Ca^{2+} exchange (see Figure 1). This second phase may be regarded as the cellular physiological response of calcium homeostasis to ischemic anoxia. Delayed functional recovery may occur after reperfusion, while ultrastructural changes such as clearing of the mitochondrial matrix, partial fragmentation of the cristae, swelling of the nuclei and sarcoplasmic reticulum are rapidly reversible[80]. Creatine phosphate levels increase rapidly to supranormal values while resynthesis and repletion of the adenine nucleotides is much slower[74,80]. It may be noted that ischemia *per se* is not associated with an appreciable increase of total calcium in the heart[78,81-84], but the observed

gradual rise of end-diastolic pressure during ischemia[85] and contracture of the sarcomeres[74] are indicative of an increase of
the cytosolic calcium concentration.

The third phase of ischemia involves the onset of metabolic
changes that culminate in irreversible tissue damage. The mechanism
and even the nature of some of these changes remain speculative,
but the consequences are depletion of the ATP content to about
1 µmol/g dry wt and ultrastructural changes such as mitochondrial
swelling, loss of the cristae, presence of large amorphous densities
in the mitochondria and small defects of the sarcolemma, together
with poor functional recovery with reflow[74,80]. A description of
the nature and time sequence of the biochemical changes that make
the difference between reversible and irreversible cell injury have
remained elusive. In particular, although it is recognized that
calcium homeostasis[78] and adenine nucleotide homeostasis[74] are both
deranged, the cause and effect relationships between defects in these
mechanisms and the possibility of exacerbation of effects in ischemia
as distinct from high-flow hypoxia due to the greater fall of the
intracellular pH[61] have yet to be ascertained. Defects of the Ca^{2+}
and other ionic pumps and of energy metabolism have been observed
by numerous investigators in organelles isolated from post ischemic
heart tissue, but it seems more reasonable to suppose that these are
contributory rather than causal factors for irreversibility. Since
the plasma membrane is responsible for maintaining intracellular
ionic homeostasis as well as providing a barrier to prevent loss
of intracellular constituents, it is reasonable to suppose that
alterations of the organization of membrane phospholipids with loss
of structural integrity would be the most probable causative factor
for irreversible loss of cellular function during ischemia, although
this may not be fully revealed until flow is restored. This is most
apparent in the so-called calcium paradox, where loss of plasma
membrane integrity is seen when Ca^{2+} is restored to the perfusion
fluid after an interval of Ca^{2+}-free perfusion[86,87].

Changes to the membrane phospholipid composition during
ischemia with development of aberrant structure-function relationships with respect to Ca^{2+} transport are probably progressive and
are likely to affect all the intracellular membranes to some degree.
Various authors have speculated on the possible changes that might
occur as a consequence of increased phospholipase activity, which
includes loss of phospholipids, the disruptive effect of lysophospholipids as well as the detergent like effects produced by high
cytosolic concentrations of fatty acids, fatty acyl-CoA and pal-
mitoylcarnitine[82,88-91]. Phospholipase A1 and/or A2 activities
have been found to be associated with most intracellular membranes
or organelles after isolation[88,89]. These activities, including
those associated with the lysosomes, are normally latent, and at
present an adequate description of the biochemical mechanisms responsible for increasing their activity is lacking. However, a

combination of three factors seem essential, namely abnormally high concentrations of Ca^{2+}, H^+ and surface active agents such as palmi-toylcarnitine. Current problems relate to loss of integrity of the lysosomal membranes with release of lysosomal phospholipases[91], the role of Ca^{2+}-activated proteases[92], and the Ca^{2+} requirement for phospholipase A_2 activation[93]. Present evidence indicates that significant Ca^{2+} activation of phospholipases occurs over the range of 0.1 to 1 mM Ca^{2+}, which is an unreasonably high estimate of the cytosolic free Ca^{2+} concentration during ischemia even when consideration is given to a decrease of the calcium concentration gradient between the static extracellular space and the cytosol. Consequently, if a primary role is envisioned for an elevated intracellular free Ca^{2+} concentration in the region of 10 μM for phospholipase activation, it is necessary to postulate a higher Ca^{2+} affinity than hitherto observed, possibly mediated by calmodulin[94] or by removal of a protein inhibitor[95].

Overt and clearly defined functional, metabolic and ultrastructural changes are evident when reflow occurs to irreversibly damaged tissue[74,80,82]. If the ischemic episode has not progressed too long, reoxygenation of the tissue permits some restoration of the mitochondrial membrane potential and oxidative phosphorylation, and the mitochondria attempt to buffer the elevated cytosolic free Ca^{2+} concentration by an increased Ca^{2+} uptake. However, the cytosolic calcium pool is now no longer restricted, as in normal calcium homeostasis, because of a defective permeability barrier of the plasma membrane to extracellular Ca^{2+} and phosphate. Consequently, the mitochondria rapidly become overloaded with calcium, with formation of calcium phosphate precipitates in the matrix[83,84]. Unlike the low energy cost of normal Ca^{2+} cycling across the mitochondrial membrane, high rates of mitochondrial Ca^{2+} uptake prevent the phosphorylation of ADP, hence ATP levels are likely to remain very low even after the onset of reoxygenation. If the damage to the plasma membrane is sufficiently severe, passive uncontrolled Ca^{2+} entry into the cell exceeds the capacity of plasma membrane Ca^{2+}-ATPase, Na^+, K^+-ATPase and Na^+-Ca^{2+} pumps to extrude Ca^{2+} and Na^+, with the result that the intracellular calcium homeostatic mechanisms are overloaded and degradative enzymic processes continue. Clearly, many changes occur almost simultaneously during ischemia, including others not mentioned in this brief synopsis, and it is difficult to distinguish between primary and secondary events that might be responsible for irreversible cell damage. The present hypothesis suggests that abnormalities of cellular calcium homeostasis may be very important in permitting irreversible changes of plasma membrane structure and integrity with the consequent inability of the cell to maintain normal ionic gradients.

ACKNOWLEDGMENTS

This work was supported by NIH grants AM-15120 and HL-14461.

REFERENCES

1. DiPOLO, R., REQUERA, J., BRINLEY, F. J.,Jr., MULLINS, L. J., SCARPA, A. and TIFFERT, T. Ionized calcium concentrations in squid axons. J. Gen. Physiol. 67, 433-467 (1976).
2. ALLEN, D. G. and BLINKS, J. R. Calcium transients in aequorin-injected frog cardiac muscle. Nature 273, 509-513 (1978).
3. MURPHY, E., COLL, K. E., RICH, T. L. and WILLIAMSON, J. R. Hormonal effects on calcium homeostasis in isolated hepatocytes. J. Biol. Chem. 255, 6600-6608 (1980).
4. MARBAN, E., RINK, T. J., TSIEN, R. W., and TSIEN, R. Y. Free calcium in heart muscle at rest and during contraction measured with Ca^{2+}-sensitive microelectrodes. Nature 286, 845-850 (1980).
5. DUBYAK, G. R. and SCARPA, A. Sarcoplasmic Ca^{2+} transients during the contractile cycle of single barnacle muscle fibres: measurements with arsenazo III-injected fibres. J. Muscle Res. Cell Motility 3, 87-112 (1982).
6. FABIATO, A. Myoplasmic free calcium concentration reached during the twitch of an intact isolated cardiac cell and during calcium-induced release of calcium from the sarcoplasmic reticulum of a skinned cardiac cell from the adult rat or rabbit ventricle. J. Gen. Physiol. 78, 457-497 (1981).
7. TSIEN, R. Y., POZZAN, T. and RINK, T. J. T-cell mitogens cause early changes in cytoplasmic free Ca^{2+} and membrane potential in lymphocytes. Nature 295, 68-71 (1982).
8. LANGER, G. A. The structure and function of the myocardial cell surface. Amer. J. Physiol. 235, H461-H468 (1978).
9. BORLE, A. B. Control, modulation and regulation of cell calcium. Rev. Physiol. Biochem. Pharmacol. 90, 13-153 (1981).
10. JOSEPH, S. K., COLL, K. E., COOPER, R. H., MARKS, J. and WILLIAMSON, J. R. Mechanisms underlying calcium homeostasis in isolated hepatocytes. J. Biol. Chem., submitted.
11. COLL, K. E., JOSEPH, S. K., CORKEY, B. E. and WILLIAMSON, J. R. Determination of the matrix free Ca^{2+} concentration and kinetics of Ca^{2+} efflux in liver and heart mitochondria. J. Biol. Chem. in press (1982).
12. MEIJER, A. J., GIMPEL, J. A., DELEEUW, G. A., TAGER, J. M. and WILLIAMSON, J. R. Role of anion translocation across the mitochondrial membrane in the regulation of urea synthesis from ammonia by isolated rat hepatocytes. J. Biol. Chem. 250, 7728-7738 (1975).
13. BERRY, M. N. and FRIEND, D. S. High yield preparation of isolated rat liver parenchymal cells: a biochemical and fine structural study. J. Cell Biology 43, 506-520 (1969).
14. VAN ROSSUM, G. D. V., SMITH, K. P. and BEETON, P. Role of mitochondria in control of calcium content of liver slices. Nature 260, 335-337 (1976).
15. WILLIAMSON, J. R., STEINMAN, R., COLL, K. E. and RICH, T. L. Energetics of citrulline synthesis by rat liver mitochondria. J. Biol. Chem. 256, 7287-7297 (1981).

16. HERBETTE, L., MARQUARDT, J., SCARPA, A. and BLASIE, J. K. A direct analysis of lamellar xray diffraction from hydrated oriented multilayers of fully functional sarcoplasmic reticulum. Biophys. J. 20, 245-272 (1977).

17. SCARPA, A. Measurements of cation transport with metallochromic indicators. Methods Enzymol. 56, 301-338 (1979).

18. NICHOLLS, D. G. The regulation of extramitochondrial free calcium ion concentration by rat liver mitochondria. Biochem. J. 176, 463-474 (1978).

19. BROWN, H. M. and RYDQVIST, B. Arsenazo III-Ca^{2+} effect of pH, ionic strength, and arsenazo III concentration on equilibrium binding evaluated with Ca^{2+} ion-sensitive electrodes and absorbance measurements. Biophys. J. 36, 117-137 (1981).

20. PORTZEHL, H., CALDWELL, P. C. and RÜEGG, J. C. The dependence of contraction and relaxation of muscle fibres from the crab Maia Squinado on the internal concentration of free calcium ions. Biochim. Biophys. Acta 79, 581-591 (1964).

21. OHNISHI, S. T. A method of estimating the amount of calcium bound to the metallochromic indicator arsenazo III. Biochim. Biophys. Acta 586, 217-230 (1979).

22. BYGRAVE, F. L. Mitochondrial calcium transport. Curr. Top. Bioenerget. 6, 259-318 (1977).

23. CHEN, J. J., BABCOCK, D. F. and LARDY, H. A. Norepinephrine, vasopressin, glucagon, and A23187 induce efflux of calcium from an exchangeable pool in isolated rat hepatocytes. Proc. Nat. Acad. Sci. USA 75, 2234-2238 (1978).

24. REUTER, H. Properties of two inward membrane currents in the heart. Ann. Rev. Physiol. 41, 413-424 (1979).

25. GARGOIUL, Y. M. Cardioactive drugs and the calcium slow channel in the heart. Trends Pharmacol. Sci. 2, 44-47 (1981).

26. RINALDI, M. L. LE PEUCH, C. J. and DEMAILLE, J. G. The epinephrine-induced activation of the cardiac slow Ca^{2+} channel is mediated by the cAMP-dependent phosphorylation of calciductin, a 23000 M_r sarcolemmal protein. FEBS Lett. 129, 277-281 (1981).

27. REEVES, J. P. and SUTKO, J. L. Sodium-calcium exchange in cardiac membrane vesicles. Proc. Natl. Acad. Sci. USA 76, 590-594 (1979).

28. PITTS, B. J. R. Stoichiometry of sodium-calcium exchange in cardiac sarcolemmal vesicles. J. Biol. Chem. 254, 6232-6235 (1979).

29. BERS, D. M., PHILIPSON, K. D. and NISHIMOTO, A. Y. Sodium-calcium exchange and sidedness of isolated sarcolemmal vesicles. Biochim. Biophys. Acta 601, 358-371 (1980).

30. CARONI, P., REINLIB, L. and CARAFOLI, E. Charge movements during the Na^+-Ca^{2+} exchange in heart sarcolemmal vesicles. Proc. Natl. Acad. Sci. USA 77, 6354-6358 (1980).

31. CARONI, P. and CARAFOLI, E. Personal communication (1982).

32. CARONI, P. and CARAFOLI, E. An ATP-dependent Ca^{2+}-pumping system in dog heart sarcolemma. Nature 283, 765-767 (1980).

33. TRUMBLE, W. R., SUTKO, J. L. and REEVES, J. P. ATP-dependent calcium transport in cardiac sarcolemmal membrane vesicles. Life. Sci. 27, 207-214 (1980).

34. CARONI, P. and CARAFOLI, E. The Ca^{2+} pumping ATPase of heart sarcolemma. J. Biol. Chem. 256, 3263-3270 (1981).

35. CARONI, P. and CARAFOLI, E. Regulation of Ca^{2+}-pumping ATPase of heart sarcolemma by a phosphorylation-dephosphorylation process. J. Biol. Chem. 256, 9371-9373 (1981).

36. ENDO, M. Calcium release from the sarcoplasmic reticulum. Physiol. Rev. 57, 71-108 (1977).

37. FABIATO, A. and FABIATO, F. Calcium and cardiac excitation-contraction coupling. Ann. Rev. Physiol. 41, 473-484 (1979).

38. LARAIA, P. J. and MARKIN, E. Adenosine 3':5'-monophosphate-dependent membrane phosphorylation. Circ. Res. 35, 298-306 (1974).

39. KIRCHBERGER, M. A., TADA, M. and KATZ, A. M. Adenosine 3':5'-monophosphate dependent protein kinase-catalyzed phosphorylation reaction and its relationship to calcium transport in cardiac sarcoplasmic reticulum. J. Biol. Chem. 249, 6166-6173 (1974).

40. LE PEUCH, C. J., HAIECH, J. and DEMAILLE, J. G. Concerted regulation of cardiac sarcoplasmic reticulum calcium transport by cyclic adenosine monophosphate dependent and calcium-calmodulin-dependent phosphorylation. Biochemistry 18, 5150-5157 (1979).

41. BILEZIKJIAN, L. M., KRANIAS, E. G., POTTER, J. D. and SCHWARTZ, A. Studies on phosphorylation of canine cardiac sarcoplasmic reticulum by calmodulin-dependent protein kinase. Circ. Res. 49, 1356-1362 (1981).

42. KIRCHBERGER, M. A. and ANTONETZ, T. Calmodulin-mediated regulation of calcium transport and ($Ca^{2+}+Mg^{2+}$)-activated ATPase activity in isolated cardiac sarcoplasmic reticulum. J. Biol. Chem. 257, 5685-5691 (1982).

43. ROBERTSON, S. P., POTTER, J. D. and ROUSLIN, W. The Ca^{2+} and Mg^{2+} dependence of Ca^{2+} uptake and respiratory function of porcine heart mitochondria. J. Biol. Chem. 257, 1743-1748 (1982).

44. SARIS, N.-E. and Åkerman, K. E. O. Uptake and release of bivalent cations in mitochondria. Curr. Top. Bioenerget. 10, 103-179 (1980).

45. NICHOLLS, D. G. and CROMPTON, M. Mitochondrial calcium transport. FEBS Lett. 111, 261-268 (1980).

46. WILLIAMSON, J. R., COOPER, R. H. and HOEK, J. B. Role of calcium in hormonal regulation of liver metabolism. Biochim. Biophys. Acta 639, 243-295 (1981).

47. CROMPTON, M., SIGEL, E., SALZMANN, M. and CARAFOLI, E. A kinetic study of the energy-linked influx of Ca^{2+} into heart mitochondria. Eur. J. Biochem. 69, 429-434 (1976).

48. BRAGADIN, M., POZZAN, T. and AZZONE, G. F. Kinetics of Ca^{2+} carrier in rat liver mitochondria. Biochemistry 18, 5972-5978 (1980).

49. AFFOLTER, H.and CARAFOLI, E. Hyperbolic kinetics of the electrophoretic carrier of Ca^{2+} uptake in liver mitochondria. J. Biochemistry 119, 199-201 (1981).

50. CARAFOLI, E. The calcium cycle of mitochondria. FEBS Lett. 104, 1-5 (1979).

51. FISKUM, G. and LEHNINGER, A. L. Regulated release of Ca^{2+} from respiring mitochondria by $Ca^{2+}/2H^+$ antiport. J. Biol. Chem. 254, 6236-6239 (1979).

52. BERNARDI, P. and AZZONE, G. F. A membrane potential-modulated pathway for Ca^{2+} efflux in rat liver mitochondria. FEBS Lett. 139, 13-16 (1982).

53. BECKER, G. L. Steady state regulation of extramitochondrial Ca^{2+} by rat liver mitochondria. Biochim. Biophys. Acta 591, 234-239 (1980).

54. HUTSON, S. M., PFEIFFER, D. R. and LARDY, H. A. Effect of cations and anions on the steady state kinetics of energy-dependent Ca^{2+} transport in rat liver mitochondria. J. Biol. Chem. 251, 5251-5258 (1976).

55. REED, K. C. and BYGRAVE, F. L. A kinetic study of mitochondrial calium transport. Eur. J. Biochem. 55, 497-504 (1975).

56. BECKER, G. L., FISKUM, G. and LEHNINGER, A. L. Regulation of free Ca^{2+} by liver mitochondria and endoplasmic reticulum. J. Biol. Chem. 255, 9009-9012 (1980).

57. BLACKMORE, P. F., HUGHES, B. P., SHUMAN, E. A. and EXTON, J. H. α-Adrenergic activation of phosphorylase in liver cells involves mobilization of intracellular calcium without influx of extra-cellular calcium. J. Biol. Chem. 257, 190-197 (1982).

58. DENTON, R. M. and McCORMACK, J. G. On the role of the calcium transport cycle in heart and other mammalian mitochondria. FEBS Lett. 119, 1-8 (1980).

59. STEENBERGEN, C., DELEEUW, G, BARLOW, C. H., CHANCE, B. and WILLIAMSON, J. R. Heterogeneity of the hypoxic state in per-fused rat heart. Circ. Res. 41, 606-615 (1977).

60. WILLIAMSON, J. R., DAVIS, K. N. and MEDINA-RAMIREZ, G. Quan-titative analysis of heterogeneous NADH fluoresence in perfused rat hearts during hypoxia and ischemia. J. Mol. Cell. Cardiol., in press (1982).

61. NAYLER, W. G., POOLE-WILSON, P. A. and WILLIAMS, A. Hypoxia and calcium. J. Mol. Cell. Cardiol. 11, 683-706 (1979).

62. NEELY, J. R., WHITMER, J. T. and ROVETTO, M. J. Effect of coronary blood flow on glycolytic flux and intracellular pH in isolated rat hearts. Circ. Res. 37, 733-741 (1975).

63. STEENBERGEN, C., DELEEUW, G., RICH, T. L. and WILLIAMSON, J. R. Effects of acidosis and ischemia on contractility and intra-cellular pH of rat heart. Circ. Res. 41, 849-858 (1977).

64. GARLICK, P. B., RADDA, G. K. and SEELEY, P. J. Studies of
    acidosis in the ischaemic heart by phosphorus nuclear magnetic
    resonance. Biochem. J. 184, 547-554 (1979).
65. CASE, R. B., FELIX, A. and CASTALLAN, F. S. Rate and rise of
    myocardial pCO_2 during early myocardial ischemia in dog.
    Circ. Res. 45, 324-330 (1979).
66. COBBE, S. M. and POOLE-WILSON, P. A. The time of onset and
    severity of acidosis in myocardial ischemia. J. Mol. Cell.
    Cardiol. 12, 745-760 (1980).
67. EBASHI, S., KITAZAWA, T., T., KOHAMA, K. and VAN EERD, P. C.
    Calcium ion in cardiac contractility. In Recent Advances in
    Studies on Cardiac Structure and Metabolism, Vol. 11,
    T. Kobayashi, T. Sano and N. S. Dhalla, Eds., pp. 93-101,
    Baltimore: University Park Press (1978).
68. FABIATO, A. and FABIATO, F. Effects of pH on the myofilaments
    and the sarcoplasmic reticulum of skinned cells from cardiac
    and skeletal muscles. J. Physiol. (Lond) 276, 233-255 (1978).
69. ROBERTSON, S. P., JOHNSON, J. D. and POTTER, J. D. The effects
    of pH on calcium binding to the Ca^{2+}-Mg^{2+} and the Ca^{2+} specific
    sites of bovine cardiac TnC. Circulation 58,supp. II 72 (1978).
70. SHIGEKAWA, M., FINEGAN, J. M. and KATZ, A. M. Calcium trans-
    port ATPase of canine cardiac sarcoplasmic reticulum: a com-
    parison with that of rabbit fast skeletal muscle sarcoplasmic
    reticulum. J. Biol. Chem. 251, 6894-6900 (1976).
71. ROVETTO, M. J., WHITMER, J. T. and NEELY, J. R. Comparison
    of the effects of anoxia and whole heart ischemia on carbo-
    hydrate utilization in isolated working rat hearts. Circ.
    Res. 32, 699-711 (1973).
72. BAILEY, I. A., RADDA, G. K., SEYMOUR, A. M. and WILLIAMS, S. R.
    The effects of insulin on myocardial metabolism and acidosis
    in normoxia and ischemia. Biochim. Biophys. Acta 720, 17-27
    (1982).
73. BERNE, R. M. and RUBIO, R. Adenine nucleotide metabolism in
    the heart. Circ. Res. 23, III 109-120 (1974).
74. JENNINGS, R. B. and REIMER, K. A. Lethal myocardial ischemic
    injury. Amer. J. Pathol. 102, 241-255 (1981).
75. WILLIAMSON, J. R. Mitochondrial function in the heart.
    Ann. Rev. Physiol. 41, 485-506 (1979).
76. KATZ, A. M. and REUTER, H. Cellular calcium and cardiac cell
    death. Amer. J. Cardiol. 44, 188-190 (1979).
77. PHILIPSON, K. D., BERSOHN, M. M. and NISHIMOTO, A. Y. Effects
    of pH on Na^{+}-Ca^{2+} exchange in canine cardiac sarcolemmal vesi-
    cles. Circ. Res. 50, 287-293 (1982).
78. NAYLER, W. G. The role of calcium in the ischemic myocardium.
    Am. J. Pathol. 102, 262-270 (1981).
79. KUBLER, W. and KATZ, A. M. Mechanism of early "pump" failure
    of the ischemic heart: possible role of adenosine triphos-
    phate depletion and inorganic phosphate accumulation. Amer.
    J. Cardiol. 40, 467-471 (1977).

80. SCHAPER, J., MULCH, J., WINKLER, B. and SCHAPER, W. Ultrastructural, functional and biochemical criteria for estimation of reversibility of ischemic injury: a study of the effects of global ischemia on the isolated dog heart. J. Mol. Cell. Cardiol. 11, 521-541 (1979).

81. WATTS, J. A., KOCH, C. D. and LANOUE, K. F. Effects of Ca^{2+} antagonism in energy metabolism: Ca^{2+} and heart function after ischemia. Am. J. Physiol. 238, H909-H916 (1980).

82. CHIEN, K. R., PFAU, R. G. and FARBER, J. L. Ischemic myocardiol cell injury. Am. J. Pathol. 97, 505-530 (1979).

83. SHEN, A. C. and JENNINGS, R. B. Myocardial calcium and magnesium in acute ischemic injury. Am. J. Pathol. 67, 417-440 (1972).

84. SHEN, A. C. and JENNINGS, R. B. Kinetics of calcium accumulation in acute myocardial ischemic injury. Am. J. Pathol. 67, 441-452 (1972).

85. HEARSE, D. J., GARLICK, P. B. and HUMPHREY, S. M. Ischemic contracture of the myocardium: mechanisms and prevention. Am. J. Cardiol. 39, 986-993 (1977).

86. GRUNWALD, P. M. and NAYLER, W. G. Calcium entry in the calcium paradox. J. Mol. Cell. Cardiol. 13, 867-880 (1981).

87. HEARSE, D. J., HUMPHREY, S. M. and BULLOCK, G. R. The oxygen paradox and the calcium paradox: two facets of the same problem? J. Mol. Cell. Cardiol. 10, 641-668 (1979).

88. KATZ, A. M. and MESSINEO, F. C. Lipid-membrane interactions and the pathogenesis of ischemic damage in the myocardium. Circ. Res. 48, 1-16 (1981).

89. CORR, P. B., LEE, B. I. and SOBEL, B. E. Electrophysical and biochemical derangements in ischemic myocardium: interactions involving the cell membrane. Acta Med. Scand. Supp. 651, 59-69 (1981).

90. CHIEN, K. R., REEVES, J. P., BUJA, L., BONTE, F., PARKEY, R. W. and WILLERSON, J. T. Phospholipid alterations in canine ischemic myocardium. Circ. Res. 48, 711-719 (1981).

91. BECKMAN, J. K., OWENS, K., KNAUER, T. E. and WEGLICKI, E. B. Hydrolysis of sarcolemma by lysosomal lipases and inhibition by chlorpromazine. Am. J. Physiol. 242, H652-H656 (1982).

92. BEINLICH, C. J., CLARK, M. G., MCKEE, E. E., LINS, J. A. and MORGAN, H. E. Neutral-alkaline proteolytic activity in rat cardiac muscle cells. J. Mol. Cell. Cardiol. 13, 23-36 (1981).

93. FREI, E. and ZAHLER, P. Phospholipase A_2 from sheep erythrocyte membranes: Ca^{2+} dependence and localization. Biochim. Biophys. Acta 550, 450-463 (1979).

94. WONG, P. Y-K. and CHEUNG, W. Y. Calmodulin stimulates human' platelet phospholipase A_2. Biochem. Biophys. Res. Commun. 90, 473-480 (1979).

95. HIRATA, F. The regulation of lipomodulin, a phospholipase inhibitory protein in rabbit neutrophils by phosphorylation. J. Biol. Chem. 256, 7730-7733 (1981).

THE ROLE OF HEART BINDING ANTIBODIES IN RHEUMATIC FEVER

John B. Zabriskie, and
Jacqueline E. Friedman

*Rockefeller University
1230 York Avenue
New York, N.Y. 10021

INTRODUCTION

It is obvious to any student of cardiology that the heart may be injured in a number of ways only some of which are immunologically mediated. However as our knowledge of cardiac pathologic mechanisms increases, it is this author's opinion that immunological mechanisms will play a much greater role in cardiac pathology than has hitherto been suspected. On this note I would like to review with you at least one example where a microbial-host immunological interaction appears to play a dominant role in causing cardiac damage. Hopefully further knowledge of this disease state may provide information concerning a number of myocardial diseases the etiology of which is still unknown.

HEART REACTIVE ANTIBODIES IN RHEUMATIC FEVER

I. Humoral Studies:

The observation that the sera of patients with rheumatic fever contain antibodies directed against components of cardiac tissue is not a new one. Using a variety of immunological techniques, a number of investigators have observed a serological reaction against heart tissue in the sera of acute rheumatic fever patients (1, 2). While the exact antigenic stimulus for the production of these antibodies was unknown, the general assumption by these authors was that these antibodies were either a result of direct toxic damage to the heart with subsequent release of cardiac antigens or the interaction of streptococcal components of products and cardiac tissue with the formation or

457

uncovering of new cardiac antigens. Kaplan's observation (7) that the antibodies raised in rabbits to streptococcal antigens bound to mammalian cardiac tissue added another parameter to the nature of the origin of these heart-reactive antibodies in rheumatic fever patients; namely, that heart-reactive antibodies in the sera of these patients in reality might be streptococcal induced.

The nature of the antigen or antigens responsible for the observed heart reactive antibodies has been a matter of some discussion. Our own data (15) indicate that one of the antigens resides in the streptococcal cell membrane while Kaplan's (8) experiments suggest that there is a second cross reactive antigen in the streptococcal cell wall which is closely associated with but not identical to the M protein moiety of the organism. Interest in the latter cross-reactive antigen has been rekindled with the observation by Manjula and Fischetti (9) that there is a strong structural homology between the M protein moiety and muscle tropomyosin. Additional evidence has been accumulated by Dale and Beachey (3) indicating that a peptic digest of the M protein moiety contains both the opsonic antigen and the heart cross reactive antigen on the same M protein moiety. Thus one can now say with some certainty that there are at least three microbial cross reactions between streptococcal antigens and tissue muscle proteins as defined by rabbit antisera. However, it should be pointed out that the sarcolemmal heart reactive staining seen in the majority of human sera was completely absorbed by membrane antigens (13, 16).

While the exact nature of the antigen(s) responsible for the observed cross-reactivity between streptococcal membranes and mammalian tissue remains somewhat clouded, these studies did serve as a springboard for our investigations into the antibodies present in the sera of patients with acute rheumatic fever. We asked ourselves three basic questions concerning the nature of these antibodies. First, how common were heart-reactive antibodies in the sera of patients with rheumatic fever and were they organ specific? Second, what was the nature of the antibodies, i.e., were they streptococcal-induced or cardiac-antigen-induced antibodies? Finally, were these antibodies cytotoxic in vitro for cardiac tissue monolayers and how did they interact with sensitized cells from rheumatic fever patients?

In order to answer the first question, namely, the incidence of heart-reactive antibodies in patients with acute rheumatic fever, the indirect or "sandwich" technique of immunofluorescent staining was used (16). Figure 1 demonstrates the type of immunofluorescent staining pattern which was observed in the majority of patients with acute rheumatic fever. As noted in the

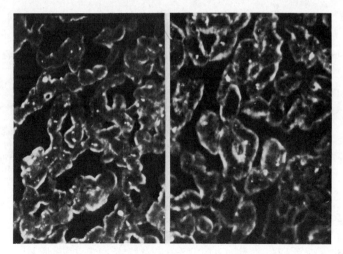

Fig. 1   Immunofluorescent staining patterns seen in microphoto-
graphs of cardiac muscle fibers. Right side panel shows
the staining of the serum of a patient with acute
rheumatic fever. Left side shows the staining   exhibited
by a rabbit serum immunized with streptococcal membrane
antigens.

photomicrograph, the most intense staining was always seen along
the sarcolemmal border of the muscle fiber, often extending down
along the membrane invaginations in the myofiber.   The right
handed side of the photomicrograph shows a similar pattern of
immunofluorescent staining when a rabbit   anti-streptococcal
membrane antiserum was used. Dr. Kaplan has also reported that
a certain percentage of rheumatics exhibited primarily   an
intermyofibrillar   pattern of immunofluorescent staining and
others gave a diffuse myofibrillar staining reaction (8).

Since the intensity of staining of the sera of patients with
acute rheumatic fever appeared to be four to five times that
observed with sera obtained from subjects with uncomplicated
streptococcal infections, the sera of a group of patients with
either documented scarlet fever or scarlet fever followed by
acute rheumatic fever were tested. Table I summarizes the
results of these studies, and it can be seen that during the
first week following the scarlet fever infection both groups had
demonstrable titers of heart-reactive antibody present in their
sera.   However, the titers in general at that stage were higher
in the rheumatic group and continued to rise to high titers with
the onset of the clinical symptoms of acute rheumatic fever. In
contrast, sera drawn from patients with uncomplicated scarlet
fever during the same time as those patients who developed rheu-

Table I

A Comparison of the Average Titers of
Cross-Reactive Antibody in Patients with Streptococcal
Infections, Their Sequelae and Other Diseases

Diagnosis	No. of patients	Dilutions of sera obtained in first 1-2 weeks			Dilutions of sera obtained at onset of rheumatic fever		
		1:5	1:10	1:20	1:5	1:10	1:20
Scarlet fever	15	++	+	0	+	0	0
Scarlet fever with rheumatic fever	15	+++	++	0	++++*	++	+
Rheumatoid arthritis	6				0**	0	0
Lupus erythematosis	4				0	0	0

*Refers to the intensity of immunofluorescent staining of
heart tissue graded from 0 - 4+.

**These sera obtained during active disease.

matic fever showed falling titers of heart-reactive antibody.

While it is conceivable that the heightened antigenic
response in the rheumatic group (as reflected in the increased
ASO titers) was responsible for the higher level of
heart-reactive antibody titers, many patients in the
uncomplicated scarlet fever group had high ASO titers (>2000),
4-6 + CRP levels and yet no heart-reactive antibody. In fact,
positive heart-reactive antibody titers >1:10 in our hands are in
general indicative of an active rheumatic process.

If there was a direct association of this antibody with the
active rheumatic process, then this antibody should disappear
during the convalescent stage and reappear with each
recrudescence of rheumatic fever. Figure 2 illustrates the
pattern of heart-reactive antibody titers in a patient who had
two attacks 11 years apart. While not typical of the rheumatic
recurrence which usually takes place within the first year or two
after the initial attack, this patient illustrates several
important points with respect to the association of heart

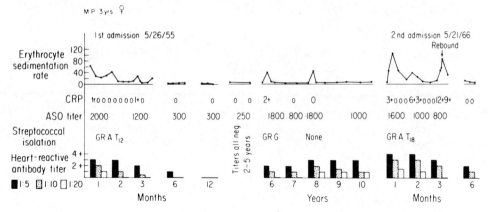

Fig. 2 The laboratory and heart reactive antibody data in patient MP who had clinical evidence of serum carditis at age 3 and a second attack of acute rheumatic fever 11 years later. Note the lack of heart reactive antibody from years 2-5 and then the reappearance of antibodies in years 6-10 associated with two intercurrent streptococcal infections (years 6 and 8).

reactive antibodies with the disease process. The initial attack was accompanied by a high ASO titer, positive CRP, elevated heart-reactive antibody titers, and definite evidence of carditis. Following a combined course of steroid and aspirin treatment, the heart-reactive antibody titers declined and were negative from the second to the fifth year. At this point the patient admitted several breaks in penicillin prophylaxis, and this was reflected in the elevation of ASO titers and clinical signs of intercurrent streptococcal infections on at least two occasions. Of interest was the associated rise in heart-reactive antibody titers to significant levels during this period. Finally, the third intercurrent infection resulted in a marked rise of heart-reactive antibody levels in the serum of the patient and clinical recurrence of the disease process.

The presence of high titers of heart-reactive antibodies in the sera of patients with acute rheumatic fever prompted an investigation as to the nature of these antibodies. Were they, in fact, streptococcal-induced heart-reactive antibodies similar to that observed in the sera of rabbits immunized with streptococcal membranes? Accordingly, the sera of 20 patients with acute rheumatic fever were appropriately diluted to give a 4+ staining over human cardiac sections. These dilutions were then absorbed with varying amounts of streptococcal membranes and human cardiac tissue. Following high-speed centrifugation the

Table II

Antigens

	No.	Control staining	Membranes 1-2 mg.	Cardiac tissue 1-2 mg.
Acute rheumatic fever	20	4+	0	0
Postcardiotomy	12	4+	4+*	0

* Same results were obtained using up to 12 mg. of streptococcal membranes.

supernatants were tested for residual immunofluorescent staining. The sera from 12 patients who had undergone cardiotomy per se for diseases unrelated to rheumatic fever and who also gave good immunofluorescent staining patterns were included as controls. In Table II it is evident that the immunofluorescent staining of the sera of patients with acute rheumatic fever is absorbed by both streptococcal membranes and cardiac tissue. In contrast, the staining of postcardiotomy sera is absorbed only by cardiac tissue and streptococcal membranes even in amounts up to 12 mg. were ineffective in blocking immunofluorescent staining. These studies strongly suggest there are two heart-reactive antibodies; one related to cross-reactivity with streptococcal structures, the other related most probably to cardiac antigen release.

Answers to the third question, namely, the interaction of the antibody with sensitized cells from the host and the role of the cytotoxicity of this antibody, are only beginning to emerge. Towards this end, monolayers of tissue cell lines of human skeletal and fetal cardiac tissue have been prepared from either biopsy material or human fetal organs. In addition, fetal rabbit cardiac monolayers have also been established. Lymphocytes obtained from rheumatic individuals were then placed on these cell monolayers, both alone and in conjunction with streptococcal antigens. While these results are preliminary, certain observations are worthy of comment. First, sensitized cells from rheumatic individuals are quite capable of specifically killing cardiac monolayers (6) (17). Of interest was the fact that serum obtained from the same rheumatic individuals effectively blocked the cytotoxic effect of lymphocytes. Antibody alone apparently had little effect on the monolayers (6).

Studies in experimental animals by Yang et al (14) tend to confirm the observations in rheumatic fever patients. Lymphocyte populations obtained from guinea pigs sensitized to streptococcal group A cell membrane antigens were specifically cytotoxic for embryonic cardiac cell monolayers. Guinea pigs sensitized to group C membranes did not kill the cardiac cell monolayers. The addition of heart reactive antibody from these guinea pigs did not enhance the killing, suggesting that the observed cytotoxicity was antibody independent.

II. Antigen Purification Studies:

The streptococcal membrane antigens responsible for the induction of heart reactive antibodies has been isolated in a highly purified state in our laboratory by Dr. van de Rijn and is a series of four closely related proteins ranging in molecular weight from 32,000-22,000 daltons and does not appear to be related to the M protein moiety (13).

The M protein cross reactive antigen apparently is restricted to only a few serologically defined streptococcal types and has been identified by Kaplan to be present predominantly in type 5 and type 19 strains. Recently, using a highly purified pepsin digested type 5 M protein preparation, Dale and Beachey (3) demonstrated that the particular segment of purified M antigen capable of inducing heart reactive antibody in certain animals was intimately related to the opsonic antibody. Thus, the absorption type specific M protein opsonic antibodies with heart antigen resulted in the loss of both the immunofluoresent staining of heart tissue and the type of specific protective antibody. These results have obvious implications concerning the potential dangers involved in the creation of streptococcal vaccines derived from these type specific M protein moieties.

During the past year our own laboratory has been concerned with the further isolation and identification of the cross reactive antigen in heart tissue which cross reacts with the streptococcal membrane antigens. Both bovine heart and human heart extracts have been used in an ELISA assay system to determine reactivity of rheumatic fever sera to these antigens. Figure 3 shows a DEAE cellulose fractionation of a saline extract of bovine heart followed by a step wise salt elution of the material. Using a reference rheumatic fever serum known to contain heart reactive antibody by the fluorescence technique in the ELISA assay, Table III shows that the fall through fraction 1 contained the majority of the reactivity against the rheumatic fever serum. Table IV shows that the reactivity to this antigen

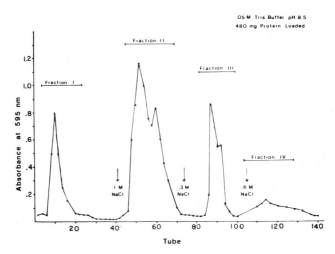

Fig. 3 Protein determinations of eluates from a DEAE cellulose
column loaded with a saline extract of bovine heart
tissue.

was significantly greater in a number of rheumatic fever sera
compared to a standard group of scarlet fever patients without
rheumatic fever. It should be pointed out that some overlap
between the groups did exist and suggests antibody reactivity to
common antigens in the two groups, a phenomenon noted by Kaplan

Table III

ELISA Assay with Bovine Heart Fractions*
and a Rheumatic Fever Patients Serum

Bovine Heart* Saline Extract	Fx 1**	Fx 2	Fx 3	Fx 4
Acute Rheumatic Fever Serum GL 37 1:50				
.161	.254	.05	.0	.0

*All fractions were diluted 1/1000 for the assay.
**Fx 1, 2 etc. were obtained from the DEAE column (Fig. 3).

Table IV

ELISA Assay Using Bovine Heart
DEAE Column Fraction I at 1:100 Dilution

Patients	Antibody Dilutions		
	1:100	1:200	1:400
Rheumatics (7)	340	219	151
Scarlet Fever (5)	228	140	94

in his earlier studies of these heart antigens (7). The antigen has been further purified on CM sepharose columns. The reactive antigen in the ELISA system appears to have a molecular weight of 43,000 daltons. Of interest was the observation that another protein of similar molecular weight appears to be equally reactive with both rheumatic and scarlet fever sera indicating that some common heart reactive antibodies are present in both groups of patients. However one of the antigens is more reactive with rheumatic fever sera than with scarlet fever sera.

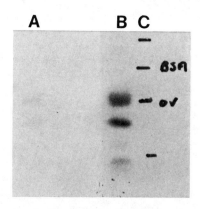

Fig. 4   A photomicrograph depicting reactive human heart antigens
         on nitrocellulose paper following transference from an
         SDS PAGE of the extracts. Antibodies which bind to the
         heart antigens were developed by radiolabelled Protein A.
         Note the presence of at least three distinct bands (lane
         B) in the sera of patients with acute rheumatic fever as
         compared to the two faint bands in lane A using scarlet
         fever sera. Lane C depicts the molecular weight
         radiolabel standards of BSA (67,000 daltons) and OVA
         (43,00 daltons).

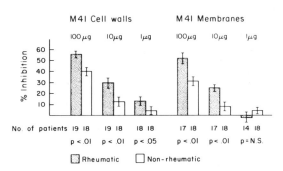

Fig. 5   Migration inhibition values to Type 41 streptococcal
         antigens in patients with acute rheumatic fever compared
         to controls. Note the increased reactivity to both cell
         wall and membrane antigens in rheumatics.

Another approach to the question of the heart reactive
antigen has been our use of the nitrocellulose transfer technique
(5) in which the antigen is first separated in gel
electrophoresis, transferred to nitrocellulose paper stained with
antibody   and   then   developed   autoradiographically   with
radiolabelled staphylococcal protein A. Using this very
sensitive technique for detection of antigens, Fig. 4
demonstrates the presence of two strong radiolabelled bands
developed by a rheumatic fever serum which were barely detected
in scarlet fever sera and are approximately 43,000 and 38,000
daltons respectively.

In summary the heart antigen purification studies appear to
be promising and it is hoped that final purification and analysis
of these muscle antigens will provide insight into the nature of
the cross reactions between streptococcal antigens and cardiac
antigens.

III. Cellular:

As mentioned previously, the question of whether or not
cellular mechanisms also play a role in the disease process has
been the subject of our continuing investigations.   Studies of
the cellular reactivity of peripheral blood mononuclear cell
populations to streptococcal antigen in acute rheumatic fever
patients in Trinidad indicate that these patients react primarily
to streptococcal membrane antigens obtained from strains
primarily associated with rheumatic fever (Fig. 5) and not to
strains associated with post streptococcal glomerulonephritis
(Fig. 6). This increased cellular reactivity appears to persist

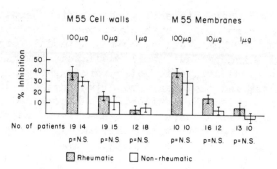

Fig. 6   Migration inhibition values to Type 55 streptococcal
         antigens in patients with acute rheumatic fever compared
         to controls.   Note the lack of heightened reactivity to
         these antigens in rheumatics.

for at least two years after the initial attack and fits well
with the concept of increased susceptibility to recurrences
during the first two years after an attack of rheumatic fever.
While not shown, a number of control antigens including group C
and D streptococcal membranes did not elicit an increased
response in those patients (11) (12).

     Concerning cellular reactivity to heart antigens   in
rheumatic patients, surprisingly few reports have appeared.
McLaughlin et al (9), using an acid extract of heart muscle
tissue were unable to detect any heightened reactivity in acute
rheumatic fever patients.   However, Gowrishanker and Agarwal (4)
using an eight molar urea extract of heart valves did demonstrate
heightened reactivity to these antigens in acute rheumatic fever
patients.   Using a crude homogenate of heart tissue our own
efforts in this respect have been unrewarding but the antigens
responsible for the binding to rheumatic fever heart reactive
antibody have not yet been used in our cellular assays.

CONCLUSIONS

     All evidence to date indicates that there is an abnormal
response on the part of the host against certain streptococcal
antigens which are cross reactive with heart and muscle tissue.
While our personal bias in the disease rheumatic fever leans
towards the streptococcal membrane antigen as the predominant

antigen responsible for the induction of heart reactive antibody, data concerning other cross reactive antigens must be carefully considered in the pathogenesis of this disease.

Perhaps the most interesting observations are concerned with the cellular response to both streptococcal and heart antigens. Data from both the human and experimental models indicates that an antibody independent cell mediated immunity is solely responsible for the cytotoxic action of lymphocytes obtained from these patients and that heart reactive antibody does not play a role in this cytopathic effect. Whether or not cellular reactivity to streptococcal antigens seen in rheumatic fever patients is cross reactive with heart antigens remains a moot point but one can at least state with some certainty that streptococcal stimulated lymphocytes do kill specific heart monolayers.

It is hoped in the context of this conference that the use of single cell and beating heart cell monolayers (either human or experimental animals) will help to resolve some of the still unanswered questions concerning host-microbe relationships in this disease. Furthermore, understanding of this disease has obvious implications for other as yet undefined diseases of cardiac origin.

REFERENCES

1) Brokman, H., Brill, J., and Frendzall, J., Komplement Ablengung mit Organ Extrackten von Rheumatikern B.B.F. - Reaktions bei sogernnetern akutern Gelenk-rheumatismus. Klin. Wehnsch, 16:502 (1937).

2) Cavelti, P.A., Autoantibodies in rheumatic fever. Proc. Soc. Exp. Biol. Med., 60:376 (1945).

3) Dale, J.B. and Beachey, E.H., Protective antibody against a peptide fragment of type 5 streptococcal M protein cross-reacts with human host tissue. Presented at the Fed. for Clinical Research, Washington, D.C., Abs. No. 565A (1982).

4) Gowrishanker, R., and Agarwal, S.C., Leucocyte migration inhibition with human heart valve glycoproteins and group A streptococcal ribonucleic acid proteins in rheumatic heart disease and post streptococcal glomerulonephritis. Clin. Exp. Immunol. 39:519-525 (1980).

5) Hall, W.W. and Choppin, P.W., Measles virus proteins in the brain tissue of patients with subacute sclerosing panencephalitis. New Engl. J. Med. 304:1152-1155 (1981).

6) Hutto, J.H., and Ayoub, E.M., Cytotoxicity of lymphocytes from patients with rheumatic carditis to cardiac cells in vitro, In "Streptococcal Diseases and the Immune Response", Eds. Read, S.E., and Zabriskie, J.B., Academic Press, NY, p. 733 (1980).

7) Kaplan, M.H., Meyeresian, M., and Kushner, I., Immunologic studies of heart tissue. IV. Serologic reactions with human heart tissue as revealed by immunofluorescent methods: isoimmune, Wasserman, and auto immune reactions. J. Exp. Med., 113:17 (1961).

8) Kaplan, M.H., and Frengley, J.D., Autoimmunity to the heart in cardiac disease. Current concepts of the relation of autoimmunity to rheumatic fever, postcardiotomy and postinfarction syndromes and cardiomyopathies. Am. J. Cardiol., 24:459 (1969).

9) Manjula, B.N. and Fischetti, V.A., Tropomyosin-like seven residue periodicity in three immunologically distinct streptococcal M proteins and its implications for the antiphagocytic property of the molecule. J. Exp. Med. 151:695-708 (1980).

10) McLaughlin, J.F., Paterson, P.Y., Harts, R.S. and Enibury, S.H., Rheumatic carditis: in vitro responses of peripheral blood leucocytes to heart and streptococcal antigens. Arth. Rheum. 15:600 (1972).

11) Read, S.E., Zabriskie, J.B., Fischetti, V.A., Utermohlen, V. and Falk, R., Cellular reactivity to streptococcal antigens in patients with streptococcal infections and their sequelae. J. Clin. Invest. 54:439-450 (1974).

12) Reid, H.F.M., Read, S.E., Poon-King, T. and Zabriskie, J.B. The cellular immune response to streptococcal antigens in patients with post streptococcal sequelae in Trinidad, In "Streptococcal Diseases and the Immune Response", S. Read and J.B. Zabriskie, eds., Academic Press, NY, p. 595 (1980).

13) van de Rijn, I., Zabriskie, J.B., and McCarty, M., Group A streptococcal antigens cross-reactive with myocardium: purification of heart-reactive antibody and isolation and characterization of the streptococcal antigen. J. Exp. Med., 146:579-599 (1977).

14) Yang, L.C., Soprey, P.R., Wittner, M.K., and Fox, E.N., Streptococcal induced cell mediated immune destruction of cardiac myofibers in vitro. J. Exp. Med., 146:344-360 (1977).

15) Zabriskie, J.B., and Freimer, E.H., An immunological relationship between the Group A streptococcus and mammalian muscle. J. Exp. Med., 124:661 (1966).

16) Zabriskie, J.B., Hsu, K.C., and Seegal, B.C. Heart-reactive antibody associated with rheumatic fever: characterization and diagnostic significance. Clin. Exp. Immunol., 7:147-159 (1970).

17) Zabriskie, J.B., Read, S.E., and Ellis, R.J., Cellular and humoral studies in diseases with heart-reactive antibodies, In "Papers in Immunology", Academic Press, NY and London, p. 213 (1971).

HUMORAL IMMUNITY AND HEART DISEASE:

POSTPERICARDIOTOMY SYNDROME

Mary Allen Engle

Stavros S. Niarchos Prof. of Pediatrics Cardiology
Director of Pediatric Cardiology
The New York Hospital-Cornell Medical Center
New York, New York 10021

INTRODUCTION

Historically it was adults with rheumatic heart disease and mitral stenosis who first suffered from the common postoperative complication of the postpericardiotomy syndrome (PPS). Fever appeared or persisted beyond the first postoperative week together with signs and symptoms of pericardial reaction: chest pain, pericardial friction rub, electrocardiographic as well as radiographic evidence of pericarditis and often of pericardial and pleural effusions, together with leukocytosis and less specific sign of inflammation. In the setting of rheumatic mitral stenosis, it was natural to assume that this postoperative illness was due to reactivation of rheumatic fever and to treat the patients with medication considered beneficial in acute rheumatic fever: salicylates or steroids.

Then the children entered the picture as closed or open heart procedures for congenital heart disease developed. We observed the identical postoperative syndrome in these patients with nonrheumatic heart disease. As we reviewed our surgical experience in children with congenital heart disease,[1,2] we found that the complication occurred only after the surgeon had widely incised the pericardium to do the operation. We realized that the common denominator for the complication in adults and children was entry in the pericardium. Therefore we proposed the descriptive term postpericardiotomy syndrome.[1,2] We thought that this reaction might represent an auto-immune response or perhaps a viral illness, but we had no opportunity to test either hypothesis until determinations for anti-heart antibody by immunofluorescent technique and for anti-viral antibody by complement fixation tests were developed.

471

MATERIAL AND METHODS

About ten years ago, we undertook a prospective, double-blind
study in children who were consecutive long-term survivors of intrapericardial surgery for congenital heart disease[3] to test the hypothesis that this was an auto-immune illness. We observed the children in the hospital and for the first three months postoperatively,
noting evidence of the syndrome and classifying it as mild, moderate
or severe. We drew blood samples the day preoperatively and at
intervals postoperatively: around the 7th-10th day and in the first,
second, and sometimes third postoperative months for determination
of heart-reactive antibody. As the study progressed, we correlated
the clinical and immunologic data.

RESULTS

We found that the incidence of the syndrome continued to be
between 25-30%, just as in the past, and that about one-third had
mild, another third moderate, and one-third severe illness. Prior
to surgery, no one had detectable anti-heart antibody (AHA). After
surgery, we found three patterns of response in AHA: no rise at all
(Negative) or a rise to 2+ or greater beginning around the 7th-10th
day with persistence for about a month or two before it declined
and disappeared (Positive) or a rise beginning at the same time but
to less than 2+ and declining earlier (Intermediate). Correlation
of results of clinical findings with AHA at regular intervals re
vealed consistently that no patient with Negative AHA had the
clinical syndrome whereas all with Positive AHA had clinical PPS and
a rare child with Intermediate AHA had mild syndrome. We interpreted
these findings to indicate that this syndrome represented an auto-
immune response in autologous heart and pericardium in response to
intrapericardial entry and the opportunity for intrapericardial
trauma and bleeding.

After the first 120 patients, we continued the study in this
manner, but in addition, we tested the hypothesis that viral illness
played a role in this syndrome. We added the determination of anti-
viral antibody (AVA) in a second and independent laboratory. A four-
fold or greater rise and then fall in AVA was considered to be consistent with viral illness. Thus, we converted the double-blind to
a triple-blind prospective study for the next 280 children.[4,5]
Correlation of data from the clinical and two laboratory studies at
intervals indicated that in the patients with no PPS, only a few
with negative AHA (7.8%) and a few more with Intermediate AHA (19.2%)
had a significant antiviral rise in titre, whereas with clinical PPS
and high AHA, 70% of patients had such a rise. This high order of
association of high AHA with change in AVA suggested that the syndrome was an immune response in association with a viral infection.

If this were so, did the changing AVA titre represent

reactivation of a latent virus from a remote infection, or a recent
illness, or perhaps a concurrently acquired viral infection? To
answer this, we analyzed the patients with and without PPS in relation to the three AHA responses and to whether AVA was or was not
detected on the day prior to surgery and according to any change
in titre postoperatively. We found that most patients with no
syndrome had no change in AVA and had negative AHA (92%) or Intermediate AHA (78%). Clinically, those with Negative AHA were indis-
tinguisable from those with Intermediate AHA since they did not have
PPS. Neither did the vast majority of them have evidence of viral
illness. On the other hand, over half (53%) of the children with
PPS and Positive AHA did have evidence of viral infection in that
they had no detectable AVA on admission but then showed a four-fold
or greater rise. This suggests that they acquired a viral infection
concurrent with their hospitalization for cardiac surgery. Another
smaller group with PPS, 16%, had a low titre of AVA on admission,
followed by a significant rise. Perhaps in these children the
trauma of surgery caused reactivation of an illness that had occurred
in the recent or remote past. Another response in AVA, noted in 10%
with PPS, was a high titre on admission, followed by a drop in titre.
These were probably convalescent from a fresh virus infection when
they entered the hospital for cardiac surgery. In 21% with PPS we
found no change in AVA titre from the preoperative sample. They
too may have shown a serologic response had we tested sera against
a larger battery of viruses than we chose for study.

     We selected the following viral agents to test in this pros-
pective study: Adenovirus, Coxsackie B 1-6, and Cytomegalovirus.
In addition, we tested for reaction against Mycoplasma pneumoniae
and found only a rare child with a rise and no correlation with PPS.
However, for the eight viruses tested, we found interesting results
as the study progressed. First, there was no single virus with rise
in complement-fixing antibody that was associated with the syndrome
Instead, we found for each virus tested, a 50% to 100% incidence of
clinical PPS and Positive AHA when a four-fold or greater rise in
titre to that agent occurred. Most patients had a rise in titre to
a single virus and rarely to more than one. Second, we found a
changing prevalence of viruses and AVA rise as the study progressed.
This change over the years was most dramatic for Coxsackie B4, but
changing prevalence was noted for each virus: a rise in AVA was
noted frequently for a couple of years and then infrequently for the
next year or two when other viruses were on the rise in frequency.
For example, with Coxsackie B4, we detected none in the first 137
patients studied, but by the cumulative analysis of the first 190
patients, there were as many with rise in AVA to this virus as to
Cytomegalovirus, which had been the agent with the greatest number
of significantly rising titres. At conclusion of the prospective
study in the children, after we had evaluated 280 in the pediatric
age group, Coxsackie B4 stood out above all others as the agent
most frequently found to cause a four-fold or more rise in titre.[5]

These observations suggested that the syndrome was associated with viruses prevalent in the community at the time of the operation. Year-by-year analysis of AVA response showed the rise and fall in the different viruses that conformed to variations known to occur in virus infections as populations develop some immunity to one virus, which then becomes quiescent as a cause of infection while others take over. In this study, Coxsackie B4 occurred in epidemic proportions in the second and third years and alerted us to the strong possibility that whatever role a virus infection plays in triggering or abetting the auto-immune response we call PPS, no single virus is implicated but instead, viruses prevalent in the community at the time of surgery.[5]

When one considers the opportunities for contact with viruses that hospitalization for surgery provides, it is evident that many exist: with operating room personnel while the patient's pericardium is open, with nurses and doctors in the intensive care unit when immune mechanisms have been somewhat comprised by anesthesia and surgery and when there is close contact of professional and patient, with other children on the pediatric floors as well as with many personnel that include technicians, nurses, students, physicians.

Of the 400 children studied, 50 had a second intrapericardial procedure. This provided an opportunity to answer the questions whether the incidence of PPS would be greater the second time around, whether occurrence of PPS after the first operation meant that it would occur the second time as well and perhaps even more severely, and whether the same high order of association of AVA-AHA rise and PPS existed in re-operations as we had found in the whole series, in which 350 were first operations.

We found first, that the incidence was no higher after the second intrapericardial procedure; it was 36%, just as for the group as a whole who were two years of age or older (see below). Second, having PPS after the first procedure did not mean that it would necessarily develop the second time or be more severe. Third, we found the same association of syndrome and viral illness as for the entire group. Among those without PPS, 15% of those with Negative AHA and 0% of those with Intermediate AHA had a four-fold rise in AVA, whereas 100% of those with Positive AHA and PPS had this significant rise. Therefore, it seems that viral reaction together with pericardiotomy are the major ingredients that relate to clinical PPS, whether the pericardium is entered for the first or for a second time.

Although all the operations performed on the 400 children in this study were intrapericardial, some operations involved muscle resection and much opportunity for myocardial trauma, opening up of

antigen-antibody binding sites and providing opportunity for viral
invasion of injured heart muscle or pericardium or for the stirring
up of a latent virus infection. So we analyzed the incidence of
PPS, Aha and AVA responses for each type of cardiac operation. Repair
of tetralogy of Fallot was the most frequently performed operation,
followed in decreasing order by atrial septal defect, simple ventricular septal defect (VSD), complex ventricular septal defect,
Mustard operation for simple transposition of the great arteries,
pulmonary valvotomy, and a miscellaneous group. For each malform-
ation clinical PPS with rise in AHA and in AVA was related just as
described for the total 400 operations. Incidence of PPS was least
(0%) for simple transposition, in which parietal pericardium is
resected, atriotomy performed, atrial septum excised, pericardial
baffle placed to reroute venous return to the heart, and the new
pulmonary venous atrium enlarged with a strip of pericardium. This
operation was performed chiefly in infants. Incidence of PPS was
highest after repair of tetralogy of Fallot (44%) and of complex
VSD (46%). Both offered the greatest opportunity for myocardial
trauma: right ventriculotomy in a hypertrophied ventricular wall
and excision of large amounts of obstructing infundibular fibro-
muscular hypertrophy in all instances of tetralogy repair and most
instances of complex VSD. So we concluded that the degree of myocardial trauma at operation bore a relation to PPS: the greater the
damage, the greater the risk of the complication.[5]

The early and mid-1970-s when this prospective study began co-
incided with the new trend in pediatric cardiac surgery to early
primary repair of congenital anomalies in infancy in preference to
delay until childhood years, and in preference to a two-staged
approach of first, palliation in infancy followed by repair in
childhood. We observed that very few of the 113 under the age of
two years had the syndrome, only 3.5%, and none of the 42 babies
under the age of six months did; whereas, in each older age group
(two up to five years, six to 10 years, 11 years and older) the
incidence was 36%. Why were the infants spared? Even though they
had the same kinds of surgery as the whole group, with the same
opportunities for myocardial trauma that ranged from extensive
(repair of tetralogy of Fallot, e.g.) to minimal (Mustard operation
for transposed great arteries), they rarely had clinical PPS or high
titre AHA or AVA.

Several explanations seem plausible and may, at least in part,
be the answer. Young infants may be protected by transplacental
transfer of maternal antibody and also by the fact that they are
babies with serious heart disease, so that they tended to be protected from contact with people known to have a respiratory or
gastrointestinal infection. Furthermore, although none of the
infants had indication of immunologic imcompetence, they were still
undergoing immunologic maturation. Perhaps a certain degree of
maturity is required before the infant can mount the kind of

auto-immune response and antiviral reaction that measurements of
AHA and AVA test. After the second birthday, however, there was no
age difference among the children through adolescence in susceptibility to syndrome.

How did adults undergoing intrapericardial surgery fare? As
we concluded the study of the 400 children and adolescents[6], we
began a similar triple-blind prospective study in adults.[6]

The incidence of PPS in 142 adults aged 21 years and older was
less than in the pediatric age group: 17.6%. We noted a declining
incidence in PPS as age advanced. Under age 40 years, the incidence
was similar to that in younger subjects: 28.6%. From 41 to 50 years
and 51 to 60 years incidence was 20% and 19.6%, respectively. In
the seventh decade, it was less: 14.3%. After age 70, it was the
least: 10%. The two decades of 51-60 and 61-70 had the greatest
numbers of operations: 46 patients were in their 50's and 49 in
their 60's.

Relative sparing of the elderly, as for the babies, may be
that they are protected because of many years of having and handling
viral illnesses and because they tend to be exposed to virus infections in their home environment less frequently than younger adults.
Possibly with aging comes some immunosenescence so that they are
less capable of mounting an immune response in association with
intrapericardial trauma and the exposure to viruses that can happen
in a hospital setting.

We found the same relation to heart-reactive antibody and
clinical syndrome in adults as we had in the children. While none
of the patients with Negative AHA (54.2%) or Intermediate AHA
(28.2%) had PPS, all of the patients with Positive AHA (17.6%) did.
In three the syndrome was severe, and two adults underwent pericardial resection before their severe and recurrent PPS subsided.
Nine had PPS of moderate severity, and 13 had mild PPS.

Just as for the children, we found a high order of association
between viral antibody, four-fold rise, and high titre AHA with the
clinical syndrome. Of the patients with no PPS and with Negative
AHA, only 5.2% had a four-fold or greater rise to one virus (usually)
or more than one (rarely), while 5.0% with Intermediate AHA and no
syndrome did, but 68% of the patients with Positive AHA and PPS had
a significant rise in antiviral antibody titre. Again, no single
virus was implicated: rising titre was detected in one, and rarely
more, of all eight viruses tested. Therefore, we concluded that
just as in the children, a fresh viral illness, or serologic reactivation of a latent one, is associated with the immune response of
the postpericardiotomy syndrome.

Operations on the adults were usually for coronary artery

bypass grafting alone (CABG) and somewhat less often for valve replacement alone. Neither operation involved as much opportunity for trauma as did repair of tetralogy of Fallot or complex VSD in the children. Incidence of PPS was 13.3% in the patients after CABG alone and 22.6% in patients after valve replacement alone, a difference that is not statistically significant.

Therapy for this self-limited condition is difficult to choose and the results are hard to evaluate. Most of the children with mild or moderate syndrome received no specific therapy except for restriction of activities and for diuretics for the pericardial and pleural effusion. Those with severe syndrome received either salicylates for several weeks or steroids for three weeks: full dose, first week; half dose, second week; quarter dose, third week. Steroid therapy effected more prompt relief of all signs and symtoms than did salicylates but had the disadvantage that some patients relapsed on withdrawal and needed one or two more courses of steroids. Adults were treated with indomethacin for about two weeks or with steroids. As in the children, both therapies rendered the patients afebrile and more comfortable, but again there were some relapses after treatment was stopped, especially so after steroid therapy. No patient, child or adult, died because of the syndrome. The greatest incapacity was related to large pericardial effusions that required pericardiocenteses or when recurrent and large, necessitated removel of the pericardium before the syndrome subsided.

CONCLUSIONS

In a prospective, blinded study we evaluated infants, children and adolescents, and adults for presence of postpericardiotomy syndrome (PPS) following intrapericardial surgery. We first tested the hypotheses that the illness represented an auto-immune response to intrapericardial trauma by looking for heart-reactive antibodies in postoperative sera, and we found a close correlation between clinical syndrome and development of strongly positive anti-heart antibodies (AHA). Next, in addition, we tested the hypothesis that the syndrome might involve a viral illness by looking in the same postoperative sera for a significant rise in antiviral antibody to one or more of eight viruses tested: Adenovirus, Coxsackie B 1-6, and Cytomegalovirus. We found that almost 70% of children and adults with such a rise had PPS and high titre of AHA. Infants under age two years and adults over age 70 years had the lowest incidence of PPS. Incidence of PPS was 27% in children and 18% in adults. We believe that this common postoperative syndrome is an immune response in association with viral illness, triggered by the trauma of intrapericardial surgery.

REFERENCES

1. Ito, T., Engle, M.A., Goldberg, H.P.: Postpericardiotomy
    syndrome following surgery for nonrheumatic heart disease.
    Circulation 17: 549, 1958.
2. Engle, M.A., Ito, T.: The postpericardiotomy syndrome.
    Am. J. Cardiol 7: 73, 1961.
3. Engle, M.A., McCabe, J.C., Ebert, P.A., Zabriskie, J.B.:
    The postpericardiotomy syndrome and antiheart antibodies.
    Circulation 49: 401, 1974.
4. Engle, M.A., Zabriskie, J.B., Senterfit, L.B., Tay, D.J.,
    Ebert, P.A.: Immunologic and virologic studies in the
    postpericardiotomy syndrome. J. Pediatr 87: 1103, 1975.
5. Engle, M.A., Zabriskie, J.B., Senterfit, L.B., Gay, W.A. Jr.,
    O'Loughlin, J.E., Ehlers, K.H.: Viral illness and the post-
    pericardiotomy syndrome. A prospective study in children.
    Circulation 62: 1151, 1980.
6. Engle, M.A., Gay, W.A. Jr., McCabe, J., Longo, E.,
    Johnson, D., Senterfit, L.B., Zabriskie, J.B.: Postperi-
    cardiotomy syndrome in adults: Incidence, autoimmunity and
    virology. Circulation 64(suppl II): II-58, 1981.

CELL-MEDIATED IMMUNE INJURY TO THE HEART

H. Friedman*, S. Specter*, A. Cerdan **, C. Cerdan **,
and K. Chang**

*Dept. of Med. Micro. and Immunol., Univ. of South
   Florida College of Med., Tampa, Florida
**Deborah Heart and Lung Hospital, Browns Mills, N.J.

Ischemic heart disease is considered a primary form of fatal cardiac disease both in the United States and many other developed countries of the world. A frequent consequence of sudden myocardial ischemia, such as that which follows coronary thrombosis, is myocardial infarction. Muscle necrosis may be prevented if collateral circulation is adequate. However, it is now widely accepted that during corrective surgical procedures cardiac antigens may be released and an autoimmune-type response may ensue. The relationship between cardiac manifestations after cardiac infarction or cardiac surgery is unresolved and controversial. Cardiac autoantibodies are often detected in the sera of patients following infarction and/or cardiotomy but the pathogenic roles of these serum factors have not been unequivocally explained. Furthermore, little attention has been directed to the nature and role of autoreactive immunocompetent cells in the autoimmune-associated cardiac type disorders.

There has been much evidence that antibodies may appear after an infarct or following cardiac surgery (1-5). Such antibodies have often been detected by immunoflurorescent procedures, agglutination tests with erythrocytes passively sensitized with cardiac-derived antigens, including myocardial proteins and enzymes, often appear in the serum following cardiac injury. It is possible that antigen-antibody complexes may be involved in the post-myocardial infarction or post-cardiotomy syndromes which occur generally 7-14 days after the initial cardiac episode. Cardiac antigens, however, may also elicit sensitized lymph cells capable of reacting specifically with the antigen. It has been observed that following sensitization of experimental animals with streptococci which share antigens with myocardial tissue, autoreactive lymphoid

479

cells develop which respond in vitro to myocardial tissue extracts
by blastogenic proliferation (6,7). In addition, there have been
some reports with experimental animals that migration inhibitory
factor, considered a correlate of cell mediated immunity, develops in lymphoid cell culture supernatants from specifically sensitized animals in the presence of the myocardial extracts. A detailed analysis of the appearance of similar sensitized leukocytes
in the peripheral blood of patients after myocardial infarct or
cardiac surgery was made in the present study in an attempt to
identify and ascertain the role of cardiac reactive cells in the
sequelae of myocardial infarction or following surgery. Results
of this study demonstrate that peripheral blood leukocytes from
patients who have had a myocardial infarct or after cardiac surgery
are capable of reacting with relatively small amounts of mitochondrial extracts prepared from human heart tissue in a direct
migration inhibitory assay in vitro. Saline extracts from cardiac
tissue was much less effective in eliciting this reaction and human
myoglobin antigen had no effect.

EXPERIMENTAL METHODS AND PROCEDURES

     Patient populations used in this study were hospitalized at
the Albert Einstein Medical Center, Philadelphia, Pennsylvania, or
the Deborah Heart and Lung Institute in Browns Mills, New Jersey
for cardiac disease. The myocardiac infarct patients were admitted because of possible acute cardiac ischemic disease and those
studied were confirmed as having a myocardial infarct. Patients
undergoing surgery were admitted for a variety of open-heart procedures including mitral valve commisurotomies, etc. The patients
ranged in age from 17 to 68. Control individuals were patients
who were hospitalized for other purposes and had no evidence of
heart disease. Peripheral blood leukocytes were obtained from the
patients on admission and at various times thereafter, usually two
or three times during the first week and at weekly intervals for
up to 6 weeks. The microagarose droplet method of Harrington and
Stastny was used for determining migration inhibition using three
types of heart antigens (8). For this purpose, heart tissue was
obtained at autopsy from individuals who had died from non-cardiac
causes. Whole saline extracts were prepared by homogenizing
200 grams of cardiac muscle in physiological saline for 2-5 minutes
with a tissue homogenizer at $4^{\circ}C$. Cellular debris was removed by
centrifugation at 2,000 x g and the soluble extract filter steril-
ized. Mitochondria were obtained from homogenized heart extract
exactly as described elsewhere by differential centrifugation (9).
Myoglobin was prepared from heart tissue extracts by ammonium
sulfate precipitation followed by chromatography. For the migration inhibition assay, 5×10^7 peripheral blood leukocytes obtained
at various times from control and cardiac patients were placed in
the agarose in microdroplets in plastic microtiter plates. To
each well was then added 0.25 ml of tissue culture medium either

without addition or containing graded amounts of the cardiac antigens, i.e. saline extracts, mitochondrial preparations or myoglobin.
As additional controls, either whole saline extracts or mitochondrial fractions of human kidneys were utilized. In all cases, the
migration of leukocytes in the agar droplet after 24 hours incubation at 37°C was determined by microscopic examination using a calibrated micrometer areas of migration. Migration of peripheral
blood leukocytes in the agar droplets without added antigen was
compared to those microdroplets containing various antigens or extracts.

EXPERIMENTAL RESULTS

     Previous studies in this laboratory have shown that patients
recovering from myocardial infarctions or after myocardial surgery
often develop significant levels of antibodies detected by an indirect hemagglutination procedure using erythrocytes sensitized
with human heart saline extracts. Peak responses usually occurred
between 2 and 4 weeks after the infarct or surgery. There was
rarely, if ever, significant antibody levels in patients who had
been admitted to the hospital with symptoms of a heart attack but
were diagnosed as not having had an infarct or myocardial ischemia.
Furthermore, approximately one-third of the patients who had undergone myocardial surgery developed circulating antibodies within
2-3 weeks after surgery. Therefore, it was of interest to determine whether similar groups of patients would show evidence of
cell-mediated immunity utilizing the migration inhibition procedure
with the patient's peripheral blood leukocytes. As is apparent in
Figure 1, there was no significant level of migration inhibition
of leukocytes from 7 normal control patients hospitalized for a
variety of non-cardiac purposes when their peripheral blood cells
were tested against the saline heart extract, mitochondria or myoglobin, regardless of concentration. The few instances of migration inhibition were usually just above the level considered significant (i.e. 20% inhibition) as compared to leukocyte migration
in the absence of antigen. In contrast, nearly two-thirds of the
14 patients examined in this study at various times after either a
diagnosed infarct or post-cardiac surgery showed significant levels
of migration inhibition (Figure 1). It is evident that the greatest levels of inhibition occurred with the mitochondria as the antigen. Much less inhibition, generally insignificant, occurred with
the highest concentration of the saline extract as antigen and only
insignificant inhibition occurred with the myoglobin. The largest
amount of mitochondrial antigen used, i.e. 500 µg, when added to
the peripheral blood leukocytes tested in vitro, resulted in the
greatest migration inhibition. As controls, kidney extracts, including mitochondrial preparations, failed to elicit such migration inhibition.

As is evident in Figure 2, there was generally similar levels of

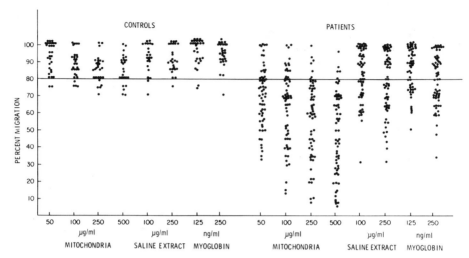

Figure 1 - Inhibition of migration of human peripheral
blood mononuclear cells. Multiple responses over several
weeks for 7 controls and 14 patients with either
myocardial infarcts or following open heart surgery.
Each point represents one test.

migration inhibition with the mitochondrial antigen using peripheral blood leukocytes from patients after either a myocardial
infarction or after cardiac surgery. In general, the greatest
inhibition of migration occurred with the 500 μg dose of antigen
and peripheral blood from patients two or three weeks after the
infarct or surgery. A few examples of the reactions observed with
selected patients are shown in Figures 3, 4 and 5. The first
patient illustrated (Figure 3) showed a marked increase of migration inhibition the second week after surgery. This was evident
mainly with the mitochondrial extract, but there was a slight effect with the saline extract and none with the myoglobin. By
the fourth week after surgery, inhibition of migration of the
patient's leukocytes decreased to normal values, but then there
was an increase during the fifth to sixth week. The largest concentration of mitochondria resulted in the largest degree of migration inhibition. By the fifth week after surgery, the patient
developed a fever and symptoms of post-myocardial infarction syndrome. Treatment at this time with cortisone reversed the symptoms and resulted in a rapid return to normal (data not shown) of
peripheral blood leukocyte responsiveness to the heart mitochondria. Results with another patient are illustrated in Figure 4;
this patient also showed some leukocyte migration inhibition at
the beginning of observation after open heart surgery with a
further increase of reactivity throughout the course of hospital-

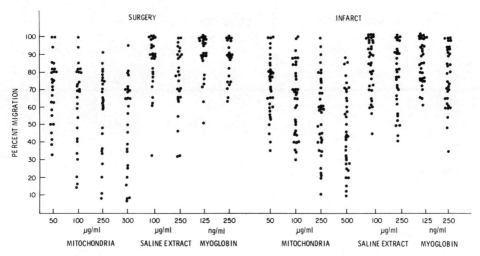

Figure 2. Inhibition of migration of human peripheral blood mononuclear cells. Separate examination of 7 surgery patients and 7 myocardial infarct patients examined during a 3 to 6 week period.

ization, but at a much lower level than some of the other patients. The pattern of migration inhibition was somewhat different in that there was no effect noted with myoglobin or saline extract, and a moderate suppression of migration with mitochondrial extracts. A third patient, illustrated in Figure 5, exhibited a marked increase in migration inhibition during the first 2-3 weeks after cardiac surgery. Two to three weeks after the surgery the mitochondrial antigen resulted in essentially no migration of leukocytes in the test system. However, there was no evidence of any clinical post-cardiotomy syndrome. Table 1 summarizes the results of the migration inhibitory assay with peripheral blood leukocytes from the post-surgical and post-myocardial infarction patients as compared to control patients. It is evident from the summation of these results that mitochondrial antigen added at a concentration of 500 µg per culture well resulted in the most consistent and re-producible reactions.

DISCUSSIONS AND CONCLUSIONS

The results of these studies support the view that CMI may be involved in post-myocardial infarction and post-myocardial sur-gical reactions. Over two-thirds of the patients who had defini-tively diagnosed myocardial ischemia and studied in a hospital situation for a month or longer revealed sensitivity of their peripheral blood leukocytes to a mitochondrial antigen prepared

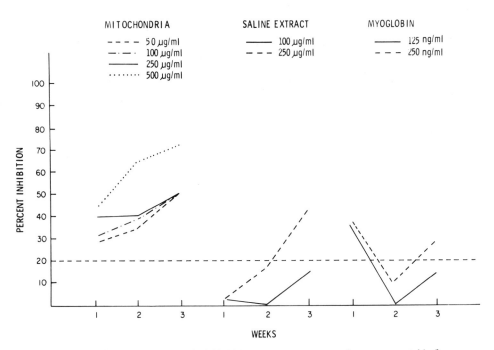

Figure 3. Migration inhibition responses of a myocardial infarct patient for 3 weeks showing increasing reactivity through the observation period.

from normal human hearts. The crude saline extracts had much less effect in eliciting a similar reaction and human myoglobin was essentially ineffective. It is important to note that in control studies it was shown that the same mitochondrial antigens had essentially no inhibitory effect on migration of peripheral blood leukocytes from normal patients without evidence of myocardial disease. Furthermore, mitochondrial extracts prepared from human kidneys failed to elicit a similar migration inhibitory reaction with peripheral blood leukocytes from those cardiac patients who evinced sensitivity to the cardiac mitochondrial antigens. In further studies, it was found the peripheral blood leukocytes from patients who had undergone open-heart surgery for a variety of purposes also evinced sensitivity to mitochondrial antigen. The cruder saline extract, or purified myoglobin had little effect in eliciting a similar migration inhibition in vitro.

The MIF assay in vitro, either a macrosystem using capillary tubes or the microsystem utilized in the present study, is considered an in vitro correlate of T cell mediated immunity. Inhibition of macrophages or granulocytes in the peripheral blood,

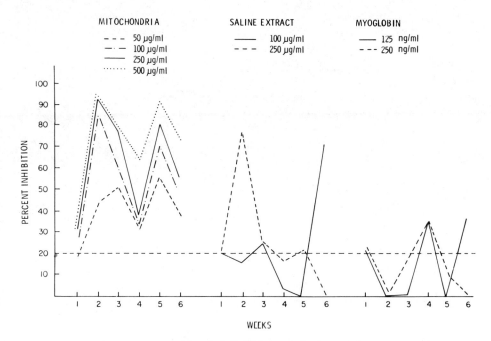

Figure 4. Migration inhibition responses for an open-
heart surgery patient. Activity peaked at week 2 and
began return to control levels through week 4; at week 5
activity increased again; this was followed a few days
later by a post-cardiotomy syndrome episode.

as well as polymorphonuclear cells, in terms of their migratory
ability through agar gel is considered a response to MIF released
by sensitized T lymphocytes responding to specific antigen (8).
Many varieties of this in vitro assay have been developed but in
general it is widely acknowledged that inhibition of migration of
leukocytes in the presence of an antigen reflects a specific immunologically mediated response. This can be ascertained, however,
only when there is a relative inhibition of migration of cells in
the presence of antigen as compared to absence of antigen. Furthermore, specificity must be demonstrated utilizing antigens to
which the individuals are putatively sensitized. In control
studies it was found that antigen extracts prepared from kidneys
failed to elicit similar migration inhibition with cardiac patients
who showed a sensitivity to the heart antigens. Since the saline
extracts from the heart were relatively poor in eliciting a response, it may be assumed that these extracts do not express sufficient specific myocardial antigen to which the patients are
sensitized or the fractionation procedures may have inactivated
the appropriate antigen. It is also of interest that the heart

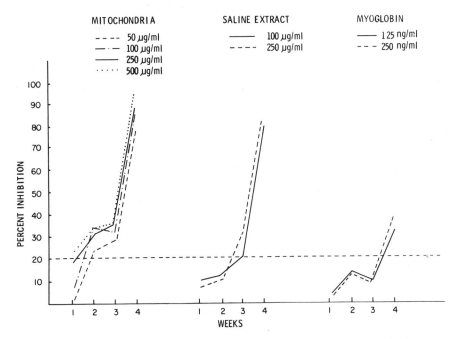

Figure 5. Migration inhibition responses for an open
heart surgery patient. High MI activity was not as-
oociated with any clinical post-cardiotomy problems.

antigens used in these studies were derived from unrelated individuals without known cardiac disease.   Thus, it would appear that
if the reaction is indeed a cell mediated immune response to myocardial antigens of the patient per se, these antigens are not
individual specific.   This is generally true in most cases of
autoimmunity where specific immune responses may be elicited with
tissue extracts from any individual of the same species, and sometimes from different species.

      The observation that patients who had underone open-heart
surgery also develop reactive lymphocytes suggests that the exposure to myocardial antigens may be sufficient to sensitize
lymphoid cells to the same or related antigens.   Since relatively
few individuals develop the post-myocardial infarction or post-
cardiotomy syndrome, it seems likely that the presence of such
sensitized lymphocytes in patients is not sufficient to elicit
the symptoms of an autoimmune response.   Nevertheless, it appears
important to be able to determine the relative degree of sensitization of individuals to cardiac antigens following injury to the
heart using in vitro assays for cellular immunity.   In this regard, there have been a number of studies in man and experimental

TABLE 1

MIGRATION INHIBITION OF PERIPHERAL BLOOD LYMPHOCYTES FROM PATIENTS
WITH HEART DISEASE USING HEART ANTIGENS

		MITOCHONDRIA[a] (μg)		HEART HOMOGENATE (μg)		MYOGLOBIN (μg)	
		100	250	500	100	250	250
Controls	x̄	86.1±1.9[b]	81.6±2.3	77.5±3.2	91.8±1.4	89.7±1.6	92.8
Coronary Artery Disease	x̄	61.2±3.4	53.5±4.0	44.2±4.0	84.2±2.8	77.0±3.4	75.1
	%	71	66	57	92	86	81
	p[c]	<0.0005	<0.0005	<0.0005	<0.05	<0.005	<0.005
Open Heart Surgery	x̄	61.7±4.9	58.8±5.0	51.6±5.2	83.6±3.2	76.2±3.8	86.0
	%	71	72	67	91	85	93
	p[c]	<0.0005	<0.0005	<0.0005	<0.05	<0.0025	<0.05

[a] 0.025 ml of medium containing antigen was added to agarose droplet containing 1×10^5 Ficoll separated peripheral blood lymphocytes.

[b] Numbers represent an average of several tests on at least 7 patients per group and are expressed as % migration of controls without antigen ± S.D.

[c] Statistical analysis performed using Student's t. test.

All groups except MYOGLOBIN 125 μg for OHS patients (data not shown) show statistical significance for heart patients vs. controls. However, if 80% migration is used as a determination point, then only the mitochondria caused significant migration inhibition.

animals over the last decade or so revealing development of serum
antibodies to heart tissue (1,3). Such studies showed that antibodies reactive to cardiac tissue may occur in patients infected
with microorganisms with cross-reactive antigens, i.e. streptococci, or other microorganisms which inflict damage to the heart,
i.e. a wide variety of bacteria, viruses, or fungi. In experimental animal models it has been shown that immunization of animals with antigenically cross-reactive microbes or even heart tissue per se elicits anti-heart antibodies detectable by a wide
variety of serologic methods. Furthermore, attempts have been
made to show development of cellular immunity in individuals infected with bacteria such as streptococci or immunized with cardiac reactive lymphoid cells which can cause cytolytic damage to
guinea pig·myocytes in vitro (10). Similarly, beating myocites
have been used in a number of studies to demonstrate that antibodies can inflict damage to the myocytes detectable by both immunologic and physiologic assays (11). Thus, it appears likely
that in both experimental models and in man antibodies as well as
sensitized lymphoid cells may appear following damage to the heart.
The results of the present study expand previous observations in
this laboratory concerning humoral immunity and demonstrate that
lymphoid cells capable of interacting with heart mitochondria
occur after myocardial infarction or surgery. The role of these
immune factors in cardiac pathology remains to be determined.

SUMMARY

     A micro in vitro procedure was utilized to assess cell-medi-
ated immunity of patients following myocardial infarction or cardiac surgery. For this purpose, peripheral blood leukocytes from
patients were tested in a microdroplet assay with antigen preparations derived from human cardiac tissue. Whereas whole saline
extract and human myoglobin preparations had little effect on the
migration of peripheral blood leukocytes in vitro, mitochondrial
preparations were markedly effective in inhibiting migration of
the leukocytes in the presence of mitochondrial extracts appeared
to reflect development of cell mediated immunity to heart antigens after the myocardial infarct or surgery. These results extend the observations that humoral antibody may appear in patient
following cardiac injury. The role of either antibody or sensitized lymphoid cells in mediation of post-myocardial infarction
or post-cardiotomy syndromes is not clear, but it appears clear
that injury to the heart induced auto-reactive responses which
may play a role in subsequent pathologic events following the
initial cardiac injury.

REFERENCES

1. Bauer, H., T.J. Water, J.V. Talano, E. Esconzia and E. Bauer.
   1970. Antimyocardial antibodies in the diagnosis and prognosis

of coronary heart disease. Circulation 42:55.

2. Fletcher, G.F. and N.K. Wenger. 1968. Autoimmune studies in patients with primary myocardial disease. Circulation 37:1032.

3. Heine, W.I., H. Friedman, M.S. Mandell and H. Goldberg. 1966. Antibodies to cardiac tissue in acute ischemic heart disease. Amer. J. Cardiol., 17:798.

4. Hess, E.V. and A. Kirsner. 1973. Immunologic studies in myocardial disease in "Myocardial Disease", N.O. Fowler, ed., Grune and Stratton, New York.

5. Laufer, A. 1975. Human and Experimental Myocarditis. Israel J. Med. Sci. 11:37.

6. Read, S.E., R.E. Falk and J.D. Zabriskie. 1971. Cellular reactivity to streptococcal antigens in rheumatic heart disease. Clin. Res. 19:786.

7. Zabriskie, J.D., S.E. Read and R.J. Ellis. 1971. Cellular and humoral studies in diseases with heart reactive antibodies in "Progress in Immunology", B. Amos, ed., Academic Press, New York.

8. Harrington, H.T.,Jr. and P. Stastny. 1973. Macrophage migration from an agarose droplet: Development of a micromethod for assay of delayed hypersensitivity. J. Immunol. 110:752.

9. Jacqua-Stewart, M.J., W.O. Read and R.P. Steffer. 1979. Isolation of pure myocardial subcellular organelles. Anal. Biochem. 96:293.

10. Yang, L.C., P.R. Soprey, M.K. Wittner and E.N. Fox. 1977. Streptococcal-induced cell-mediated immune destruction of cardiac myofibrils in vitro. J. Exp. Med. 146:344.

11. Friedman, I. and A. Laufer. 1976. Electron microscopical studies of the effect of antiheart antibodihs and complement on beating heart cells in culture. J. Mol. Cell. Cardiol. 8:641.

CELLULAR IMMUNE MECHANISMS IN COXSACKIEVIRUS GROUP B, TYPE 3 INDUCED MYOCARDITIS IN BALB/C MICE

Sally A. Huber, and Lilian P. Job

Department of Pathology
University of Vermont
Burlington, Vermont 05405

SUMMARY

Coxsackie B viruses are a common cause of viral myocarditis in humans. A murine model of the human disease has been developed using Coxsackievirus group B, type 3 and inbred Balb/c mice. Infection of T lymphocyte deficient mice does not result in significant myocarditis indicating the importance of T cells in this disease. The virus can be isolated from the hearts of T cell deficient and normal mice in equal concentrations. Virus elimination presumably is mediated by virus specific neutralizing antibody induced in both groups. T lymphocytes, natural killer cells and macrophage obtained from normal virus infected mice are all capable of lysing myofibers in vitro. Maximum lysis is obtained with the cytolytic T cells. When these cell populations or Coxsackievirus immune antibody were adoptively transferred into T lymphocyte deficient animals infected with the virus, only animals given T cells developed significant myocarditis.

INTRODUCTION

Coxsackie B viruses are small, nonbudding viruses which are a major etiologic factor in human myocarditis. Virus infections involving the heart result first in scattered hypereosinophilic myofibers with few inflammatory cells. Later in infection, degeneration and necrosis of the myofibers are usually accompanied by extensive mononuclear cell infiltration.[7,15,23] Manifestations of Coxsackie B viral infections in mice closely resemble those in humans, providing a convenient model for the disease.[9-12,23]

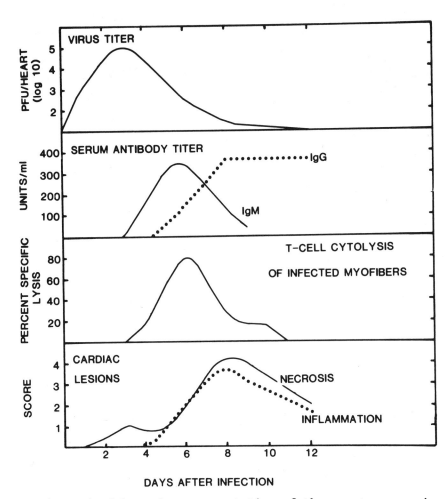

Figure 1. Schematic representation of the events occurring
in the heart after Coxsackievirus B-3 infection.

Investigations in this laboratory have resulted in a good
understanding of the importance of the immune system in producing
cardiac injury in animals in vivo.[9-12]   A schematic
representation of the events in virus infection in Balb/c mice
and the cellular and humoral responses subsequent to that

infection are given in Figure 1. Maximum cardiac injury
correlates temporally with the development of T cell medicated
cytolytic activity in peripheral lymphoid organs and to the IgG
antibody response. Myocarditis does not correspond to periods of
maximum virus concentrations in the heart.[23]   Further evidence of
the importance of T cells in this disease comes from the failure
of T lymphocyte deficient mice to develop significant
inflammation and necrosis after infection, despite normal virus
replication and elimination in the heart.[24]   Elimination of the
virus from the heart presumably is mediated by induction of an
IgM virus neutralizing antibody response.[18,19,24]

    Although T lymphocytes are clearly involved in the induction
of myocardial injury, it is not clear what mechanism(s) are
involved. T cells have a number of functions in the immune
response. One function is to act as helper cells in the
production of IgG antibody. Antibody in the presence of either
complement or K cells and macrophage (effectors of antibody
dependent cell medicated cytotoxicity, ADCC) may cause
destruction of myofiber target cells.[5,13]   A second function of
T cells is as effectors of direct cytotoxicity of infected
cells.[4,9,10]

    In addition, localized immune T cells, or antibody
activated complement and ADCC effectors may produce chemotactic
factors drawing cells capable of nonspecifically inducing cardiac
injury to the inflammatory site.[6,20]   Examples of such cells are
natural killer cells, polymorphonuclear (PMN) cells and macrophage.[5,6,8,11,13,21]

    The purpose of this paper is to characterize the various
components of the complex cellular immune response of the host to
Coxsackie B-3 virus infection in relationship to their importance
in myocarditis.

MATERIALS AND METHODS

Animals

Balb/c mice were purchased originally from Cumberland Farms,
Clinton, Tenn. CBA mice were originally obtained from Jackson
Laboratories, Bar Harbor, Maine. Neonates and 6- to 8-week-old
adult males were obtained from colonies maintained at the Cornell
University Medical College.

Virus preparation and purification

A "myocarditic" Coxsackievirus B-3 (Nancy strain), was
adapted to the heart by Dr. J.F. Woodruff and was passaged three
times in HeLa cell monolayers (Gey strain; Flow Laboratories,
McLean, Va.) and thereafter grown in HeLa cell suspensions
(Mandel strain; courtesy of Richard Crowell) by a previously
described technique.[3] Encephalomyocarditis (EMC) virus, the M
variant, was obtained from Dr. J.E. Craighead (University of
Vermont, Burlington, Vermont) and grown in L cells. The
maintenance medium was Joklik's modified minimal essential medium
(Flow Laboratories) containing double-strength essential amino
acids and vitamins in Hanks basic salt solution, 5% fetal calf
serum (FCS), and antibiotics (100 ug of streptomycin per ml and
100 U of penicillin per ml). Virus purification was performed by
using CsCl gradients according to the method of Oberg and
Phillipson.[16] The titers of purified virus ranged from 9-10 x
10^{10} plaque-forming units (PFU) per ml; samples were stored at
$-70°C$ in phosphate-buffered saline (PBS) without Ca^{2+} and Mg^{2+}.
Purified virus was used in all experiments.

Infection of mice

Each animal was infected by intraperitoneal inoculation of 0.5 ml
PBS containing 1-3 x 10^4 PFU of purified coxsackievirus B-3.

Titration of virus in organs and neutralizing antibody in the serum.

Organ virus titers were obtained by homogenization of the organs
in minimal essential medium, centrifugation of the cellular
debris, and titration of the viruses by plaque formation on
monolayers of HeLa cells as described previously.[24] For serum
neutralizing antibody titrations, blood was obtained from the
heart, the serum harvested, heat inactivated at 56°C for 30
minutes and stored at -20°C. Samples from individual animals
were assayed by incubation of twofold dilutions of the serum with
100 plaque forming units (PFU) Coxsackie B-3 virus for 45 minutes
prior to addition to monolayers of HeLa cells in the PFU assay.[12]
A 50% reduction of PFU was taken as the end point.

Spleen cell suspensions

Spleens were teased in cold basal medium Eagle (BME) containing
5% FCS, 100 ug of streptomycin per ml, and 100 U of penicillin
per ml. The cells were washed twice (300 x g for 10 minutes),
suspended in medium and layered on a Ficoll-hypaque gradient
(Pharmacia Fine Chemicals Inc., Piscataway N.J.) centrifuged at
178 x g for 10 minutes and the cells at the interface removed and
then washed with medium. Adherent cells were removed by

incubating spleen cells in plastic petri dishes (60 x 15 mm; Falcon Plastics, Oxnard, California) at a concentration of 20 x 10^6 cells per ml for 1 hour at 37°C. The nonadherent cells were harvested, washed once, and suspended in BME containing FCS at a concentration of 10^7 viable nucleated cells per ml. The adherent, macrophage enriched cell population was recovered by incubation of the petri dishes with PBS containing 20 mg/100ml ethylenediaminetetracetic acid (EDTA).

Preparation of cell populations enriched for Natural Killer or T cells

Spleen cells from mice infected 3 or 6 days earlier were depleted of red blood cells and macrophage as described above. A total of 3×10^7 cells were then suspended in 3 ml of BME - 5% FCS and incubated with 0.1 g nylon wool (Fenwal Laboratories, Morton Grove, Ill.) for 30 minutes at 37°C. The nonadherent cells were recovered by washing the nylon wool with 30 ml medium. To obtain NK cells from day 3 immune spleen cells, the recovered nonadherent cells were treated with anti thy 1.2 and anti mouse Ig serum and complement as described below. T cell enriched populations were obtained from nonadherent day 6 immune cells treated with antibody to mouse Ig and complement.

Anti-thy 1.2 and anti Ig serum treatment of spleen cells

Monoclonal anti-thy 1.2 serum (OLAC Ltd., Blackthorn, England) was titrated as described previously.[12] The antiserum used in these experiments had a cytotoxicity titer against 1.25×10^6 Balb/c thymocytes of 1.5×10^5. Lysis of thy 1.2 positive cells was performed as described previously.[10,11] using a 1:1,000 dilution of anti-thy 1.2 serum and a 1:5 dilution of guinea pig complement (GIBCO) which had been absorbed with Balb/c thymocytes. This treatment increased the percentage of immunoglobulin-containing spleen cells from 43 to 91%.

Affinity purified rabbit anti mouse immunoglobulin serum (Bionetics Laboratories, Kensington, MD) was used at a 1/10 dilution. This treatment increased the percentage of thy 1.2 positive cells in the spleen from 23 to 57%.

Preparation, culture, and characterization of myofibers

Hearts were removed aseptically from Balb/c mice within 48 hr of birth. Single-cell suspensions of myofibers were prepared by using a modification of the procedure of Bollon et al.[1] Briefly, hearts were minced and then subjected to stepwise enzymatic digestion with 0.25% pancreatin (GIBCO Laboratories, Grand Island, N.Y.). The isolated cells were washed with BME containing penicillin, streptomycin, 5% FCS, 10% horse serum, 0.2

mg of crystalline insulin, and 20 mM HEPES
(N-2-hydroxyethylpiperazine-N'-2-ethanesulfonic acid) buffer
(complete BME) per 100 ml of medium and then depleted of
endothelial cells and fibroblasts by two sequential 1-hr
adsorptions in 25-cm^2 plastic flasks (Falcon Plastics) at 37°C.
The nonadherent myofibers were recovered, washed once,
resuspended in complete BME, and then dispensed into 6-mm tissue
culture well (Linbro Chemical Co., Hamden, Conn.). After 48
hours (the time needed for these cells to become firmly adherent
to plastic), the myofibers were used in the cytotoxicity assay.

In a sparate experiment 2 x 10^6 myocardial cells in complete
BME were seeded onto cover slips (9 by 22 mm) and maintained in
Leighton tubes (16 x 100 mm; T.C. Wheaton Co., Millville, N.J.)
for examination by light microscopy. At 48 hours the cultures
contained individual cells and cell clusters which contracted
rhythmically (50 to 80 beats per min.). In addition, 90% or more
of the cells were identified as muscle fibers after staining with
phosphotungstic acid-hematoxylin; sarcomeres were observed under
light microscopy.

Cytotoxicity assay

The technique has been described in previous reports.[9-12]
Briefly, 7 x 10^4 neonatal myofibers in 0.2 ml of complete BME
were dispensed into 6-mm plastic tissue culture wells and
incubated at 37°C in a humidified atmosphere containing 5% CO_2.
After 48 hours the cells were infected with 100 PFU of virus per
cell, a dose known to result in infection of 75% of the myofibers
by 16 hours. After 1 hour unabsorbed virus was removed by
washing the monolayers. Target cells not exposed to virus were
processed in identical fashion. Myofibers were then labeled by
adding 5 μ Ci of ^{51}Cr to each well (Na$_2$[51]CrO$_4$; Amersham/Searle,
Arlington Heights, Ill.). After 45 to 60 minutes at 37°C, the
monolayers were washed three times and overlaid with 0.2 ml of
immune or nonimmune spleen cells in BME-FCS or with medium alone.
The cultures were incubated at 37°C for 18 hours at a spleen cells
to target cell ration of 150:1. The ^{51}Cr levels in the supernatants and in the cells were determined as described previously;[9-12]
radioactivity was measured by using an Intertechnique CG 4000 gamma
counter. [51]Cr release was calculated by using the following expression: [(counts per minute in supernatant)/(counts per minute
in supernatant + counts per minute in cells)] x 100.

Cytotoxicity was expressed as the percentage of lysis, as
calculated by the following expression:

$$\frac{E - C}{F - C} \times 100$$

where E represents the percentage of ^{51}Cr released from the
      experimental
      group;
   C represents the percentage of ^{51}Cr released from myofibers
      incubated in
      medium alone
   F represents the maximum ^{51}Cr releasable from the target
      cells.

The percentage of specific lysis represented the percentage of
lysis by sensitized hymphocytes minus the perentage of lysis by
nonimmune lymphocytes.

T lymphocyte deprived mice

At 3 weeks of age, Balb/c mice were thymectomized by opening the
anterior mediastinum through an incision in the neck and sternum
extending to the second rib. The thymus was aspirated. One week
later the animals were exposed to 800 R using a Gamma Industries
Setheratron Jr. Cobalt-60 teletherapy machine. On the same day,
3 to 5 x 10^6 syngeneic bone marrow cells obtained from donor mice
by flushing the tibia and femoral shafts with BME were injected
i.v. into recipient mice through the tail vein. Mice were
maintained for 5 weeks on drinking water containing tetracycline
(125 mg/liter).[24]

Phytohemagglutinin stimulation of spleen cells

Gross examination of the mediastinum was done on all TXBM mice
at the end of each experiment. In addition, spleen cells from
all TXBM mice were stimulated with the T cell mitogen, phyto-
hemagglutinin (PHA). 1 x 10^5 spleen lymphocytes were cultured
with 1 μl PHA-M (GIBCO) in 200 ul RPMI 1640 medium containing
5% FCS in microtiter wells. After 4 days, 2 μ Ci methyl-^{3}H-
thymidine, specific activity 15 Ci/mM (amersham - Searle,
Arlington Heights, Ill.) was added to each culture and the
cells were harvested onto fiberglass filter strips using a
Multiple Automated Sample Harvester (MASH)(Belco Glass Inc.,
Vineland, N.J.) 24 hours later. The strips were air dried and
the sections containing the radioactive material were placed into
scintillation vials containing 4 ml Econofluor (New England
Nuclear Co. Boston, Mass.). The vials were counted in a Packard
Tricarb liquid scintillation counter. All TXBM mice were
demonstrated to be negative for residual thymus and PHA
stimulation.

Histology

Organs were fixed in 10% buffered formalin fixative and stained with hematoxylin and eosin (H & E). The extent of myocardial necrosis and inflammation was graded on a scale of 0 to 4 as described in detail elsewhere.[24] Briefly, for necrosis a score of 0 indicates no necrotic or hypereosinophilic myofibers per section, whereas a score of 4 indicates widespread frank necrosis of myofibers/section. Inflammation was scored on the basis of the number of foci of inflammatory cells per section, with 0 indicating no inflammation and 4 denoting more than 90 foci. The mean score for myocardial necrosis and inflammation per group of animals was calculated from the scores of the individual animals.

Statistical Analysis

The Student t test was used to analyze the significance of differences between groups.

RESULTS

The first experiment was designed to characterize Coxsackievirus B-3 infections in T lymphocyte deficient and sufficient animals. TXBM and normal animals were infected with 1 x 10^4 PFU virus. At various times from 1 to 39 days later, the animals were sacrificed and examined for virus, inflammation and necrosis in the heart and virus neutralizing antibody in the serum. A separate group of 24 TXBM and 24 normal mice were infected and followed for cumulative mortality. As shown in Table 1, TXBM mice had considerably less cardiac damage and animal mortality compared to normal animals. Virus concentrations in the heart and serum antibody titers were identical until the twelfth day when antibody levels in TXBM mice were significantly lower due to the absence of the IgG response.

The spleens of the normal animals were assayed for cytolytic activity to both uninfected and Coxsackievirus B-3 infected myofibers during the first 2 weeks after infection (Figure 2). Cytotoxicity develops rapidly after infection and peaks on days 5 to 7, decreasing thereafter. Early cytolytic activity (up to day 4) is directed equally to both target cells while activity observed after day 4 is mainly directed to virus infected targets. The early (day 3) and later (day 6) cytolytic activity was characterized as to the effector cells most probably involved (Table 2). The early effector cells apparently are natural killer cell based the nonspecificity of the cytolysis. The day 3 spleen cell population lysed myofibers infected with the noncrossreactive encephalomyocarditis (EMC) virus as well as allogeneic CBA myofibers. In addition, the cytolytic activity was not removed by treatment of the spleen cells with anti thy 1.2 and anti mouse Ig plus complement or by passage of the cell

TABLE 1 - Characterization of Coxsackievirus B-3 infection in intact and TXBM male Balb/c mice.

Day after Virus injection [a]	Virus titers in Heart [b] normal ♂	TXBM ♂	Serum Neutralizing antibody [c] normal ♂	TXBM ♂	Cardiac lesions (N/I) [d] normal ♂	TXBM ♂	Percent cumulative mortality [e] normal ♂	TXBM ♂
1	1.5 ± 0.8	1.8 ± 0.5	< 40	<40	0.0	0.0	0	0
3	10.4 ± 2.5	12.4 ± 0.9	<40	<40	0.3 ± 0.2 / 0.5 ± 0.3	0.4 ± 0.2 / 0.3 ± 0.3	4	13
6	3.1 ± 1.3	5.5 ± 1.7	410 ± 35	465 ± 70	1.3 ± 0.1 / 1.6 ± 0.4	0.8 ± 0.5 / 0.5 ± 0.5	29	13
9	0.15 ± 0.04	0.3 ± 0.1	289 ± 60	150 ± 90	3.7 ± 0.8 / 2.7 ± 0.6	0.9 ± 0.6 / 0.9 ± 0.3	54	17
12	0.003 ± 0.0	0.005 ± 0.0	390 ± 85	125 ± 30	3.1 ± 0.7 / 1.9 ± 0.9	0.7 ± 0.2 / 0.8 ± 0.5	75	21
17	0 ± 0	0 ± 0	250 ± 50	70 ± 70	2.4 ± 0.5 / 1.3 ± 0.6	1.0 ± 0.5 / 0.3 ± 0.3	92	29
39	0 ± 0	0 ± 0	ND	ND	3.0 ± 0.6 / 1.0 ± 0.5	0.5 ± 0.4 / 0 ± 0	96	33

[a] Mice were inoculated with 3×10^4 PFU i.p. in 0.5 ml PBS, 2 to 12 animals were used/group

[b] PFU virus $\times 10^4$/heart ± SEM

[c] Reciprocal of arithemetic mean ± SEM

[d] Graded on a scale of 0 to 4. Mean score ± SEM

[e] Twenty-four mice

TABLE 2 - Identification of potential cytolytic mechanisms for myofibers in Coxsackievirus B-3 (CVB 3) infections.

Percent Specific Lysis[a]

Potential Cytolytic Mechanism	Source of Effector[g]	Syngeneic Target Cells			Allogeneic Target Cells	
		CVB 3 Infected Balb/c Myofibers	EMC Virus Infected Balb/c Myofibers	Uninfected Balb/c Myofibers	CVB 3 Infected CBA Myofibers	Uninfected CBA Myofiber
"Natural Killer" (null) Cell	Day 3 immune spleen (anti thy 1,2 and anti Ig+ complement treated)	28.1 ± 5.2[c]	20.8 ± 6.3	35.2 ± 3.3	30.9 ± 2.9	29.8 ± 4.5
T cytolytic Effector Cell	Day 6 immune spleen	65.7 ± 7.8	10.9 ± 3.7	35.5 ± 5.9	17.1 ± 8.1	13.4 ± 1.3
	Day 6 immune spleen (anti thy 1,2+ complement treated)	7.1 ± 1.2	8.3 ± 5.1	5.7 ± 2.3	9.0 ± 5.3	9.8 ± 2.9
	Day 6 immune spleen (anti Ig+ complement treated)	73.2 ± 8.1	5.0 ± 1.0	51.0 ± 1.5	9.3 ± 2.5	10.2 ± 4.5
Macrophage	Day 6 immune spleen (plastic adherent cells)	21.0 ± 9.4	15.9 ± 2.8	18.3 ± 1.7	ND	ND
Antibody Dependent Cell mediated Cytotoxicity	Day 6 immune spleen (plastic adherent cells) Plus:					
	(1) normal mouse serum	20.9 ± 3.8	12.8 ± 5.9	19.2 ± 2.0	ND	ND
	(2) Day 12 Coxsackievirus B-3 immune mouse serum	27.3 ± 4.1	17.9 ± 0.8	20.5 ± 3.3	ND	ND
	(3) hyperimmune rabbit anti Coxsackievirus B-3 serum	22.2 ± 2.0	19.5 ± 1.4	20.6 ± 2.1	ND	ND
Antibody dependent Complement mediated lysis	(1) normal mouse serum	-1.3 ± 2.5	0.9 ± 3.0	0.0 ± 1.0	ND	ND
	(2) Day 12 Coxsackievirus B-3 immune serum	8.4 ± 0.5	3.3 ± 2.5	1.9 ± 1.9	ND	ND

[a] Approximately 2×10^4 myofibers were cultured in 6mm diameter wells of tissue culture plates. The cells in some wells were incubated with 100 PFU Coxsackievirus B-3 (CVB 3) or encephalomyocarditis (EMC) virus for 1 hour, then all cultures were labelled with ^{51}Cr for 1 hour. Effector cells were added at an effector/target cell ratio of 150:1 and the cultures were harvested at 18 hours. In cultures assaying ADCC and antibody dependent complement medium lysis, 10 ul normal serum or Coxsackievirus immune serum was added to the culture medium for a final concentration of 1:20.

[b] Male Balb/c mice were inoculated ip with 1×10^4 PFU virus. The spleens were removed 3 or 6 days later, depleted of red blood cells on Ficoll: hypaque gradients and of macrophage by adsorption to plastic petri dishes. Macrophage enriched cells were recovered by incubating the plastic adherent cells with PBS containing 20 mg/100ml EDTA. T and/or B cells were depleted by treatment with antibody to thy 1.2 and mouse Ig + complement.

[c] Results represent the mean percent specific lysis ± SEM of 3 experiments. Spontaneous ^{51}Cr release for the target cells ranged from 25.1 to 41.9% and percent lysis in the presence of normal spleen cells ranged from -11.1 to 5.7%.

population through nylon wool (not shown).[8,11,21] In contrast,
cytolytic activity present in day 6 immune spleen cells is
predominantly mediated by T lymphocytes as determined by
sensitivity of the effector cells to anti thy 1.2 antibody and
complement and by virus and allotype specificity of killing.[4,9]
Removal of B cells by treatment of the spleen population with
anti mouse Ig and complement had no effect on cytotoxicity.

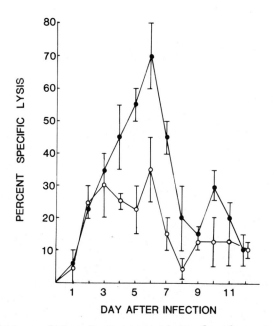

Figure 2. Kinetics of in vivo generation of male cytotoxicity
          against Coxsackievirus infected (o) and uninfected (o)
          myofibers using an effector: target cell ratio of
          150:1 and an incubation period of 18 hours.
          Spontaneous ^{51}Cr release from infected and uninfected
          targets was 29.2 and 31.5% and percent lysis with
          normal lymphocytes was 37.9 and 30.3% respectively.
          The results represent the mean percent specific lysis
          of 3 experiments ± SEM.

Table 3. Demonstration of the ability of immune cells and serum
to induce myocarditis in T lymphocyte deficient mice.

Cells or Serum Tranferred into TBXM Infected Mice[a]	Cardiac Lesions (I/N)[b]	Percent Mortality[c]
None	0.9 ± 0.3	17
Normal spleen cells	1.2 ± 0.1	17
Day 3 immune NK-like spleen cells	0.7 ± 0.5	8
Day 6 macrophage enriched cells	1.2 ± 0.2	25
Day 6 immune T cells	2.7 ± 0.3	63
Day 6 macrophage + irradiated T cells	1.5 ± 0.4	42
Day 12 immune mouse serum	0.0 ± 0.4	0
Normal mouse serum	0.5 ± 0.5	25
Normal T cell sufficient mice	3.7 + 0.7	75

[a] TXBM male Balb/c mice were infected with 1 x 10^4 PFU virus.
Three days later, mice were intravenously transfused with 4 x
10^6 normal syngeneic spleen cells/mouse, or with a similar
number of macrophage or T lymphocyte enriched cells obtained
from the spleens of mice 6 days after infection. One group
received 4 x 10^6 macrophage and 4 x 10^6 T cells (irradiated
1000R). Other groups received 1 x 10^6 NK enriched cells
obtained from mice 3 days after infection or with 0.5 ml normal
or day 12 Coxsackie- virus immune serum. Controls consisted of
infected normal and TXBM infected mice. All animals were
sacrificed 7 days after infection (4 days after receiving cells
or serum) and the hearts examined for inflammation and
necrosis.
[b] Inflammation/Necrosis graded on a scale of 0 to 4. Mean score
± SEM of 6-10 mice/group
[c] 12 mice/group. Mortality measured to 10 days post infection.

Macrophage isolated from the spleen cell population produced
minimal and nonspecific myofiber cytolysis. There was a
suggestion that an equivalent number of macrophage showed
enhanced cytotoxicity of the infected myofibers in the presence
of hyperimmune or day 12 antibody to Coxsackie B-3 virus, but the
amount of increased killing was nonsignificant. Antibody to the
virus was also directly slightly lytic to Coxsackie virus B-3
infected myofibers in the presence of guinea pig complement.

The evidence from the in vitro experiments described above
indicate that the only major cytolytic mediators of myofiber
destruction appeared to be T lymphocytes. However, in the heart,
large numbers of macrophage and virus immune serum either in the
presence of complement or macrophage may result in significant
accummulative damage while being only minimally effective in
vitro. In an attempt to determine whether these effectors can
induce myocarditis in vivo, TXBM mice were infected with 1×10^4
PFU virus and on the third day adoptively transfused i.v. with
highly enriched populations of macrophage (4.0×10^6 cells/mouse)
and cytolytic T cells (4.0×10^6 cells/mouse) NK cell enriched
populations (1×10^6 cells/mouse) or with 0.5 ml Coxsackievirus
immune serum. Control animals consisted of infected normal and
TXBM animals, and TXBM animals given 4.0×10^6 normal spleen
cells or serum. All mice were sacrificed 4 days later and the
hearts were examined for inflammation and necrosis. As can be
seen in Table 3, only the spleen cell population enriched for
cytolytic cells T cells restored myocarditis in TXBM mice.

DISCUSSION

Picornaviruses, especially Coxsackie and ECHO viruses, are
commonly identified agents causing virus heart disease in humans.
Virus induced heart disease is relatively common in the general
population. Estimates based on large studies of sequential
autopsies place the incidence at 2.3 to 5 % of the general
population. This incidence increases in infected populations
during known picornavirus epidemics. Coxsackie virus infections
rarely result in death in adults although children, especially
during the neonatal period, are at significantly greater risk.
Even in nonfatal cases, however, cardiac damage may result in
permanently or temporarily reduced work capacity due to pleural
effusion, arrhythmias, cardiomegaly, dilated cardiomyopathy, ventricular aneurisms and congestive heart failure[15,23]. The potential for
severe sequela of viral myocarditis emphasizes the importance of understanding the mechanisms of cardiac injury in this disease.

Cardiac injury in viral myocarditis may result from either
of two basic mechanisms. Myofiber necrosis unassociated with
inflammation may occur in individuals due to viral infection and

replication in the myofiber ultimately resulting in cytopathic alterations and cell death. Early in murine infections, scattered hypereosinophilic and necrotic myofibers are observed in the heart at times correlating to maximum virus concentrations. In addition, the virus is capable of infecting and lysing cultures of myofibers, fibroblasts and endothelial cells in vitro.[9,23]

Based on observations in the murine model, direct virus mediated damage of infected tissues is minimal.[24] Following the third day of infection in mice virus titers decrease rapidly concurrently with rising virus neutralizing antibody titers. The temporal inverse association between virus concentrations and antibody in the animals suggests that the antibody is the major mechanism of viral clearance. This view is supported by the ability to protect mice from severe Coxsackieviral disease by adoptive transfer of specific antibody prior to or within 24 hours after infection.[19] However, other experimental evidence indicates that macrophage/monocytes are also involved in viral elimination. Infection of suckling mice with Coxsackievirus usually is lethal. Yet adoptive transfer of syngeneic macrophage from uninfected adults protects these animals. Protection is enhanced when both antibody and macrophage are given.[17] Secondly, cortisone treatment of mice prior to infection inhibits the development of inflammatory lesions without affecting virus neutralizing antibody titers. Yet immunosuppressed animals have persistant and enhanced virus titers in target organs associated with marked parenchymal damage and tissue necrosis.[22]

The second mechanism of myocardial damage in Coxsackieviral infections is T cell associated immune damage. Maximum inflammation and necrosis in the heart correlates with the development of a virus specific cytolytic T cell response in the animals. In addition, T lymphocyte deficient animals fail to develop significant myocarditis, myofiber necrosis or mortality subsequent to infection, compared to normal, infected mice, despite the presence of equivalent virus concentrations in target organs. The fact that virus elimination occurs normally in TXBM mice indicates that T cells are not involved in this aspect of the disease.[9,23,24]

It is tempting to correlate myofiber destruction in the inflammatory lesions directly to the cytolytic T cell. However, T cells have a number of functions in immunity which may influence inflammation.[2,14] The production of IgG antibodies may result in direct complement mediated or antibody dependent cell mediated lysis of the myofibers.[5,17] In the results presented here, virus specific antibody had little effect on virus infected myofibers cultured in vitro nor did the adoptive transfer of the antibody into T cell deficient animals induce myocarditis in

vivo. It seems unlikely, therefore, that either of these
mechanisms play an important role in this disease.

A second possible role of T cells is the chemotactic
attraction and activation of macrophage to the inflammatory
site.[5,6,20] The hypothesis that the major mediator of myofiber
damage is a nonspecific cytolytic cell such as macrophage or
natural killer cell is attractive for two reasons. First, the
Coxsackie virus itself is lysogenic to infected cells.
Therefore, if only infected cells could act as targets for virus
specific cytolytic mediators, it is reasonable to assume that
these cells would have died anyway from the infection alone.
Secondly, most of the inflammation and necrosis in the heart
occurs when virus concentrations are rapidly diminishing or no
longer detected in the heart. At this time, few virus infected
cells would be available as targets for the antigen-specific
cytolytic effectors and cardiac damage resulting from elimination
of infected myofibers would presumably be minimal. In the
present experiments, highly enriched populatons of macrophage
were shown to be only slightly cytolytic to myofibers in vitro.
Still, in sufficient numbers, these cells could presumably
induce damage in vivo. Adoptive transfer of macrophage alone
obtained from immune animals were unable to induce myocarditis
in T cell deficient hosts. This could be explained by the
necessity of a small number of specifically immune T cells
localizing in the lesion first. However, adoptive transfer
of a limited number of irradiated immune T cells with the
macrophage still induced only minimal myocarditis. These results
do not give strong evidence for the involvement of macrophage in
direct myofiber destruction, nor do they conclusively disprove
macrophage involvement. Further work must be done to clarify
this point.

As with macrophage, there is no evidence that natural killer-
like cells present early after infection play a significant role
in myocarditis. These cells are cytolytic to both infected and
uninfected target cells but are not observed consistently in male
mice after the fourth to fifth day of infection. Therefore, the
disappearance of NK-like activity precedes by one or more days
the development of cardiac lesions. In addition, the NK cell
activity in female mice is significantly greater than in male
animals, yet females do not develop severe myocarditis.[11,12] The
lack of correlation between NK-like cell activity and myocarditis
is in agreement with our inability to induce the cardiac lesions
with adoptively transferred NK-enriched cells.

In summary, the results obtained to date strongly implicate
the cytolytic T cell as the major source of cardiac injury in
this model. Interestingly, the in vitro cell mediated
cytotoxicity assay clearly shows that the T cell population is

lytic primarily to infected myofibers, but also produces
significant lysis of uninfected target cells as well. It is well
known that immune T cells recognize infected targets by both
virus specific and major histocompatibility antigens.[4] The same
effector T cell may lyse both targets, presumably by the
recognition of H-2 antigens on the cell surface. In this
instance, myocarditis could be considered an autoimmune disease.

ACKNOWLEDGEMENTS

    This work was supported in part by PHS Grants-in-Aid HL
27976 and HL/AI 28480 from the National Institutes of Health and
an American Heart Association Grant-In-Aid 81-1158.

    The authors wish to thank Mrs. Jacqueline Marceau for help
in preparing this manuscript.

REFERENCES

1. Bollon, A.P., Nath, K. and Shay, J.W. Establishment of
      contracting heart muscle cell culture. Tissue Culture
      Association Manual 3,637-640 (1977)
2. Cantor, H. and Boyse E.A. Functional subclasses of T
      lymphocytes bearing different Ly antigens.I. The
      generation of functionally distinct T-cell subclasses
      is a differentiation process independent of antigen.
      Journal Experimental Medicine 141,1376-1399 (1975)
3. Crowell, R.L. and Syverton, J.T. The mammalian cell-virus
      relationship. VI Sustained infection of HeLa cells by
      Coxsackie B-3 virus and effect on superinfection.
      Journal Experimental Medicine 113, 419-435 (1961)
4. Doherty, P.C., Blanden, R.V. and Zinkernagel, R.M.
      Specificity of virus-immune effector T cells for H-2K
      or H-2D compatible interactions: Implications for
      H-antigen diversity. Transplantation Review 29, 89-124
      (1976)
5. Evans, R. and Alexander, P. Mechanisms of immunologically
      specific killing of tumor cells by macrophages. Nature
      236, 168-170 (1972)
6. Fidler, I.J. Activation in vitro of mouse macrophages by
      syngeneic, allogeneic or xenogeneic lymphocyte
      supernatants. Journal of National Cancer Institute
      55,1159-1163 (1975)
7. Godman, G.C. The cytopathology of enteroviral infection.
      International Review of Experimental Pathology 5,67-110
      (1966)
8. Herberman, R.B., Nunn, M.F. and Lavren, D.H. Natural
      cytotoxic reactivity of mouse lymphoid cells against

syngeneic and allogeneic tumor. II Characterization of
effector cells. International Journal Cancer 16,
230-239 (1975)
9. Huber, S.A., Job, L.P. and Woodruff, J.F. Lysis of infected
myofibers by Coxsackievirus B-3-immune T lymphocytes.
American Journal of Pathology 98,681-694 (1980)
10. Huber, S.A., Job, L.P. and Woodruff, J.F. Sex-related
differences in the pattern of Coxsackievirus
B-3-induced immune spleen cell cytotoxicity against
virus infected myofibers. Infection and Immunity
32,68-73 (1981)
11. Huber, S.A., Job, L.P., Auld, K.R. and Woodruff, J.F.
Sex-related differences in the rapid production of
cytotoxic spleen cells active against uninfected
myofibers during Coxsackievirus B-3 infection. Journal
of Immunology 126,1336-1340 (1981)
12. Huber, S.A., Job, L.P. and Auld, K.R. Influence of sex
hormones on Coxsackie B-3 virus infection in Balb/c
mice. Cellular Immunology 67,173-189 (1982)
13. Kim, Y-B, Huk, N.D., Koren, H.S. and Amos, D.B. Natural
killing (NK) and antibody-dependent cellular
cytotoxicity (ADCC) in specific pathogen-free (SPF)
miniature swine and germ-free piglets. I comparison of
NK and ADCC. Journal of Immunology 125,755-762 (1980).
14. Kisielow, P., Hirst, J.A., Shiku, M., Beverley, P.C.L.,
Boyse, E.A. and Oettegen, H.F. Ly antigens as markers
for functionally distinct subpopulations of
thymus-derived lymphocytes of the mouse. Nature
253,219-220 (1975)
15. Lerner, A.M. and Wilson, F.M. Virus myocaridopathy.
Progress in Medical Virology 15,63-91 (1973)
16. Oberg, B and Phillipson, L. Replication of Poliovirus RNA
studied by gel filtration and electrophoresis.
European Journal Biochemistry 11,305-315 (1969)
17. Oldstone, M.B.A. Virus neutralization and virus-induced
immune complex disease. Progress in Medical Virology
19,84-119 (1975)
18. Rager-Zisman, B. and Allison, A.C. The role of antibody and
host cells in the resistance of mice against infection
with Coxsackie B-3 virus. Journal of General Virology
19,329-338 (1973)
19. Rager-Zisman, B. and Allison, A.C. Effects of
immunosuppression on Coxsackie B-3 virus infection in
mice, and passive protection by circulating antibody.
Journal of General Virology 19,339-351 (1973)
20. Ruddle, N.H. Delayed hypersensitivity to soluble antigens
in mice II analysis in vitro. International Archives
Allergy Applied Immunology 58,44-52 (1979)
21. Welsh, R.M. Cytotoxic cells induced during lymphocytic
choriomeningitis virus infection of mice.

I.Characterization of natural killer cell induction.
Journal of Experimental Medicine 148,163-181 (1978)
22. Woodruff, J.F. Lack of correlation between neutralizing
    antibody production and suppression of Coxsackievirus
    B-3 replication in target organs: Evidence for
    involvement of mononuclear inflammatory cells in host
    defense. Journal of Immunology 123,31-36 (1979)
23. Woodruff, J.F. Viral myocarditis. American Journal of
    Pathology 101,425-484 (1980)
24. Woodruff, J.F. and Woodruff, J.J. Involvement of T
    lymphocytes in the pathogenesis of Coxsackie virus B-3
    heart disease. Journal of Immunology 113,1726-1734
    (1974)

A MOLECULAR BIOLOGIC APPROACH TO CARDIAC TOXICOLOGY

Elwood O. Titus

Division of Drug Biology
Bureau of Drugs, Food and Drug Administration
Washington, D.C. 20204

Molecular biology seeks to depict biological function in terms of discrete events, individually accessible to biochemical study. With the myocardial cell this approach has had some success. The affinity of receptors for a variety of drugs, the ionic basis for signal transmission across the sarcolemmal membrane, and the enzymatic components of the various membranes that control internal calcium, have been studied and provide a rationale for at least some of the reversible, pharmacologically induced dysfunctions that represent the side effects of conventional drugs on this cell. This symposium, however, deals largely with chemical agents which initiate sequences of incompletely understood events that lead ultimately to irreversible tissue damage and cell death. Among these effects, the myocardial necrosis produced by suprapharmacological concentrations of isoproterenol has been of special interest because its production may have some elements in common with infarction or ischemic damage and because it induces resistance to further chemical damage. Selye [31] showed some years ago that coronary occlusion with infarct protects against isoproterenol necrosis and the mechanism may well be related to that by which isoproterenol induces resistance to its own effects [1]. Clarification of the mechanism of the initial steps in generation of the isoproterenol lesion would be of interest and the purpose of this paper is to offer a few speculative remarks on the subject. Two recurrent themes in discussions about cardiac damage are the possible role of increased intracellular calcium and the possible involvement of free radical damage to cell membranes. Some of the discussion

509

will therefore be devoted to a few techniques, already familiar
but still incompletely developed, for studying these factors.

Of the several cation concentration gradients which the
myocardial cell must maintain for viability, that for calcium is
the steepest, varying from about 250 to 1200 (outside/inside) in
systole and diastole, respectively [2]. Calcium influx is thus
an early consequence of any damage to the sarcolemmal membrane
barrier as well as of the specific pharmacological activation of
calcium channels. Influx sustained sufficiently to increase
cytosolic calcium levels places significant demands on the ATP
required for actomyosin ATPase and for the energy-requiring
sequestration and outpumping mechanisms that maintain the
gradient. As cytosolic levels begin to approach equilibrium
with external concentrations, calcium will inhibit mitochondrial
ATP synthesis [29]. (See the review by Bloom [2] for earlier
literature references.) There is thus available a
calcium-mediated, self-reinforcing mechanism for irreversible
cell damage once the barrier to external calcium has been
breached. This plus the presence of beta-adrenergically
activated calcium channels in the sarcolemma give intuitive
appeal to the hypothesis of Fleckenstein et al. [10] that
calcium overload, followed ultimately by reduction of ATP to
levels insufficient to sustain cell viability, is the mechanism
by which grossly suprapharmacological levels of isoproterenol
initiate myocardial necrosis. Evidence for the early cellular
uptake of calcium required by this mechanism has been obtained
and the process is inhibited by verapamil [3]. Lehr [19] has
pointed out, however, that inhibition of calcium uptake by
parathyroidectomy in rats does not protect against isoproterenol
and that verapamil has to be used in concentrations considerably
in excess of those required to block calcium uptake.

An ischemic model is preferred by Lehr [19], in which
reduction of coronary flow by isoproterenol would reduce
mitochondrial ATP production in the myocardial cell to levels
insufficient to maintain membrane integrity. Calcium uptake
would now occur secondarily to the resulting sarcolemmal damage,
and the late appearance of a large calcium influx may be a
consequence of cell death [4]. Lehr et al. [20] have reviewed
the evidence that depletion of cellular magnesium may be the
common biochemical denominator in myocardial necrosis of any
etiology. Such depletion would then result in the inability to
sustain the phosphate transfer reactions that involve magnesium
as a cofactor and in a generalized perturbation of sarcolemmal
ionic fluxes involving loss of phosphate and potassium and
uptake of sodium and calcium. Whatever the mechanism of the
later damage, selection of ischemia or the pharmacological
effect of isoproterenol on the sarcolemma as the initiating

insult is difficult, since ischemia is known to stimulate
catecholamine release and beta blockers can reduce not only the
calcium uptake after isoproterenol but also the resting calcium
levels and the calcium uptake after ischemia [21,27]. There is
always the possibility for circular arguments.

If hypoxia is indeed a factor in isoproterenol
cardiotoxicity, there is some possibility that oxygen-centered
free radicals, by inducing lipid peroxidation, SH oxidation,
etc., may be a cause of tissue damage. Kappus and Sies [16], in
a discussion of hypoxic effects, point out that a number of
exogenous and endogenous compounds can be reduced by cellular
reductases that involve one electron transfer. The reduction of
ubiquinone to the semiquinone is an obvious example. The
product, being a free radical, can react directly with oxygen to
produce the superoxide radical and regenerate the quinone.
Enzymatic re-reduction of the substrate permits the cycle to be
repeated with continuous consumption of oxygen and continuous
production of superoxide radicals. The mitochondrial electron
transport chain can itself be a source of superoxide radicals.
Although the system should fully reduce oxygen to water via the
terminal cytochrome oxidase, intermediate components can be
leaky. Some of the semiquinone form of ubiquinone, for example,
becomes accessible for direct oxygenation, and it has been
estimated that as much as 1% of the electron flow through the
system may leak off by this route to generate superoxides [22].
Demopoulos et al. [7], in a recent review devoted to the
initiation of ischemic damage in the central nervous system,
have noted that one of the consequences of inadequate energy
production is an increasing dissociation of the ubiquinone from
its usual tight association with the mitochondrial system, so
that leakage through the superoxide-generating system is even
further enhanced. Thus a hypoxic environment in which enough
oxygen still remains to drive the cycle can be seriously
detrimental. At the moment it is not clear whether the
hypothetical model for ischemic damage to the brain is operative
in the heart.

A number of enzymes, including aldehyde oxidase,
dihydro-orotic dehydrogenase, and xanthine oxidase, produce
superoxide during normal turnover. Xanthane oxidase is involved
in a second model system for ischemic injury, in this case
mucosal lesions in the small intestine [26]. Intestinal
xanthine oxidase, normally in the D form which reduces NAD^+,
is stated [30] to be rapidly converted by ischemia to the O
form, which reduces oxygen [36] with concomitant production of
superoxide radicals. The conversion would appear to be effected
by a calmodulin-dependent protease. Alleviation of the injury
by superoxide dismutase and partial prevention by allopurinol

have been taken as evidence for a free radical mechanism
involving xanthine oxidase. In the heart, allopurinol was
observed to protect partially against isoproterenol-induced
myocardial necrosis. These experiments, however, were not
designed to test a free radical theory but were primarily
concerned with the purine- sparing action of the drug [37]. The
superoxide radical will damage membranes and kill cells, but
there is considerable work to suggest that other free radicals
produced in the chain of reaction products derived from
superoxide are the major sources of damage [22]. Superoxide
will react with itself in a pH-dependent reaction that yields
peroxide. The spontaneous reaction is slow but it is catalyzed
by the ubiquitous superoxide dismutase. Peroxide in turn will
react further with superoxide to yield oxygen and water plus the
extremely reactive free OH radical. This reaction is catalyzed
by traces of bound iron found in tissue (transferrin is, for
example, very effective), and an analogous reaction will also
generate free hydroxyl radical from lipid peroxides without a
catalyst. Thus once lipid peroxides have been produced by
attack of the oxidizing substances in the above chain, the
opportunity arises for free radical chain reactions.

Because of the above sequence of reactions and because of
its existence in an oxygen atmosphere, the eucaryotic cell is
always at risk of free radical damage generated by its own
metabolism, not to mention the chemical insults of interest
here. It is not surprising that protective enzymes are
ubiquitous in mammalian cells [16]. Reduction of the amount of
superoxide entering the reaction chain is achieved by superoxide
dismutase. Hydrogen peroxide is reduced to water by catalase
when it is at high levels or by glutathione peroxidase at lower
levels. If lipid peroxides have formed, they can also serve as
substrates for this enzyme and both the selenium-requiring and
selenium-independent forms of glutathione peroxidase can reduce
them to alcohols.

Although the role of free radicals in the early stages of
isoproterenol-induced damage is speculative, the free radicals
are obviously important mediators of the cardiotoxicity of
another substance discussed in this symposium, doxorubicin.
This anthraquinone appears to be reducible by several
flavin-dependent oxidoreductases to a semiquinone radical [11]
which can then participate in the cyclic reduction of oxygen to
superoxide, as in the model discussed earlier [16]. The role of
free radicals in the doxorubicin-induced chronic cardiomyopathy
in the rabbit was confirmed by the ameliorative effects of free
radical scavengers [34]. The anatomical and morphological
aspects of doxorubicin cardiomyopathy have been reviewed
recently by Herman [12]. Given the differences in chemistry,

pharmacology, and tissue distribution of the two drugs, it is
not surprising that doxorubicin and isoproterenol do not produce
morphologically similar effects. Nevertheless, doxorubicin
should provide a useful model with which to study the effects of
a known initiator of free radical damage on some of the membrane
functions relevant to this discussion. In pharmacological
studies with isolated electrically driven rabbit papillary
muscle, the effects of doxorubicin were consistent with
inhibition of both the release and reuptake of stored calcium,
presumably reflecting acute oxidative damage to sarcoplasmic
reticular membranes by free radicals [25]. In a chronic study,
three of eight rabbits receiving doxorubicin developed
cardiomyopathy, and calcium levels in the hearts of these three
were about 2.7 times those of controls and 1.8 times those of
non-responding treated animals [24]. Verapamil has been
reported to diminish the cardiac effects of doxorubicin [5], but
neither this drug nor nifedipine had such an effect in other
tests [17]. Efforts to determine whether repeated assault by
doxorubicin-generated free radicals has any major effect on the
intracellular calcium economy have thus been rather
inconclusive. Efforts to explain the relatively high
sensitivity of the heart to doxorubicin, however, have disclosed
that the endogenous protective mechanisms against
oxygen-centered radicals are markedly deficient [8]. In the
mouse heart, superoxide dismutase and catalase levels were about
27 and 1.3%, respectively, of those in liver.
Selenium-dependent glutathione oxidase was not significantly
different from that in liver. Doxorubicin, although it was
without effect on superoxide dismutase, did in part enhance its
own toxicity by reducing glutathione peroxidase to about 63% of
normal.

It is clear from the above that the myocardium should be
particularly susceptible to damage from the various
oxygen-centered radicals which derive from superoxide. Should
it develop from further research that radical mechanisms are
likely to be important in the chemical induction of necrosis, it
will become of theoretical interest to identify those radical
initiators and intermediates which are generated in the tissue
subject to chemical insult. In theory it should be possible to
detect radicals directly by electron paramagnetic resonance
(EPR) spectroscopy. Although experiments in vivo are not
practical, except for special cases as noted below, the physical
dimensions of the cavities in current spectrometers should
permit work with small tissue samples, isolated cell
suspensions, or membrane preparations in vitro. Unfortunately
the oxygen-centered radicals are so reactive that they never
achieve steady-state levels sufficient for detection, but spin
trapping techniques can in theory overcome this problem and may

become of increasing interest to toxicologists as their
biological applications develop. The method was developed
largely in the laboratory of Janzen [14], who has recently
reviewed the technique and some of its emerging biological
applications. A useful introduction to the principles has been
published by Evans [9]. The method takes advantage of the
ability of sterically hindered nitroso compounds or nitrones to
react covalently with an unstable free radical such as the
hydroxyl radical to form a stable, long-lived nitroxide radical
that can be observed at room temperature in an EPR
spectrometer. Since the stable free radical accumulates as more
oxygen-centered radical is generated, the method is more
sensitive than those which measure only steady-state
concentrations of free radical. Because the hyperfine splitting
constants that govern the separation of the characteristic
3-line nitroxide spectrum are to some extent sensitive to the
structure of the radical moiety acquired by the spin-trap, the
spectra can aid in the identification of the original radical.
In order that the trapping rate be maximized with respect to
competing reaction paths for radicals, it is necessary to
maintain high concentrations of trapping reagent in the
incubation mixtures. For biological preparations the more
water-soluble traps such as 5,5-dimethyl-1-pyrroline-1-oxide
(DMPO) and N-t-butyl-alpha-4-pyridyl nitrone-1-oxide (POBN) are
therefore useful. POBN is especially useful for the hydroxyl
radical, with which it gives a well characterized adduct, stable
at physiological pH [15]. Although most biological applications
to date have been in vitro, free radicals have been trapped in
vivo with N-t-butyl-alpha-4-pyridyl-1-oxide. When administered
to animals, this lipophilic trap is sequestered in hepatic
lipids, where it is available to react with free radical
intermediates in the breakdown of CCl_4. Upon sacrifice of the
animals, a stable free radical adduct could be extracted from
hepatic lipids for spectral analysis [18].

Spin trapping is not without its pitfalls. Unequivocal
assignment of the EPR signal to the correct structure of the
spin-adduct is important. There may be kinetic problems, e.g.,
spin-adducts are not always stable and trapping rates can
occasionally be slow compared to other pathways for the radical,
but the method promises to be increasingly useful biologically.
Papers on the kinetics of breakdown of adducts with oxygen
center radicals [6] and on the detection of radicals generated
during microsomal lipid peroxidation [28] offer some examples of
the practical problems in application of the technique.

Since the role of altered calcium fluxes in triggering
necrotic change will be of continuing interest, toxicologists
may find increasing use for a series of new calcium indicators

designed to give fast quantitative measurements of intracellular
calcium concentrations. The rationale for development of these
indicators has been described by Tsien [32]. The compounds are
derivatives of EGTA [ethylene glycol bis (beta-aminoethyl ether)-
N,N,N',N'-tetraacetic acid], and thus have a binding cavity that
accommodates calcium but cannot constrict sufficiently to
chelate magnesium. The key to successful development of the
indicators has been incorporation of the carbons of the
aminoethyl moiety into aromatic rings. This has two useful
consequences. First, the basicity of the nitrogens in EGTA is
reduced, thus reducing the strong dependence of binding on pH
variations near 7 and markedly increasing the rate of binding.
With the parent EGTA the necessity of displacing bound protons
to form the calcium chelate makes binding relatively slow.
Second, the conjugation of nitrogen electron pairs with aromatic
rings becomes sensitive to the orientation of those chains
bearing the carboxyl groups. As a consequence of this, the
intensity of ultraviolet absorption diminishes and band shapes
change as the nitrogens and their attached side chains move to
envelop a calcium ion. When the aromatic rings are also
fluorophores the fluorescence becomes very sensitive to calcium
concentrations. In an ingenious adaptation, the carboxyl groups
of these probes have been converted to acetoxymethyl esters,
which rapidly pass through cell membranes and are hydrolyzed
intracellularly to the parent indicator [33]. Indicators useful
at the calcium concentrations occurring intracellularly and with
selectivity for calcium over magnesium of the order of 2×10^4
have been obtained.

   Finally it is worth mentioning another reagent, palytoxin,
which may be of interest in studying calcium fluxes in
myocardial cells. The structures of several variants of this
extremely potent, non-protein toxin have been published recently
by Moore and Bartolini [23], and an overall survey of its
toxicity has appeared [35]. Because it produces rapid coronary
occlusion in minute doses the substance is unlikely to be useful
in vivo, but its pharmacological properties suggest that it may
have some utility in manipulating calcium fluxes in the
membranes of in vitro or isolated organ preparations. It would
appear to be either a calcium ionophore or a specific opener of
calcium channels and is of interest because of its remarkable
affinity for the membrane. Its application is somewhat
complicated by the production of increased sodium permeability,
at least partially inhibitable by tetrodotoxin. These
properties are exemplified in a study by Ito et al. [13] of the
effects of palytoxin on the electrical and mechanical responses
of guinea pig papillary muscle.

REFERENCES

1. BALAZS, T., OHTAKE, S. & NOBLE, J.F. The development of resistance to the ischemic cardiopathic effect of isoproterenol. Toxicology and Applied Pharmacology 21, 200-213 (1972).

2. BLOOM, S. Reversible and irreversible injury: Calcium as a major determinant. In Cardiac Toxicology, Vol. 1, T. Balazs, Ed., pp. 179-201. Boca Raton: CRC Press (1981).

3. BLOOM, S. & CANCILLA, P. Myocytolysis and mitochondrial calcification in rat myocardium after low doses of isoproterenol. American Journal of Pathology 54, 373-391 (1969).

4. BLOOM, S. & DAVIS, D. Calcium as mediator of isoproterenol-induced myocardial necrosis. American Journal of Pathology 69, 459-470 (1972).

5. BRISTOW, M.R., MASON, J.W., BILLINGHAM, M.E. & DANIELS, J.R. Doxorubicin cardiomyopathy: Evaluation by phonocardiography, endomyocardial biopsy, and cardiac catheterization. Annals of Internal Medicine 88, 168-175 (1978).

6. BUETTNER, G.R. & OBERLEY, L.W. Considerations in the spin trapping of superoxide and hydroxyl radical in aqueous systems using 5,5-dimethyl-1-pyrroline-1-oxide. Biochemical and Biophysical Research Communications 83, 69-74 (1978).

7. DEMOPOULOS, H.B., FLAMM, E.S., PIETRONIGRO, D.D. & SELIGMAN, M.L. The free radical pathology and the microcirculation in the major central nervous system disorders. Acta Physiologica Scandinavica Supplementum 492, 91-119 (1980).

8. DOROSHOW, J.H., LOCKER, G.Y. & MYERS, G.E. Enzymatic defenses of the mouse heart against reactive oxygen metabolites: Alterations produced by doxorubicin. Journal of Clinical Investigation 65, 128-135 (1980).

9. EVANS, C.A. Spin trapping. Aldrichimica Acta 12, 23-29 (1979).

10. FLECKENSTEIN, A., JANKE, J., DORING, H. & LEDER, O. Myocardial fiber necrosis due to intracellular calcium overload - a new principle in cardiac pathophysiology. Recent Advances in Studies on Cardiac Structure and Metabolism 4, 563-580 (1974).

11. GOODMAN, J. & HOCHSTEIN, P. Generation of free radicals and lipid peroxidation by redox cycling of adriamycin and daunomycin. Biochemical and Biophysical Research Communications 77, 797-803 (1977).

12. HERMAN, E. Cardiotoxicity of anti-neoplastic drugs. In Cardiac Toxicology, Vol. 2, T. Balazs, Ed., pp. 165-189. Boca Raton: CRC Press (1981).

13. ITO, K., KARAKI, H. & URAKAWA, N. Effects of palytoxin on mechanical and electrical activities of guinea pig papillary muscle. Japanese Journal of Pharmacology 29, 467-476 (1979).

14. JANZEN, E.G. A critical review of spin trapping in biological systems. In Free Radicals in Biology, Vol. 4, W.A. Pryor, Ed., pp. 115-154. New York: Academic Press (1980).

15. JANZEN, E.G., WANG, Y.Y. & SHETTY, R.V. Spin trapping with α-pyridyl-1-oxide N-tert-butyl nitrones in aqueous solution. A unique electron spin resonance spectrum for the hydroxyl radical adduct. Journal of the American Chemical Society 100, 2923-2925 (1978).

16. KAPPUS, H. & SIES, H. Toxic drug effects associated with oxygen metabolism: Redox cycling and lipid peroxidation. Experientia 37, 1233-1241 (1981).

17. KLUGMANN, S., BARTOLI KLUGMANN, F., DECORTI, G., GORI, D., SYLVESTRI, F. & CAMERINI, F. Adriamycin experimental cardiomyopathy in Swiss mice. Different effects of two calcium antagonistic drugs on ADM-induced cardiomyopathy. Pharmacological Research Communications 13, 769-776 (1981).

18. LAI, E.K., McKAY. P.B., NOGUCHI, T. & FONG, K. In vivo spin trapping of trichloromethyl radicals formed from CCl4. Biochemical Pharmacology 28, 2231-2235 (1979).

19. LEHR, D. Studies on the cardiotoxicity of alpha and beta adrenergic amines. In Cardiac Toxicology, Vol. 2, T. Balazs, Ed., pp. 75-113. Boca Raton: CRC Press (1981).

20. LEHR, D., CHAU, R. & IRENE, S. Possible role of magnesium loss in the pathogenesis of myocardial fiber necrosis. Recent Advances in Studies on Cardiac Structure and Metabolism 6, 95-109 (1975).

21. LUCCHESI, B., BURNREISTER, W., LOMAS, T. & ABRAMS, G. Ischemic changes in the canine heart as affected by the dimethyl quaternary analog of propranolol, UM 272. Journal of Pharmacology and Experimental Therapeutics 199, 310-328 (1976).

22. McCORD, J.M. Superoxide, superoxide dismutase and oxygen toxicity. In Reviews in Biochemical Toxicology, Vol. 1., E. Hodgson, J.R. Bend & R.M. Philpot, Eds., pp. 109-124. New York: Elsevier/North Holland (1979).

23. MOORE, R.E. & BARTOLINI, G. Structure of palytoxin. Journal of the American Chemical Society 103, 2491-2494 (1981).

24. OLSON, H.M., YOUNG, D.M., PRIEUR, D.J., LeROY, A.F. & REAGAN, R.L. Electrolyte and morphologic alterations of myocardium in adriamycin-treated rabbits. American Journal of Pathology 77, 439-454 (1974).

25. OLSON, R.D., BOERTH, R.C., GERBER, J.G. & NILES, A.S.
    Mechanism of adriamycin cardiotoxicity: Evidence for
    oxidative stress. Life Sciences 29, 1393-1401 (1981).
26. PARKS, D.A., BULKLEY, G.B., GRANGER, D.N., HAMILTON, S.R. &
    McCORD, J.M. Ischemic injury in the cat small intestine:
    Role of superoxide radicals. Gastroenterology 82, 9-15
    (1982).
27. REIMER, K.A., RASMUSSEN, M.M. & JENNINGS, R.B. On the
    nature of protection by propranolol against myocardial
    necrosis after temporary coronary occlusion in dogs.
    American Journal of Cardiology 37, 520-527 (1976).
28. ROSEN, G.M. & RAUCKMAN, E.J. Spin trapping of free
    radicals during hepatic microsomal lipid peroxidation.
    Proceedings of the National Academy of Sciences, USA 78,
    7346-7349 (1981).
29. ROSSI, C.S. & LEHNINGER, A.L. Stoichiometric relationships
    between accumulation of ions by mitochondria and the
    energy-coupling sites in the respiratory chain.
    Biochemische Zeitschrift 338, 698-713 (1963).
30. ROY, R.S. & McCORD, J.M. Ischemic-induced conversion of
    xanthine dehydrogenase to xanthine oxidase. Federation
    Proceedings 41, 767 (1982).
31. SELYE, H. The Chemical Prevention of Necrosis. New York:
    Ronald Press (1958).
32. TSIEN, R.Y. New calcium indicators and buffers with high
    selectivity against magnesium and protons. Design,
    synthesis, and properties of prototype structures.
    Biochemistry 19, 2396-2404 (1980).
33. TSIEN, R.Y. A non-disruptive technique for loading calcium
    buffers and indicators into cells. Nature 290, 527
    (1981).
34. VAN VLEET, J.F., GREENWOOD, L., FERRANS, V.J. & REBAR,
    A.H. Effect of selenium-vitamin E on adriamycin-induced
    cardiomyopathy in rabbits. American Journal of Veterinary
    Research 39, 997-1010 (1978).
35. VICK, J.A. & WILES, J.S. The mechanism of action and
    treatment of palytoxin poisoning. Toxicology and Applied
    Pharmacology 34, 214-223 (1975).
36. WAUD, W.R. & RAJAGOPALAN, K.V. The mechanism of conversion
    of rat liver xanthine dehydrogenase from an
    NAD^+-dependent form (type D) to an O_2-dependent form
    (type O). Archives of Biochemistry and Biophysics 172,
    365-379 (1976).
37. WEXLER, B.C. & McMURTRY, J.P. Allopurinol amelioration of
    the pathophysiology of acute myocardial infarction in
    rats. Atherosclerosis 39, 71-87 (1981).

ANTHRACYCLINE CARDIOTOXICITY

Victor J. Ferrans

Pathology Branch, National Heart, Lung, and Blood
Institute, National Institutes of Health
Bethesda, Maryland 20205

The clinical and pathological features of the cardiotoxicity
produced by antineoplastic antibiotics of the anthracycline type
are reviewed. The mechanisms by which these changes are produced
are discussed, and new data concerning the prevention of this
cardiotoxicity are presented.

INTRODUCTION

The practical therapeutic use of daunorubicin and doxorubicin,
two antineoplastic drugs of the anthracycline family, is limited
by the cardiotoxic effects of these agents. These effects can be
subdivided into acute, subacute and chronic depending upon their
temporal relationship to the administration of the drugs. The
acute effects consist of hypotension, tachycardia and arrhythmias,
and develop within minutes after intravenous administration. The
subacute effects are characterized by fibrinous pericarditis or
myocardial dysfunction, and occur within four weeks of the first
or second dose of the drug. The chronic effects become evident
only after several weeks or months of treatment, and are manifested
by the insidious onset of severe, often fatal congestive heart
failure.

Anthracyclines induce multiple, complex biochemical changes
in myocardium. Among these are: 1) binding of anthracyclines
(intercalation) to nuclear and mitochondrial DNA, leading to
inhibition of DNA, RNA and protein synthesis, to fragmentation of
DNA and to inhibition of DNA repair; 2) binding of anthracyclines
to membranes, resulting in interference with various functions of
membranes, including Na-K-dependent ATPase activity, calcium trans-

port and intracellular electrolyte balance; 3) inhibition of
reactions utilizing coenzyme Q; 4) chelation of divalent cations,
including calcium, iron and copper; 5) decrease in the activity of
glutathione peroxidase, and 6) promotion of complex peroxidative
phenomena by means of reactions mediated by free radicals (57).

ACUTE CARDIOTOXICITY OF ANTHRACYCLINES

The peripheral vascular effects of anthracyclines are consequences of histamine release, which in turn causes a secondary
release of catecholamines. This concept is supported by the results
of studies showing: a) that the intravenous injection of doxorubicin or daunorubicin increases the plasma levels of histamine
and catecholamines (6, 34); b) that the hypotension caused by these
agents can be almost completely prevented by pretreatment with
compound 48/80, which releases histamine by degranulating mast
cells (34), and c) that rat peritoneal mast cells are rapidly
degranulated by exposure to doxorubicin (45). Morphologic changes
related to the acute arrhythmias remain to be determined, although
it is known that in chronic anthracycline toxicity, the specialized
cardiac conducting cells of the rabbit, pig and dog show lesions
similar to those in ordinary working myocardium (26, 31, 33). The
only cardiac morphologic change that has been found to occur very
shortly after administration of doxorubicin is fragmentation of the
nucleolonema, with subsequent development of nucleolar segregation,
which takes place in mouse myocardium as early as 10 minutes after
a single injection of 10 mg/kg (37). Nucleolar segregation also
occurs in mouse and rat hepatocytes and in rat ventricular myocardium after the administration of large, single doses of doxorubicin
(39) and in Novikoff hepatoma cells treated with doxorubicin,
carminomycin or marcellomycin (14). This change is also produced
by other drugs, such as actinomycin D, which bind to DNA (47).
Doxorubicin and daunorubicin penetrate rapidly into nuclei, to
which they impart a reddish fluorescence (9, 15). Thus, these
observations show that anthracyclines produce acute, toxic effects
on nuclei. The long-term significance of nucleolar segregation is
unclear, because the morphology of nucleoli returns to normal by
14 hours after administration of doxorubicin (37).

Nuclear lesions have been observed only in a small percentage
of cardiac muscle cells in patients dying of chronic anthracycline
toxicity (9, 10). These lesions consist of various degrees of
unraveling of chromatin fibers into fine fibrils and filaments.
These changes are not specific for anthracycline toxicity (10). We
have not consistently observed these changes in experimental
animals given anthracyclines _in vivo_, although we have reproduced
them in monkey myocardium incubated _in vitro_ with anthracycline-
containing solutions (10). Thus, cumulative damage to DNA in

cardiac muscle cells (which are not capable of reproducing themselves, thereby diluting the damage to the genetic material) can result from the administration of repeated doses of anthracyclines. Such damage (including breaks in DNA) may not be properly repaired by cardiac muscle cells, and may lead to severe interference with protein synthetic processes. This is also shown by the fact that treatment with anthracyclines causes an acute, considerable decrease in cardiac weight in experimental animals. In our experience, this acute decrease in cardiac weight is not accompanied by qualitative changes in the morphology of the myocytes. Since the half-life of contractile proteins in cardiac muscle is in the range of one to two weeks, these effects may be of crucial importance in the pathogenesis of anthracycline-induced cardiomyopathy.

SUBACUTE CARDIOTOXICITY OF ANTHRACYCLINES

Bristow et al. (7) described eight patients in whom cardiac dysfunction developed within four weeks of receiving their first or second course of daunorubicin or doxorubicin. Four patients presented with pericarditis; three of these also had evidence of myocardial dysfunction. Cardiac morphologic findings in one of these patients consisted of: chronic anthracycline-type lesions (see below), focal myocardial necroses (the patient died in cardiogenic shock), fibrinous pericarditis, and infiltration of the epicardium with lymphocytes and polymorphonuclear leukocytes. The latter finding was in contrast with the more chronic lesions produced by anthracyclines, in which an inflammatory reaction is usually absent. An additional four patients presented with signs and symptoms of congestive heart failure. These patients either were elderly or had evidence of previous heart disease. One of these patients suffered a myocardial infarction 24 hours after receiving 60 mg/m^2 of daunorubicin; earlier doses in the same course had been associated with evidence of myocardial ischemia. Necropsy study in this patient showed no morphologic evidence of anthracycline cardiotoxicity. Bristow et al. (7) concluded that anthracyclines may manifest clinically significant cardiotoxicity at total cumulative doses much lower than those which have been associated with chronic cardiomyopathy.

CHRONIC CARDIOTOXICITY OF ANTHRACYCLINES

The morphologic changes (Figures 1 and 2) observed in chronic cardiotoxicity of anthracyclines (3, 7, 9, 10, 13, 20, 27, 28, 30, 33, 38, 40, 55) consist of: a) cardiac dilatation and, occasionally, mural thrombosis; b) degeneration and atrophy of cardiac myocytes, and c) interstitial edema and fibrosis. Valvular and vascular lesions are not present. The cardiac dilatation and mural thrombosis resemble those seen in patients with idiopathic congestive or

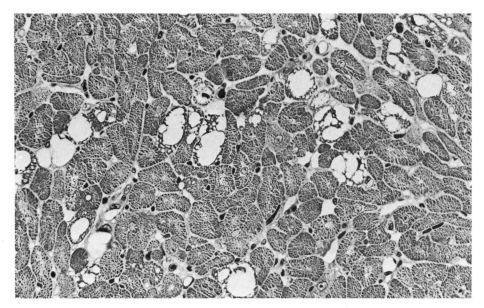

Figure 1. Light micrograph of one-micron-thick plastic section of myocardium of dog given 16 mg/kg of doxorubicin, showing typical vacuolization of cytoplasm. Alkaline toluidine blue stain, X 350.

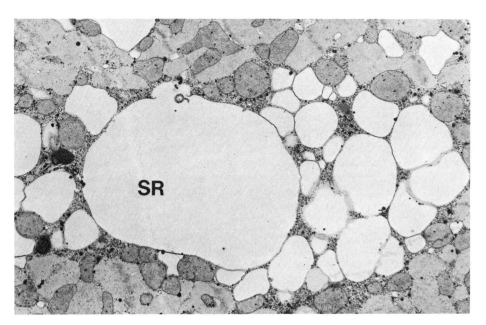

Figure 2. Electron micrograph showing dilated tubules of sarcoplasmic reticulum (SR) and electron-dense lamellae in damaged cardiac muscle cell of dog given 16 mg/kg of doxorubicin. X 13,000.

ventricular-dilated cardiomyopathy. The degeneration of cardiac
muscle cells assumes two forms: the first is characterized by myofibrillar loss, so that by light microscopy the affected cells
appear pale-staining but nonvacuolated; the second type is manifested by marked cytoplasmic vacuolization, usually associated
with myofibrillar loss. The reasons for these variations in the
response of individual cells to the same stimulus remain unknown.
One micron-thick sections of tissues embedded in glycolmethacrylate
resin and stained with hematoxylin-eosin or toluidine blue offer
considerable greater histologic detail than do sections of paraffin-
embedded tissues and provide a practical alternative to the use of
electron microscopy for the morphologic evaluation of anthracycline
cardiotoxicity. The degeneration of cardiac muscle cells in chronic
anthracycline toxicity is associated with ultrastructural changes
involving the myofibrils, the nuclei, the mitochondria and the
membrane systems of the T-tubules, the sarcoplasmic reticulum and
the intercellular junctions (9, 10, 12, 20, 33, 36, 44, 46). The
myofibrils show disruption, with lysis of the myofilaments. These
changes account for at least part of the cellular atrophy. The
cytoplasmic vacuolization is due mainly to pronounced swelling of
the tubules and cisterns of sarcoplasmic reticulum. Accumulation of
lipid and dilatation of tubules of the T-system also can contribute
to the vacuolated appearance. Dilated T-tubules are recognized by
their lining layer of basal lamina material. This layer is absent
from dilated tubules of sarcoplasmic reticulum, which have clear
lumina (21). Dilatation of the sarcoplasmic reticulum is a
nonspecific change that occurs in a number of conditions in which
cardiac myocytes become edematous (21). It should be pointed out,
however, that the most vacuolated myocytes in chronic anthracycline
toxicity do not show diffuse cytoplasmic swelling; in such cells
the distension of the sarcoplasmic reticulum is a sharply localized
phenomenon.

The intercellular junctions of damaged myocytes undergo dissociation, with formation of hemidesmosomes, intracytoplasmic junctions
and spherical microparticles. None of these changes is specific.
The hemidesmosomes are derived from the dissociation of desmosomes
(8). The intracytoplasmic junctions are formed by the specialized
apposition of two parts of the plasma membrane of the same cell,
and probably result from the rearrangement of remnants of specialized components of previously present intercellular junctions (8).
The spherical microparticles are related to the remodeling of
plasma membranes, especially in areas of cellular dissociation (24).

The mitochondria show a variety of changes, including pleo-
morphism, decrease in overall size, alterations in matrix density,
and formation of electron-dense concentric lamellae. Mitochondrial
inclusions have been observed in human myocardium obtained at
necropsy; however, such inclusions are of the amorphous density or
flocculent type and are related to postmortem autolysis (9).

Calcific inclusions have not been demonstrated in mitochondria of
anthracycline-treated animals. Some of the dense, concentric
lamellae are associated with dense bodies which probably are derived
from lysosomes. Mitochondrial changes are more prominent in acute
than in chronic toxicity; the reverse is true of alterations in
sarcoplasmic reticulum. It is surprising that mitochondrial morphology can be normal in cells showing severe changes in the sarcoplasmic
reticulum.

Cardiac tissues in anthracycline toxicity have an increased
content of calcium, sodium and water (44). These changes probably
result from increased permeability of damaged membranes, with subsequent calcium overload and increases in the tissue content of
sodium and water. The inhibition of Na-K-dependent ATPase may be
important in this respect (29). The interstitial fibrosis is difficult to evaluate because the edema and the cellular atrophy
exaggerate the prominence of the interstitial connective tissue.
Endothelial damage has been observed in some animal species (12),
but is not considered to be a feature of the toxicity in humans (3).

The morphologic features of chronic anthracycline cardiotoxicity
are basically the same in humans and in the rat (12), mouse (37, 46),
dog (52), pig (53) and rabbit (36) models. These changes are related
to the total cumulative dose and to the time scheduling of individual
doses. For a given cumulative dose, they tend to be less marked
when the drug is given in smaller individual doses (57). In mouse
myocardium, such changes begin to develop within 24 hours after the
administration of a large, single dose of doxorubicin (37). When
smaller, repeated doses are given, the changes may take several
weeks or months to develop. The main target organs in very acute
toxicity are the gastrointestinal tract and the bone marrow, lesions
in which can cause death before the typical cardiac morphologic
changes develop. For this reason, it is important to determine
whether or not improvements in mortality rates in acute toxicity
studies of protective agents are mediated through cardiac effects.
There is significant variation in the severity of morphologic changes
demonstrated by different patients or experimental animals in
response to a given dose level. For this reason, careful statistical
analysis is needed to evaluate the effects of potential protective
agents. It should also be noted that the early lesions are focal,
becoming more diffuse as their severity increases.

The relation between total cumulative dose of anthracyclines,
the development of cardiac morphologic changes and the occurrence
of congestive heart failure is of great clinical interest. Bristow
et al. (5) have shown that the morphologic findings in endomyocardial
biopsy can be used to guide additional therapy in patients in whom
either the clinical findings or the total cumulative dose suggest
a high risk of development of anthracycline cardiomyopathy.

Isner et al (35) evaluated the relationship between clinical evidence and histologic signs of anthracycline toxicity by reviewing the clinical and pathologic findings in 64 patients studied at necropsy, all of whom had received doxorubicin or daunorubicin chemotherapy. Twenty (31%) of the 64 patients had documented clinical toxicity consisting of impaired left ventricular systolic performance: in 7 (35%) of these 20 patients, histologic signs of toxicity were absent. In the remaining 13 patients, histologic signs of toxicity ranged from mild to severe. Of the 44 (69%) patients without clinical signs of drug toxicity, 21 (48%) had no histologic signs of cardiotoxicity; however, in 23 (52%) of the patients without clinical toxicity, morphologic signs of toxicity were present, mild in most patients, but extensive in four. Signs of severe histologic toxicity were found in 19 (30%) of the 64 patients and were associated with large doses (over 450 mg/m^2) of drug, mediastinal irradiation, and age over 70 years. The results of this study suggest that attempts to monitor cardiotoxicity by the evaluation of cardiac morphologic changes in patients undergoing anthracycline therapy may be limited by the fact that clinical evidence of cardiotoxicity may be present without accompanying histologic changes; likewise, histologic changes of anthracycline toxicity may be present without clinical evidence of toxicity.

PATHOGENESIS OF CARDIAC MORPHOLOGIC CHANGES INDUCED BY ANTHRACYCLINES

The pathogenesis of the changes enumerated above has not been fully elucidated, but it seems likely that several different drugs effects are important. We believe that the myofibrillar loss results mainly from interference with protein synthesis; the nuclear changes, from the binding of the drugs to nuclear DNA, and the changes involving the membrane systems (sarcoplasmic reticulum and plasma membranes) from peroxidative phenomena. It seems likely that calcium overloading contributes to the development of anthracycline-induced lesions, as it does in other types of cellular damage; however, treatment with calcium antagonists fails to protect against this cardiotoxicity (6). The possibility that the lesions in chronic anthracycline cardiotoxicity are due to release of histamine and catecholamines has been suggested by studies showing that pharmacologic blocking of catecholamine and histamine receptors (α, β, H_1 and H_2 receptors) reduces the severity of chronic anthracycline-induced lesions (6). The mechanisms by which this protection is exerted are not clear, as the doses of blocking agents used in this study were rather high; thus, it is possible that effects other than receptor blockade may be involved. Furthermore, the cardiac lesions produced by catecholamines (22, 23) and histamine (25) consist of focal necroses which differ considerably from the chronic degenerative lesions produced by anthracyclines. Thus,

we believe that histamine and catecholamines have only a contributory
role in the pathogenesis of anthracycline cardiomyopathy.

Anthracyclines can initiate peroxidative phenomena by facilitat-
ing the transfer of electrons from endogenous compounds such as
NADPH to oxygen, resulting in the formation of superoxides that can
decompose to hydroxy radicals, peroxy radicals and hydrogen
peroxide. These in turn can oxidize unsaturated fatty acids and
other constituents of membranes (57). A number of studies, the
results of which are summarized below, suggest that the morphologic
features of the toxicity produced by peroxidative and free radical
phenomena vary according to the nature, mechanism of formation and
site of release of the offending compounds. These observations
also suggest that differences in the ability to provide metabolic
defenses against free radical damage may be the cause of variations in the sensitivity response of individual patients to the
cardiotoxic effects of anthracyclines.

Two observations indicate that lipid peroxidation plays a
role in the pathogenesis of anthracycline toxicity: the first is
that the administration of very large doses of α-tocopherol,
(vitamin E, a free radical scavenger) reduces significantly the
acute toxicity and mortality produced by large doses of doxorubicin
in mice, and the second is that malondialdehyde, a product of peroxidation and decomposition of unsaturated fatty acids, is readily
detectable in the hearts of mice for two to six days after administration of doxorubicin, but not in the hearts of control mice or
mice treated with both doxorubicin and α-tocopherol (42, 43).
Nevertheless, several studies from different laboratories have shown
that α-tocopherol provides only very modest protection against the
chronic cardiotoxicity of doxorubicin in several species of
animals (4, 48, 49, 54, 56). In none of these species has it been
possible to show that α-tocopherol induces a dramatic qualitative
or quantitative change in the morphology of the cardiac lesions.

Ubiquinone, which acts as a free radical scavenger and as an
antagonist to the inhibitory effects of anthracyclines on reactions
mediated by coenzyme Q, also has been reported to ameliorate the
acute and chronic toxicity of doxorubicin (1), again suggesting
that such a toxicity is related to peroxidative phenomena. It is
of interest to note that animals exposed to high concentrations
of oxygen develop skeletal and cardiac muscle lesions which in
several ways (including dilatation of sarcoplasmic reticulum)
resemble those produced by anthracyclines (11). It is possible
that such lesions are mediated by peroxidative changes.

In contrast to their similarity to changes produced by oxygen
toxicity, the changes produced by anthracyclines differ from those
occurring in radiation injury and in deficiency of selenium and
vitamin E (Se-E), two conditions in which cardiac damage is known

to be mediated by peroxidative and free radical phenomena. In radiation injury to the heart (19), the initial damage is most prominent in capillary endothelial cells, which become edematous or necrotic; platelet and fibrin thrombi are frequent. In later stages there is severe interstitial fibrosis; however, at no time do the cardiac myocytes show changes similar to those in anthracycline cardiotoxicity. The combined administration of doxorubicin and radiation to rabbits results in the superimposition of lesions typical of each of these two agents and in significant enhancement of the cardiotoxicity of doxorubicin (17, 18). This enhancement, and a "recall phenomenon" for previous radiation, also have been demonstrated in humans (2).

Comparisons of the pathologic changes produced by anthracyclines and by Se-E deficiency are of interest because selenium and vitamin E, in conjunction with glutathione peroxidase, form an antioxidant system which prevents the peroxidation of membrane lipids and other cellular constituents. Cardiac lesions in Se-E deficiency have been best characterized in the pig (50, 51) and consist of: 1) multiple foci of necrosis, with hyalinization or with hypercontraction bands and mitochondrial swelling, disruption and calcification; 2) intramyocardial hemorrhage ("mulberry heart"); 3) fibrinoid necrosis of small intramural coronary arteries, and 4) capillary microthrombi composed of fibrin and platelets. The alterations cited above differ clearly from those in anthracycline toxicity, which in the pig induces (50, 51) changes similar to those in humans and in other species.

In humans, deficiency of selenium has been identified as the factor responsible for the occurrence of Keshan disease, a type of congestive cardiomyopathy which is endemic in certain regions of China. The reason for the occurrence of this deficiency is the extremely low content of selenium in the soil. Beause of this, the selenium content of foods grown in these areas is very low, and dietary deficiency eventually develops. This cardiomyopathy is characterized by large foci of myocytolysis and subsequent fibrosis; however, vascular lesions do not occur in myocardium in this disease, thus distinguishing it from the selenium-vitamin E deficiency in pigs (21). The nutritional status of Keshan disease patients with respect to vitamin E has not been determined. Of special interest is the fact that we have found (unpublished observations) that the lesions produced by doxorubicin in rats are worsened by deficiency of selenium, even in the presence of adequate intake of vitamin E.

As discussed above, the administration of large doses of selenium and vitamin E provides only minimal protection against chronic anthracycline cardiotoxicity (4, 48, 49, 54, 56). Furthermore, it has been shown (41) that ferric or ferrous ions can form with doxorubicin a complex which catalyzes the reduction of oxygen by both cysteine and glutathione, producing superoxide and hydrogen

peroxide. This complex also binds in vitro to human erythrocyte
ghost membranes and causes them to be destroyed in the presence of
glutathione. These results may provide an explanation for the
findings of Herman et al., who showed that ICRF 187 (razoxane),
probably acting as an iron chelator, markedly reduces the chronic
cardiotoxicity of doxorubicin or daunorubicin in experimental
animals (31-33). This compound, which has an antineoplastic effect
of its own, appears to provide a useful means of reducing the
chronic cardiotoxicity of anthracyclines. It seems likely that
the peroxidative damage which is associated with the chronic
cardiotoxicity of anthracyclines is catalyzed by the iron-doxo-
rubicin complex, and that ICRF 187 can interfere with the formation
of this complex. ICRF 187 also is beneficial in the toxicity
produced by acetaminophen in liver (unpublished observations) and
by alloxan in pancreatic β cells (16). Both of these toxicities
are mediated by the iron-catalyzed formation of free radicals.
Thus, ICRF 187 offers a new approach to the pharmacological
prevention of cellular damage produced by peroxidative phenomena.

REFERENCES

1. Bertazzoli, C., Sala, L., Solcia, E., & Ghione M. Experimental
   adriamycin cardiotoxicity prevented by ubiquinone in vivo in
   rabbits. *IRCS Journal of Medical Science* 3, 468 (1975).
2. Billingham, M. E., Bristow, M. R., Glatstein, E., Mason, J. W.,
   Masek, M. A. & Daniels, J. R. Adriamycin cardiotoxicity:
   endomyocardial biopsy evidence of enhancement by irradiation.
   American Journal of Surgical Pathology 1, 17-23 (1977).
3. Billingham, M. E., Mason, J. W., Bristow, M. R. & Daniels, J.
   R. Anthracycline cardiomyopathy monitored by morphologic changes.
   Cancer Treatment Reports 62, 865-872 (1978).
4. Breed, J. G. S., Zimmerman, A. N. E., Dormans, J. A. M., &
   Pinedo, H. M. Failure of the antioxidant vitamin E to protect
   against adriamycin-induced cardiotoxicity in the rabbit.
   Cancer Research 40, 2033-2038 (1980).
5. Bristow, M. R., Mason, J. W., Billingham, M. E., & Daniels, J.
   R. Doxorubicin cardiomyopathy. Evaluation by phonocardiography,
   endomyocardial biopsy, and cardiac catheterization. *Annals of
   Internal Medicine* 88, 168-175 (1978).
6. Bristow, M. R., Minobe, W. A., Billingham, M. E., Marmor, J. B.
   Johnson, G. A., Ishimoto, B. M., Sageman, W. S. & Daniels, J.
   R. Anthracycline-associated cardiac and renal damage in
   rabbits: evidence for mediation by vasoactive substances.
   Laboratory Investigation 45, 157-168 (1981).
7. Bristow, M. R., Thompson, P. D., Martin, R. P., Mason, J. W.,
   Billingham, M. E. & Harrison, D. C. Early anthracycline cardio-
   toxicity. *American Journal of Medicine* 65, 823-832 (1978).

8. Buja, L. M., Ferrans, V. J., & Maron, B. J. Intracytoplasmic junctions in cardiac muscle cells. *American Journal of Pathology* 74, 613–648 (1974).
9. Buja, L. M., Ferrans, V. J., Mayer, R. J., Roberts, W. C. & Henderson, E. S. Cardiac ultrastructural changes induced by daunorubicin therapy. *Cancer* 32, 771–788 (1973).
10. Buja, L. M., Ferrans, V. J. & Rabson, A. S. Letter: Unusual nuclear alterations. *Lancet* 1, 402–403 (1974).
11. Caulfield, J. B., Shelton, R. W. & Burke, J. F. Cytotoxic effects of oxygen on striated muscle. *Archives of Pathology* 94, 127–132 (1972).
12. Chalcroft, S. C. W., Gavin, J. B. & Herdson, P. B. Fine structural changes in rat myocardium induced by daunorubicin. *Pathology* 5, 99–105 (1973).
13. Cortes, E. P., Lutman, G., Wanka, J., Wang, J. J., Pickren, J., Wallace, J. & Holland, J. F. Adriamycin (NSC–123127) cardiotoxicity. A clinicopathologic correlation. *Cancer Treatment Reports* 6, 215–225 (1975).
14. Daskal, Y., Woodard, C., Crooke, S. T. & Busch, H. Comparative ultrastructural studies of nucleoli of tumor cells treated with Adriamycin and the newer anthracyclines, Carminomycin and Marcellomycin. *Cancer Research* 38, 467–473 (1978).
15. Egorin, M. J., Hildebrand, R. C., Cimino, E. F. & Bachur, N. R. Cytofluorescence localization of adriamycin and daunorubicin. *Cancer Research* 34, 2243–2245 (1974).
16. El-Hage, A. N., Herman, E. H. & Ferrans, V. J. Reduction in the diabetogenic effect of alloxan in mice by treatment with the antineoplastic agent ICRF-187. *Research Communications in Chemical Pathology and Pharmacology* 33, 509–523 (1981).
17. Eltringham, J. R., Fajardo, L. F. & Stewart R. Adriamycin cardiomyopathy: enhanced cardiac damage in rabbits with combined drug and cardiac irradiation. *Radiology* 115, 471–472 (1975).
18. Fajardo, L. F., Eltringham, J. R. & Stewart, J. R. Combined cardiotoxicity of Adriamycin and X-radiation. *Laboratory Investigation* 34, 86–96 (1976).
19. Fajardo, L. F. & Stewart, J. R. Pathogenesis of radiation-induced myocardial fibrosis. *Laboratory Investigation* 29, 244–257 (1973).
20. Ferrans, V. J. Overview of cardiac pathology in relation to anthracycline cardiotoxicity. *Cancer Treatment Reports* 62, 955–961 (1978).
21. Ferrans, V. J. & Butany, J. W. Ultrastructural pathology of the heart. In *Diagnostic Electron Microscopy*, Vol. 4. B. Trump & R. Jones, Eds. New York: John Wiley & Sons, Inc. (in press, 1982).
22. Ferrans, V. J., Hibbs, R. G., Walsh, J. J. & Burch, G. E. Histochemical and electron microscopical studies on the cardiac necroses produced by sympathomimetic agents. *Annals of the New York Academy of Sciences* 156, 309–332 (1969).

23. Ferrans, V. J., Hibbs, R. G., Weily, H. S., Weilbaecher, D. G., Walsh, J. J. & Burch, G. E. A histochemical and electron microscopic study of epinephrine-induced myocardial necrosis. *Journal of Molecular and Cellular Cardiology* 1, 11-22 (1970).

24. Ferrans, V. J., Thiedemann, K.-U., Maron, B. J. & Roberts, W. C. Spherical microparticles in human myocardium. An ultrastructural study. *Laboratory Investigation* 35, 349-368 (1976).

25. Franco-Browder, S., Guerrero, M., Gorodezky, M., Bravo, L. M. & Aceves, S. Lesiones miocárdicas producidas por liberadores de histamina en ratas. *Archivos del Instituto de Cardiología de México* 30, 720-728 (1960).

26. Gandolfi, A. Cardiotossicità cronica da adriamicina: studio morfologico ultrastrutturale sul miocardio ventricolare e sul sistema di conduzione del cuore di coniglio. *Ateneo Parmense. Sezione 1. Acta Bio-Medica* 47, 69-78 (1976).

27. Gilladoga, A. C., Manuel, C., Tan, C. C., Wollner, N. & Murphy, M. L. Cardiotoxicity of adriamycin (NSC-123127) in children. *Cancer Chemotherapy Reports* 6, 209-214 (1975).

28. Gilladoga, A. C., Manuel, C., Tan, C., Wollner, N., Sternberg, S. S. & Murphy, M. L. The cardiotoxicity of adriamycin and daunomycin in children. *Cancer* 37, 1070-1078 (1976).

29. Gosalvez, M., van Rossum, G. D. V., & Blanco, M. F. Inhibition of sodium-potassium-activated adenosine 5'-triphosphatase and ion transport by Adriamycin. *Cancer Research* 39, 257-261 (1979).

30. Halazun, J. F., Wagner, H. R., Gaeta, J. F. & Sinks, L. F. Daunorubicin cardiac toxicity in children with acute lymphocytic leukemia. *Cancer* 33, 545-554 (1974).

31. Herman, E. H. & Ferrans, V. J. Reduction of chronic doxorubicin cardiotoxicity in dogs by pretreatment with (±)-1,2-Bis (3,5-dioxopiperazinyl-1-yl) propane (ICRF-187). *Cancer Research* 41, 3436-3440 (1981).

32. Herman, E. H. & Ferrans, V. J. ICRF-187 reduction of chronic daunorubicin and doxorubicin cardiotoxicity in rabbits and beagle dogs. *Chemioterapia Oncologica* 5, 37-41 (1981).

33. Herman, E. H., Ferrans, V. J., Jordan, W. & Ardalan, B. Reduction of chronic daunorubicin cardiotoxicity by ICRF-187 in rabbits. *Research Communications in Chemical Pathology and Pharmacology* 31, 85-97 (1981).

34. Herman, E., Young, R., & Krop, S. Doxorubicin-induced hypotension in the Beagle dog. *Agents and Actions* 8, 551-557 (1978)

35. Isner, J. M., Ferrans, V. J., Cohen, S. R., Witkind, B. G., Virmani, R., Gottdiener, J. S. & Roberts, W. C. Variability of cardiac histologic toxicity in patients treated with anthracycline chemotherapy. *American Journal of Cardiology* 45, 396 (1980).

36. Jaenke, R. S. An anthracycline antibiotic-induced cardiomyopathy in rabbits. *Laboratory Investigation* 30, 292-304 (1974).

37. Lambertenghi-Deliliers, G., Zanon, P. L., Pozzoli, E. F. &
    Bellini, O. Myocardial injury induced by a single dose of
    adriamycin: an electron microscopic study. *Tumori* 62, 517-529
    (1976).
38. Lefrak, E. A., Pitha, J., Rosenheim, S. & Gottlieb, J. A clini-
    copathologic analysis of adriamycin cardiotoxicity. *Cancer*
    32, 302-314 (1973).
39. Merski, A., Daskal, I., & Busch, H. Effects of adriamycin on
    ultrastructure of nucleoli in the heart and liver cells of the
    rat. *Cancer Research* 36, 1580-1584 (1976).
40. Minow, R. A., Benjamin, R. S., Lee, E. T. & Gottlieb, J. A.
    Adriamycin cardiomyopathy-risk factors. *Cancer* 39, 1397-1402
    (1977).
41. Myers, C. E., Gianni, L., Simone, C. B., Hendrickson, M.,
    Klecker, R.& Greene, R. Oxidative destruction of erythrocyte
    ghost membranes catalyzed by the doxorubicin-iron complex.
    Biochemistry (in press, 1982).
42. Myers, C. E., McGuire, W. P., Liss, R. H., Ifrim, I., Grot-
    zinger, K., & Young, R. C. Adriamycin: the role of lipid
    peroxidation in cardiac toxicity and tumor response. *Science*
    197, 165-167 (1977).
43. Myers, C. E., McGuire, W. P., & Young, R. C. Adriamycin:
    amelioration of toxicity by α-tocopherol. *Cancer Treatment
    Reports* 60, 961-962 (1976).
44. Olson, H. M., Young, D. M., Prieur, D. J., LeRoy, A. F. &
    Reagan, R. L. Electrolyte and morphologic alterations of
    myocardium in adriamycin-treated rabbits. *American Journal of
    Pathology* 77, 439-454 (1974).
45. Regal, E., Kaliner, M.; El-Hage, A., Ferrans, V. J., Kawanami,
    O., & Herman, E. H. Anthracycline-induced histamine release
    from rat mast cells. *Agents and Actions* (in press, 1982).
46. Rosenoff, S. H., Olson, H. M., Young, D. M., Bostick, F. &
    Young, R. C. Adriamycin-induced cardiac damage in the mouse.
    A small animal model of cardiotoxicity. *JNCI. Journal of the
    National Cancer Institute* 55, 191-194 (1975).
47. Unuma, T., Senda, R., & Muramatsu, M. Mechanism of nucleolar
    segregation-differences in effects of actinomycin D and
    cycloheximide on nucleoli of rat liver cells. *Journal of
    Electron Microscopy (Tokyo)* 22, 205-216 (1973).
48. VanVleet, J. F. & Ferrans, V. J. Cutaneous lesions and hemato-
    logic alterations in chronic adriamycin intoxication in dogs
    with and without vitamin E and selenium supplementation.
    American Journal of Veterinary Research 41, 691-699 (1980).
49. VanVleet, J. F. & Ferrans, V. J. Evaluation of vitamin E and
    selenium protection against chronic adriamycin toxicity in
    rabbits. *Cancer Treatment Reports* 64, 315-317 (1980).
50. VanVleet, J. F., Ferrans, V. J. & Ruth, G. R. Ultrastructural
    alterations in nutritional cardiomyopathy of selenium-vitamin E
    deficient swine. I. Fiber lesions. *Laboratory Investigation*
    37, 188-200 (1977).

51. VanVleet, J. F., Ferrans, V. J. & Ruth, G. R. Ultrastructural alterations in nutritional cardiomyopathy of selenium-vitamin E deficient swine. II. Vascular lesions. *Laboratory Investigation* 37, 201-211 (1977).
52. VanVleet, J. F., Ferrans, V. J. & Weirich, W. E. Cardiac disease induced by chronic adriamycin administration in dogs and an evaluation of vitamin E and selenium as cardioprotectants. *American Journal of Pathology* 99, 13-42 (1980).
53. VanVleet, J. F., Greenwood, L. A., & Ferrans, V. J. Pathologic features of adriamycin toxicosis in young pigs: nonskeletal lesions. *American Journal of Veterinary Research* 40, 1537-1552 (1979).
54. VanVleet, J. F., Greenwood, L., Ferrans, V. J. & Rebar, A. H. Effect of selenium-vitamin E on adriamycin-induced cardiomyopathy in rabbits. *American Journal of Veterinary Research* 39, 997-1010 (1978).
55. Von Hoff, D. D., Rozencweig, M., Layard, M., Slavik, M. & Muggia, F. M. Daunomycin-induced cardiotoxicity in children and adults. A review of 110 cases. *American Journal of Medicine* 62, 200-208 (1977)
56. Wang, Y., Madanat, F. F., Kimball, J. C., Gleiser, C. A., Ali, M. K., Kaufman, M. W. & Van Eys, J. Effect of vitamin E against adriamycin-induced toxicity in rabbits. *Cancer Research* 40, 1022-1027 (1980).
57. Young, R. C., Ozols, R. F. & Myers, C. E. The anthracycline antineoplastic drugs. *New England Journal of Medicine* 305, 139-153 (1981).

ALLYLAMINE CARDIOTOXICITY: METABOLISM AND MECHANISM

Paul J. Boor

Department of Pathology, Chemical Pathology Laboratory
University of Texas Medical Branch
Galveston, Texas

Allylamine (CH_2=CH-CH_2NH_2) is an unsaturated aliphatic amine which is used in the production of drugs, antiseptics, and plastics. Although many investigators have studied the potent and relatively specific cardiovascular toxicity of allylamine, the mechanism of its toxic action remains obscure.

This brief review will summarize previous work on allylamine-induced vascular and myocardial lesions, and will focus on our laboratory's recent studies of the cardiovascular metabolism of this interesting toxin.

MORPHOLOGY

When given in food [1,2] or drinking water [3] for a period of weeks to months, allylamine causes severe myocardial fibrosis that is generally more severe at the cardiac apex and is often transmural (Fig. 1). Microscopically, the fibrosis is initially subendocardial, spares a few layers of subendocardial myocytes, and is associated with bizarre endocardial alterations [4] such as bony and cartilagenous metaplasia of trabeculae carnae (Fig. 2). In addition, cartilagenous metaplasia of the aortic arch [5] and medial hypertrophy of coronary arteries [2] occur after prolonged administration of allylamine.

Although several investigators have implicated coronary arterial lesions as the cause of this striking myocardial fibrosis [1,2,6], our study of the sequence of these pathologic events demonstrates that acute myocardial necrosis occurs before significant vascular lesions [3].

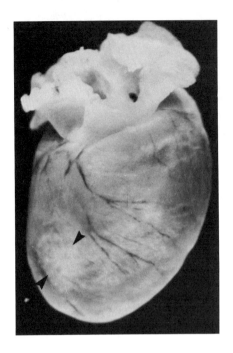

Figure 1: A posterior view of heart of allylamine treated rat shows extensive fibrosis seen as white streaks. Focally, the fibrosis near the apex is trans-mural (arrows). Rat given 0.1% allylamine in drinking water for 21 days; X8 (approx.).

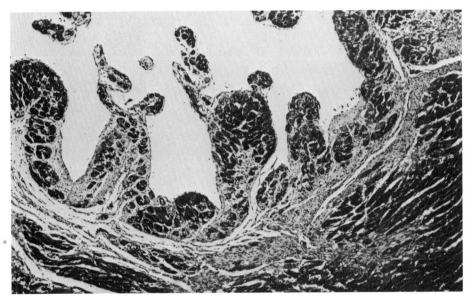

Figure 2: Microscopic view of rat heart shows subendocardial fibrosis that spares a few layers of subendocardial myocytes. Rat treated as in Figure 1; Masson Trichrome stain; X290.

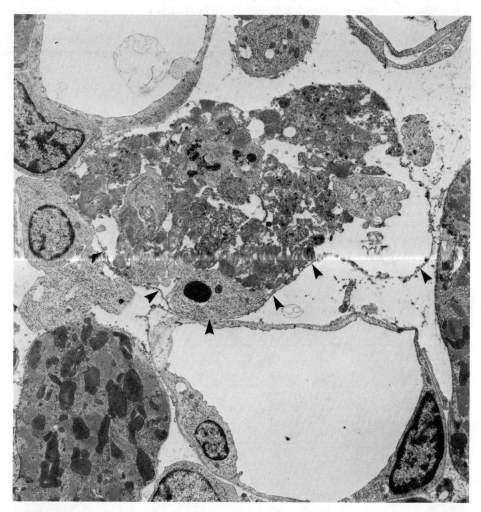

Figure 3: Electronmicrograph of acute allylamine toxicity shows single myocyte undergoing advanced necrosis, with clumped myofibrils, electron dense mitochondrial deposits, and lysis of cell. Note macrophage processes invading along the remnants of basal lamina (arrows). Rat given 2 gavage doses of 150 mg/kg, 24 hours apart; X59,000.

Indeed, ultrastructural lesions occur after one or two gavage doses of allylamine [7]. These ultrastructural myocyte lesions are characterized by focal myofibrillar degeneration, lipid droplet accumulation, and Z-line distortion and dissolution followed by myocyte necrosis and rapid infiltration by macrophages associated with eosinophilic granulocytes (Fig. 3). Vascular lesions or thrombi are not seen acutely. A peculiar nuclear activation of interstitial and endothelial cells is also manifest early during acute allylamine intoxication. These morphologic findings suggest a direct toxic effect of allylamine or a metabolite on the myocardial cell, and argue against vascular damage as a cause of myocardial necrosis.

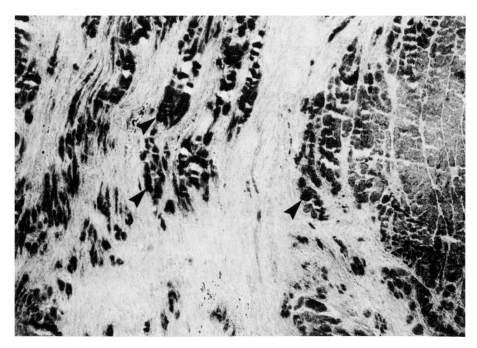

Figure 4: Histochemical MAO stain of allylamine-induced scar in rat myocardium shows intense staining of myocytes in and near fibrous tissue (arrows), when compared to myocardium at right of photomicrograph. Rat treated as in Figure 1; X290.

INVOLVEMENT OF AMINE OXIDASE

Two pieces of experimental evidence have suggested that a form of amine oxidase is involved in the toxicity of allylamine. First, allylamine-induced lesions may be prevented by the administration of hydralazine [5] or semicarbazide [8]. These compounds are weak inhibitors of monoamine oxidase (MAO) and potent inhibitors of a recently studied [9-11] separate form of amine oxidase, benzylamine oxidase (BzAO).

Secondly, histochemical [4] and biochemical [8,12] in vivo studies of the MAO system during allylamine intoxication indicate that systemic MAO is profoundly altered by allylamine. Myocyte MAO staining greatly increases in intensity near allylamine-induced fibrous tissue (Fig. 4); apical and subendocardial myocytes also show a moderate, diffuse increase which seems to precede myocardial necrosis [4]. In addition, myocardial MAO, measured biochemically in the whole rat heart, undergoes dramatic and paradoxical alterations which are directly related to the histologic degree of myocardial damage [8].

METABOLISM

The evidence suggesting involvement of some form of amine oxidase in allylamine toxicity led us to the hypothesis [13] that allylamine is metabolized by an amine oxidase to a toxic intermediate which is directly responsible for cellular damage, i.e. a distal or ultimate toxin. A likely toxic intermediate would be the aldehyde, acrolein, which has been isolated as an in vitro product of metabolism of allyl alcohol [14]. The proposed oxidation would also be expected to liberate peroxide:

$$CH_2=CH-CH_2NH_2 \xrightarrow[\text{(O)}]{\text{(amine oxidase)}} CH_2=CH-CHO \quad + \quad H_2O_2$$

We tested this hypothesis in homogenates of several rat organs, and isolated acrolein as the reaction product [15]. The different organs examined showed a wide range of activities; metabolism of allylamine to acrolein was particularly vigorous in aorta.

Table 1. Metabolism of Allylamine to Acrolein
          by Rat Tissue Homogenates[a]

Sample	Acrolein (% conversion)
Aorta	80
Lung	22
Skeletal Muscle	8
Heart	5
Liver	0
Brain	0
Plasma	0

[a]Homogenates incubated with 0.3 mM allylamine for
6 hr; acrolein was detected fluorometrically after
distillation; for details see Ref. 15.

The enzyme responsible for allylamine metabolism is unknown.
Inhibitor studies performed in rat heart homogenate, however, suggest that the enzyme active in allylamine conversion to acrolein
is BzAO. This recently studied amine oxidase appears to have widespread distribution in experimental animals and man [9-11] and also
exhibits an organ distribution which is strikingly similar to the
activity of various organs in converting allylamine to acrolein
(see Ref. 9 compared to Table 1). Therefore, we strongly suspect
that BzAO is responsible for the metabolism of allylamine, and
experiments to test this hypothesis in vivo are underway.

Table 2. Effect of Inhibitors on Acrolein Formation
          in Rat Heart Homogenate[b]

Inhibitor	Type of Inhibition	% Inhibition	
		1 M	50 M
Clorgyline	"A" MAO	0	0
Depreyl	"B" MAO	0	13
Isoniazid	"A" + "B" MAO	0	0
Semicarbazide	BzAO	0	92
Procarbazine	BzAO	74	100
Hydralazine	BzAO + "plasma" AO	71	100

[b]Reaction mixtures were preincubated with indicated
concentration of inhibitor. See Ref. 15 for details.

MECHANISM

The mechanism by which the distal toxin, acrolein, causes myocellular and vascular damage during allylamine intoxication is unknown. Two mechanisms seem likely, however.

First, acrolein might act upon the small or medium-sized intramyocardial arteries to cause spasm and resultant temporary occlusion. Vascular spasm, as a factor in human myocardial infarction, has recently received great clinical and experimental attention [16]. The morphology of allylamine-induced myocardial necrosis is consistent with ischemic damage followed by reflow, and - hypothetically - spasm might not result in any morphologic damage to vessels in acute allylamine intoxication. During subsequent chronic intoxication, cellular damage of smooth muscle cells and vascular endothelium by acrolein could result in the intimal smooth muscle cell proliferation [2] and bizarre endo-thelial alterations noted in cardiac vessels and aorta.

A second possible mechanism of allylamine's injurious effects could be that the ultimate toxin, acrolein, exerts a direct toxic effect on myocardial cells acutely causing cellular necrosis, and only chronically effecting vessels.

In conclusion, it is highly likely that the metabolism of allylamine is closely related to its toxic effects. The experi-mental evidence surrounding allylamine cardiotoxicity supports the concept that cardiovascular organs act as metabolic tissues capable of biotransforming foreign substances through their own characteristic enzymatic pathways.

ACKNOWLEDGMENTS

This work has been supported by Young Investigator Award HL-21327, Research Career Development Award HL-00929, and Grants HL-21327 and HL-26189 from the National Heart, Lung and Blood Institute. The assistance of Ms. Diane Pugh in the preparation of the manuscript is gratefully appreciated.

REFERENCES

1. Lalich, J.J.: Coronary artery hyalinosis in rats fed allylamine. Exp. Mol. Pathol. 10:14, 1969.

2. Lalich, J.J., Allen, J.R. and Paik, W.C.W.: Myocardial fibrosis and smooth muscle cell hyperplasia in coronary arteries of allylamine-fed rats. Am. J. Pathol. 66:225, 1972.

3. Boor, P.J., Moslen, M.T. and Reynolds, E.S.: Allylamine cardiotoxicity. I. Sequence of pathologic events. Toxicol. Appl. Pharmacol. 50:581, 1979.

4. Boor, P.J., Nelson, T.J. and Chieco, P.: Allylamine cardiotoxicity. II. Histopathology and histochemistry. Am. J. Pathol. 100:739, 1980.

5. Lalich, J.J. and Paik, W.C.W.: Influence of hydralazine consumption on allylamine-induced myocardial fibrosis and hypertrophy in rats. Exp. Mol. Pathol. 21:29, 1974.

6. Will, J.A., Rowe, G.G., Olson, C. and Crumpton, C.W.: A chemically induced acute model of myocardial damage in intact calves. Res. Commun. Chem. Pathol. Pharmacol. 2:61, 1971.

7. Boor, P.J. and Ferrans, V.J.: Ultrastructural alterations in allylamine-induced cardiomyopathy. Lab. Invest., 47(1): (In Press), 1982.

8. Boor, P.J. and Nelson, T.J.: Allylamine cardiotoxocity: III. Protection by semicarbazide and in vivo derangements of monoamine oxidase. Toxicology 18:87-102, 1980.

9. Lewinsohn, R., Bohm, K.-H., Glover, V. and Sandler, M.: A benzylamine oxidase distinct from monoamine oxidase B - widespread distribution in man and rat. Biochem. Pharmacol. 27:1857, 1978

10. Lyles, G.A. and Callingham, B.A.: Evidence for a clorgyline-resistant monoamine metabolizing activity in the rat heart. J. Pharm. Pharmac. 27:682, 1975.

11. Bhansali, K.G., Hayes, B.E. and Clarke, D.E.: Benzylamine oxidase in rabbit lung. Fed. Proc. 41:1056, 1982.

12. Valiev, A.G.: Influence expected by some aliphatic amines on the monoamine oxidase activity in rats. Farmakol. Tosikol. (Moscow) 31:238, 1968.

13. Boor, P.J., Reynolds, E.S., Dammin, G.J. and Bailey, K.A.: Allylamine-induced myocardial damage: Protection by monoamine oxidase inhibitors. Fed. Proc. 36:397, 1977.

14. Serafini-Cessi, F.: Conversion of allyl alcohol into acrolein by rat liver. Biochem. J. 128:1103, 1962.

15. Nelson, T.J. and Boor, P.J.:   Allylamine cardiotoxicity.
     IV.   Metabolism to acrolein by cardiovascular tissues.
     Biochem. Pharmacol. 31:509-514, 1982.

16. Luchi, R.J., Chahine, R.A. and Raizner, A.E.:   Coronary
     Artery Spasm. Ann. Intern. Med., 91:441, 1979.

CARDIOVASCULAR TOXICITY OF IONOPHORES USED AS FEED ADDITIVES

Berton C. Pressman and Mohammad Fahim

Department of Pharmacology
University of Miami
Miami, FL 33101

INTRODUCTION

Formidable quantities of microbial metabolites belonging to the class of <u>ionophores</u> are currently being fed to poultry and cattle raised for human consumption. Most fryers and broilers in the United States received 120 ppm monensin in their feed to control coccidiosis[1] while beef cattle are fed 30 ppm monensin which, possibly by exerting a favorable effect on the flora of the rumen,[2] promotes a more efficient fermentation of cellulose and subsequent conversion of feed to meat.[3]

Several questions must be considered when man's food supply is exposed to a new biologically active agent: (1) what are its qualitative and quantitative physiological properties; (2) what are its predictable toxicological consequences; (3) to what quantities is man likely to be exposed; (4) what are the overall toxicological hazards the substance poses for man.

METHODS AND RESULTS

Physiological Effects of Monensin

This paper will deal mainly with the specific ionophore monensin since this is the major ionophore in agricultural use at the moment. It is a member of the <u>carboxylic</u> subclass of ionophores, virtually all of which have similar physiological properties and are accordingly either being actively developed as feed additives or else have this potentiality.

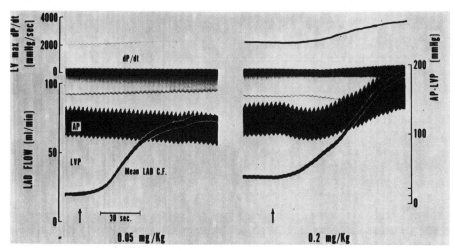

Fig. 1.   Typical response of instrumented anesthetized dog to in-
          injected bolus of monensin. Aortic pressure obtained from
          catheter in aorta connected to pressure transducer; dP/dt
          obtained by electronic differentiation of signal from
          pressure-tipped manometer in left ventricle; coronary flow
          recorded from electromagnetic flow probe placed around the
          left anterior descending coronary artery dissected free of
          the myocardium. Pentobarbital was used as anesthetic.

     The principal hemodynamic effects of monensin on anesthetized,
instrumented dogs are indicated in Fig. 1. A low dose, 0.050 mg/kg,
(left panel) produces a rapid and powerful increase in coronary
flow,indicative of coronary dilatation without any accompanying
alterations of blood pressure or cardiac contractility as measured
by the index dP/dt.[4,5] At this dose level some effects on contractility eventually occur, peaking at about 10 min after monensin injection. At a higher dose, 0.20 mg/kg, (right panel) a transient
drop in aortic pressure appears, indicative of a drop in total peripheral resistance, followed by a rise in pressure which is related to increasing cardiac contractility and cardiac output. Very
similar cardiovascular effects have been reported with lasalocid,
salinomycin, and other carboxylic ionophores.[4,6-8]

     Since the cardiovascular function most sensitive to monensin
is coronary resistance, this can be considered as the appropriate
threshold parameter for evaluating monensin toxicity. According
to Fig. 2, a dose of about 2.5 µg/kg doubles coronary flow[9] from
which we may extrapolate that a threshold dose is about 1 µg/kg.
To place this in proper perspective, a 1 kg chicken consuming 8.5%
of its weight daily of feed containing 120 ppm monensin would take
in 10,000 µg/day of ionophore.

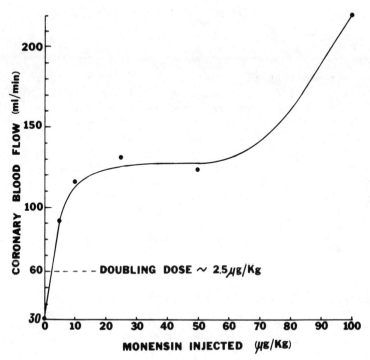

Fig. 2. Dose–response curve of coronary flow of anesthetized dog
         to monensin. Peak responses were obtained 5 min after
         injection of each indicated dose of monensin on different
         sets of dogs.

        Although drug induced coronary vasodilatation presents no
threat to normal individuals, it poses special problems to victims
of coronary disease. If a given coronary vessel becomes partially
occluded through disease, the resultant flow impairment would produce some degree of hypoxia which would trigger the autoregulatory
process causing the vessel to dilate. Such a vessel, if dilated
close to its limit, cannot respond further to a coronary vasodilator
to the same degree as normal, unoccluded vessels possessing normal
tone. Thus, dilatation by a coronary vasodilator of normal vessels
in parallel with less responsive occluded vessels would divert blood

flow away from the latter to the normal vessels, thereby exacerbat-
ing hypoxia in the myocardium fed by the occluded vessels. This
phenomenon, termed coronary steal, has been well studied in connection with the coronary vasodilatory drug dipyridamole.[10]

Since an appreciable fraction of the population at large suf-
fers from some degree of coronary disease, ingestion of even small
amounts of dietary monensin could produce an appreciable incidence
of adverse effects such as hypoxia with attendant angina. Such
responses to dietary monensin might well escape clinical detection
as they would be swamped by the spontaneous incidence of adverse
episodes among victims of coronary disease. Moreover, coronary
steal would not present a problem to the large segment of the popu-
ation not predisposed to a deleterious response by coronary disease.
Nevertheless, in view of the significant incidence of coronary disease within the population at large, and the number of people who
consume poultry (perhaps beef should also be considered), the incidence of adverse human reactions to dietary monensin may be appreciable. A number of human adverse reactions to monensin are already
on file with the FDA* although these may represent mainly industrial
exposure to younger workers and not be directly pertinent to the
hazards posed to the older population by dietary monensin.

Molecular Basis of Biological Properties of Monensin

The molecular properties of ionophores have been studied in
considerable detail. This has provided us with not only a rational
mechanism for their physiological and toxicological properties, but
also an understanding of their unique chemical and physical properties. The latter in turn have supplied a rationale for an unusual
tissue assay procedure for ionophores which will be described
shortly.

The structure of monensin is illustrated in Fig. 3. The
generic characteristic of ionophores is their ability to form lipid
soluble complexes with cations by liganding them to a system of
oxygen atoms (in rare instances nitrogen atoms as well).

The molecular backbone serves two specific functions. In its
complexation conformation it focuses the oxygen atoms in space to
form a cavity which accommodates the complexed cation. In this
configuration the polar groups as well as the polar cation occupy
the interior of a spheroid with the non-polar, alkyl groups deployed
about the exterior where they present themselves to the molecular
environment. This renders the complex as a whole soluble in low

---

*FDA Adverse Reaction Reports Form 2025, obtainable from the FDA,
5600 Fishers Lane, Rockville, MD 20857.

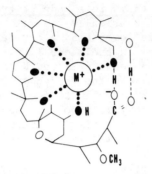

Fig. 3. Structure of monensin. Oxygen atoms directly involved in
liganding are filled in black.

polarity media including organic solvents as well as the lipid bilayer of biomembranes. The second function of the backbone is to
facilitate complexation-decomplexation kinetics which enables ionophores to act as extremely efficient transporters of cations across
biological membranes with turnover numbers attaining several
hundred/sec. This is related to the ability of the ionophore backbone to assume an alternate "defocused" conformation which releases
its complexed ion and retains the empty ionophore at the polar membrane interface until it can capture another cation and reassume
its lipid soluble conformation.[11]

These conformational attributes of ionophores have been studied
at the molecular level by X-ray crystallography, nuclear magnetic
resonance (NMR), circular dichroism (CD), and molecular modeling by
computer, and are consequently understood in considerable depth.
For the investigator who wants to pursue the structures of available
ionophores and their physicochemical and biological properties, in
greater detail, a number of reviews and monographs are available.[12-15]

Neutral ionophores, such as valinomycin, which transport ions across biological membranes along with their net charge, severely disrupt electrophysiological processes and are consequently exceedingly toxic to animals. Carboxylic ionophores, such as monensin, on the other hand transport cations as electrically neutral zwitterions, utilizing the anionic charge of their terminal carboxyl (cf. Fig. 3) to offset the positive charge of the transported cation. In electrophysiological terms this mode of transport is termed exchange-diffusion, is electrically neutral, perturbs membrane potentials minimally and is tolerated rather well by animals. A striking feature of ionophores is their equilibrium selectivity for cations, e.g. valinomycin prefers to ligand K^+ over Na^+ by a ratio of about 10,000.[13] Nevertheless the thermodynamic driving force of the normally prevailing transcellular ion gradients dictate that a monovalent selective carboxylic ionophore such as monensin ($Na^+:K^+ > 10$) would catalyze a rise in intracellular Na^+ in exchange for the release of an approximately equivalent amount of K^+.

Mechanism of Biological Effects of Carboxylic Ionophores

The biological effects of an ionophore-mediated rise in intracellular Na^+ appear to be best explained in terms of a displacement and liberation of intracellularly bound Ca^{2+}, increasing its access to intracellular Ca^{2+} receptor sites.[13,14] Thus, the effect of monensin on cardiac contractility would be due at least in part to increasing the availability of intracellular Ca^{2+} to troponin C during a contraction. Another effect of raising intracellular Ca^{2+} is the stimulation of exocytotic secretion. Monensin has been shown to release catecholamines from isolated adrenal chromaffin cells, even in the absence of extracellular Ca^{2+}.[16] Monensin-induced release of catecholamines from the adrenals and possibly nerve endings presumably accounts for the partial sensitivity of monensin-induced stimulation of contractility to β-adrenergic blockade.[17] In analogous fashion, the rise in plasma glucose induced by monensin could be attributed to the endocytotic release of glucagon from the pancreatic α cells.

Monensin-induced Ca^{2+} elevation cannot be the direct cause of coronary vasodilatation, i.e. smooth muscle relaxation. This can be accounted for, however, by a Ca^{2+}-induced exocytotic release of adenosine[17] from storage granules[18], activating the adenosinergic receptors of the coronary arteries[19] possibly aided by Ca^{2+}-induced prostaglandin synthesis.[20] These autocoids could dilate the coronary by stimulating an outwardly directed Ca^{2+} pump in the coronary smooth muscle.[21]

Ionophore-Mediated Cation Transport Across Erythrocyte Membrane

The ability of monensin to transport alkali ions across a plasma membrane is conveniently monitored by ion selective electrodes[22] with human erythrocytes suspended in mock plasma (Fig. 4).

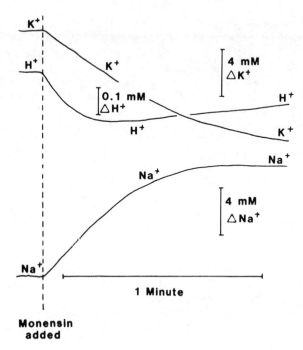

Fig. 4. Effect of monensin on fresh human erythrocyte cations. Erythrocytes washed with 140 mM NaCl, 5 mM KCl with 25 mM HEPES buffer, pH 7.4. Na^+ trace obtained from Microelectrode Inc. Na^+ electrode MI-40, K^+ trace from Beckman cationic electrode 39047 and pH from A.H. Thomas combination pH electrode which supplied the common reference electrode. The method is described in further detail in Ref. 22.

Since the electrodes sense ion concentration changes in the medium, they reflect the converse of the ion changes taking place within the erythrocytes. Monensin initiates a marked influx of Na^+ into the erythrocytes counterbalanced by a slower efflux of K^+. The electro-

static imbalance between Na$^+$ and K$^+$ gives rise to a compensatory
movement of H$^+$ which can be tracked as a drop in pH of the medium.
As the Na$^+$ influx slows up and the pH gradient rises, the latter in
turn supplies the driving force to continue the K$^+$ efflux until net
K$^+$ efflux approximately equals the net Na$^+$ influx.[16]

The initial imbalance between Na$^+$ influx and K$^+$ efflux is a result of the marked selectivity of monensin for Na$^+$ over K$^+$ and its
ability to transport H$^+$ in the form of its protonated carboxyl (cf.
Fig. 3). If a K$^+$-over-Na$^+$ selective ionophore, e.g. nigericin, were
added to the system, the initial rate of K$^+$ efflux would have exceeded that of Na$^+$ influx, the difference again being made up by H$^+$
transport, in this case an H$^+$ efflux. The final equilibrium, however, would relax to more or less the same point as that induced by
monensin.[3,11] Thus, although the wide variation of ion selectivities
among the carboxylic ionophores is striking, it does not affect the
ultimate ionic equilibrium they promote across the cell membrane.[13]
As shall be seen, the ion selectivity of ionophores does influence
the nature of the radiochemical assay required to detect a given
ionophore.

Development of Radiochemical Assay for Carboxylic Ionophores

The ability of ionophores to form lipid soluble complexes has
been exploited for development of a sensitive radiochemical assay
for ionophores. Thus, under selected conditions a lipid soluble
ionophore will cause the migration of a normally highly polar radioactive alkali cation from a polar aqueous phase to a nonpolar organic
phase. A similar technique has previously been used to determine the
affinity of ionophores for different cations.[23]

The tissue (2 g) is homogenized in 7 ml methanol containing
0.1 N acetic acid which extracts the ionophore in its uncomplexed
protonated form together with only a small fraction of the total
lipids. The homogenate is heated briefly (5 min) to 70° to coagulate
the protein and centrifuged. Four ml of the clear methanolic extract
is removed, 6 ml water added to increase its polarity, and then the
monensin counterextracted into 3 ml of hexane. A 2 ml aliquot of
the hexane extract is transferred into a 1 dram (4.5 ml) screw top
vial and shaken against an aqueous solution containing: Ba(OH)$_2$,
5 mM, with enough CAPS (Cyclohexylaminopropane sulfonate) to bring
its pH down to 9.5; 1 µCi ^{22}Na$^+$; 10^{-5} M carrier NaCl. The vials are
tightly capped and thoroughly shaken for about 30 sec and then centrifuged to clear the upper hexane layer of microdroplets from the
lower phase. A 1 ml aliquot of the upper phase is then carefully
removed for β-liquid scintillation counting in a standard toluene-
PPO-diMePOPOP cocktail. The amount of radioactivity in the upper
phase is an index of the amount of lipid soluble monensin-Na$^+$ complex
formed and is calibrated by running appropriate blanks, standards and
recoveries with known quantities of monensin. Because of its low

lipid content, for plasma the methanol extraction procedure is not
required; it is sufficient to acidify the plasma with acetic acid
and extract the ionophore directly into heptane.[24]

Despite its relatively high cost and inconveniently long half
life (2.6 y), $^{22}Na^+$ is required for the monensin assay because of
the strong preference of this particular ionophore for Na^+ over Rb^+.[23]
Most other ionophores have a preference for Rb^+ over Na^+ (Table 1)
and the assay can be adapted for them by replacing the $^{22}Na^+$ and NaCl
with the less expensive $^{86}Rb^+$ ($t_{\frac{1}{2}}$ = 18d) and RbCl. Thus the assay
should be universal for detecting carboxylic ionophores in tissues.
This is significant in that all carboxylic ionophores evaluated have
equivalent effects on poultry and cattle growth and it is possible
that some of them might compete with monensin commercially in the
future. Use can also be made of the $^{22}Na^+$:$^{86}Rb^+$ binding ratio,
diagnostic for each ionophore, to identify an unknown ionophore and
distinguish ionophore complexation of radionuclides from nonspecific
nonselective ion pairing with lipophilic anions such as phospholipids.

Applications of Radiochemical Monensin Assay to Dogs and Rabbits

The radiochemical assay was applied to dogs in order to compare
the effects of oral and i.v. administration of monensin on plasma
levels.[9,24] Fig. 5 depicts the effect of an i.v. injection of 100
µg/kg monensin on the heart rate, femoral arterial pressure and
plasma glucose and monensin levels. Plasma monensin fell rapidly
with a $t_{\frac{1}{2}}$ of about 2.5 min indicating rapid absorption into the
tissues. Femoral blood pressure rose following a transient dip,
plateauing 1 min after monensin injection and returning to base
levels after 2 hrs. Heart rate also rose rapidly and returned to
control values within 20 min. The persistence of cardiac responses
after the disappearance of monensin from the plasma suggests that
the cardiac tissue took up and retained the ionophore; this is supported by perfusion experiments on the isolated rabbit heart which
rapidly takes up monensin and releases it with a $t_{\frac{1}{2}}$ of 10 min.[25]
Another response parameter which characterizes the systemic effects
of monensin and other carboxylic ionophores is a delayed but persistent rise in plasma glucose.[24] Preliminary results indicate this
is due principally to the direct effects of carboxylic ionophores in
stimulating glucagon secretion and inhibiting the secretion of
insulin.

The time course of the response of dogs to i.v. monensin has
been compared to the response to a larger dose of monensin administered orally as a capsule to unanesthetized animals (Fig. 6). As
expected plasma monensin rose more slowly but was more persistent
as a steady state was achieved between monensin entering the blood
from the gastrointestinal tract and subsequently being absorbed by

Table 1. Na^+/Rb^+ Complexation Ratios of Ionophores

Ionophore	Heptane	70% Toluene:30% Butanol
Monensin	> 500	110
Salinomycin	2.3	0.17
Narasin	3.0	0.26
Lasalocid	0.03	0.08
Nigericin	1.0	0.66

The data are the ratios of the two phase K_A's of aqueous solutions of $^{22}NaCl$ or $^{86}RbCl$, pH 9.5 equilibrated against the indicated organic solvent.[23] Note that the ratios differ considerably between solvents confirming that ionophore selectivity is not a constant property of the ionophore but is modified by solvent polarity.

the tissues and/or eliminated. It can be shown that the plasma level-time integral for a drug is proportional to the net amount which passes through the blood. In order to estimate the absolute amount of orally ingested monensin absorbed, the proportionality constant can be determined by comparision with the plasma level-time integral of the disappearance of a known amount of the drug injected directly into the blood. The plasma-monensin-time curve in Fig. 5 provides this calibration standard. Its integral is about 1/20 that of Fig. 6 which corresponds to the ratio of administered doses, 2 mg/kg oral vs. 100 µg/kg i.v. This indicates that in the dog virtually all monensin orally ingested passes through the gastrointestinal tract into the blood from which it is absorbed by tissues and/or eliminated (cf. Refs. 9,24).

In the rabbit, orally ingested monensin (10 mg/kg) passes into the blood stream considerably more slowly (Fig. 7). It requires about 4 hrs for a significant level to appear in the plasma although only 1.5 hrs are required for a significant elevation of the pulse rate. Plasma levels continue to rise for 16 hrs at which time sacrificed animals show considerable monensin levels (0.2-0.7 ppm) in the tissues. As in the dog, orally ingested monensin also causes rises in arterial pressure and plasma glucose. The fact that the rabbit absorbs orally ingested monensin more slowly but more persistently than the dog presumably reflects general differences in the digestive tracts between carnivores and herbivores. We have also observed cardiovascular responses including coronary vaso-

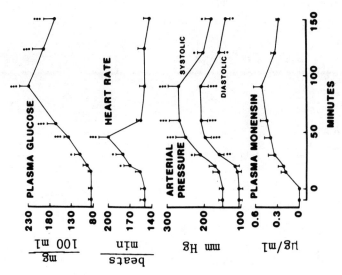

Fig. 6. Effect of orally injested monensin (2 mg/kg) on conscious dogs. Dogs (N=5) were maintained suspended in sling. Data obtained in same manner as Fig. 5.

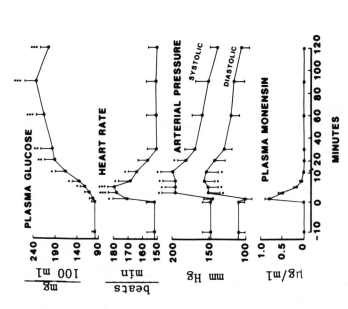

Fig. 5. Effect of intravenous injection of monensin (100 μg/kg) on anesthetized dogs. Heart rate was obtained from EKG recording, pressure was obtained from catheter in femoral artery, plasma glucose from glucose oxidase assay and plasma monensin from radiochemical assay described in text. * indicates $P < 0.05$ from control values, **, $P < 0.01$, ***, $P < 0.001$ (paired t-test), N=10.

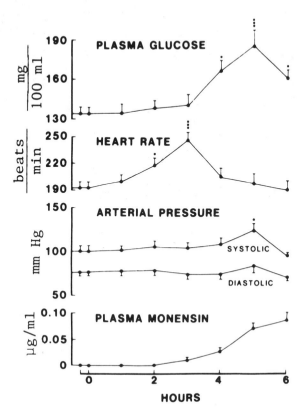

Fig. 7.   Effect of orally ingested bolus of monensin (10 mg/kg) on
          conscious rabbits.   Arterial pressure obtained from cathe-
          ter in ear artery.   Other data obtained by same methods as
          in Fig. 5 (N=6).

dilatation a few seconds after injecting alcoholic monensin into
the stomach of instrumented, anesthetized dogs and sheep. Thus, on
the basis of appearance of orally ingested monensin in the blood,
together with the appearance of cardiovascular responses typical of
those induced by the ionophore, it is evident that monensin is easily
absorbed in active form from the gastrointestinal tract in the dog,
rabbit and sheep and presumably a wide diversity of animal species.
Thus, inferences, from the appearance of dietary monensin in the
feces of chickens[26] and cattle[27], that the ionophore passes through
the gastrointestinal tract without affording the tissues opportunity

to absorb it, must be carefully re-examined. In this regard one
would expect on the basis of its polarity that monensin is similar
to most drugs which easily pass across biological membranes and hence
are susceptible to oral absorption[28].

Application of Radiochemical Monensin Assay to Chickens

Bearing in mind that an increase in $^{22}Na^+$ binding capacity of
tissue extracts is presumptive rather than definitive evidence for
the presence of monensin, the effect of feeding chickens diets containing 110 ppm monensin on the $^{22}Na^+$ binding capacity of extracts
obtained as outlined previously is shown in Table 2. Some questions
might be raised over the relatively large binding of $^{22}Na^+$ by tissues
from animals fed diets free of monensin, the "controls", compared to
tissue-free blanks but this can reasonably be accounted for as non-
specific ion pairing with lipophilic anions such as phospholipids.
What is overwhelmingly apparent is that extracts of tissues from
birds fed monensin supplements bind several fold more $^{22}Na^+$ than the
control series. It is obvious that ingesting monensin affected the
level of some Na^+-binding tissue components. If these are not exclusively monensin per se at the very least they are most likely other
lipid soluble $^{22}Na^+$-binding metabolites of monensin. In view of the
mechanism of action of monensin discussed earlier, one would predict
equivalent biological properties including coronary vasodilatation
for any tissue components capable of forming lipid soluble Na^+ complexes. Hence, the tissues of birds fed monensin contain material
which is likely to be physiologically active if ingested by man,
regardless of whether or not it is monensin per se. Furthermore,
appreciable quantities of the $^{22}Na^+$-binding material are retained
after withdrawing monensin from the diet for 24 hr. Other series we
have run have detected low levels of residual $^{22}Na^+$-binding above
controls as long as 5 days after monensin withdrawal.

Precise quantitation of the monensin or equivalent metabolites
indicated by the assay is complicated by the fact that differing
lipid components from different tissues could affect the stability
of monensin-Na^+ complex. In order to make the assay quantitative it
is necessary to run appropriate calibration recoveries as was done
in Table 3. In this series the raw counts found in the muscle were
appreciably less than found in the liver, cf. Table 2, however this
could be accounted for by differences in the age and variety of
chickens. For both liver and muscle the monensin-fed chicks showed
a three fold increase in $^{22}Na^+$ binding in both liver and muscle. The
recovery series for both organs showed graded responses to "spikes"
of 1.5 and 3.0 µg of monensin, although the effect of the 3.0 µg
spike was slightly less than twice that of the 1.5 µg spike. The
$^{22}Na^+$-binding increment of the monensin fed series was used to calculate the equivalent increase in monensin represented by the increase in $^{22}Na^+$ produced by incorporating monensin (120 ppm) in the
diet which were 0.68 and 0.60 ppm for liver and muscle, respectively.

Table 2. Effect of Dietary Monensin (120 ppm) on
Binding of ^{22}Na$^+$ by Hexane Extracts of
Chicken Tissues

Tissue	Control cpm	7 Day Monensin cpm	7 Day Monensin 1 Day Purged cpm
Plasma	180 ± 40	450 ± 50	110 ± 50
Muscle	2100 ± 240	6400 ± 800	3200 ± 150
Liver	2000 ± 160	10300 ± 630	3500 ± 400
Crop	1300 ± 240	6400 ± 940	2000 ± 200
Heart	1300	3800	1900
Lung	380	1700	370
Kidney	1400	5000	2000
Brain	1400	6400	2500
Spleen	900	4800	2700
RBC	1000	4800	2700

Procedure for obtaining hexane extracts and binding of
^{22}Na$^+$ described in assay in text. "No tissue" chemical
control values were 35 cpm. Where N=8 standard deviations are given; where standard deviations are not
given N=4.

After one day of purging with a monensin-free diet the chickens retained 0.10 and 0.11 ppm in liver and muscle.

DISCUSSION

     In order to set up rational standards for protecting man against
ingesting potentially harmful levels of monensin in poultry and beef,
the hazards and dose-response characteristics of the drug must be
known and a reliable assay be available capable of detecting the material in the range of physiological significance. Based on our
experience with dogs, about 1 μg/kg monensin i.v. is the threshold
for producing coronary responses. If "unpurged" chickens accidently
come to market we see from Table 3 that under one limited experimental
set of conditions about 0.6-0.7 ppm or 600-700 μg/kg can accumulate in
poultry muscle and liver, hence if the assay is accurate a 70 kg man
eating 250 g poultry consumes 150-175 μg monensin or about twice the
threshold dose in the dog. Although the threshold dose for orally

Table 3. Effect of Dietary Monensin (120 ppm) on Binding of $^{22}Na^+$ by Hexane Extracts of Chicken Muscle and Liver

Sample	% of Activity of Aqueous Phase Entering Hexane Extract		
	Control	7 Day Monensin	Calculated Tissue Monensin
Liver	0.45%	1.45%	0.68 ppm
+ 1.5 µg monensin	2.10	2.55	
+ 3.0 µg monensin	3.05	3.55	
Muscle	0.15	0.56	0.60 ppm
+ 1.5 µg monensin	.70	1.07	
+ 3.0 µg monensin	1.00	1.50	

Each extract was repeated in duplicate on unspiked tissue and on same tissue spiked with 1.5 µg and 3.0 µg monensin for each 2 g tissue sample.

ingested monensin in man might be somewhat higher due to slow absorption, we believe it would be prudent to incorporate a safety factor of 10-100 to allow for individual differences in sensitivity to monensin among the major segment of the population who regularly consume poultry and beef.

A large number of adverse reaction reports on file with the FDA concerned with accidental overdosing of animals due to errors in mixing feed or feeding properly compounded feed to the wrong species, e.g. poultry feed to turkeys, cattle feed to horses, are a source of added concern for the possibility of exposing man to detrimental doses of monensin.* Indeed several adverse reaction

*FDA Adverse Reaction Reports Form 2025, obtainable from the FDA, 5600 Fishers Lane, Rockville, MD 20857.

reports to date actually document exposure to monensin of men, presumably industrial workers concerned with ionophore production, who
developed headache, nausea, nosebleed and skin rash. Concern with
the possibility of man ingesting toxic levels of monensin would
appear more warranted than the currently prevalent concern for adverse reactions to such substances as saccharine or cyclamate based
on extrapolations from chronically feeding animals heroic levels.

We have concentrated in this report on the danger posed to man
of the coronary vasodilatory properties of monensin. The drug presents other hazards which are more difficult to assess quantitatively.
The direct inotropic effects of monensin associated with increase of
intracellular Na^+ may exacerbate the toxicity of digitalis[30] which
also appears to work by raising intracellular Na^+. The ability of
monensin to release catecholamines from chromaffin cells[16] or nerve
endings may affect people with hypertension adversely. Lastly, the
effect of monensin on pancreatic α and β cells may be deleterious to
diabetics.

Current permissible levels of monensin in meat appear to have
been arrived at on the basis of the sensitivity of the presently
available "bioautographic" assay[31] and prior to the availability of
information about the levels of ionophore which produce identifiable
physiological effects. This assay is based on the zone of inhibition
of bacterial growth on a plate in contact with a thin layer chromato-
gram of a sample purified extensively by prior solvent extraction
procedures. Our radiochemical assay is simpler, more rapid, and at
this stage of development has comparable sensitivity to the bioautographical assay although the results obtained differ. The radiochemical assay is based on the special molecular properties of ionophores to complex cations which have been studied intensively by
ourselves and others for over 18 years[12-15,32] and is based on
principles at least as sound as those of the bioautographical assay
currently preferred by the FDA. In view of the ability of the radiochemical assay to detect both monensin and monensin-like compounds
which the bioautographical assay may not, the discrepancy between
the two assays is an issue which must be resolved and cannot be
lightly dismissed. The levels reported in Table 3 exceed the maximal
levels suggested by the FDA for meat destined for human consumption,
0.05 ppm,[33] even after one day of purging with monensin-free feed.
The three day purging period currently in practice may have to be
lengthened to provide a greater safety margin, and compliance with
the recommended purging regimen may have to be more strictly monitored. Clearly, a more rapid, reliable and sensitive assay for ionophores in meat at the marketplace is desirable.

Recently we have had some encouraging preliminary results by
purifying the hexane tissue extract by simple silica gel chromatography. This eliminates the annoying high $^{22}Na^+$ binding background
material apparent in the control samples of Tables 2 and 3. The

chromatographic procedure also enables us to process ten or more times as much tissue for each two phase partition vial which promises to increase sensitivity to about 0.005 ppm monensin in tissue. The processed samples are clean enough to be placed directly on a reversed phase high pressure liquid chromatography column which, coupled with the radiochemical assay, should enable us to distinguish monensin definitively from any ion complexing metabolites which may form in tissues. Thus we believe the discrepancy between the radiochemical and bioautographical monensin assays will be resolved shortly.

ACKNOWLEDGEMENTS

We wish to thank F.A. Lattanzio, Jr., G.R. Painter and Miss G. del Valle for help with various phases of the experimental work. The work was supported in part by NIH Grant HL-23932.

REFERENCES

1. R. F. Shumard and M.E. Callender, Monensin, a new biologically active compound. VI. Anticoccidial activity, Antimicrob. Agents Chemother. 7:369 (1968).
2. L. F. Richardson, A. P. Raun, E. L. Potter, C. O. Cooley, and R. P. Rathmacher, Effect of monensin on rumen fermentation in vitro and in vivo, J. Anim. Sci. 43:657 (1976).
3. A.P. Raun, C.O. Cooley, E. L. Potter, R. P. Rathmacher, and L. F. Richardson, Effect of monensin on feed efficiency of feed lot cattle, J. Anim. Sci. 43:670 (1976).
4. B. C. Pressman and N. T. deGuzman, Biological applications of ionophores: theory and practice, Ann. N.Y. Acad. Sci. 264: 373 (1975).
5. R. K. Saini, R. K. Hester, P. Somani, and B. C. Pressman, Characterization of the coronary vasodilator and hemodynamic actions of monensin, a carboxylic ionophore, J. Cardiovasc. Pharmacol. 1:123 (1979).
6. N. T. deGuzman and B. C. Pressman, The inotropic effects of the calcium ionophore X-537A in the anesthetized dog, Circulation 44:1072 (1974).
7. R. W. Watkins, P. Somani, and B. C. Pressman, Cardiovascular actions of salinomycin, a new carboxylic ionophore, Fed. Proc. 37:864 (1978).
8. N. Moins, P. Gachon, and P. Duchene-Marullaz, Effects of two monocarboxylic ionophores, grisorixin and alborixin, on cardiovascular functions and plasma cation concentrations in the anesthetized dog, J. Cardiovasc. Pharmacol. 1:659 (1979).
9. B. C. Pressman, G. Painter, and M. Fahim, Molecular and biological properties of ionophores, in: "Inorganic Chemistry in Biology and Medicine, (ACS Symp. Ser. 140), A. E. Martell, ed., Am. Chem. Soc., Washington, D.C. (1980).

10. L. C. Becker, Conditions for vasodilator-induced coronary steal in experimental myocardial ischemia, Circulation 57:1103 (1978).

11. G. R. Painter and B. C. Pressman, Dynamic aspects of ionophore mediated membrane transport, in: "Topics in Current Chemistry" Vol. 101, Springer-Verlag, Berlin, Heidelberg (1982).

12. Yu.A. Ovchinnikov, V. T. Ivanov, and A. M. Shkrob, "Membrane Active Complexones", B.B.A. Library Vol. 12, Elsevier, New York (1974).

13. B. C. Pressman, Biological applications of ionophores, Ann. Rev. Biochem. 45:501 (1976).

14. B. C. Pressman and M. Fahim, Pharmacology and toxicology of the monovalent carboxylic ionophores, Ann. Rev. Pharmacol. Toxicol. 22:465 (1982).

15. M. Dobler, "Ionophores and their Structures", Wiley-Interscience, New York (1982).

16. S. J. Suchard, F. A. Lattanzio, Jr., R. W. Rubin, and B. C. Pressman, Stimulation of catecholamine secretion from cultured chromaffin cells by an ionophore-mediated rise in intracellular sodium, J. Cell. Biol., In press.

17. B. C. Pressman and F. A. Lattanzio, Jr., Cardiovascular effects of ionophores, in: "Frontiers of Biological Energetics", P. L. Dutton, J. S. Leigh and A. Scarpa, eds., Academic Press, New York (1978).

18. R. A. Olsson, D. Saito, D. G. Nixon, and R. B. Vomacka, Compartmentation of the cardiac adenosine pool, Fed. Proc. 40:564 (1982).

19. F. A. Lattanzio, M. Fahim, R. Koos, M. Clark, and B. C. Pressman, The effects of prostaglandin release by ionophores on cardiovascular responses in the intact dog, Fed. Proc. 41:1766 (1982).

20. R. M. Berne, Cardiac nucleotides in hypoxia: possible role in regulation of coronary blood flow, Am. J. Physiol. 204:317 (1963).

21. C. van Breemen, P. Aaronson, and R. Loutzenhiser, Sodium-calcium interactions in mammalian smooth muscle, Pharmacol. Rev. 30:167 (1979).

22. B. C. Pressman, Biological applications of ion specific electrodes, Methods in Enzymol. 10:714 (1967).

23. B. C. Pressman, Ionophorous antibiotics as models for biological transport, Fed. Proc. 27:1283 (1968).

24. M. Fahim and B. C. Pressman, Cardiovascular effects and pharmacokinetics of the carboxylic ionophore monensin in dogs and rabbits, Life Sci. 29:1959 (1981).

25. F. A. Lattanzio, Jr., A study of the effects of carboxylic ionophores on the isolated rabbit heart, M.S. Thesis, Univ. of Miami, FL (1981).

26. R. J. Herberg and R. L. Van Duyn, Excretion and tissue distribution studies in chickens fed ^{3}H monensin (Na salt), J. Agric. Food Chem. 17:853 (1969).

27. A. Donoho, J. Manthey, J. Occolowitz, and L. Zornes, Metabolism
     of monensin in the steer and rat, J. Agric. Food Chem. 26:
     1090 (1978).
28. C. Hansch, Chap. 2, Quantitative structure-activity relationships
     in drug design, in: "Medicinal Chemistry" Vol. 1, E. J.
     Ariëns, ed., Academic Press, New York (1971).
29. B. C. Pressman, M. Fahim, F. A. Lattanzio, Jr., G. Painter, and
     G. del Valle, Pharmacologically active residues of monensin
     in food, Fed. Proc. 40:663 (1981).
30. M. Shlafer and P. Kane, Subcellular actions and potential adverse
     cardiac effects of the cardiotonic ionophore monensin, J.
     Pharmacol. Exp. Ther. 214:567 (1980).
31. A. L. Donoho and R. M. Kline, Monensin, a new biologically active
     compound. VII. Thin-layer bioautographic assay for monensin in
     chick tissues, Antimic. Agents Chemother., p. 763 (1968).
32. C. Moore and B. C. Pressman, Mechanism of action of valinomycin
     on mitochondria, Biochem. Biophys. Res. Commun. 15:562 (1964).
33. S. E. Feinman and J. C. Matheson, Draft Environmental Impact
     Statement: Subtherapeutic Antibacterial Agents in Animal
     Feed (1968), Available from FDA, 5600 Fishers Lane, Rockville,
     MD   20857

SENSITIVITY AND RESISTANCE OF THE MYOCARDIUM TO THE TOXICITY OF ISOPROTERENOL IN RATS

T. Balazs, G. Johnson, X. Joseph, S. Ehrreich, and S. Bloom*
Bureau of Drugs, Food and Drug Administration
Washington, D.C. 20204
*George Washington University Medical Center
Washington, D.C. 20037

1. INTRODUCTION

The toxicity of a chemical is not a colligative property of a substance; it is a function of the susceptibility of the organism upon which the chemical acts. The susceptibility is determined by the physiological state of the organism, as illustrated by the cardiotoxicity of isoproterenol.

Various conditions influence the sensitivity of the rat to the cardiotoxicity of the beta-adrenergic agent isoproterenol [3,20]. An increased sensitivity manifests itself by an extraordinary decrease in the lethal dose, with deaths occurring within 1 h after subcutaneous (sc) injection, or by an increase in the severity of myocardial necrosis that develops within 24 h after a single treatment. A decreased sensitivity (resistance) is shown by a great increase in the lethal dose and a decrease in severity of the lesion. The cardiotoxicity of isoproterenol is the result of cardiovascular pharmacologic effects, since propranolol, a beta-receptor blocking agent, protects against both events [11]. To assess whether the differences in the cardiotoxicity are due to a variation in the degree of pharmacological effects, we measured some of these effects in both sensitive and resistant animals. The pharmacological effects, tachycardia and hypotension, lead to myocardial hypoxia as evidenced, e.g., by the increased lactate levels in the coronary sinus blood [14]. Thus factors such as variation in the myocardial sensitivity to hypoxia or to other metabolic consequences may determine the severity of cardiotoxic effects. Data from our experiments are suggestive of such a mechanism.

2. Isoproterenol-Induced Sudden Cardiac Death

The median lethal dose (LD_{50}) of isoproterenol is influenced by a variety of physiological conditions.

The LD_{50} of isoproterenol HCl injected sc is about 1 g/kg in the male Sprague-Dawley rat weighing 150 to 200 g and 0.3 to 0.6 mg/kg in those weighing 300 to 500 g. When the weight of rats was reduced from an average of 560 g to 430 g by feeding a calorically restricted diet during a 5-week period, the LD_{50} was increased to 900 mg/kg. The LD_{50} of their ad libitum-fed controls, which weighed an average of 600 g, was 0.35 mg/kg [5].

We compared the mortality and cause of deaths in Sprague-Dawley male rats weighing 150-200 g or about 500 g. Animals were injected under identical conditions on the same day with isoproterenol HCl in graded doses from 0.1 to 1000 mg/kg. No deaths occurred at any dose in the group of the light rats, but a dose-related mortality was observed in the heavy rats. LD_{50} values determined by injecting additional groups of rats were 1300 mg/kg in the light rats and 0.66 mg/kg in the heavy rats. Although deaths occurred in 1 to 2 h in the heavy rats, they occurred beyond the 6-h observation period in the light rats.

In additional groups of animals, electrocardiograms were recorded after administration of various sc doses of isoproterenol. Unrestrained rats were placed in individual plastic cages. Electrodes were implanted sc and recordings were taken at 10-min intervals and when clinical signs indicated that they should be taken. Premature ventricular contractions occurred within 15 to 30 min; in some instances they were followed by ventricular tachycardia and subsequent fibrillation in the heavy rats. Fibrillation and convulsions preceded death, which occurred within 1 hour. Arrhythmias were not seen in the light rats; deaths due to respiratory arrest occurred later. Pretreatment with aminophylline (given sc 20 min before isoproterenol) potentiated the incidence of ventricular fibrillation and death in the heavy rats; it did not cause fibrillation but increased the mortality in the light rats (Table 1).

Results of these experiments indicated that the increased susceptibility of the heavy rat to the lethal toxicity of isoproterenol is related to the development of ventricular fibrillation.

TABLE 1.   Incidence of fibrillation and death in rats ($\underline{n}$ = 10) treated with isoproterenol (ISO)

Weight, g	Treatment	Dose, mg/kg	No. of rats Fibrillated	Died
150-200	ISO	700	0	3
500-600	ISO	0.1	4	4
500-600	ISO	0.3	8	8
150-200	ISO + Aminophylline	700 75	0	10
500-600	ISO + Aminophylline	0.1 75	10	8
500-600	ISO + Aminophylline	0.1 37.5	10	3
500-600	Aminophylline	75	0	0

To substantiate the role of body weight versus age in this event, groups of rats weighing an average of 526 g were fed a calorically restricted diet. After 1 week they had lost 10% of their weight, and were then injected sc with isoproterenol at doses of 1.0 or 100 mg/kg.   One of four rats in the restricted diet group and three of four in the ad libitum group fibrillated and died after the 1 mg/kg dose.   None of the four in the restricted group died, but three in the control group died after the 100 mg/kg dose.   Deaths were preceded by fibrillation in two of these rats.   Previously untreated rats of both groups received food ad libitum thereafter.   When their weights were about 540 g, they were injected with 1 mg of isoproterenol/kg.   Five of six rats in each group fibrillated and died.

The 4- to 5-month-old male Sprague-Dawley rat is inherently obese [7].   This condition results in an increased cardiac output, which requires a greater oxygen supply.   It is unlikely that this would be met during the response to isoproterenol, which further increases the oxygen demand.   Thus a myocardial hypoxia develops, which impairs the energy supply and consequently the normal electrical activity of the cell. Increased concentration of intracellular calcium - a consequence of hypoxia - has been particularly implicated in the genesis of ventricular fibrillation [8].   Isoproterenol increases the plasma free fatty acid level (more so in obese than in lean rats) and increases myocardial cyclic AMP.   These changes can contribute to the development of fibrillation [16] as also shown by the potentiating effect of aminophylline.

The incidence of fibrillation was lower at high dose levels (100 to 1000 mg/kg) in the heavy rats. This might be attributed to the ability of isoproterenol to act as an agonist on the alpha receptors, which may ameliorate the beta effects.

3. Sensitization to the Isoproterenol-Induced Cardiac Lesion

Suprapharmacological doses of isoproterenol produce myocardial necrosis. The positive chronotropic and inotropic effects increase the demand for substrate and oxygen, which may not be sufficient in the area of lowest perfusion, e.g., in the left ventricular subendocardium. The low perfusion is shown by the fact that during the early period of the isoproterenol effect the transcapillary passage of fine structural protein tracers is completely inhibited [19]. The beta-adrenergic receptor blocking agent, propranolol, which inhibits the pharmacological effects of isoproterenol, reduces the extent of the lesion [11]. Thus production of the lesion is attributable to the exaggerated cardiovascular pharmacological effects. The extent of the lesion is known to be influenced by the body weight [18]. We tested the pharmacological effect as a function of this variable.

Three groups of Sprague-Dawley male rats weighing 70 to 80 g (4 weeks old), 140 to 150 g (6 weeks old), and 320 to 360 g (9 weeks old) were used. Although pretreatment heart rates decreased with age, the maximal heart rates were comparable after isoproterenol was given in the range of 1.0 to 1000 mg/kg. Consequently the incremental effect of the compound on the heart rate was greater in older and heavier rats. The duration of tachycardia was comparable in each age group at the various dose levels. Deaths occurred at each dose level in the 9-week-old rats, but only one rat died at the highest dose of the 6-week-old group and none died in the 4-week-old group. Ventricular fibrillation occurred only at the 1 and 10 mg/kg doses in 9-week-old rats; deaths occurring at higher doses were somewhat delayed and were not preceded by fibrillation (Table 2).

The dose responses for myocardial lesions in survivors killed 24 h posttreatment indicated that the 9-week-old rats had the greatest sensitivity. The body fat content of Sprague-Dawley male rats weighing 360 g is about 20% of their total body weight. This value is greater than those measured in rats fed obesogenic diets for 3 months [7]. The role of body fat in the sensitization to the cardiac lesion-inducing effect of isoproterenol is reflected by the influence of the body weight loss on the extent of the lesion.

TABLE 2. Comparative study on the effects of isoproterenol in rats of different weights

Isoproterenol mg/kg, sc	Weight g Age, days			Heart rate pretreatment* Age, days			Heart rate maximum† Age, days			Heart rate 180 min post treatment Age, days			Mortality			Score of necrosis		
	26-28	34-41	62-63	26-28	34-41	62-63	26-28	34-41	62-63	26-28	34-41	62-63	26-28	34-41	62-63	26-28	34-41	62-63
0 (Saline)‡	103 ±4 (6)	203 ±5 (6)	339 ±7 (6)	412 ±5 (6)	349 ±12 (6)	333 ±11 (6)	464 ±19 (6)	371 ±11 (6)	385 ±21 (6)	457 ±17 (6)	331 ±8 (6)	320 ±11 (6)	0	0	0	0	0	0
0.1	-	-	356 ±8 (3)	-	-	335 ±6 (3)	-	-	500 ±11 (3)	-	-	339 ±9 (3)	0	0	1/3			1.0 (2)
1.0	78 ±9 (4)	146 ±2 (6)	331 ±7 (6)	485 ±22 (4)	407 ±7 (6)	346 ±6 (6)	596 ±5 (4)	566 ±8 (6)	539 ±5 (6)	443 ±15 (4)	489 ±21 (6)	408 ±7 (6)	0	0	3/6	0 (4)	0.9 ±0.2 (6)	2.7 ±0.9 (3)
10	71 ±5 (4)	138 ±8 (6)	338 ±13 (6)	458 ±30 (4)	410 ±20 (6)	342 ±12 (6)	585 ±14 (4)	565 ±4 (6)	538 ±14 (6)	551 ±5 (4)	554 ±7 (6)	537 ±19 (6)	0	0	2/6	0.2 ±0.2 (4)	1.5 ±0.4 (6)	2.2 ±0.4 (4)
100	78 ±8 (4)	140 ±6 (6)	341 ±6 (6)	449 ±25 (4)	408 ±17 (6)	325 ±5 (6)	597 ±4 (4)	589 ±13 (6)	608 ±22 (6)	570 ±9 (4)	573 ±16 (6)	588 ±31 (6)	0	0	3/6	0.7 ±0.1 (4)	1.1 ±0.2 (6)	2.5 ±0.8 (3)
1000	80 ±4 (5)	148 ±5 (5)	318 ±9 (3)	446 ±19 (5)	414 ±15 (5)	338 ±13 (3)	613 ±10 (5)	646 ±16 (5)	626 ±11 (3)	613 ±10 (5)	646 ±16 (5)	0	0	1/5	3/3	1.6 ±0.4 (5)	1.4 ±0.5 (4)	0

Values are given as means ± SE, with the number of rats in parentheses.
*Average heart rate over a 30-min period immediately before treatment.
†Maximum heart rate excluding the first (5 min) reading.
‡Age of saline controls = 30 days, 44 days, and 65 days.

The effects of weight reduction on the isoproterenol-induced heart lesion was examined in groups of rats ($\underline{n}$ = 6) weighing about 500 g. One group was fed calorically restricted diets for 2 weeks and lost 18% of their weight. These rats and ad libitum-fed controls were injected with a single sc dose of 0.1 mg of isoproterenol/kg, and 24 h later they were killed for histologic evaluation of the extent of lesions. The extent of necrosis was estimated, using a scale of 0 to 3. While the ad libitum-fed group had a score of 1.6 $\pm$ 0.5 (SE) and another ad libitum-fed group 1.2 $\pm$ 0.6, the lesion score of the group fed the restricted diet was 0.4 $\pm$ 0.25.

We also examined the influence of age/weight on sensitivity to the cardiotoxicity of isoproterenol in mice. Three groups of CD-1 mice 4, 8, and 16 weeks of age, weighing an average of 26, 33, and 38 g were used; the LD_{50} values of isoproterenol given intraperitoneally (ip) were 206, 214, and 192 mg/kg, respectively. Ten mice of each of the three groups were injected ip with 1/10 of the LD_{50} dose; they were killed 48 h later and the hearts were examined histologically. Lesions were graded on a scale of 0 to 3. The average lesion score was 0.6 $\pm$ 0.21 for the 4-week-old mice, 0.62 $\pm$ 0.17 for the 8-week-old mice, and 1.9 $\pm$ 0.35 for the 16-week-old mice. In another experiment, mice 16 weeks of age were fed a calorically reduced diet until they lost 10 to 15% of their weight. They were injected ip with a single dose of isoproterenol as above. The score of myocardial lesion was 0.3 $\pm$ 0.21 and that of their pair-injected controls was 1.9 $\pm$ 0.42.

Results of these experiments substantiated the role of excess body fat in sensitizing to the cardiac necrosis-inducing effect of isoproterenol in both species. A greater sensitivity to the metabolic consequences, rather than to the tachycardia per se, seems to be responsible for the more extensive myocardial necrosis in the heavy rats. Since hypoxia is considered to be the primary mediator in the mechanism of isoproterenol cardiotoxicity, the greater susceptibility of the heavy rats, compared with that of light rats or of those that lost weight, can be attributed to its a priori increased cardiac metabolic demand.

4. Development of Resistance to the Cardiotoxicity of Isoproterenol

Previous studies have indicated that after the development of the myocardial necrosis induced by isoproterenol,

sensitivity of the myocardium to the lesion-inducing effect of
a subsequent isoproterenol challenge decreases [6]. Since the
lesion is attributed to the exaggerated pharmacological
effects, the diminished sensitivity could be attributed to a
decreasing intensity of these effects.

We have compared cardiovascular pharmacological effects of
sc isoproterenol in rats following acute and repeated
treatments. Four groups of 15 to 20 male Sprague-Dawley rats
weighing 225 to 300 g were used. They received 0.1 mg/kg on 2
consecutive days; 0.5 mg/kg on 2 consecutive days; 0.1 mg/kg
for 9 consecutive days; or 0.5 mg/kg on 3 days during week 1, 4
days during week 2, and 2 days during week 3.

At the end of each treatment period, dose responses on the
effects of heart rate and blood pressure to 0.00062 to 3.2 µg
of isoproterenol/kg were determined in three or four treated
rats and in controls. For detection of receptor densities,
specific binding of [^{3}H]dihydroalprenolol was measured [2].
The extent of necrotic and healed lesions were quantitatively
estimated from the apical sections stained by trichrome. The
image was projected onto graph paper, and the number of grid
intersections that overlapped normal, inflamed, or scarred
regions was used to calculate the percentage of the area
showing recent or healed injuries.

No differences could be detected in the intensity of
pharmacological effects or in the maximum number of binding
sites to [^{3}H]dihydroalprenolol between rats of the various
groups (Figures 1-3). Although 12 to 16% of the cut surface
showed fresh lesions after acute (2-day) treatments, only 1 to
2% had lesions after the subacute treatment, with 15 to 17% of
the scar occupying primarily the subendocardial area of the
left ventricle.

Results of this experiment indicated that the decrease in
the size of the lesion, a manifestation of the resistance, can
not be attributed to an alteration of the intensity of
pharmacological effects.

Data from a recent study by Nomura et al. [15] showed that
isoproterenol (0.01 or 0.1 mg/kg, twice daily, ip) given for 10
days to rats resulted in a decrease in the number of beta
receptors and an increase in the number of muscarinic
acetylcholine receptors. The ED_{50} value for the inotropic
response to isoproterenol in the isolated atria from these rats
was 9.0-fold higher than that from their untreated controls.

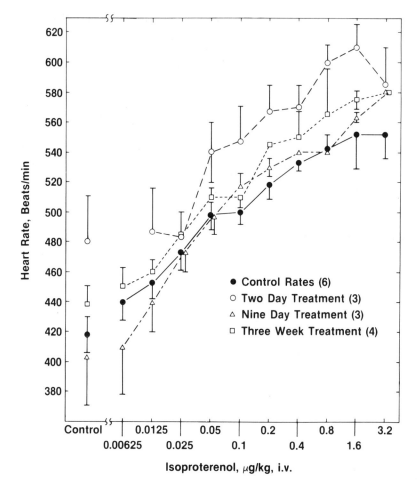

FIGURE 1.   Heart rate responses to isoproterenol in
concious rats previously challenged with isoproterenol (sc).

It is unlikely that the down-regulation of receptor would
result in a long-lasting change such as that which
characterizes the resistance described above.   Moreover,
evidence has been presented that even after 90% of the cardiac
beta receptors had been inactivated the maximum inotropic
response to isoproterenol was not reduced [21].

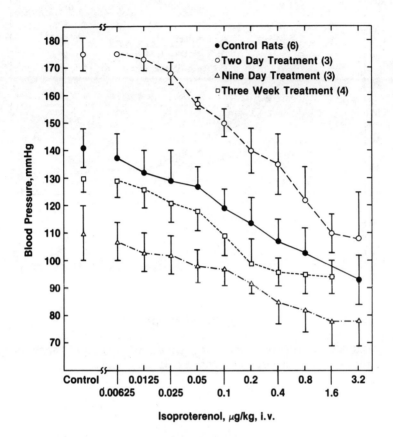

FIGURE 2.   Blood pressure responses to isoproterenol in concious rats previously challenged with isoproterenol (sc).

Another cause of the resistance could be related to the elimination of the most sensitive subendocardial area by the preceding insults. To test this possibility, we treated groups of Sprague-Dawley male rats weighing 400 to 450 g with repeated or single doses of isoproterenol. One group of rats received daily doses of 50 µg/kg for 10 days. Other groups

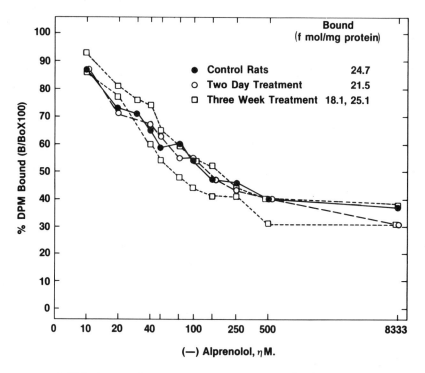

FIGURE 3. Effect of isoproterenol (sc) challenge on myocardial beta-receptor binding of alprenolol.

received single doses of 50, 5, or 0.5 µg/kg. The first group and a control group were challenged with 50 µg/kg of the drug on 2 consecutive days 21 days after the end of the 10-day treatment. The other three groups and controls were challenged 21 days after treatment with a single dose of 50 µg of isoproterenol/kg. Hearts were processed and lesions were evaluated as described above. Increased resistance was demonstrated by the decrease in size of the fresh lesion after the challenge.

The area of the scar was about 20% of the cut surface in the first group pretreated for 10 days. There was no acute lesion following the challenge. Although the extent of scarring was only about 5% in the group pretreated with a single dose of 50 µg of isoproterenol/kg, the acute lesion of the rechallenge represented less than 1%. The area of scarring was only about 1% after a single preparatory dose of 5 µg/kg, and the extent of the fresh lesion after the challenge was 2%. The latter was 5 and 7% in the controls and those pretreated with 0.5 µg/kg, respectively (Table 3). Thus an increased resistance manifested itself even if the scar occupied only a small fraction of the area most susceptible to the lesion. A single injection of 0.5 µg/kg failed to increase the resistance. This dose produced an increase in the heart rate but the duration was only 30 min.

The pretreatment-induced resistance also influenced the acute toxicity of isoproterenol. The LD_{50} was measured in 600-g rats 10 days after the end of a preparatory treatment with 50 µg of isoproterenol/kg for 10 days. The LD_{50} of sc isoproterenol was 9 mg/kg, but was 0.1 to 0.3 mg/kg in controls. Deaths were preceded by fibrillation in each rat of the control group but in only 50% of the resistant animals.

Results of these experiments confirmed that the development of resistance is a real, adaptive phenomenon. Evidence has been presented that the isoproterenol-induced lesion also protected against hypobaric pressure-induced myocardial necrosis and also against coronary ligation-reperfusion injury [1].

TABLE 3.   The extent of myocardial lesions in rats pretreated with various dosing regimens of isoproterenol and challenged 21 days later

Group No.*	Pretreatment		Challenge		Lesion scores (%+SE)	
	Dose (µg/kg)	Duration (days)	Dose (µg/kg)	Duration (days)	Acute	Scar
1	50	10	50	2	0.05+0.05	20.2+5.1
2	0		50	2	13.8+3.1	0.03+0.03
3	50	1	50	1	0.8+0.3	5.3+1.4
4	0		50	1	5.2+1.2	0.9+0.3
5	5	1	50	1	1.9+0.7	1.0+0.1
6	0.5	1	50	1	7.0+2.1	0.7+0.1
7	0		50		5.5+2.2	1.3+0.4

*Each group was comprised of 8-10 rats.

Evidence of an adaptation to the hypoxia in the
isoproterenol-treated rat heart has been demonstrated by a
change in the lactic dehydrogenase (LDH) isoenzyme pattern
[22]. LDH activity temporarily increased after a single dose
of isoproterenol, returning to the control value by the tenth
day. Although the cardiac isoenzyme (LDH-H) decreased, the
skeletal muscle isoenzyme (LDH-M) increased. It is conceivable
that the altered metabolic environment induced these changes.
Hypoxia has been found to alter the LDH isoenzyme pattern of
cultured heart cells in a similar manner [9]. Fetal heart,
which is relatively resistant to anoxia, contains mostly LDH-M
units [13]. The dominance of an anaerobic glycolytic pathway
has also been demonstrated histoenzymatically in the hearts of
rats following coronary ligation [12]. This was accompanied by
ultrastructural changes resembling those of the fetal heart
cells. Events such as stimulation of the pentose phosphate
pathway or reversion to an embryonic-type tissue have also been
postulated to be a factor in the increased resistance of
regenerating epithelium following exposure to noxious agents
[4].

5. Conclusions

Results of the studies presented here reveal the lack of
differences in the intensity of cardiac or cardiovascular
pharmacological effects of isoproterenol in rats having greatly
different sensitivities to the cardiotoxic effects of the
compound. It is likely that the cardiotoxic effects, the
fibrillation and the lesion, have a common determinant, since
both develop in heavy rats and are absent or diminished in
young rats of light body weight, in heavy rats after weight
reduction, and in rats having an induced, preexisting lesion.
Hypoxia, the consequence of the exaggerated cardiovascular
effects, could be the common mediator in the pathogenesis of
the fibrillation as well as the lesion. Thus their occurrence
is a function of the degree of sensitivity or resistance of the
myocardium to hypoxia. The great sensitivity of the heavy,
obese rats to isoproterenol-induced hypoxia can be attributed
to its a priori increased cardiac metabolic demand. An
adaptation to hypoxia or to its consequences, e.g.,
intracellular calcium overload in the rat with preexisting
lesion, can be inferred. The mechanisms of these events remain
to be determined.

The saga of the experimental cardiotoxicity of
isoproterenol demonstrates the complexities of preclinical
safety evaluation. The influence of various factors on the

cardiotoxicity of isoproterenol may explain why myocardial necroses were not detected during the initial subacute toxicity studies performed by Dertinger et al. [10]. These investigators used weaned rats, which are not sensitive to the cardiotoxic effect of the 100 mg/kg dose used, and if any lesion developed, it most likely produced resistance.

Although our activity has been an exercise in experimental toxicology, it may be of interest to human medicine. It seems to be appropriate to remember the work of the late Dr. W. Raab, a pioneer in the research on the role of catecholamines in hypoxic myocardial disease. In his description of the cardiotoxic effect of catecholamines in humans, Dr. Raab emphasized the significance of various factors that increase myocardial vulnerability as well as the development of resistance through repeated application of catecholamine-liberating stresses [22]. A morphological correlate of adaptation, the reversion of the heart cells to a fetal type, has been observed in the rat both during isoproterenol-induced resistance and following forced exercise or restraint [12]. The molecular mechanisms of the resistance or the sensitivity of various degrees, however, remain to be investigated.

Acknowledgement

Dr. J. Kenimer of the Food and Drug Administration performed the receptor binding studies.

REFERENCES

1. ABRI, O. & HECHT, A. The influence of long-term application of isoproterenol. Experimental Pathology 20, 146-152 (1981).
2. ALEXANDER, R.W., WILLIAMS, L.T. & LEFKOWITZ, R.J. Identification of cardiac beta-adrenergic receptors by (-) [^{3}H]alprenolol binding. Proceedings of the National Academy of Sciences, USA, 72, 1564-1568 (1975).
3. BALAZS, T. Cardiotoxicity of isoproterenol in experimental animals. Influence of stress, obesity and repeated dosing. In Recent Advances in Studies on Cardiac Structure and Metabolism, Vol. 1. E. Bajusz & G. Rona, Eds., pp. 770-778. Baltimore: University Park Press, (1972).
4. BALAZS, T. Development of tissue resistance to toxic effects of chemicals. Toxicology 2, 247-255 (1974).

5. BALAZS, T., ARENA, E. & BARRON, G.N. Protection against
    the cardiotoxic effect of isoproterenol HCl by restricted
    food intake in rats. Toxicology and Applied Pharmacology
    21, 237-243 (1972).
6. BALAZS, T., OHTAKE, S. & NOBLE, J.F. The development of
    resistance to the ischemic cardiopathic effect of
    isoproterenol. Toxicology and Applied Pharmacology 21,
    200-213 (1972).
7. BALAZS, T., SAHASRABUDHE, M.R. & GRICE, H.C. The
    influence of excess body fat on the cardiotoxicity of
    isoproterenol in rats. Toxicology and Applied
    Pharmacology 4, 613-620 (1962).
8. CLUSIN, W.T., BRISTOW, M.R., KARAGUEUZIAN, H.S., KATZUNG,
    B.G. & SCHROEDER, J.S. Do calcium-dependent ionic
    currents mediate ischemic ventricular fibrillation?
    American Journal of Cardiology 49, 606-612 (1982).
9. DAWSON, D.M., GOODFRIEND, T.L. & KAPLAN, N.O. Lactic
    dehydrogenases: Functions of the two types. Science 143,
    929-933, (1964).
10. DERTINGER, B.L., BEAVER, D.C. & LANDS, A.H. Toxicity of
    1-(3,4-dihydroxyphenyl)-2-isopropylamino ethanol
    hydrochloride (Isuprel). Proceedings of the Society for
    Experimental Biology and Medicine 68, 501-507 (1948).
11. DORIGOTTI, L., GAETAN, M., & GLASSER, A.H. & TUROLLA, E.
    Competitive antagonism of isoprenaline induced cardiac
    necroses by ß-adrenoreceptor blocking agents. Journal of
    Pharmacy and Pharmacology 21, 188-191 (1969).
12. DUSEK, J., RONA, G. & KAHN, D.S. Healing process in the
    marginal zone of an experimental myocardial infarct.
    American Journal of Pathology 62, 321-332 (1971).
13. KAPLAN, N.O. Effect of hormones and environmental factors
    on lactic dehydrogenases. Journal of Cellular and
    Comparative Physiology 66 (Suppl. 1), 1-10 (1965).
14. KRASNOW, N. and ROHL, D. Validity of isoproterenol-
    induced myocardial lactate production: An internal
    control. American Heart Journal 83, 143-144 (1972).
15. NOMURA, Y., KAJIYAMA, H. & SEGAWA, T. Alteration in
    sensitivity to isoproterenol and acetylcholine in the rat
    heart after repeated administration of isoproterenol.
    Journal of Pharmacology and Experimental Therapeutics 220,
    411-416 (1982).
16. OPIE, L.H., NATHAN, D. & LUBBE, W.F. Biochemical aspects
    of arrhythmogenesis and ventricular fibrillation.
    American Journal of Cardiology 43, 131-148 (1979).
17. RAAB, W. Neurogenic multifocal destruction of myocardial
    tissue (pathologenic mechanism and its prevention).
    Reviews in Canadian Biology 22, 217-239 (1963).

18. RONA, G., CHAPPEL, C.I., BALAZS, T. & GAUDRY, R. The
     effect of breed, age and sex on myocardial necrosis
     produced by isoproterenol in the rat. Journal of
     Gerontology 14, 169-173 (1959).
19. RONA, G., HUTTNER, T. & BOUTET, M. Microcirculatory
     changes in myocardium with particular reference to
     catecholamine-induced cardiac muscle cell injury. In
     Handbuch der Allgemeinen Pathologie, Vol. III/7. H.
     Messen, Ed., pp. 791-888. Berlin: Springer Verlag
     (1977).
20. RONA, G., KAHN, D.S. & CHAPPEL, C.I. Studies on
     infarct-like myocardial necrosis produced by
     isoproterenol: A review. Reviews in Canadian Biology 22,
     241-255 (1963).
21. VENTER, J.C. High efficiency coupling between
     beta-adrenergic receptors and cardiac contractivity.
     Direct evidence for "spare" beta-adrenergic receptors.
     Molecular Pharmacology 16, 429-440 (1979).
22. WENZEL, D.G. & LYON, J.P. Sympathomimetic amines and
     heart lactic dehydrogenase isoenzymes. Toxicology and
     Applied Pharmacology 11, 215-228 (1967).

ELECTROCARDIOGRAPHIC MONITORING IN TOXICOLOGICAL

STUDIES: PRINCIPLES AND INTERPRETATIONS

David K. Detweiler

University of Pennsylvania
Sch. Vet. Med. 3800 Spruce Street
Philadelphia, PA   19104

I. INTRODUCTION

After a long period when reviews of cardiovascular toxicology were sporadic (Böhle, 1966; Wenzel, 1967; Selye, 1970: Chung and Dean, 1972; Davies and Gold, 1977) the literature has been dramatically enriched during the past 18 months by the appearance of three monographs devoted to cardiotoxicity (Bristow, 1980; Balazs, 1981; Van Stee, 1982). Although there is some sharing of authors and, of course, topics in these three works, they are not excessively repetitious and each collection of articles makes its own unique contribution.

The various effects of drugs and electrolytes on the electrocardiogram have been reviewed by Scherf and Schott, 1973; Bellet, 1963, 1972; Surawicz and Lasseter, 1970; Surawicz, 1967, 1972, and the large literature on the electrophysiologic effects of antiarrhythmic agents and various toxins is under almost constant review (Vaughan Williams, 1975; Singh et al., 1980; Harrison, 1981; Lazdunski and Renaud, 1982). Recently, two publications have appeared on the use of electrocardiographic monitoring of dogs (Detweiler, 1981a) and rats (Budden et al., 1981) in experimental toxicity studies.

Electrophysiological alterations are a principal manifestation of cardiotoxicity. This mandates electrocardiographic monitoring in preclinical testing. To maximize the effectiveness of this non-invasive method attention to recording schedules, lead systems, species selection, and proper interpretation is required.

II. AIMS OF ELECTROCARDIOGRAPHIC MONITORING

The aims of electrocardiography in drug studies differ somewhat in emphasis from those of clinical electrocardiography. The objectives include:

1. Early recognition of electrocardiographic changes that indicate the presence of a drug action before frank electrocardiographic abnormalities are produced.

2. Detection of effects on conduction and action potential duration that, if progressive, can lead to significant functional effects.

3. Separation of direct (primary) from indirect (secondary; e.g., reflex, electrolyte imbalances) actions on the heart.

4. Monitoring the onset, course and possible disappearance of drug effects on the heart during continued drug administration.

5. Determining that the test agent has no electrocardiographic effects indicating cardiac actions or that those present represent innocuous actions.

6. Finding electrocardiographic evidence of cardiotoxicity.

The use of pretest records, control groups, various dose groups, escalating doses, and recovery records increase the odds that these objectives can be achieved.

III. RATIONALE AND JUSTIFICATION

In the past, several drugs were introduced for use in man before it was discovered that they could produce possibly dangerous cardiac electrophysiological effects or frank myocardial damage. Examples of this are the anthracycline antibiotics, cobalt salts (used as a foam stabilizer in beer), sympathomimetic bronchodilators, vasodilating antihypertensive agents, phenothiazine and butyrophenone derivative tranquilizers, and tricyclic antidepressants (Balazs and Herman, 1976; Robinson and Barker, 1976; Holden and Itil, 1977). In each instance, evidence of untoward cardiac effects with these agents could be demonstrated in electrocardiograms from experimental animals studied subsequently.

There are several cogent reasons that justify electrocardiographic monitoring in all toxicity trials:

1. The three most important manifestations of cardiac injury are: alterations in electrical properties, alterations in contractility and death (Bloom, 1981). The electrical

property alterations often precede the last two and can
be monitored non-invasively. Electrocardiographic monitoring is therefore obligatory in toxicity studies.

2. The electrocardiogram contributes to the information on
the general health of the animal.

3. Pretest electrocardiograms can identify certain cardiac
abnormalities so that affected animals can be eliminated
when this is justified and desirable.

4. The electrocardiogram may provide the only evidence of
cardiotoxicity with drugs that damage the heart during the
early days of a trial period and then confer an immunity
to further toxic effect with continued administration
(Balazs, 1974).

5. Many drugs produce electrocardiographic abnormalities
without producing detectable myocardial lesions.

6. In trials with drugs that produce cardiac lesions seen
at necropsy, electrocardiographic monitoring may make
it possible to identify the time of onset and follow the
course of the toxic effect.

7. Drugs that cause no toxic arrhythmias or myocardial lesions
may, nevertheless, produce electrophysiological effects
that can be detected in the electrocardiogram.

IV. APPARATUS

Electrocardiographs minimally should satisfy the standards
established by the American Heart Association (Pipberger, 1975)
and fidelity should be checked by the manufacturers representative
or equivalent at least every 6 months. Frequency response should
be well beyond 100 Hz for dog and large monkey electrocardiograms
and approach 200 Hz for small laboratory species such as rats.
Three channel electrocardiographs especially those that can be
programmed to register up to 12 leads on a short strip are preferred for reasons detailed previously (Detweiler, 1981a, 1981b).

V. TECHNIQUE

A. Restraint

With all quadrupeds forelimb and scapula positioning must be
standardized to obtain consistent orientation of electrocardiographic vectors in normal serial records (Hill, 1969, Detweiler,
1981b). This difficulty is obviated with thoracic leads. Torso
position should also be kept consistent, although the effect on

limb lead vectors is not great provided limb position relative,
the torso is not changed. In toxicity studies sedatives and anad
thetics to facilitate restraint should be avoided whenever posation,
With the common laboratory species (dog, cat, guinea pig, rabbitv.
and rat) simple manual restraint is satisfactory and preferred.
Monkeys ordinarily require physical restraint in a chair or other
type holder (Osborne, 1973) or sedation (e.g., Sernylan).

B. Leads and Lead Systems

For dogs the conventional 10 lead system is recommended,
consisting of limb leads I, II, III, aVR, aVL, aVF and thoracic
leads rV_2 (5th right intercostal space at the edge of the sternum),
V_2 (6th left intercostal space at the edge of the sternum), V_4
(6th left intercostal space at the costochondral junction) and
V_{10} (over the dorsal spinal process of the 7th thoracic vertebra).
This system may also be used for cats.

For rhesus monkeys the systems used include standard and augmented unipolar limb leads combined with the precordial leads of
Atta and Vanace (1960), (MV_1, 4th right intercostal space at the
midclavicular line; MV_2, 4th left intercostal space at the midclavicular line; MV_3, 5th left intercostal space at the left mid-
axillary line) or corresponding to V_1, V_3, and V_5 in man, (Malinow,
1966); and V_{10}. The lead system used by Wolf et al. (1969) has
been found satisfactory for squirrel monkeys: standard and augmented
unipolar limb leads with chest leads designated V_1 (over the 3rd
rib one cm. to the right of the midline), V_4 (over the 9th rib, one
cm. to the left of the midline), V_6 (over the 8th rib at the mid-
axillary line) and V_{10}. For further papers and bibliographies on
primate electrocardiograms see Grauwiler, 1965; Hamlin et al., 1961;
Malinow and DeLannoy, 1967; Singh et al.,; Toback et al., 1978;
Osborne 1978; Malinow et al., 1974.

For rats, rabbits, and guinea pigs the lead system adopted by
Spörri (1944) for quadrupeds, reminiscent of the heart triangle of
W. Nehb (Lepeschkin, 1951), consists of bipolar leads from the
right dorsal scapular region to the sacral area (lead D or dorsal);
right dorsal scapular region to cardiac apex region (lead A or
axial); and sacral area to cardiac apex region (lead I or inferior).
Employing the conventional limb lead electrodes in this system, lead D,
consists of RA-LA electrodes (lead I electrodes) lead A the RA-
LF electrodes (lead II electrodes), and lead I the LA-LF electrodes
(lead III electrodes). The advantages of this system are that only
three electrodes are required, forelimb position has virtually
no effect on the records, the animals can remain in their usual
position when restrained, and ventricular ectopic beats are usually
clearly aberrant in at least one of these leads (Detweiler, 1981b).

Duration of Recording

Electrocardiographic changes such as interval prolongation,
ᵗain conduction disorders, and ST segment deviation are usually
ᵉsent steadily in a record in contrast with arrhythmias that are
ᵘally intermittent. Abnormal arrhythmias are often the only
ᵉvidence of cardiotoxicity, but, on the other hand also occur
ᵖpontaneously in control records from otherwise normal animals.
Ectopic beats are fairly rare in pretest records from experimental
dogs but are more frequent in monkeys, rats, and minipigs, especially when they experience the restraint required for electrocardiography for the first time. This creates the same dilemma in
evaluating records as that encountered in studying antiarrhythmic
drugs in human patients (Morganroth, 1981; Rydén et al., 1975).
There is no easy solution to this problem short of monitoring the
electrocardiogram for impractically long periods of time. On the
other hand, unequal duration of recording periods per animal can
only decrease the comparability of the incidence of arrhythmias
between individual subjects. Accordingly, each animal should be
monitored for the same period at each recording session. As an
attempt at standardization for unanesthetized subjects it is
recommended that for dogs the period of recording should be 1.0
full minute, during which all leads are to be taken. For monkeys,
cats, rabbits and guinea pigs with more rapid heart rates this
period should be 30 seconds and for rats and mice with still faster
rates, 15 seconds. These time periods are based on the following
considerations:

1. The number of consecutive heart beats recorded from the
   different species will generally fall within the same
   range of about 75 to 150 beats per recording period.

2. The period of restraint required is feasible for unanesthetized subjects.

Unfortunately, however, such brief periods of recording are
insufficient for reliable detection of the true prevalence of
arrhythmias in groups of animals. As in man, intermittent electrocardiographic sampling is generally an unsuitable method for arrhythmia detection for evaluation of arrhythmogenic or antiarrhythmic actions of drugs (Rydén et al., 1975).

VI. PROTOCOL DESIGN

The frequency at which electrocardiograms should be taken is
the first decision required. This should be often enough pretest
to detect and confirm the presence of abnormalities in the test
animals, at appropriate intervals during the drug trial to identify the onset and course of drug related changes, and at appropriate intervals following drug withdrawal (recovery period)
to determine after effects. The following information on the

agent is useful if known: pharmacological, electrocardiographic
and cardiotoxic actions anticipated; time of peak drug action ar
its duration: pharmacokinetics. In the face of limited informa
the protocol must consider all possible patterns of cardiotoxicit

A. Pretest Tracings

A minimum of two pretest records should be taken about one
week apart not longer than two weeks before the drug trial is to be
initiated.

B. General Protocol During Drug Administration

The time course of cardiotoxicity follows three general
patterns: 1) early effects during the first week or two of dosing;
2) delayed effects developing during the first 4 to 8 weeks of drug
administration and 3) late effects requiring weeks or months to
become apparent.

Drugs such as beta adrenergic agonists and antihypertensive
agents induce cardiomyopathies that become apparent shortly after·
drug administration. Typically, after the initial insult, the myocardium becomes resistant to the effect, additional lesions are
not induced by continued dosing, and no lesions may found at necropsy.
Electrocardiographic changes, chiefly ventricular extrasystoles, are
likely to appear during the first week of dosing and then disappear for the duration of the study. This may be the only evidence
of this sort of cardiotoxicity. Drugs that modify the electrophysiologic properties of myocardial cells (antiarrhythmic agents)
ordinarily produce their electrocardiographic effects promptly and
they persist as long as dosing continues. Agents such as psychotropic drugs, depending on dose levels, may not affect the electrocardiogram immediately and their action may be progressive (i.e.,
the electrocardiographic changes become more pronounced in degree
and the number of affected animals per dose group increases) during
the first four to eight weeks of administration and then plateau.

While it is rare for cardiotoxicity to develop first after the
initial three months of a drug trial, the anthracycline derivative
antineoplastic drugs are well knwon to induce cardiomyopathy some
weeks or months after treatment.

To accommodate these three patterns of cardiotoxicity in
chronic (three to twelve months or longer) toxicity studies, the
minimal protocol recommended is: Two pretest records (seven to ten
days apart); records during week one, at month one, at three month
intervals thereafter, and at days one and three and weeks one and
two in recovery animals.

In dose range finding studies of, say, one to two weeks du-

ration two pretest records followed by daily records at one, three
and five or one, four and seven hours, and at twenty-four hours
(i.e., predose on the next day) after the first daily dose makes it
possible to detect and follow the course of any electrocardiographic
effects.

In subchronic toxicity trials (three to four weeks) two pretest
records seven to ten days apart may be followed by daily records
when an electrocardiographic effect is anticipated or at weekly
intervals when electrocardiographic changes are unlikely.

To discover any electrocardiographic effects that disappear
as the drug level declines, electrocardiograms should be recorded
at the time of peak drug action after dosing. To determine whether
the effects persist or if there are any after effects, electrocardiograms should be taken as long as possible after drug administration, e.g., twenty-four hours later, just before the next daily
dose in the case of single dose per day administration.

Because diurnal environmental influences can affect heart rates
and other electrocardiographic features, it is best to record by
replicates made up of animals from each dose group, rather than by
dose groups in sequence.

Obviously, all contingencies cannot be anticipated in designing
protocols. It is important that the study plan be flexible and
interactive with the investigator as events unfold. It may be
desirable to avoid death by lowering cardiotoxic dose levels or to
raise dose levels when agents known to have cardiotoxic effects are
to be compared with other drugs of the same type. The important
aim is to identify the chief target organs of a toxic dose, but not,
necessarily, to terminate the trial too early through fatal cardiac
effects, before other organ toxicity can be identified as well.
Finally, one must be constantly on the lookout for the rare spontaneous intercurrent disease (e.g., cardiomyopathy) that can con-
found interpretation.

VII. ACUTE PHARMACOLOGY AND TOXICOLOGY

Electrocardiograms are usually recorded routinely in acute
pharmacological and toxicological studies with the larger laboratory
species and, more recently, in similar studies with rats, often
with computer assisted analysis of the electrocardiographic time
intervals (Budden et al. 1981). In addition to the value of these
data in their own right, they often provide useful guidance regarding dose levels expected to cause cardiotoxicity in subacute
and chronic toxicity trials. A single lead is usually employed
and this is generally satisfactory since time interval and rhythm
changes are adequately detected. The advantages of computer analysis

are too self-evident to require discussion. Technics and results
from computer assisted analyses of rat electrocardiographic data
from acute experiments have been detailed in a recent monograph
(Budden et al., 1981).

VIII.   ANALYSIS OF THE ELECTROCARDIOGRAM

A. General

Presently, in subacute and chronic toxicity trials, the
electrocardiographer considers electrocardiographic characteristics
of serial records from individual animals assigned to control and
various dose groups. A subjective value is attached to each relevant
aspect of the electrocardiographic findings. A decision as to
whether there is reliable electrocardiographic evidence of a
drug effect is then arrived at, based on a knowledge of the electrocardiographic characteristics of the species involved. A prior
knowledge of species differences, prevalence of spontaneous abnormalities and normal variants is required. Speed and accuracy are
heavily dependent on previous experience and constant practice.
Needless to say, because of the subjective component and reliance
on past experience, interpretations may vary crucially from electrocardiographer to electrocardiographer. There is considerable
need to standardize and codify this decision making process to increase its sensitivity, specificity and consistency. This problem
urgently requires attention and approaches are now available that
only need implementation. The coding of drug-induced ST-T complex
changes is central to electrocardiographic analysis in drug work.
This has just recently been employed for the computer-assisted
analysis of exercise electrocardiograms in man (Ellestad, 1981).
Multivariate analysis, applied to the interpretation of exercise
electrocardiograms in man (Greenberg et al., 1980), will greatly
extend the usefulness of electrocardiography in drug studies too.

B. Comparison of Records

The availability of pretest records, from each animal and the
grouping of animals into control and dose groups is of great
advantage because comparisons can be made in serial records and by
dose groups. Drug induced electrocardiographic changes do not
necessarily produce abnormal records, but changes in serial records
that are clustered in particular dose groups may have sufficient
significance to identify a drug effect. For example, the effects
of some tranquilizers and certain antiarrhythmic drugs on the ST-T
complex is such as to cause these contours to become similar in the
various thoracic leads in most of the dogs in a given dose group,
even though the individual records remain within normal limits.

C. Information Recorded

A statement should be noted for each record examined indicating
whether or not it is within normal limits of rate, electrocardiographic time intervals, rhythm, and configuration. Any noteworthy
changes should be described, abnormal or not, for each animal and
by dose group. Abnormal electrocardiograms should be described
and a specific electrocardiographic diagnosis of the abnormality recorded. It is useful to devise arbitrary scoring systems based on
drug induced changes observed, to indicate the degree to which the
electrocardiograms from different animals have been modified.
(Fillmore and Detweiler, 1973; Teske et al., 1976).

D. Quality Control

The quality of the finished electrocardiogram is determined
by instrument performance and technician competence in avoiding
errors and artifacts. Instrument reliability will usually be
assured by routine check-ups by manufacturer's service personnel.
To avoid poor quality records it is desirable to provide an evaluation method and goals for adequate achievement for those taking
the records. For this purpose a quality check list and classification system have been devised for grading the adequacy of electrocardiograms in animal studies (Detweiler, 1981a).

E. Computer Assisted Analysis

There has been over 20 years of well-documented experience
in computer-assisted electrocardiographic diagnosis of human electrocardiograms (Caceres, 1978; Hagen et al., 1978; Rautaharju
et al., 1978). This approach for pharmacological and toxicological
studies in animals is particularly timely now. Over the years
several individual laboratories have used computerized methods to
determine electrocardiographic time intervals and such methods
are applied in several laboratories for rat electrocardiograms
(Budden et al., 1981). The programming effort involved is considerable. To date no diagnostic programs have been developed
specifically for drug action detection and there are no central
facilities for multiuser use of a successful analysis program.
Accordingly the benefits of computer technology have not been generally available for electrocardiographic monitoring in toxicity
trials and pharmacological studies on unanesthetized subjects. The
numbers of animal electrocardiograms now being generated by the
drug industry alone has not been assessed, but the total is very
large. It is predictable that more activity in this area will be
seen in the near future.

IX. NORMAL ELECTROCARDIOGRAMS

A. General

Because pretest and control records are essential, each laboratory is in a position to develop its own individual data base.
Recently, this became necessary when cynomolgus monkeys were introduced on a fairly large scale, and there were few data available
on this species electrocardiogram. The literature on Beagle
(Detweiler, 1981a) and rat (Budden et al., 1981) electrocardiograms
have been reviewed in detail. The standard work for the older
literature on animal electrocardiograms is the aforementioned
monograph by Grauwiler (1965); see also Lepeschkin, 1951 and Zuckermann, 1959. For papers since that time on laboratory animals the
following may be consulted: monkeys (Macaca mulatta: Malinow,
1966; Singh et al., 1970; Macaca fuscata, Malinow and DeLannoy, 1967;
Macaca fascicularis, Toback et al., 1978; Saimiri sciureus, Wolf
et al., 1969); swine (v. Mickwitz, 1967; Bohn u. Henner, 1968;
Dukes and Szabuniewicz, 1969; Thielscher, 1969); rabbits (Szabuniewicz et al., 1971; Jacotot, 1965); hamsters (Glassman and Angelakos,
1965); and mice (Goldberg et al., 1968).

B. Classification of Mammalian Electrocardiograms

The types of adult mammalian electrocardiograms are depicted
in Fig. 1. There are three chief species differences: 1) duration
of the QT interval relative to mechanical systole; 2) disparity in
the direction and sense of the QRS vectors; and 3) inequality in
the degree of T wave lability.

1. QT duration and ST segment. Many rodents, insectivores
and kangeroos have short QT intervals relative to mechanical systole
(Grauwiler and Spörri, 1960) and there is no true ST segment. This
is related to the absence of a plateau in the transmembrane action
potential (Detweiler, 1981b).

2. QRS vector direction and sense. The ventricular activation
patterns fall into two general types (Hamlin and Smith, 1965;
Roshchevsky, 1978). In Group A (dog, man, monkey, cat, rat, etc.)
the QRS vectors generally produce a large negative deflection in
lead V_{10} and a positive deflection in lead aVF. Group B (hoofed
mammals, dolphins, etc.) have QRS vectors that, generally, produce
a largely positive deflection in lead V_{10} and a negative deflection
in lead aVF. These pattern differences are associated with the
distributive characteristics of the Purkinje network: In group A
animals it is largely a subendocardial network while in group B it
is more elaborate and penetrates deeply into the ventricular myocardium.

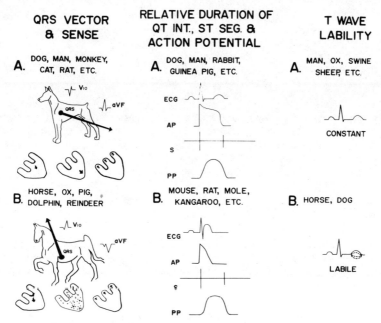

Fig. 1. The chief species differences in mammalian electrocardiograms are illustrated. Left panel: the QRS vector and
sense differs characteristically between two groups: A.
primates, dogs etc., in which the major QRS vector is toward
the hind limbs: and B. hoofed mammals etc., in which the
major QRS vector is directed ventro-dorsally from sternum
toward the spine. Middle panel: the action potential duration relative to mechanical contraction duration is about
equal in group A (dog, man etc.,), but much shorter in group
B (rat, kangaroo etc.), in which there is also no ST segment. Right panel: T-waves are fairly stable in polarity
in group A animals (man, ox, etc.), but labile in group B
(horse, dog). ECG, electrocardiogram; AP, action potential;
A, heart sounds; PP, left ventricular pressure pulse.

    3. T-wave lability. In most mammals (man, primates, hoofed
mammals) the limb lead T-waves are fairly constant in amplitude
and polarity. In dogs and horses the T-wave vectors are quite
labile in polarity and amplitude in limb and some thoracic leads.

In dogs T-waves in all except two of the conventional leads may vary
in polarity in serial records. These two exceptional leads are
rV_2 and V_{10} in which T is normally positive (rV_2) or negative (V_{10})
in about 90 percent of individuals. (Hill, 1968a, 1968b).

X. ELECTROCARDIOGRAPHIC FEATURES OF PRETEST AND CONTROL RECORDS

A. General

The pretest and control records are from ostensibly normal
animals. Ordinarily, only a very small percentage of such animals
are found to have verifiable spontaneous heart disease. A larger
number, however, have atypical electrocardiograms. Some of these
are definitely abnormal while others represent normal variants.

1. Normal versus abnormal electrocardiograms. The initial
task is to classify records as normal or abnormal.

Normal: An electrocardiogram is normal if all its variables
(heart rate, time intervals, amplitude and polarity of waves in all
leads, and rhythm) fall within the specified ranges or limits for
a given species.

Abnormal: Any electrocardiographic feature that is outside normal limits and is definitely more prevalent in the presence
of cardiac toxicity or other disease.

2. Normal variant. A number of electrocardiographic charcter-
istics are sufficiently rare or puzzling to attract attention in
electrocardiograms from control animals not known to have cardiac
disease. These are considered normal variants until proven otherwise. Some of these, however, can be induced by drug action. Their
presence can attain significance if they newly arise in serial
records of animals in specific dose groups. Examples for Beagles
include: first and second degree heart block; broad S-waves exceeding 40 per cent of the QRS duration; dome-dart ST-T complexes
without QT prolongation; U-waves > 0.05 mv.; P-wave reversal; to
mention only a few of some 25 or more that have been identified.

3. Arrhythmias and conduction disorders. As mentioned previously, the brief period during which an electrocardiogram is taken
will not give a true estimate of the prevalence of intermittent
events such as arrhythmias. Nevertheless, arrhythmias occur sporadi-
cally among control records. Examples that are fairly common are:
first and second degree atrioventricular block and ventricular extrasystoles in dogs; ventricular extrasystoles and apparent right
bundle branch block in monkeys; ventricular extrasystoles and premature sinus beats with aberrant ventricular conduction in minipigs;
atrioventricular dissocation in excited cats; sinus arrhythmia,
second degree atrioventricular block, and ventricular extrasystoles

in rats. Respiratory sinus arrhythmia, of course, is ubiquitous in
resting dogs.

The presence of these abnormalities in control records raises
two questions: 1) do they represent myocardial disease and, if not,
2) should the animals be excluded from a study? In most cases
sporadic arrhythmias have been found to be transient when serial
records were taken and heart disease could not be established at
necropsy. The right bundle branch block pattern appears to be
a normal variant in monkeys. In rats, pigs, and monkeys ventricular
extrasystoles appear to be induced with the excitement and struggling
caused by restraint, because their incidence decreases with training
and because their appearance will continue or occur in a few additional subjects during a study in which serial records are taken over
a sustained period. In dogs this is less common. Accordingly, it
is usual to exclude dogs from a study when extrasystoles are present
in pretest records. In rats and minipigs when this is done, other
individuals are likely to exhibit extrasystoles later on with little
change in the overall prevalence rate. The question of exclusion
has not been settled: some investigators feel it is unscientific
to do so, while others feel all animals with abnormal records should
be excluded, even though this may not alter the prevalence rate as
a study progresses. Individual preference prevails at the moment.

4. Intercurrent diseases. The only diseases that have affected
substantial numbers of animals in experimental groups appear to have
been related to viral infections. An outbreak of sialodacryoadenitis
in rats was associated with a high incidence of ventricular extrasystoles during a drug trial (Detweiler et al., 1981) and a cardiomyopathy in Beagles previously exposed to parvovirus caused severe
arrhythmias and other electrocardiographic abnormalities (Cimprich
et al., 1981; Detweiler et al., 1982). Except for these recent observations, intercurrent disease with unsuspected cardiac effects
has not been an important problem.

XI. DRUG INDUCED ELECTROCARDIOGRAPHIC CHANGES

A. Functional versus Morphological Effects

Electrocardiographic changes caused by chemicals may result
from myocardial cell membrane effects, unaccompanied by known
structural lesions. These functional effects produce conduction changes
and alterations in the transmembrane action potentials that relate
to the electrocardiographic changes (see Surawicz and Lasseter,
1970; Surawicz, 1967, 1972, Detweiler, 1981a). A variety of drugs
and certain chronic electrolyte and nutritional imbalances cause cell
degeneration and necrosis as seen with beta adrenergic agonists,
digitalis and potassium or magnesium deficiency (Detweiler, 1981a).

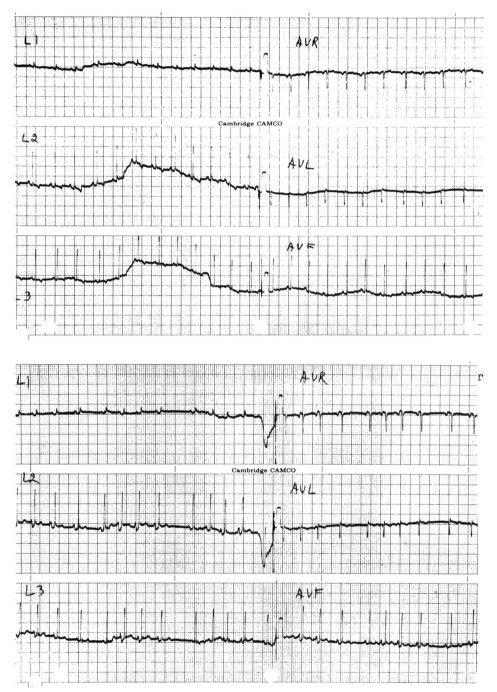

Fig. 2. The pretest (top) and treatment (bottom) record of a

dog receiving large doses of a vehicle consisting of poly-
thylene glycol, 50%; propylene glycol, 40% and ethanol,
10%. There were no effects on the electrocardiogram other
than marked increase in the amplitude of the atrial T (Ta)
wave, most pronounced in leads II, aVF and aVR (bottom).

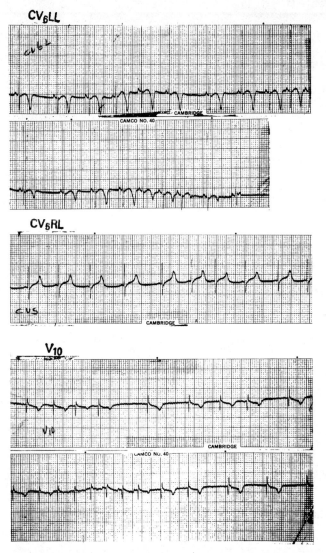

Fig. 3. Record from a Beagle receiving a phenothiazine derivative
neuroleptic drug. The QT intervals are variable and prolonged (from 0.30 to 0.34 sec.). Dome-dart ST-T complexes
are present in lead CV_5RL (rV_2) and deep, negative T-waves
in lead CV_6LL (V_2).

B. Some Examples of Drug Induced Electrocardiographic Changes.

The effects of various drugs on the dog electrocardiogram were reviewed recently (Detweiler, 1981a). They are generally similar in the other species including the rat, although the latter is resistant to digitalis glycoside effects. Much of the information about the drugs involved is confidential so that only the general classification of the agents involved can be given in most cases.

In Fig. 2 the effect of an alcoholic vehicle exclusively on the atrial T-wave (Ta) of the electrocardiogram is illustrated. The solvent mixture was made up of polyethylene glycol, 50 per cent; propylene glycol, 40 per cent; and ethanol, 10 per cent. This underscores the possible deleterious effects of alcohols used as vehicles and the importance of including vehicle control groups in toxicity studies. Polyethylene glycols are known to enhance the arrhythmogenic effect of digitalis and cause depression of atrial conduction (Rubin and Rubin 1981). Propylene glycol was found to be even more potent than polyethylene glycol in converting digitalis glycoside induced ventricular tachycardia to ventricular fibrillation in cats (Van Stee, 1982). Ethanol in high doses (e.g., up to 36% of total caloric intake) is well known to have deleterious effects on the dog heart including QRS and QT prolongation and arrhythmogenesis (Regan and Haider, 1980).

Any agent affecting the electro-physiological properties of the heart is almost certain to change the contour or duration of the cellular action potentials and thus affect the ST-T complex of the electrocardiograms. Examples are given in Figs. 3 through 8. These kind of changes are non-specific in the sense that the variety of contour changes is limited no matter what the cause. For example, the dome-dart ST-T configuration exhibited in Fig. 3 from a phenothiazine tranquilizer and in Fig. 4 from a thyromimetic agent, is also seen with various drugs that also have local anesthetic actions as is the case, for example, with some antihistaminic agents. The electrocardiographic effects of hyperkalemia are rather more specific when uncomplicated by other electrolyte changes or drug action (Fig. 5). The classical inversion of T-waves caused by digitalis glycosides is shown in Fig. 6 where the usually positive TrV_2 is negative. QT interval prolongation is often associated with ventricular arrhythmias, presumably owing to re-entrant beats (Fig. 7). Drugs with catecholamine actions are often arrhythmogenic and may produce isoproterenol-like cardiomyopathy (Fig. 8). An unusual effect is the appearance of distinct afterpotentials that may result in supposedly triggered extrasystoles, as seen in Fig. 9.

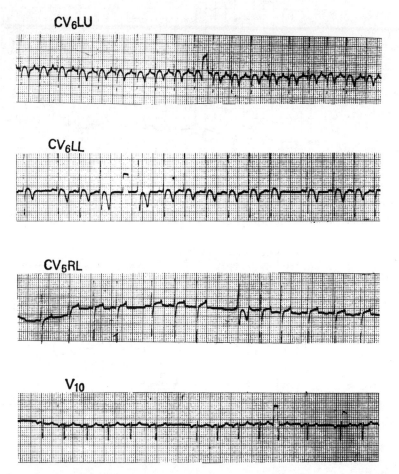

Fig. 4.   Record from a Beagle receiving a thyromimetic agent that
caused myocardial damage. The arrhythmia was identified
as ventricular parasystole in a longer record. There
are dome-dart ST-T complexes in lead CV_5RL (rV_2), TV_{10}
is positive and the T-wave in CV_6LU (V_4) and CV_6LL (V_2)
deeply negative and variable.

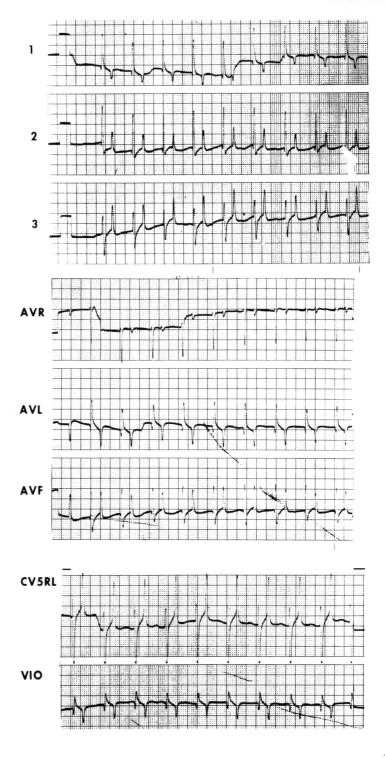

Fig. 5.   Electrocardiogram from a dog receiving an angiotensin
          converting enzyme blocker combined with a thiazide diuretic.
          Uremia developed with high serum potassium levels (10.6
          mEq./l.).   The changes are typical of hyperkalemia with high
          amplitude, "tented" T-waves in several leads, absence of
          P-waves (sino-ventricular rhythm), and prolongation of QRS
          and QT intervals.

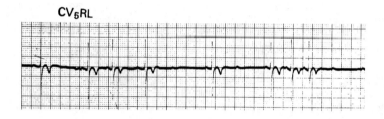

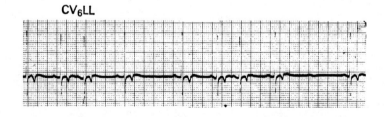

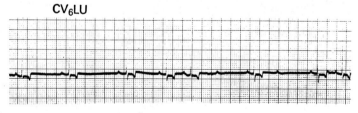

Fig. 6.   Second degree AV block and T reversal in chest leads
          including CV_5RL (rV_2) in a Beagle, caused by digitalis
          toxicosis.

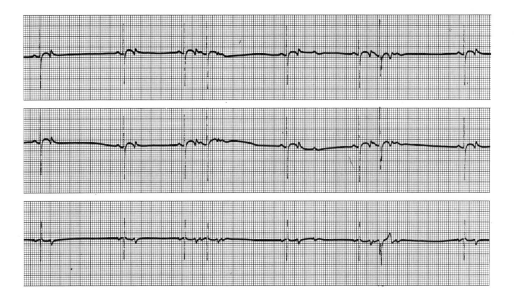

Fig. 7. Leads rV$_2$, V$_2$, V$_{10}$, from top to bottom. This dog received
a neuroleptic compound that caused bradycardia (heart rate
50 to 55/min.) QT prolongation (0.28 sec.), second degree
AV block, and ventricular extrasystoles. The diphasic
(-/+) T-waves are abnormal for lead rV$_2$ (top).

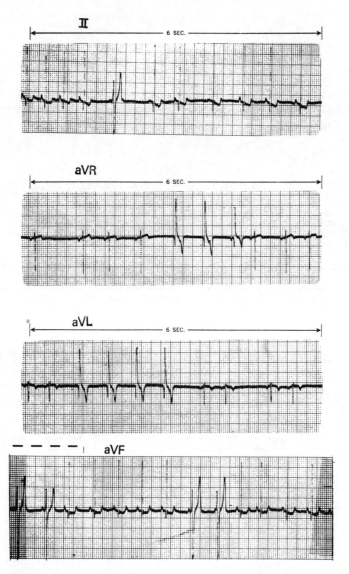

Fig. 8.   Electrocardiogram from a Beagle receiving a bronchodilator
          compound. The nomotopic rhythm is irregular (sinus
          arrhythmia) at a rate varying between 85 and 115 beats/
          min.   The RR intervals of successive ectopic beats varied
          from 0.5 to 0.6 sec. (corresponding to heart rates of 100-
          120 beats/min.) and when separated by nomotopic beats were
          approximate multiples of RR intervals of 0.6 sec.   In lead
          aVR the third ectopic beat is considered a fusion beat.
          The coupling intervals were variable. Ventricular parasys-
          tole was confirmed in a longer record.

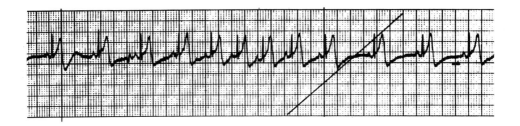

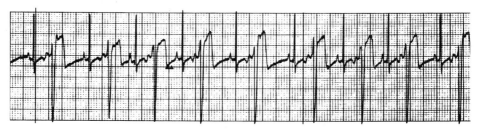

Fig. 9.   This drug, an antibiotic, produced symmetrical, high
amplitude T-waves and after-potentials with a rate of rise
of 2.5 mv./sec. (top record), culminating in ventricular
bigeminy, probably the result of triggered extrasystoles
(bottom record).   Lead aVF.

C. Communicating Electrocardiographic Results

    1. Cautionary views. It is important to remember that con-
clusions about the electrophysiologic mechanisms explaining electrocardiographic changes are speculative unless confirmed by invasive
electrophysiological studies. The value of the electrocardiogram
should not be overrated; it is merely one component of the laboratory
data on which inferences regarding toxicity are based. While
an electrocardiographer may not be misled by a dogmatic diagnostic
statement in ECG jargon that implies a specific anatomical lesion or
physiological state, one not well versed may be confounded. The
electrocardiographic report should not contain evaluations of
functions beyond the compass of electrocardiography (e.g., myocardial
inotropy, hemodynamics) and should not be dogmatic about suspected
organic myocardial damage.

    2. Statements of interpretation. Once the electrocardiograms
have been examined and any changes noted, their toxicological significance must be decided and expressed. These interpretative
statements cover three general areas:

        a. the probable electrophysiologic mechanisms responsible
for the electrocardiographic changes. For example, QT interval
prolongation may be attributable to lenthening of cellular action
potential durations, slowing of intraventricular conduction, fusing
of the T and U-waves, or some combination of such factors.

        b. the degree of likelihood that the changes may have
resulted from actual myocardial damage, such as necrosis, rather
than electrophysiological effects unaccompanied by detectable lesions.
For example, in dogs simple time interval prolongations, with or
without coupled ventricular extrasystoles are seldom associated
with demonstrable myocardial lesions, whereas reversal of T-waves
in leads rV_2 and V_{10} accompanied by multifocal ventricular extrasystoles are often signs of myocardial damage.

        c. explanation of electrocardiographic changes that may
or may not be related to drug action on the heart. Examples are
non-specific ST segment and T-wave changes, increases in P-wave
amplitude, and rate changes. Their significance is ordinarily
unknown or of a low order, but a relationship may be found with the
clinical state of the animal. For example, in dogs subject to non-
specific stresses such as long periods of restraint(e.g., 12 or 24
hours in a sling during infusions) trauma, or focal infections deep
negative T-waves may appear in leads I, II, III, aVF, V_2, V_4, and
V_{10}.

    These statements must be framed with great care, lest they
be misunderstood in the context of the final toxicological report.
Their speculative nature and the degree of uncertainty about

conclusions from the electrocardiogram alone, not documentable by non-electrocardiographic data (e.g., necropsy, serum enzyme changes etc.), must be emphasized. That electrocardiographic changes are symptoms, not diseases, is only too often forgotten.

The important question as to whether a cardiotoxic effect results from a direct effect on the heart alone or is caused indirectly by drug induced alterations in other tissues and organs can only be decided from the results of multidisciplinary study. Cardioactive drugs of various types (e.g., antiarrhythmic and positive inotropic agents) have direct cardiotoxic effects as an expected extension of their pharmacologic action. This sort of cardiotoxicity is of little consequence as long as there is evidence of a safe therapeutic index. Other agents have unexpected direct or indirect cardiotoxic effects that may or may not be a part of desired actions on other tissues (Bristow, 1980). The antineoplastic anthracyclines produce some direct cardiac damage at therapeutic levels that appears to be part of their desired chemotherapeutic effect on neoplastic cells. They also damage the heart indirectly by releasing vasoactive substances (histamines, catecholamines and prostaglandins). Antihypertensive agents may produce cardiomyopathy indirectly by causing repeated bouts of tachycardia and poor coronary artery perfusion during daily dose induced hypotension (Balazs and Herman, 1976). Some drugs prove to be cardiotoxic quite unexpectedly in ways that must be unrelated to their intended therapeutic actions (e.g., the arrhythmogenic effects of certain antibiotics). The complicated nature of most cardiotoxicities prevents complete understanding of mechanisms even after extensive study. This underlines the need to resist drawing far reaching conclusions from electrocardiographic changes alone.

XII. SUMMARY

Since electrophysiological alterations are a principal manifestation of cardiotoxicity, electrocardiographic monitoring is mandated in preclinical drug testing. This permits early detection of the electrophysiologic precursors of cardiotoxicity and monitoring their continued course. In addition to the limb leads, thoracic leads established for the various laboratory species are indispensible. The scheduling for electrocardiogram recording should be flexible. A minimal protocol that is appropriate for most types of cardiotoxic agents is: two pretest records; records during week one, at month one, at three month intervals thereafter, and at days one and three and weeks one and two in recovery animals. In analyzing the records, the availability of pretest and serial electrocardiograms from control and treated animals of different dose groups makes it possible to detect induced changes, even though the records themselves remain within normal limits.

Mammalian electrocardiograms exhibit typical species differ-

ences and are classified in accordance with: 1) duration of the QT
interval relative to mechanical systole (rats, kangaroos etc.
have short QT intervals and no ST segment); 2) differences in the
direction of QRS vectors (the major QRS vector is directed from
sternum toward the spine in hoofed mammals etc. and caudally toward the rear limbs in primates, carnivores, etc.); and 3) T-wave
lability (T-waves are fairly consistent in most species except dogs
and horses in which they are markedly labile).

A small percentage of experimental animals have abnormal or
variant electrocardiograms. Those that have features falling outside normal limits and which are definitely more prevalent in the
presence of cardiac toxicity or disease should be classified as
abnormal. Other atypical records are usually classified as normal
variants if they are present in predictable numbers in groups of
animals. Arrhythmias and conduction disorders that occur sporadic-
ally in control records are: for dogs; first and second degree atrioventricular block, ventricular extrasystoles; for monkeys, ventricular extrasystoles, apparent right bundle branch block; for
minipigs, ventricular extrasystoles, premature sinus beats with
aberrant ventricular conduction; for cats, atrioventricular dissociation; for rats, sinus arrhythmia, second degree atrioventricular
block, ventricular extrasystoles. Whether or not to eliminate
animals with these abnormalities or normal variants from studies
remains undecided.

Intercurrent disease rarely complicates cardiotoxicity studies,
although sialodacryoadenitis in rats and cardiomyopathy in parvovirus exposed dogs have recently been associated with electrocardiographic abnormalities.

Examples of drug induced electrocardiographic changes include:
arrhythmias and conduction disorders, reversal of T-waves in leads
where they are normally stable, dome-dart ST-T complexes, after-
potentials, exaggeration of Ta, and time interval prolongations.

Electrocardiographic reports must be couched in generally
understood terms, not jargon, and should not extend speculatively
beyond the scope of electrocardiography into areas such as hemodynamics. Final decision as to whether a cardiotoxic effect is
direct or indirect always depends on the results of multidisciplinary study.

XIII. CONCLUSIONS

Serial electrocardiograms provide an indispensable diagnostic
component needed for the detection and analysis of untoward cardiac
effects in toxicity trials. Optimizing the effectiveness of this
method requires adequate apparatus, the use of multilead systems,
serial records in treated and control groups, appropriate recording

schedules and reasoned interpretation correlated with other preclinical observations.

REFERENCES

Atta, A.G. and Vanace, P.W., 1960, Electrocardiographic studies
    in the Macaca mulatta monkey, Ann. N.Y. Acad, Sci. 85:811.
Balazs, T., 1974, Development of tissue resistance to toxic effects
    of chemicals, Toxicology, 2:247.
Balazs, T. and Hermann, E.H., 1976, Toxic cardiomyopathies, Ann.
    Clin. Lab. Sci. 6:467.
Balazs, T. (ed.), 1981, "Cardiac Toxicology", Vol. I. II. III.
    CRC Press, Boxa Raton, FL.
Bellet, S., 1963, Clinical Disorders of the Heart Beat, Lea &
    Febiger, Philadelphia.
Bellet, S., 1972, Essentials of Cardiac Arrhythmias, W.B. Saunders,
    Philadelphia.
Bloom, S., 1981, Reversible and irreversible injury: calcium as a
    major determinant, in: "Cardiac Toxicology", Vol. 1, T.
    Balazs, ed., CRC Press, Boca Raton, FL., 179-199.
Böhle, E., 1966, Blutgefässe, in: "Erkrankungen durch Arzneimittel",
    R. Heinz (ed.), Thieme, Stuttgart, 170-187.
Bohn, F.K. und Henner, S., 1968, Elektrokardiographische Unter-
    suchungen bei Miniaturschweinen, Ztschr. ges. exper. Med.,
    145:365.
Bristow, M.R. (ed.), 1980, "Drug Induced Heart Disease", Elsevier,
    Amsterdam.
Budden, R., Detweiler, D.K., and Zbinden, G. (eds.), 1981, "The Rat
    Electrocardiogram in Pharmacology and Toxicology", Pergamon,
    Oxford.
Caceres, C.A., 1978, Present status of computer interpretation of the
    electrocardiogram. A 20-year overview, Am. J. Cardiol., 41:
    121.
Chung, E.K. and Dean, H.M., 1972, Diseases of the heart and vascular
    system due to drugs, in: L. Meyler and H.M. Peck (eds.), "Drug
    Induced Diseases", Vol. 4., Excerpt. Med., Amsterdam, 345-380.
Cimprich, R.E., Robertson, J.L., Kutz, S.A., Struve, P.S., Detweiler,
    D.K., DeBaecke, P.J. and Street, C.S., 1981, Degenerative car-
    diomyopathy in experimental Beagles following parvovirus ex-
    posure. Toxicol. Pathol., 9:19.
Davies, D.M. and Gold, R.G., 1977, Cardiac disorders, in: "Textbook
    of Adverse Drug Reactions", D.M. Davies, (ed.), Oxford Univ.
    Oxford, 82:102.
Detweiler, D.K., 1981a, The use of electrocardiography in toxico-
    logical studies with Beagle dogs. In, Balazs, T. (ed.)
    Cardiac Toxicology. Vol. III, CRC Press, Boca Raton, FL. 33-82.
Detweiler, D.K., 1981b, The use of electrocardiography in toxico-
    logical studies with rats, in: R. Budden, D.K. Detweiler, and
    G. Zbinden, (eds.), "The Rat Electrocardiogram in Pharmacology
    and Toxicology", Pergamon Press, Oxford, 83-115.

Detweiler, D.K., Saatman, R.A., and DeBaecke, P.J., 1981, Cardiac
    arrhythmias accompanying sialodacryoadenitis in the rat, in:
    R. Budden, D.K. Detweiler, and G. Zbinden (eds.), "The Rat
    Electrocardiogram in Pharmacology and Toxicology", Pergamon
    Press, Oxford, 129.
Detweiler, D.K., Cimprich, R.E., DeBaecke, P.J., Kutz, S.A., Robert-
    son, J.L., Street, C.S., and Struve, P.S., 1982, Cardiomyopathy
    in parvvirus exposed experimental Beagles. Trends Pharmacol.
    Sciences. 3:4.
Dukes, T.W., and Szabuniewicz, M., 1969, The electrocardiogram of
    conventional and miniature swine (S. Scropa). Can. J. Comp.
    Med. 33:118.
Ellestad, M.H., 1981, Ellestad stress test analyzer. Del Mar
    Avionics, Irvine, CA.
Friedman, H.H., 1971, "Diagnostic Electrocardiography and Vector-
    cardiography", McGraw-Hill, N.Y.
Fillmore, G.E., and Detweiler, D.K., 1973, Maintenance of subacute
    digoxin toxicosis in normal beagles, Toxicol. Appl. Pharma-
    col., 25:418.
Glassman, P.M., and Angelakos, E.T., 1965, Electrocardiogram of the
    golden hamster, Am. J. Med. Electronics, 4:42.
Goldbarg, A.N., Hellerstein, H.K., Bruell, J.H., and Daroczy, A.F.,
    1968, Electrocardiogram of the normal mouse, Mus musculus:
    General Considerations and Genetic Aspects. Cardiovasc.
    Res. 2:93.
Grauwiler, J., and Spörri, H., 1960, Fehlen der ST-Strecke im
    Elektrokardiogramm von verschiedenen Säugetierarten.
    Helv. Physiol. Acta, 18:C77-C78.
Grauwiler, J., 1965, "Herz und Kreislauf der Säugetiere", Birk-
    hauser, Basel.
Greenberg, P.S., Cangliano, B., Leamy, L., and Ellestad, M.H.,
    1980, Use of the multivariate approach to enhance the diag-
    nostic accuracy of the treadmill stress test, J. Electro-
    cardiol., 13:277
Hagen, A. et al., 1978, Task Force IA: Development of a data base
    for electrocardiographic use, Am. J. Cardiol., 41:145.
Hamlin, R.L., Robinson, F.R., and Smith, C.R., 1961, Electrocar-
    diogram and vectorcardiogram of Macaca mulatta in various
    postures, Am. J. Physiol., 201:1083.
Hamlin, R.L., and Smith, C.R., 1965, Categorization of common
    domestic mammals based upon their ventricular activation
    process, Ann. N.Y. Acad. Sci. 127:195.
Harrison, D.G. (ed.), 1981, "Cardiac Arrhythmias", Hall, Boston.
Hill, J.D., 1968a, The electrocardiogram in dogs with standardized
    body and limb positions, J. Electrocardiol., 1:175
Hill, J.D., 1968b, The significance of foreleg position in the
    interpretation of electrocardiograms and vectorcardiograms
    from research animals, Am. Heart J., 75:518

Holden, M. and Itil, T., 1977/78, Electrocardiographic changes with psychotropic drugs, in, "Stress and the Heart", D. Wheatley, (ed.) Raven Press, N.Y., 87.

Jacotot, B., 1965, L'electrocardiogramme du lapin. Analyse des traces de 75 animaux sains, Rec. Med. Vet. 141:1095.

Lazdunski, M., and Renaud, J.F., 1982, The action of cardiotoxins on cardiac plasma membranes, in I.S. Edelman (ed.) Ann. Rev. Physiol. 44:463.

Lepeschkin, E., 1951, "Modern Electrocardiography", Williams and Wilkins, Baltimore.

Malinow, M.R., and DeLannoy, C.W.,Jr., 1967, The electrocardiogram of Macaca fuscata, Folia primat., 7:284.

Malinow, M.R., Hill, J.D., and Ochsner, A.J., III, 1974, The heart rate in caged rhesus monkeys (Macaca mulatta), Lab. Anim. Sci., 24:537.

v. Mickwitz, G., 1967, Herz- und Kreislaufuntersuchungen beim Schwein mit Berücksichtigung des Elektrokardiogramms und des Phono-kardiogramms, Habilitationsschr. Tierärztl. Hochschule Hannover, West-Germany.

Morganroth, J., 1981, Ambulatory monitoring: The impact of sponta-neous variability of simple and complex ventricular ectopy, in, D.G. Harrison, (ed.) "Cardiac Arrhythmias", Hall, Boston 479.

Osborne, B.E., 1973, A restraining device for use when recording electrocardiograms in monkeys, Lab. Animals, 7:289.

Pipberger, H.V., Arzbaecher, R.C., Berson, A.S., Briller, S.A., Brody, D.A., Flowers, N.C., Geselowitz, D.B., Lepeschkin, E., Oliver, G.C., Schmitt, O.H., and Spach, M., 1975, Recommen-dations for standardization of leads and of specifications for instruments in electrocardiography and vectorcardiography, Circulation, 52:11.

Rautaharju, P.M. et al., 1978, Task Force III. Computer in diagnostic electrocardiography, Am. J. Cardiol. 41:158.

Regan, T.J., and Haider, B., 1980, Pathophysiological effects of ethanol on cardiac tissue, in: "Drug Induced Heart Disease", M.R. Bristow (ed.) Elsevier, Amsterdam, 175.

Richtarck, A., Woolsey, T.A., and Valdivia, E., 1965, Method for recording ECG's in unanesthetized guinea pigs, J. Appl. Physiol 20:1091.

Robinson, D.S., and Barker, E., 1976, Tricyclic antidepressant car-diotoxicity, J. Am. Med. Assn., 236:2089.

Roshchevsky, M.P., 1978, "Elektrokardiologia Kopytnych Zyvotnych", Nauka, Leningrad.

Rubin, J.I., and Rubin, E., 1982, Myocardial toxicity of alcohols, aldehydes, and glycols, including alcoholic cardiomyopathy in: "Cardiovascular Toxicology", E.W. Van Stee, (ed.) Raven Press, N.Y., 353.

Rydén, L., Waldenström, A., and Holmberg, S., 1975, The reliability of intermittent ECG sampling in arrhythmia detection, Circ. 52:540.

Scherf, D. and Schott, A., 1973, "Extrasystoles and Allied Arrhyth-
    mias", Year Book Medical Publishing, Chicago.
Selye, H., 1970, "Experimental Cardiovascular Diseases", Vol. 1 and
    2, Springer, Berlin.
Singh, R., Chakravarti, R.N., Chhuttani, P.N., and Wahi, P.L., 1970,
    Electrocardiographic studies in rhesus monkeys, J. Appl.
    Physiol. 28:346.
Singh, B.N., Collett, J.J., and Chew, C.Y.C., 1980, New perspectives
    in the pharmacologic therapy of cardiac arrhythmias. Prog.
    Cardiovasc. Dis. 22:243.
Spörri, H., 1944, Der Einfluss der Tuberkulose auf das Elektrokardio-
    gramm. Untersuchungen an Meerschweinchen und Rindern. Arch.
    wiss. prak. Tierheilk. 79:57.
Surawicz, B., 1967, Relationship between electrocardiogram and electro-
    lytes, Am. Heart J., 73:814.
Surawicz, B., 1972, The pathogenesis and clinical significance of
    primary T-wave abnormalities, in: "Advances in Electrocardio-
    graphy", R.D. Schlant, and I.W. Hurst, (eds.) Grune & Stratton,
    N.Y.
Surawicz, B., and Lasseter, K.C., 1970, Effect of drugs on the electro-
    cardiogram, Prog. Cardiovasc. Dis., 13:26.
Szabuniewicz, M., Hightower, D., and Kyzar, J.R., 1971, The electro-
    cardiogram, vectorcardiogram and spatiocardiogram in the rabbit,
    Can. J. Comp. Med., 35:107.
Teske, R.H., Bishop, S.P., Righter, H.F., and Detweiler, D.K., 1976,
    Subacute digoxin in toxicosis in the Beagle dog, Toxicol. Appl.
    Pharmacol., 35:283.
Thielscher, H.H., 1969, Elektrokardiographische Untersuchungen an
    deutschen veredelten Landschweinen der Landeszucht und der
    Herdbuchzucht, Zentralblatt der Vet. med., A. 16:370.
Toback, J.M., Clark, J.C., and Mooreman, W.J., 1978, The electrocar-
    diogram of Macaca fascicularis, 28:182.
Van Stee, E.W., (ed.), 1982, "Cardiovascular Toxicology", Raven Press,
    N.Y.
Van Stee, E.W., 1982, Cardiovascular Toxicology: foundations and
    scope, in: "Cardiovascular Toxicology", E.W. Van Stee, (ed.),
    Raven Press, N.Y. 1.
Vaughan, Williams, E.M., 1975, Classification of antidysrhythmic
    drugs, Pharmacol. Therapy B., 1, 115.
Wenzel, D.G., 1967, Drug induced cardiomyopathies, J. Pharmaceut.
    Sci., 56:1209.
Wolf, R.H., Lehner, N.D.M., Miller, E.C., and Clarkson, T.B., 1969,
    Electrocardiogram of the squirrel monkey, Saimiri sciureus,
    J. Appl. Physiol., 26:346.
Zuckermann, R., 1959, "Grundriss und Atlas der Elektrokardiographie",
    Thieme, Leipzig.

     This work was supported, in part, by National Institutes of Health
Grant Number LM 01660 and by the Smith, Kline and French Laboratories,
Philadelphia, PA.

ATP content of myocytes, 219
Acetylcholine receptor, 143
Acrolein, 537
Action potential upstroke, 82
Activation-unloading shortening, 207
Adenine nucleotide pool, 403
Adenosine, 408
Adenosine monophosphate, 408
Adenylate
  cyclase, 144
  regulation, 91
Adrenergic receptors, 425
Adult myocyte, 217, 231, 249
Agonist regulation, 115
Allylamine, 533
Alpha adrenergic receptors, 100
Alpha-tocopherol, 526
Amine oxidase, 536
Anaerobic glycolysis, 403
Antibiotic, 580
Anti-heart antibody, 471
Antihypertensive drugs, 580
Anti-viral antibody, 471
Aortic pressure, 317
Arachidonic acid, 365
Arrhythmia, 393
Atrial natriuretic factor, 226
Autoimmunity, 479
Autonomic innervation, 184
Autoregulation, 327
Auxotonic contraction, 211
Beta adrenergic receptors, 92
Bidirectional block, 72
Benzylamine oxidase, 537
Ca^{2+} flux regulation in heart, 433

Ca^{2+}-Mg^{2+} ATPase, 377
CP content of myocytes, 219
Cable model, 79
Cable properties of cardiac
    muscle, 3
Calcium, 421, 509
  homeostasis and heart failure, 447
  paradox, 235, 305
  transport, 378
Canine right heart failure, 179
Cardiac
  damage, 457
  hypertrophy, 180
  muscle, 25, 249
Cardiomyopathy, 391, 521
Cardiotoxicity
  electrocardiogram, 579
Catecholamines, 182, 391
Cation
  complexation, 546
  transport, 548
Cell
  culture, 259
  division, 251
  hypertrophy, 250
  proliferation, 250
Cellular immunity, 491
Cerebral microcirculation, 366
Chemical activation, 213
Choline acetyltransferase, 159, 179
Chronotropic regulation of the
    heart, 117
Computer simulations, 211
Conductional velocity, 82
Connexons, 28

Coronary
  flow, 544
  steal, 546
Cortical microcirculation, 327
Coxsackie B-3 virus, 491
Cytoskeleton, 243
Cytosolic free Ca^{2+} concentration, 444
Cytotoxicity, 496
DNA replication, 250
Daunorubicin, 519
Decremental conduction, 61
Desmosomes, 25
Differentiation, 251
Discontinuities, 70
Discontinuous propagation, 70, 79
Distal toxin, 537
Dopamine β-hydroxylase, 160, 179
Down regulation, 148
Doxorubicin, 512, 519
ELISA assay, 463
Effective axial resistivity, 73
Electrical field interactions, 4
Electrical anistropy of cardiac muscle, 3
Electrocardiogram, 579
  mammalian, 588
  normal, 588
Electrocardiography
  drugs, 579
  cardiotoxicity, 579
Electron microscopy, 30, 523
Electron probe x-ray microanalysis, 423
Electronic spread of current, 4
Embryonic chick, 144
Endoplasmic reticulum calcium, 444
Energy production in ischemia, 408
Equivalent dipole sources, 86
Excitability, 72
  properties, 204
Excitation-contraction coupling, 377
Exocytosis, 548
FDA, 546
Fasciae adherentes, 25
Fibrosis, 533

5'hydroxytryptamine, 327
5'nucleotidase, 413
Force-sarcomere length, 211
Free radicals, 347, 396, 509, 537
Freeze fracture, 30
GTP-binding proteins, 91
Gap junction, 25, 37, 79
Glucose oxidation, 218
Glutathione peroxidase, 347
Guanyl nucleotides, 144
Guinea pig
  heart, 162
  right heart failure, 179
Heart
  antibodies, 457
  antigens, 457
  disease, 391
  failure, 180
  fibers, 38
  muscle, 250
  myocytes, 231
    from diabetic rats, 221
    properties, 234
    transport reactions, 233
  myofibrils, 306
  sarcolemma, 307, 391
Isolated myocardial cells, 200, 217
High energy phosphate, 307, 393
  in ischemia, 403
High resistance coupling, 10
Hydrogen ion, 377
Hydroperoxy-eicotetraenoic acid, 366
Hydroxyl radical, 365, 380
Hypercontracture of myocytes, 240
Hypothermia, 413
Hypoxia, 421, 511
  and substrate oxidation, 226
Injury, 28
Input resistance, 4
Intercalated disc, 1, 28, 79
Intercellular junctions, 25
Intracellular calcium
  distribution, 435
  overload, 305
Intraventricular pressure, 319
Ion selective electrodes, 548
Ionophore, 543
Irreversible injury, 403

Ischemia, 377, 421
Ischemic injury, 44, 403, 477
Isoproterenol, 510, 563
   LD$_{50}$, 564
Junctional
   permeability, 45
   potentials, 7
   transmission, 7
Keshan disease, 527
Lactate oxidation, 218
Lanthanum, 421
Leakage resistance, 80
Left ventricular
   performance, 271
   wall motion, 272
Length constant, 3
Lipid peroxide, 347, 391
Lipoprotein lipase, 224
Maculae adherentes, 25
Membrane ATPase, 308
Membranes, 421
Methacholine perfusion, 171
Migration inhibition, 480
Mitochondrial
   calcium, 437, 438
   set point, 438
Mitochondrial extracts, 480
Mitochondrial free Ca^{2+}, 442
Modulation, 50
Monensin, 543
Monoamine oxidase, 537
Muscarinic receptor, 113, 152,
      165
Myocardial
   infarct, 347, 479
   ischemia, 347
   necrosis, 536
Myocarditis, 491
Myocardium, 423
Myofibrillar ATPase, 305
Myoglobin, 480
Myokinase, 412
Myopathic hamsters, 179
Na$^+$ - K$^+$ ATPase, 308, 421
Negative chronotropy, 149
Nexuses, 25
Norepinephrine, 184
O$_2$ consumption by myocytes, 218
Obesity, 564
Ontogenesis, 152

Oxidative phosphorylation, 306
Oxygen
   consumption, 323
   paradox, 240
   radicals, 365
Palmitate oxidation, 218
Permeability of myocytes, 233
Peroxidation, 526
Phenothiazine tranquilizer, 580
Phospholipids, 427
Postpericardiotomy syndrome, 471
Potassium
   accumulation, 10
   permeability, 113
Pressure-volume index, 286
Propagation mechanisms in heart,
      13
Protein synthesis, 317
Prostaglandins, 365
Pulmonary artery constriction,
      181
Quinones, 397
Quinuclidinyl benzilate, 179
Radiochemical assay, 550
Radionuclide ventriculograms, 267
Razoxane, 528
Receptor affinity, 94
   down regulation, 171
   endocytosis, 129
   regulation, 152
Reentry, 61
Regulation of cytosolic free
      Ca^{2+}, 441
Resistance development, 568
Rheumatic fever, 457
Saltatory
   conduction, 86
   propagation, 70
Sarcoplasmic reticulum, 377, 525
Scopolamine, 173
Sino atrial node, 162
Streptococcal antigens, 457
Superoxide, 347, 365, 378
T lymphocytes, 491
Thyromimetic agent, 595
Tissue resistivity, 2
Transmission between myocardial
      cells, 11
Tyrozine hydroxylase, 160, 179
Uncoupling, 28

Unidirectional block, 69
Unloaded sarcomere
    lengthening, 200
    shortening, 200
    velocity, 205
Vascular
    permeability, 327
    sarcoplasmic reticulum, 366
    spasm, 328

Vasodilation, 367
Ventricular
    ejection fraction, 285
    fibrillation, 564
    function, 267
Viral infection, 491
Vitamin E, 393
Working hearts, 317